Neale's Common Foot Disorders
Diagnosis and Management

For Churchill Livingstone

Editorial director: Mary Law
Project manager: Valerie Burgess
Project development editor: Dinah Thom
Design direction: Judith Wright
Project controller: Pat Miller
Copy editor: Adam Campbell
Sales promotion executive: Hilary Brown

Neale's Common Foot Disorders

Diagnosis and Management

Edited by

Donald L. Lorimer BEd MChS DPodM

Former Head of the Durham School of Podiatric Medicine; Immediate Past Chairman of Council,
Society of Chiropodists and Podiatrists; Dean of the Faculty of Undergraduate Education,
Society of Chiropodists and Podiatrists, UK

Gwen French MChS DPodM

President, International Federation of Podology and Podiatry (FIPP); Formerly Head of Chiropody Department,
Greenwich District Hospital, London; Formerly Principal Lecturer in Podiatry, University of Westminster, London;
Past Chairman of Council, Society of Chiropodists and Podiatrists; Honorary Senior Teacher, London Foot Hospital, UK

Steve West BSc FChS MPodA MIPEMS

Dean and Professor of the Faculty of Health and Social Care, University of the West of England, Bristol, UK

FIFTH EDITION

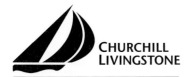

CHURCHILL
LIVINGSTONE

NEW YORK EDINBURGH LONDON MADRID MELBOURNE SAN FRANCISCO TOKYO 1997

CHURCHILL LIVINGSTONE
Medical Division of Pearson Professional Limited

Distributed in the United States of America by Churchill
Livingstone, 650 Avenue of the Americas, New York, N.Y.
10011, and by associated companies, branches and
representatives throughout the world.

First edition 1981
Second edition 1985
Third edition 1989
Fourth edition 1993
Fifth edition 1997

ISBN 0 443 05258 1

British Library Cataloguing in Publication Data
A catalogue record for this book is available from the British
Library.

Library of Congress Cataloging in Publication Data
A catalog record for this book is available from the Library of
Congress.

Note
Medical knowledge is constantly changing. As new
information becomes available, changes in treatment,
procedures, equipment and the use of drugs become
necessary. The editors/authors/contributors and the
publishers have, as far as it is possible, taken care to ensure
that the information given in this text is accurate and up-to-
date. However, readers are strongly advised to confirm that
the information, especially with regard to drug usage,
complies with latest legislation and standards of practice.

The
publisher's
policy is to use
**paper manufactured
from sustainable forests**

Produced by Longman Singapore Publishers (Pte) Ltd.
Printed in Singapore

Contents

Contributors

Eric G. Anderson MB ChB MSc FRCS(Edin) FRCS(Glas) FCh S
Consultant Orthopaedic Surgeon, Western Infirmary, Glasgow, UK

Sol W. Balkin DPM
Attending staff member, Department of Orthopaedics/Podiatry Section, Los Angeles County University of Southern California Medical Center, Los Angeles, California, USA

Alan S. Banks DPM BSc
Podiatrist, Peachtree Podiatry Group, Atlanta, Georgia, USA

Alison M. Barlow MSc MChS DPodM
Lecturer in Podiatry, University of Salford, Salford, UK

James A. Black MChS DPodM
Podiatrist, Orthopaedic Foot Clinic, Western Infirmary, Glasgow, UK

Richard J. Bogdan MS DPM FACFO
Sports Podiatrist, Concord, California, USA

Patricia M. Boyd BApplSc(Pod) DPodM
Lecturer, Queen Margaret College, Edinburgh; Podiatrist Fitness Assessment and Sports Injury Centre, University of Edinburgh, Edinburgh, UK

Susan J. Braid MSc FChS DPodM
Senior Lecturer in Podiatry, University of Salford, Salford, UK

P. D. Brash MB ChB MRCP
Senior Registrar, Department of Endocrinology, The General Infirmary at Leeds, Leeds, UK

Niall E. F. Cartlidge MB BS FRCP
Consultant Neurologist and Senior Lecturer in Neurology, Division of Neuroscience, The Medical School, University of Newcastle, Newcastle upon Tyne, UK

Alistair J. Clark BSc MChS DPodM
Senior Lecturer in Podiatry, Durham School of Podiatric Medicine, New College, Durham, UK

Hugh A. Cross BSc(Podiatry) PhD
Podiatrist, Nepal Leprosy Trust, Lalgadh, India

Gloria Dunlop MSc MChS DPodM CertFEd
Lecturer in Podiatry, Queen Margaret College, Edinburgh, UK

Michael E. Edmonds MB BS FRCP
Consultant Physician, Diabetic Department, King's College Hospital, London, UK

Manesty S. K. Forster MPhil BSc MChS DPodM
Senior Lecturer in Podiatry, Durham School of Podiatric Medicine, New College, Durham, UK

Gwen French MChS DPodM
President, International Federation of Podology and Podiatry (FIPP); Formerly Head of Chiropody Department, Greenwich District Hospital, London; Formerly Principal Lecturer in Podiatry, University of Westminster, London; Past Chairman of Council, Society of Chiropodists and Podiatrists; Honorary Senior Teacher, London Foot Hospital, UK

Colin J. Fullerton BSc MMedSci FPodA MChS DPodM
Senior Podiatrist, Centre for Podiatric Medicine, The Queen's University of Belfast, Belfast, UK

Ian Haslock MD MRCP
Consultant Rheumatologist, South Tees Acute Hospitals Trust, Middlesbrough; Visiting Professor in Clinical Bioengineering, University of Durham, Durham, UK

Margaret Johnson PhD MChS DPodM
Principal Lecturer and Head of School, Durham
School of Podiatric Medicine, New College, Durham,
UK

Donald L. Lorimer BEd MChS DPodM
Former Head of School, Durham School of Podiatric
Medicine, New College, Durham; Immediate Past
Chairman of Council, Society of Chiropodists and
Podiatrists; Dean of the Faculty of Undergraduate
Education, Society of Chiropodists and Podiatrists, UK

John C. McDermott PhD BSc
Senior Lecturer in Microbiology, Department of
Dietetics and Nutrition, Queen Margaret College,
Edinburgh, UK

E. Dalton McGlamry DPM DSc
Podiatrist, Peachtree Podiatry Group, Atlanta,
Georgia, USA

Iain M. M. Macmillan MB ChB MRCGP
Ladywell Medical Centre, Edinburgh, UK

Philip Milsom FSFCP MChS DPodM
Specialist in Podiatric Surgery, Essex Rivers
Healthcare, Colchester, UK

Rae M. Morgan BSc(Pharm) PhD MRPharmS
Reader in Pharmacology, School of Health Sciences,
University of Sunderland, Sunderland, UK

Donald E. Neale OBE FChS
Formerly Principal, Edinburgh Foot Clinic and School
of Chiropody, Edinburgh, UK

Maureen O'Donnell BSc FChS DPodM SRCh
Lecturer in Podiatry, Division of Podiatry, Glasgow
Caledonian University, Glasgow, UK

Sandy J. A. Raeburn MB ChB PhD FRCP(Edin)
Professor of Clinical Genetics, University of
Nottingham; Clinical Director, Genetics Directorate,
Nottingham Genetic Services, Nottingham, UK

George C. Rendall BSc MChS DPodM
Formerly Lecturer in Podiatry, Queen Margaret
College, Edinburgh; Private Practitioner, Orkney
Podiatry Services, Kirkwall, UK

Susan J. Ritchie MB ChB DRCOG
Clinical Assistant, Clinical Genetic Service,
Nottingham, UK

Colin E. Thomson BSc MChS DPodM FSFCP
Lecturer, Department of Podiatry and Radiography,
Queen Margaret College, Edinburgh, UK

John E. Tooke MA MSc BM BCh DM FRCP
Consultant Physician and Professor of Vascular
Medicine, Royal Devon and Exeter Hospital, Exeter, UK

Barbara Wall MSc BSc FChS DPodM
Senior Teacher, London Foot Hospital and School of
Podiatric Medicine, London, UK

Steve West BSc FChS MPodA MIPEMS
Dean and Professor of the Faculty of Health and
Social Care, University of the West of England,
Bristol, UK

Michael F. Whiting MA DPhil FChS FRSH DPodM
Dean of the Faculty of Health and Scholl Professor,
Faculty of Health, University of Brighton, Brighton,
UK

Ann Williams GradDipPhys MCSP
Lecturer in Physiotherapy, School of Biological and
Health Studies, University of Westminster, London;
Private Practice, London, UK

Preface to the fifth edition

In preparing the fifth edition of *Neale's Common Foot Disorders*, I have been joined by Gwen French and Steve West as co-editors to deal with the ever-increasing range of subject areas necessary to continue and develop the concept started in 1981 by Donald Neale. In this edition, much of the material has been changed by the inclusion of new contributors, who have rewritten many of the chapters, updating and extending the knowledge base. New areas have been included, such as a chapter on radiology which discusses this important area and relates it directly to the practice of podiatry, and a chapter on health promotion and education of patients which has been introduced to enhance awareness of education, enabling the podiatrist to become a more effective educator. A new chapter on injectable silicones also makes an important addition, particularly at a time when extensive trials are being carried out in the UK on the material, and it seems possible that changes are to be made in access to prescription-only medicines for podiatrists. A chapter on Hansen's disease has also been included because of the important role which the skills of the podiatrist have been shown to play in improving the life of so many sufferers in the developing world. The inclusion of these four chapters results from the steadily expanding demands for the skills of the podiatrist and the continual need to examine the basis of our practice. Podiatrists have shown, in the last 50 years, how important their unique contribution to medical care can be and this is set to expand with the advent of the graduate profession.

The chapter dealing with aspects of surgery has been subject to a review and is now divided into three topic areas. Each new chapter deals with different aspects of podiatric surgery, with the first concentrating on radical treatment for the nails, which is now a standard part of the practice of the State Registered Practitioner in the UK (and elsewhere in the world, in growing numbers). The excellent work on digital surgery, by Banks and McGlamry, is now a separate chapter, and has been complemented by an additional chapter on other surgical techniques written by a British podiatrist.

The chapters dealing with aspects of systemic disease have also been revised extensively, mostly by new contributors. The chapter on rheumatology has been totally rewritten and reflects current thinking on the team approach to management. The chapters on circulatory disease, neurological conditions, the effects of genetic factors, and metabolic disorders, have also been radically reviewed, and the latest thinking on patient management has been included. These major revisions in such very important chapters focus attention on the external influences which may affect the foot and lower limb and which can have profound influences on the ability of the podiatrist to operate effectively in health care teams.

The chapter on the structure and function of the foot has been extensively revised by the original authors to take account of current developments. They were also responsible, with an additional contributor, for the much revised chapter on disorders of the foot. Both of these chapters relate structure and function to the pathological changes found in patients. The chapter on clinical therapeutics has also been revised by an additional contributor, who has subjected the original material to a critical review, resulting in a wide-ranging update. Further advice was also sought on the section dealing with electrosurgery, a technique which has given promising results in the treatment of intractable plantar lesions. The need to include additional contributors in the revision of most chapters underlines the growing complexity of the practice of podiatry.

The other contributors have also made substantial alterations to the chapters for which they are responsible, making this the largest review of the subject material in the 15 years of the life of the text.

In this edition there has been an increase in the number of colour illustrations, the inclusion of which in the fourth edition was much appreciated by a large number of readers. Colour plates are included to aid the practitioner in recognising a condition and, in general, there is an increase in illustrations of all types.

Another innovation is the inclusion of key words and a contents list at the beginning of each chapter, which is of considerable assistance in locating information in the chapters. Wherever possible, short case histories have been added to help to illustrate the application of the theory.

Durham, 1996   D. L. L.

Preface to the first edition

Most books about the feet have naturally enough been written by medical authors for medical readers and they have dealt mainly with the major deformities and acute traumatic injuries and with their surgical management. Most everyday foot troubles, however, develop from biomechanical anomalies which only gradually become symptomatic, though they may ultimately be quite disabling in their cumulative effects. They only seldom reach the physician or surgeon and are generally treated by chiropodists, for whom there has recently been a relative dearth of literature. This book has been compiled to help to fill that need and it has been written with a clinical orientation.

There is abundant evidence that the common foot disorders cause a great deal of pain and disability. Numerous surveys have shown how prevalent they are among all groups of the population from school children to the elderly. They require specialised knowledge and skills for their effective management. The evolution and development of a chiropodial profession specialising in this field is sufficient testimony to the need.

In the UK, the training of a state registered chiropodist is broadly based on the medical sciences. It equips him/her to provide a comprehensive service of diagnosis and treatment virtually from the cradle to the grave and to identify those cases which require medical or surgical investigation and treatment. The scope of practice of the chiropodist has steadily enlarged within recent years and his/her therapeutic methods have become more efficient and durable. Developments in the field of mechanical therapy and the capacity to undertake minor surgical procedures under local anaesthesia have particularly increased his/her range and effectiveness.

It is in the public interest that this expansion should continue since it is a wasteful use of other costly skills and facilities if physicians and surgeons are unnecessarily burdened with cases within the competence of chiropodists. Heavy demands on hospital beds and operating theatres place a premium on effective methods of foot care which obviate or postpone the need for admission to hospital or which enhance post-operating care.

The diagnosis and management of the common foot disorders require the application of a variety of manual skills which cannot be taught or learnt solely from books. Such practical techniques as clinical examination, operating, and applying dressings can be mastered only through repeated practice under the guidance of clinical teachers. While they are all necessarily based on scientific principles, their application to individual cases is more art than science. There is no way of acquiring such skills other than by instruction from expert clinicians and practice in the techniques involved. It is impracticable to attempt to include much detailed instruction of that kind in a general text and it is properly left to the clinical teacher who has the dominant role in establishing the required levels of practical expertise.

This book attempts no more than to encapsulate current concepts on the origins, diagnosis and conservative management of the common foot disorders, while relating this particular field to the general medical and surgical conditions which bear directly upon it. The willing cooperation of so many different disciplines in its preparation is indicative of such collaboration in the clinical field.

Edinburgh, 1981   D. N.

Acknowledgements

The preparation of the fifth edition has been greatly facilitated by strengthening the editorial team with Gwen French and Steve West. This has spread the load of carrying forward the complex task started by Donald Neale. A text which ranges widely over the expanding scope of the practice of podiatry requires an ever greater effort to continue to keep it abreast of the changes.

In this fifth edition much has been revised and added, and the editors are indebted to the authors who have spent so much time in revising their work:

Miss Pat Boyd and Mr George Rendall revised the chapter which is now Chapter 1, and were joined by Mr Colin Thomson in carrying out a major revision of Chapter 5.

Mr Eric Anderson and Mr Jim Black have also carried out revisions to the chapters for which they are responsible together and on their own.

In the chapter on genetic disorders, Professor Raeburn has been joined by Dr Ritchie.

New authors have taken over a number of chapters and we are much indebted to Dr Ian Haslock for his chapter on rheumatology, Dr Mike Edmonds for his chapter on metabolic disorders, Professor Tooke and Dr Brash for their chapter on circulatory disorders and Dr Cartlidge for his chapter on neurological disorders.

Dr Sol Balkin has produced a comprehensive chapter on injectable silicones which will greatly add to the knowledge available on this important form of treatment. In preparing the work, Dr Balkin wishes to acknowledge the invaluable writing assistance of his wife, Janelle Balkin.

Four new chapters written by podiatrists are included in this edition: health education and communication, written by Mrs Gloria Dunlop; Hansen's disease, written by Mr Hugh Cross; metatarsal surgery, written by Mr Philip Milsom; and a chapter on radiology for podiatrists, written by Mr Colin Fullerton.

Once again, acknowledgement has to be made to Mrs Manesty Forster's contribution in many aspects of the production of this edition, but, in particular, for her assistance with the section on electrosurgery. Grateful thanks are due to all the staff members of the schools who offered useful advice.

I am also indebted to the assistance given by my wife, Eileen Lorimer, in the massive task of proof reading and the compilation of the index.

Finally, the editors would wish to place on record their appreciation of the help and advice given by the staff of Churchill Livingstone.

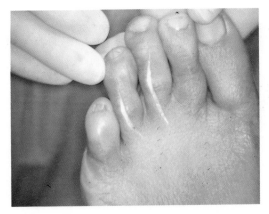

A

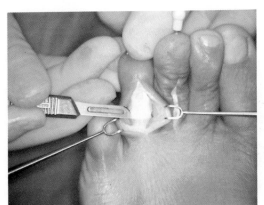

B

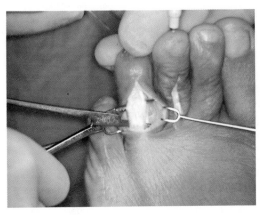

C

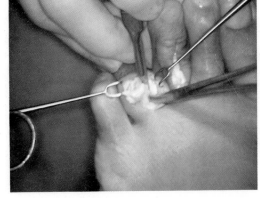

D

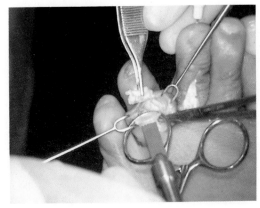

E

Plate 1 (See also Fig. 20.4) Arthroplasty. A: Midline dorsal longitudinal skin incision affords excellent exposure of the toe while avoiding neurovascular structures. (From McGlamry E D (ed) 1987 *Comprehensive textbook of foot surgery*, with permission from Williams and Wilkins, Baltimore.) B, C, D: An alternative technique to transecting the tendon is demonstrated, with undermining and retraction. Collateral ligaments are then cut to deliver the phalangeal head. E: Bone is resected with either a power saw or bone forceps.

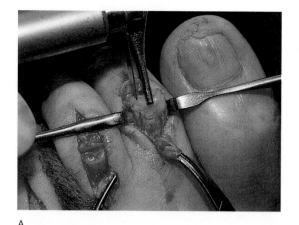

A

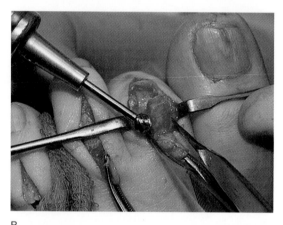

B

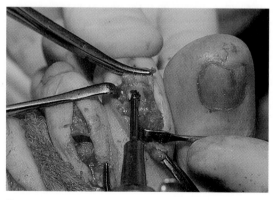

C

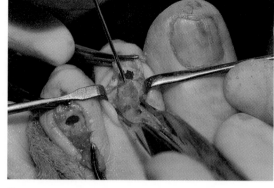

D

E

Plate 2 (See also Fig. 20.6) Peg-in-hole arthrodesis. A: The medial, lateral and plantar condyles are resected, as well as the distal articular cartilage. The dorsal cortex is carefully preserved. B: A ball burr is then used to contour the phalanx into a suitable peg. C: Starting with a very small ball burr or a side cutting burr, the initial hole is made in the base of the middle phalanx. Progressively larger ball burrs are used to ream the middle phalanx into a satisfactory receptacle. D: A hand-held Kirschner wire is used to identify the medullary canal of the proximal phalanx. Note the fully developed hole in the middle of the phalanx. E: The Kirschner wire is then introduced into the middle phalanx and directed distally through the tip of the toe. The surgeon holds the distal aspect of the toe rectus or in slight hyperextension. The wire driver is then moved to the end of the toes and the wire is retrograded across the arthrodesis site into the proximal phalanx. Fixation of the peg-in-hole arthrodesis is not mandatory, but enhances the overall stability.

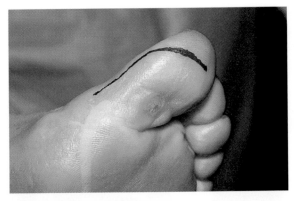

A

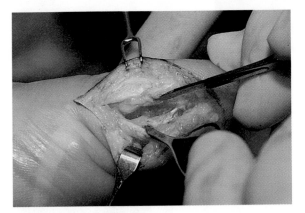

B

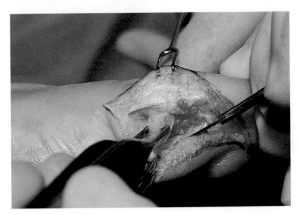

C

Plate 3   (See also Fig. 20.13) A: Skin incision for access to the medial and plantar aspects of the hallux interphalangeal joint. Note the lesion plantar to the location of the interphalangeal joint. B: Capsule opened and flexor tendon retracted plantarly, exposing sesamoid. C: Note the thickness of the sesamoid.

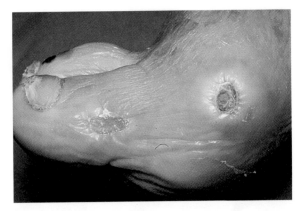

Plate 4   (See also Fig. 10.6) Ischaemic ulceration in the elderly patient.

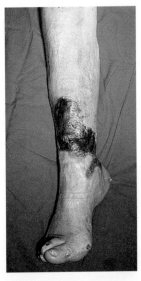

Plate 5   (See also Fig. 10.7) Onset of gangrene in the same patient as in Plate 4 following injudicious handling of the limb at risk.

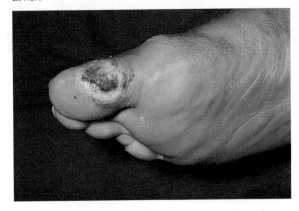

Plate 6   (See also Fig. 10.8) Neuropathic ulceration of diabetes.

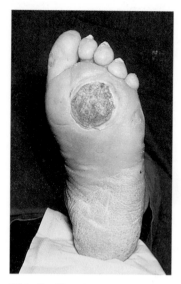

Plate 7 (See also Fig. 10.9) Basal cell epithelioma after reduction of plantar callosity.

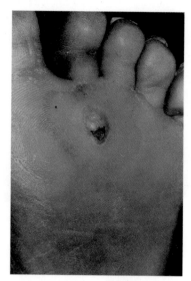

Plate 8 (See also Fig. 28.3) The undermined edges of active ulcers are a characteristic feature of the active phase of ulceration in Hansen's disease. The second metatarsal head is a common site for the first ulcer.

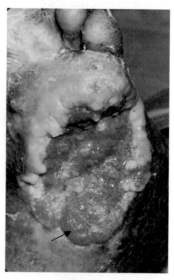

Plate 9 (See also Fig. 28.4) Complicated ulcer (in Hansen's disease). The hypergranulating surface suggests the involvement of necrotic bone.

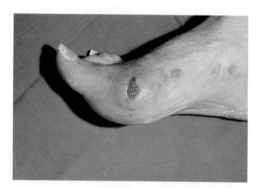

Plate 10 (See also Fig. 26.11) Rheumatoid arthritis. Skin loss caused by pressure over the first metatarsophalangeal joint in this case led to sepsis in the underlying joint.

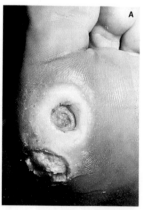

Plate 11 (See also Fig. 22.10) A: A 58-year-old woman with a painless diabetic ulcer at the site of prior callus. B: 4.9 ml of silicone implanted after healing in 1966 prevented ulcer recurrence for 16 years, during which time no special shoes or in-shoe devices were worn. (Reproduced with permission from Balkin S W 1984. The fluid silicone prosthesis. In: Weil L S (ed) Clinics in Podiatry. WB Saunders, Philadelphia.)

1

Structure and function

G. C. Rendall
P. M. Boyd

Keywords

Abduction
Adduction
Body planes
Eversion
Ground reaction forces
Inversion
Joint movement
Laws of motion
Muscle action
Postural stability
Pronation
Propulsion
Stance
Subtalar neutral
Supination
Walking

THE BIOMECHANICS OF STANCE AND GAIT

Terms of reference

In order to describe human movement it is necessary to create a universal frame of reference. This is equivalent to the lines of longitude and latitude on a world map, only in this case it is movement rather than position that is being recorded. The most universally used frame of reference involves bisecting the body with three orthogonal planes. If these planes are placed in the middle of the body, they would divide it into front and back (the *frontal* or *coronal* plane), top and bottom halves (the *transverse* plane), and right and left sides (the *sagittal* plane) (Fig. 1.1).

The movements that occur in these planes are mainly rotations around joint axes.

Movements in the frontal plane are lateral rotation of the head and trunk, abduction and adduction of the limbs,

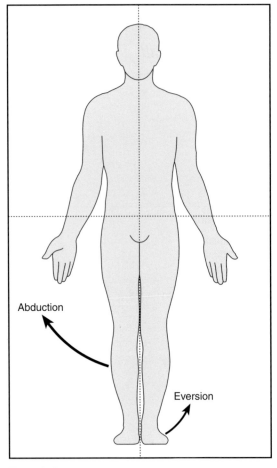

Frontal plane
Movements in the frontal plane are lateral rotation of the head and trunk, abduction and adduction of the limbs and eversion and inversion of the foot.

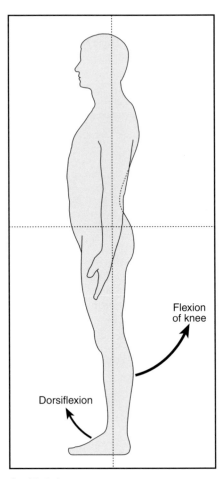

Sagittal plane
Movements in the sagittal plane are dorsiflexion and plantarflexion of the ankle and extension and flexion of all other joints.

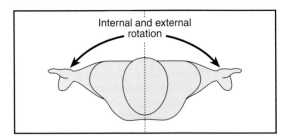

Transverse plane
Movements in the transverse plane are transverse rotation of the head and trunk, external and internal rotation of the limbs and adduction of the foot.

Figure 1.1   Movement in three cardinal body planes.

and eversion and inversion of the foot. Abduction and eversion are movements away from the midline of the body, i.e. the sole of the foot will aim outwards. Adduction and inversion are movements towards the midline of the body, i.e. the sole of the foot will aim inwards.

Movements in the transverse plane are transverse rotation of the head and trunk, external and internal rotation of the limbs, and abduction and adduction of the foot. External rotation and abduction in the transverse plane move the big toe away from the midline of the body. Internal rotation and adduction in the transverse plane move the big toe towards the midline of the body.

Movements in the sagittal plane are dorsiflexion and plantarflexion of the ankle, and extension and flexion of all other joints. Extension and dorsiflexion of the joints of the knee and foot move the toes upwards. Flexion and plantarflexion of the joints of the knee and foot move the toes downwards. Flexion of the hip, trunk and head moves the superior portion forwards relative to the inferior portion.

FORCES, MOMENTS AND SIR ISAAC NEWTON

In order to understand the function of the foot it is essential to have an understanding of simple Newtonian mechanics. Sir Isaac Newton's laws (Box 1.1) provide the basis for mathematical descriptions of mechanical concepts. It is, however, quite possible to develop a rudimentary understanding of the mechanics without using any mathematics. Indeed, we are already intuitively aware of the mechanical interactions between ourselves and our environment.

Box 1.1 Newton's laws of motion

- First law, *the law of inertia*
  A body will continue in a state of rest or in a straight line of uniform motion unless acted on by an external force. The amount of force required to change motion is directly related to the mass of the body in question.
- Second law, *the law of acceleration*
  Force = mass (kg) $\times$ acceleration (ms^{-2})
- Third law, *the law of reaction*
  If a body exerts a force on another body then the second body will apply an equal and opposite force on the first.

Forces and motion

A force is something which changes or attempts to change the state of motion of a body in space. Bodies without net forces applied will therefore not change their state of motion. In practice it is impossible to have no forces applied, but Newton's first law, *the law of inertia*, also applies to the situation where forces are in balance, for example in a tug of war where no side has the advantage. In this situation there are no resultant forces, so the forces are in equilibrium and the state of motion of the two tug-of-war teams remains

unchanged. A body's tendency to resist a change in its state of motion is described as its *inertia*. The heavier a body is, the more difficult it will be to move, i.e. the greater will be its inertia.

Newton's second law defines force as mass $\times$ acceleration. This means that in describing a force there will be two components, the size of the body applying the force and the rate at which it changes its velocity. It is easy to see that, all else being equal, a large heavy object will apply a greater force than a small light one, and that an object that travels fast will have more force than one that travels slowly. It should be clear to most readers that a large fast object carries the potential for greater force than a small slow one (e.g. a charging elephant carries a far greater threat than a charging tortoise). It is not the velocity that creates the force but the acceleration (i.e. the rate of change of velocity). The faster the velocity changes, the higher will be the force. Alternatively, the longer the period of time over which velocity changes, the smaller will be the force. If the charging elephant slows down over a sufficiently long period then the force might be quite small. In theory it is possible to have the tortoise accelerate over such a short time that it carries the greater force. Whilst this theoretical example may be difficult to envisage there are countless practical examples of using time to reduce force, such as moving the hands with the ball as a catch is made, braking gently to a stop in a car rather than slamming on the brakes, and having a crash mat in a pole vaulting competition. The foot is adept at reducing force by extending the period over which the body decelerates in gait.

Newton's third law, *the law of reaction*, is generally paraphrased as 'for every action there is an equal and opposite reaction'. Returning to the elephant, whilst it is true that the charging elephant may induce terror, it is unlikely to cause harm until there is contact. As it makes contact it causes our state of motion to be changed very rapidly by applying a large force. This force has two components, mass and acceleration. The elephant has such a large mass that its rate of change of velocity can be quite small to create a large force. Newton's third law, however, dictates that as the elephant exerts a force on us, so we exert an equal and opposite force on the elephant. This force will be of the same magnitude but in the opposite direction and through the same line of action. As the elephant hits us it is slowed down a little, i.e. it decelerates. As we strike the elephant, we accelerate in the opposite direction and with far greater magnitude. We clearly have a far smaller mass than the elephant, so that we would need to change our velocity far more rapidly to create an equivalent force. The difference between our acceleration and the elephant's will be the inverse of the difference between our mass and the elephant's mass.

Similarly, when our foot strikes the ground, the ground exerts an equal and opposite force on our foot. This *ground reaction force* is determined not only by our weight, but also by our rate of movement and by the actions taken by our limbs to alter the rate of acceleration. The foot is particularly well adapted to optimise the use of forces in walking.

Moments of force

Linear forces can push or pull and, if of sufficient magnitude, will create motion. The type of motion created by linear forces is translation. A drawer sliding open and a skier gliding downhill are examples of translatory motion. In human gait, however, the dominant form of movement is not translation but rotation around joints. The type of force that creates rotation is a moment. Moments are forces applied at a perpendicular distance from a centre of rotation (fulcrum). The mathematics of moments is surprisingly simple. A moment is equal to the force multiplied by the perpendicular distance from the fulcrum (see Box 1.2). This means that there is an absolute correlation between force and distance and the moment (the amount of turning power). If we double the force we double the turning power (torque); if we double the length to the centre of rotation we also double the turning power. Most of us already apply the principle of moments in our daily lives, perhaps when using a screwdriver to lever open a tin of paint. Indeed our environment is designed according to this simple principle. Door handles are a good example, attached as far from the hinge (fulcrum) as possible to minimise the amount of force required to open a door. The moment required to open the door is a constant. Attaching the door handle close to the hinge side would mean that a far greater force would be needed to create the same torque, i.e. we would have to pull harder to open the door.

Another means of reducing a moment is to alter the angle at which a force is applied to a lever. The moment will be greatest when a force is applied at right angles to the lever. As the line of application moves away from the perpendicular, the force begins to develop different properties. Instead of merely rotating the lever around the fulcrum, it will now also either push or pull the lever along its length. The closer the force comes to being parallel with the lever, the greater will be its pushing or pulling force and the smaller will be the turning force. This is used to advantage in the gait cycle. The axes of motion of the ankle, subtalar and midtarsal joints are all rotated away from

---

Box 1.2 Relationship between forces and moments

Moments or turning forces are a product of force and perpendicular distance (the length of the lever arm). Moments can therefore be changed by altering either the force or the length of the lever arm. For example, 500 Newtons × 0.20 m = 100 Nm; 500 Newtons × 0.10 m = 50 Nm; i.e. the moment reduces in direct relation to the length of the lever.

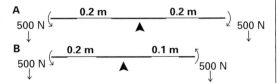

In A, the clockwise and anticlockwise moments are equal, i.e. there is equilibrium.

In B, shortening the clockwise moment arm by half reduces the resultant moment by half, therefore the lever will turn in an anticlockwise direction.

---

the sagittal plane during the early part of the stance phase, maximising the rotational component of force, so giving maximum flexibility in response to sagittal plane ground reaction forces. During the propulsive phase, as the leg externally rotates, these axes are rotated towards the sagittal plane. This minimises the rotational component of the ground reaction forces on the joints and maximises the compressional component. This assists the foot to be a rigid lever during propulsion, when sagittal plane forces through the foot are at their highest.

Most gait activity is rotational and is governed by the requirement to create a sufficiently large moment to balance or overcome given resistance. In gait, the forces involved are generated by muscles and ligaments, and the lever arms are the bones. The positions and angles of insertion of muscles have a major influence on the body's ability to ambulate efficiently.

FUNCTIONAL ANATOMY

The function of the foot is to act as an interface between the body and supporting surface in stance and gait. It is the platform upon which the body rests in standing, walking and running, and is ideally designed to cope with the range of stresses imposed upon it by human locomotory activity. Foot function in gait must vary, both to accommodate these stresses and to permit efficient locomotion. Ideally the foot is, at appropriate times, a shock absorber, a mobile adapter and a rigid lever.

The stability and behaviour of the weight-bearing foot are considerably influenced by the manner in which the body weight is transmitted to it by the tibia through the trochlear surface of the talus. The body weight is transmitted to the foot through this articulation and, from the talus, plantarly to the calcaneus and lateral column and anteriorly to the navicular and medial column. Any movements occurring in the tibia are also transmitted into the foot.

Although the plantar surface of the foot is in firm contact with the ground, movement within the foot, principally pronation and supination, can occur, allowing the body and lower limb to move above it. *Pronation* within the foot is a triplanar movement involving *abduction* (transverse plane), *eversion* (frontal plane) and *dorsiflexion* (sagittal plane). *Supination* also occurs in three planes, its components being adduction, inversion and plantarflexion. These movements take place at the *subtalar* and *midtarsal* joints in response to ground reaction forces from below, transverse and frontal plane motions of the tibia and femur from above, and eccentric and concentric contraction of muscles. Therefore the joint acts as a torque converter.

Ground reaction occurs in three planes and is entirely dependent on the force applied by the foot above. This will vary with the mass of the patient, the speed of walking, the stability/mobility of the contact limb and the interaction of the foot with the supporting surface (e.g. concrete will tend to give higher ground reaction forces than sponge rubber). Ideally, reaction forces are minimised at heel strike and maximised in propulsion. Rotational forces act with ground reaction to influence the positions of joints in the foot. In the early part of the gait cycle, internal rotation of the tibia causes the talus to adduct and plantarflex, inducing calcaneal eversion and thus producing pronation of the subtalar joint. Frontal plane ground reaction forces under the first ray supinate the forefoot, around the longitudinal axis of the midtarsal joint, maintaining a plantargrade and adaptable foot. Transverse and sagittal plane reaction forces pronate the oblique axis of the midtarsal joint. The overall effect of internal tibial rotation is to enhance forefoot adaptability and shock absorption. During propulsion, external rotation of the tibia helps to supinate the subtalar joint. Transverse plane reaction forces adduct the forefoot, supinating the oblique axis of the midtarsal joint. Abduction and dorsiflexion of the talus induce calcaneal inversion, thereby prompting lateral ground reaction forces that pronate the forefoot around the longitudinal axis of the midtarsal joint. External rotation helps to lock the forefoot, making it a rigid lever for propulsion.

Ground reaction and internal rotation are a passive result of the effect of gravity. Muscle contraction and external rotation are antigravitational. Muscles may contract eccentrically, to act as a brake, slowing down and controlling movements, or concentrically, to initiate movement or change its direction, particularly against the influence of gravity. These features combine to form a complex mechanism that allows for alterations in body posture whilst maintaining a plantargrade foot as a base upon which to stand, walk and run.

Standing

The function of the foot in standing is to act as a base, to support the body above it, and to maintain intrinsic and postural stability with the minimum of energy expenditure. Intrinsic stability is achieved by interlocking the joints under the influence of opposing forces of body weight and ground reaction forces. To achieve postural stability it is necessary to maintain the centre of mass within the base of stance.

Postural stability

The *base of stance* is that area of the body in contact with the supporting surface plus all the area contained within its margin. In quadrupedal stance a very large area is contained within the four feet, so it produces a very wide base of stance. In bipedal stance the base consists of the feet and the ground between them. The foot as a base of stance is predominantly a rigid structure acted upon by the muscles of the leg.

The *centre of gravity* is that part of a body around which all of its mass acts. During stance in humans, the centre of gravity lies within the pelvic girdle. A plumb line dropped from the centre of mass in stance would hang between the feet and slightly ahead of the tibia, through which the body mass is transmitted to the feet (Fig. 1.2). The foot extends well beyond this point and loading is principally on the heel and forefoot. The centre of gravity lies fairly centrally within the base of stance, slightly ahead of the ankle joint's axis of motion and also ahead of the knee joint. This gives clear advantages in terms of stability and energy conservation. Forward movement, which may threaten stability, is easily countered by the triceps surae contracting to pull the tibia back behind the centre of gravity. This large muscle group undergoes frequent minimal contracture (postural tone) to maintain postural stability. As long as the centre of gravity remains in front of the ankle and knee joint axes, other groups, including the anterior muscles of the leg and thigh, should remain at rest.

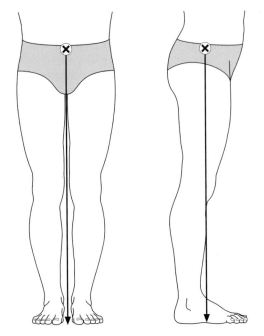

Figure 1.2 Centre of gravity in standing.

Human balance mechanisms are highly refined and thus balance maintenance seems effortless in spite of a relatively narrow base of stance. When balance systems fail it is necessary to apply these principles of static stance in order to prevent falling. Use of a walking stick or frame increases stability in such cases by substantially increasing the margins of the base of stance.

Intrinsic stability and subtalar neutral position

In stance, the foot is normally a rigid structure with the subtalar joint in its neutral position and the midtarsal joint locked. The simplest definition of subtalar joint neutral position is 'that position of the joint in which the foot is neither supinated nor pronated' (Root et al 1977). This definition, whilst unambiguous, is rather opaque and there is considerable debate over precisely how to identify subtalar neutral. Quantifying by range has been attempted. Root et al (1977) suggested that neutral lies in a position around which one-third of the total available range of motion will be pronation and two-thirds will be supination. This has been widely quoted but is at best a broad generalisation for the majority and is by no means a reliable method of accurately finding subtalar neutral for all subjects. Other methods involve finding the position by visually creating symmetry in the soft tissues beneath the medial

and lateral malleoli, and palpating the medial and lateral sides of the head of the talus until it disappears into the socket created by the midtarsal joint. These methods of determining subtalar neutral have been shown to be reliable when used by the same examiner but not when used by different examiners. In essence, whilst subtalar neutral is acceptable as a broad concept, as a precise position it clearly means different things to different people. Functionally, there is less difficulty: the subtalar joint is neutral when the articular facets of the talus and calcaneus are congruous. This approximates a position in which the normal foot will, in standing, have a forefoot and rearfoot that are parallel to each other and to a flat supporting surface. In using the term subtalar neutral, this chapter utilises this gross functional definition.

Functional rigidity is achieved by locking the midtarsal joint in maximal pronation when the subtalar joint is either neutral or supinated. Normally, at this time, the planes of the hindfoot and forefoot are parallel. Ideally, a bisection line of the posterior surface of the calcaneus is vertical when the subtalar joint is in the neutral position. This position is also achieved in walking when the weight-bearing foot reaches the end of midstance. Variations from vertical, either inverted or everted, show some mechanical anomaly that may lead to symptoms of pain or deformity (see Ch. 5).

Locking of the midtarsal joint is achieved through a combination of controlled loading from above and ground reaction forces from below. Sagittal plane ground reaction forces create a dorsiflexion moment to lock out the oblique axis of the midtarsal joint. Frontal plane ground reaction forces create an evertory moment to lock out the longitudinal axis of the midtarsal joint. Normal postural tone in triceps surae balances these forces through plantarflexion of the ankle (sagittal plane) and inversion of the calcaneus (frontal plane). Stability is achieved when all forces and moments within the foot are in equilibrium.

Walking

Steindler (1964) described the lower limb as a kinetic chain, a series of links that are free to move on each other but which are capable of combining into a stable column to support the body. The chain is said to be open when the distal link is free to move and closed when it is fixed, as in weight-bearing. When open, the distal links move on the proximal; when closed, the proximal links move on the distal. During the stance phase, the loaded limb is a closed kinetic chain in which the foot is a fixed base around which the supporting limb and the rest of the body are swung forward. During the swing phase, the unloaded lower limb is an open kinetic chain with its segments swinging freely forward in relation to the body above it.

The foot is required to be a stable base during stance. This may also be said of walking, but in walking foot function must vary throughout the gait cycle. This variability permits the foot to reduce the force of impact, adapt to variations in its relationship with the body above and the supporting surface below, and maximise efficient transference of energy.

For purposes of analysis it is convenient to divide the walking gait cycle into four distinct but consecutive phases. These are *contact*, *midstance* and *propulsion* (which together form the stance phase), and the *swing* phase. The foot functions as a shock absorber in contact and as a rigid lever in propulsion. Midstance is a period of functional transfer and stabilisation as the centre of mass passes over the loaded foot (Fig. 1.3).

Contact

Heel strike signals the end of the swing phase and the beginning of the contact phase. Force reduction in contact is essential to minimise the potentially harmful effects of impact, so the foot and lower limb act as a shock absorber during this period. Contact force is reduced by a combination of factors. The subtalar joint pronates 4–6°, the tibia internally rotates, the ankle plantarflexes, the knee flexes and the contralateral

(swing side) pelvis drops slightly in the frontal plane. The heel pad and elastic plantar components of the foot—plantar aponeurosis, deltoid, spring, long and short plantar ligaments—all assist in absorbing shock. These factors reduce force by extending the period of deceleration as the foot strikes the ground (Fig. 1.4).

The major shock-absorbing features within the foot are controlled pronation of the subtalar joint and controlled plantarflexion of the ankle joint. Pronation occurs as a result of lateral ground reaction force at heel strike creating an evertory moment around the subtalar joint. Plantarflexion occurs as a result of posterior reaction forces on contact creating a plantarflexion moment around the ankle joint. Control is given by medial and anterior resistance from contraction of tibialis anterior (creating an invertory and dorsiflexion moment). Moments, as described earlier (see Box 1.2), are turning forces that rotate levers (e.g. the bones of the foot and leg) around axes (in this case the centres of rotation of the joints). Rotation will continue to occur until moments in a certain direction equal moments in the opposite direction (e.g. clockwise = anticlockwise) at which time they are in *equilibrium*. In gait, equilibrium is normally achieved when the foot is flat on the supporting surface, at which time it is said to be *plantargrade*.

Midstance

The midstance phase begins as the metatarsals make

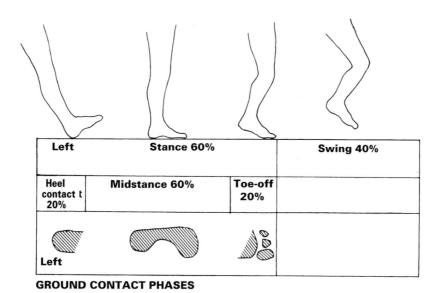

Figure 1.3 The walking cycle, showing stance and swing phases and the weight-bearing areas of the plantar surface.

Force (N) = mass (kg) $\times$ acceleration (m s^{-2})

Acceleration (m s^{-2}) = $\dfrac{\text{change in velocty (m s}^{-1})}{\text{Time (s)}}$

e.g. $\dfrac{50 \text{ kg} \times 10 \text{ m s}^{-1}}{1 \text{ s}}$ = 500 N

$\dfrac{50 \text{ kg} \times 10 \text{ m s}^{-1}}{2 \text{ s}}$ = 250 N

The components of force are mass, change in velocity and time. Increasing mass or change in velocity increases force. Increasing time reduces force.

Figure 1.4   Factors which alter forces

contact and become fully weight-bearing, and the opposite foot leaves the ground. The foot in early midstance is a mobile adapter capable of achieving stability despite variations in loading between the body and the walking surface. This is facilitated to a large degree by pronation of the subtalar joint and the associated movements of the talus and calcaneus. With subtalar pronation, the talus adducts and plantarflexes and the calcaneus everts. Elftmann (1960) suggested that this changed the alignment of the axes of motion of the calcaneocuboid and talonavicular joints. These become increasingly parallel with subtalar pronation, enabling the calcaneocuboid and talonavicular joints to move as one and thereby increasing the available range of motion. This unlocks the oblique axis of the midtarsal joint (see 'subtalar joint' and 'midtarsal joint' sections, p. 11).

Eversion of the calcaneus twists the medial side of the forefoot against the ground to produce inversion, unlocking the longitudinal axis of the midtarsal joint. Talar and calcaneal movements also destabilise the medial and lateral columns so that the forefoot is generally more able to adapt to variations in underlying terrain body position. Shock absorption continues into early midstance as muscles and ligaments lengthen under tension to control yielding motions at the knee, ankle, tarsal and midtarsal joints.

In the second half of the midstance phase, foot function changes and the need for stability and, ultimately, rigidity supplants that for adaptability and shock absorption. Towards the end of midstance, the subtalar joint resupinates, achieving subtalar neutral at around the time of heel lift. The body passes over and forward of the foot as it prepares for propulsion. The ankle joint dorsiflexes 10°, coinciding with a similar amount of hip extension. This allows the centre of gravity to pass ahead of the base of support whilst the heel remains in ground contact. Resupination is assisted by the increasing tension on the triceps surae and tibialis posterior and by external rotation of the femur and tibia. These rotations, initiated by forward rotation of the swing side of the pelvis, are transferred to the talus and on to the foot. Ground reaction forces in the transverse plane facilitate supination of the subtalar joint and locking of the oblique axis of the midtarsal joint.

Midstance should therefore be considered as a transfer phase that enables the post-contact mobile shock-absorbing foot to become a pre-propulsive rigid lever.

Propulsion

In the propulsive stage, rigidity is essential to maximise efficient transfer of energy and minimise risk of injury to joints. As the heel leaves the ground, the subtalar joint supinates rapidly due to muscular contraction by triceps surae and tibialis posterior and due to external rotation of the leg and plantarflexion of the first ray. The planes of rotation around the two articular facets of the midtarsal joint become less parallel, reducing mobility in the oblique axis of the midtarsal joint. The lateral border of the forefoot is twisted against the ground, reducing mobility in the longitudinal axis. The forefoot becomes locked to the rearfoot (see section on midtarsal joint, p. 11). Subtalar and midtarsal joint axes also rotate towards the sagittal plane to minimise their vulnerability to reaction moments (Fig. 1.5). Heel lift and calcaneal inversion also facilitate plantarflexion of the first ray, which occurs as a combined result of contraction of peroneus longus and operation of the Hicks' windlass (Fig. 1.6). This brings the medial side of the forefoot into contact, despite heel inversion, and stabilises the medial column, to maximise propulsive stability. As a result of these adaptations, during propulsion the foot is rigid, the arch height increases and loading is concentrated on the metatarsal heads and the distal pads of the toes. This area of contact provides the fulcrum for 'toe off'. The foot then leaves the ground and the swing phase begins (Fig. 1.7).

Swing

During the swing phase the foot is clear of the ground as the limb swings past its neighbour, preparing to resume weight-bearing at heel strike, and so the gait cycle is repeated. The swing phase affords the swinging limb the opportunity to recover in preparation for

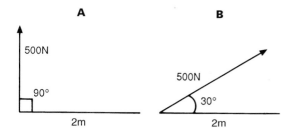

In diagram A, the 500 N clockwise force pulls at 90° 2 m from the fulcrum, giving a moment of 500 N × 2 m = 1000 Nm.

In diagram B, the 500 N clockwise force pulls at only 30° from parallel, reducing its vertical pull and therefore its moment. In this case we find the vertical component by the calculation:

$$500 \text{ N} \times 2 \text{ m} \times \sin 30° = 1000 \text{ Nm} \times 0.5 \text{ (i.e. } \sin 30°\text{)} = 500 \text{ Nm.}$$

Thus the moment *reduces* as the line of action of a force moves away from the perpendicular to the lever.

This is used to advantage in the gait cycle. Turning the axis of rotation of a joint toward the reaction forces *reduces* perpendicularity to these forces, and therefore reduces resultant moments around joints. The effect is to reduce joint stress and increase stability in propulsion.

Figure 1.5   Lever length can be changed by altering the angle of application of the force. The further the angle of application is from 90°, the smaller will be the perpendicular (turning) component of the force.

the stance phase and helps to move the centre of gravity over the stance foot. The pelvic rotation that accompanies the swinging limb also initiates the external rotation that is so important to the stance phase limb in late midstance and propulsion.

At toe-off and heel strike, both feet are simultaneously in ground contact for approximately 10% of the walking cycle. This period of double support becomes shorter with increased speed of walking until eventually in running there is no *double support phase* and both feet are off the ground in *float phase*.

Muscle action

During these alternating phases, the muscles of the lower limb act from both their proximal to their distal attachments and vice versa, according to need. A muscle may act by shortening and bringing its attachments closer together (isotonic/concentric contraction), by maintaining its length unchanged and its attachments stable under stress (isometric contraction), or by a controlled elongation that damps down and checks the moving part of its attachments under tensile force

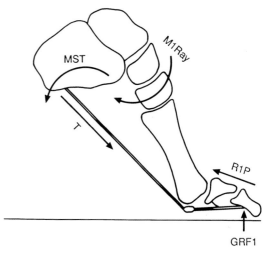

Figure 1.6   Hicks' windlass. Hicks (1954) described a mechanism by which pivoting around the metatarsal heads raises the medial longitudinal arch. Ground reaction force (GRF1) anterior to the metatarsal heads dorsiflects the first toe, creating tension in the plantar aponeurosis (T). This pulls the toe back, producing a reaction force at the first metatarsophalangeal joint (R1P) and a plantarflexion moment around the joints of the first ray (M1Ray). Tension in the aponeurosis produces a supinatory moment around the subtalar joint (MST).

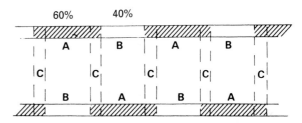

Figure 1.7   The walking cycle, showing (A) successive left and right stance phases (60%); (B) successive right and left swing phases (40%); (C) successive periods of double support (10%).

(eccentric contraction). Collectively, the muscles of the lower limb effect and control movement in the following ways:

1. *Prime movers* contract isotonically to move a part, e.g. the triceps surae muscle group acts on the calcaneus from the lower leg to plantarflex the foot.

2. *Antagonists* resist the pull of the prime movers, thus checking and controlling the movements, e.g. the quadriceps extend the knee in late swing while the hamstrings check this action immediately before heel strike.

3. *Synergists* stabilise the attachments from which the prime movers and antagonists are acting, e.g. the short digital flexors fix the toes firmly to the ground and so provide a stable base from which the long extensors and flexors can act.

4. *Fixators* stabilise intervening joints to ensure that the desired movement occurs at the appropriate articulation, e.g. the triceps surae stabilise the ankle once the leg has begun to swing forward. This action prevents further dorsiflexion at the ankle while the extensors dorsiflex the toes at the metatarsophalangeal joints.

Biomechanically, the act of walking is a repeated series of muscular actions designed to keep the body's centre of gravity off-balance just forward of its base, represented by each foot alternately. The swinging limb and the force of gravity are used to assist forward momentum and this minimises expenditure of energy. In locomotion, the contractural tone of muscles powerfully reinforces the inert tension of ligaments in binding together the parts of the foot and restraining hypermobility of joints. The tendons of tibialis posterior and peroneus longus undersling the tarsus mediolaterally and so provide a dynamic tarsal cradle. The plantar intrinsic muscles similarly provide tensile support longitudinally against the thrust of weight-bearing forces. The transverse head of the adductor hallucis reinforces and guards the transverse intermetatarsal ligaments. The peroneus longus also stabilises the first metatarsal. Muscles thus assist in maintaining structural stability under maximum load while simultaneously initiating and controlling movements.

Joint movements in the lower limb

During the gait cycle the body's centre of gravity is translated through space in a smooth undulating line of progression. Joint motions and muscle action work together to produce an energy-efficient and smooth pattern of gait. The major displacements of the limbs occur in the sagittal plane as the limbs move backwards and forwards. Most of the muscle activity occurs to control these motions and thus muscles tend to fire at the beginning and end of the stance and swing phases. The muscles also control the subtler movements of pelvic tilt and rotation, and the transverse and frontal plane motions of the lower limb and foot.

The pelvis. The pelvis pivots in the transverse plane, giving length to the stride and allowing first one leg and then the other to swing forward. The abductor muscles of the weight-bearing hip support the pelvis, allowing the swinging limb ground clearance to follow through and minimising the vertical displacement of the centre of gravity. The pelvis also rotates forward with the swinging limb and, as it does so, the weight-bearing hip is stabilised in the transverse plane by its external rotators. In this way, pelvic rotation assists external rotation of the weight-bearing lower limb in the second half of the stance phase. Pelvic rotation also helps to lengthen the limb in order to minimise vertical drop of the centre of gravity and conserve energy.

The hip. The hip extends as the limb begins to bear weight, and continues to extend as the body passes over the foot in stance phase, then flexes during swing phase. Flexion is initiated by the iliopsoas and the tensor fascia latae. Frontal plane motion in the hip complements pelvic tilt. The hip joint adducts rapidly in the contact phase in order to reduce shock by permitting downward tilt of the pelvis. It then abducts as the opposite foot comes into contact, helping to shift the centre of gravity onto the opposite foot. Hip rotation in the transverse plane is rather complicated, as the point of reference, the pelvis, is externally rotating throughout almost the whole stance phase, whilst the hip joint internally rotates during this time. This is because, in this closed chain state, the pelvis pivots on the hip joint. The pelvis and hip rotations occur at different rates. This means that while the hip joint rotates faster than the pelvis, the femur appears to rotate internally, and when the pelvis rotates faster than the hip joint, the femur appears to rotate externally. Fortunately it is much simpler, and perfectly acceptable, to consider femoral rotation relative to the line of progression, rather than hip rotation relative to the pelvis. The femur internally rotates during the first 12–15% of the gait cycle and externally rotates for the remainder of the stance phase, before internally rotating in swing. Rapid internal rotation in the contact phase assists shock absorption. External rotation restores the alignment of the knee joint so that it can work in the sagittal plane during the propulsive phase. Transverse plane reaction forces resist external rotation (abduction) of the foot, assisting supination of the subtalar joint and the oblique axis of the midtarsal joint.

The knee. The knee joint flexes and extends twice in the gait cycle. Flexion occurs just after heel contact, to absorb shock, and again during swing, to allow for foot clearance. Extension occurs immediately prior to heel strike and during midstance, as the body passes directly over the weight-bearing limb. Flexion of the knee is retarded by the quadriceps after contact, until the centre of gravity moves forward of the knee joint. Simultaneously, the knee flexes to aid clearance of the foot during swing. The swinging limb is controlled by the hamstrings as it prepares for contact. The knee joint also rotates slightly on its vertical axis, internally as it flexes and externally as it extends. In the closed chain state, the tibia and knee tend to follow the talus in the transverse plane, so that as the subtalar joint pronates, and the talus adducts, the tibia will internally rotate. Pronation of the subtalar joint induces internal rotation of the tibia and femur which, along with knee flexion, produce shock absorption as the limb becomes loaded in early stance.

The ankle. The ankle joint moves through rapid plantar flexion at heel contact. The movement is controlled by the tibialis anterior muscle contracting eccentrically to prevent foot slap and to reduce the force of impact. The ankle then dorsiflexes as the body passes over the weight-bearing limb, reaching 10° beyond the vertical. Rapid plantar flexion follows, with heel lift initiated by contraction of the triceps surae group. Once again dorsiflexion of the ankle occurs to give toe clearance during swing. The tibialis anterior muscles again facilitate this movement, this time contracting concentrically.

The subtalar joint. The subtalar joint is a triplane joint with substantial frontal and transverse plane and limited sagittal plane motion. The movements available are pronation and supination. In gait, from a position of slight supination at heel strike, the subtalar joint rapidly pronates in the contact and early midstance phases. Pronation is instigated by lateral ground reaction force. When it is combined with plantarflexion of the ankle and resisted by eccentric contracture of the tibialis anterior, subtalar joint pronation increases the period of deceleration that occurs in the transition from swing to stance. This has the direct effect of reducing contact forces (i.e. shock absorption). From about 25% of the stance phase the subtalar joint slowly resupinates, reaching neutral shortly after the swing and stance limbs pass each other at approximately 50% of the stance phase. The subtalar joint continues to supinate, and at approximately 60% of the stance phase, when gastrocnemius contracts and the heel lifts, the calcaneus becomes markedly inverted. The effect of calcaneal supination is to encourage rigidity in propulsion, principally through its relationship with the midtarsal joint. The subtalar joint might be considered the key to foot function throughout the stance phase of the gait cycle. Subtalar joint motion, unlike the relatively independent ankle joint, tends to have a major influence on other joints within the foot, particularly the midtarsal joint and the first and fifth rays. It also influences the transverse plane alignment of the leg. Subtalar joint pronation increases midtarsal

and forefoot mobility, enhancing the mobile adaptability needed in early midstance.

The midtarsal joint. The midtarsal joint is a triplanar joint with two axes and therefore two degrees of freedom. The longitudinal axis of the midtarsal joint runs close to the sagittal and transverse planes and permits motion primarily in the frontal plane (i.e. inversion/eversion). The oblique axis runs diagonally across all three planes allowing most of its motion in the transverse and sagittal planes. As the ankle and subtalar joint are the interface between the foot and the rest of the body so the midtarsal joint interfaces the rearfoot and forefoot. Midtarsal joint function is crucially important for propulsive stability as the forefoot is the contact zone during the propulsive phase. Midtarsal joint function is also highly dependent on subtalar joint function. Subtalar joint pronation leads to adduction and plantarflexion of the talus and eversion of the calcaneus. This increases forefoot adaptability in a number of ways:

1. The talus becomes less congruous with the navicular, reducing the stability of the medial column.
2. The oblique axis of motion of the midtarsal joint is lowered, increasing the sagittal plane component of its range of motion.
3. The planes of motion of the talonavicular and calcaneocuboid joints are normally opposed when the subtalar joint is in the neutral position. Talocalcaneal movements associated with subtalar joint pronation increase the parallelism of the planes of motion of these two joints and thereby increase their freedom to move in parallel. This is described as 'unlocking' the oblique axis of the midtarsal joint.

From early midstance onwards, the subtalar joint gradually moves out of pronation into supination. At about 60% of the stance phase the calcaneus becomes inverted by the contracting triceps surae. Calcaneal inversion at heel lift twists the lateral side of the forefoot against the ground, effecting an evertory reaction force. These opposing moments (inversion of the calcaneus, eversion of the lateral column) screw the foot tight at the calcaneocuboid joint. This is often described as 'locking' the longitudinal axis of the midtarsal joint in pronation. External rotation of the leg in propulsion encourages subtalar joint supination by adducting the talus. This effects a transverse plane ground reaction force (adduction) in the forefoot. Adduction twists the forefoot against the abducting talus, 'locking out' the oblique axis of the midtarsal joint in supination.

The forefoot. The ankle joint plantarflexes at contact and then dorsiflexes until such time as triceps surae contracts to plantarflex the ankle joint, lift the heel and begin the propulsive phase. This normally occurs with the ankle in about 10° of dorsiflexion. Plantarflexion of the ankle in propulsion leads to the foot pivoting around a fulcrum at the interface of the metatarsal heads and the supporting surface. This leads to digital dorsiflexion, and the reaction to this, by means of the windlass mechanism described by Hicks (1953), is metatarsal plantarflexion. The loaded first metatarsal slides back on the sesamoids assisted by contraction of the peroneus longus muscle, which inserts into its base. Eccentric contraction of flexor hallucis longus helps to stabilise the first ray and the medial column. Hicks (1953) also suggested that variable plantarflexion of the metatarsals may permit the forefoot to remain plantargrade as the heel pivots. This can be simulated by laying your hand on the table in the shape of a snooker or pool bridge. The wrist can now be twisted whilst the fingers remain on the table. This is facilitated principally by sagittal plane motion of the fingers (Fig. 1.8).

Weight distribution in locomotion

Weight distribution through the foot in locomotion is determined by the skeletal structure of the foot and its relationship to the moving body above and the ground below.

The ankle, knee and hip joints provide for extension and flexion of the limb in the sagittal plane. The hip and peritalar joints facilitate rotatory motions, the former for internal and external rotation of the thigh and leg on a vertical axis, and the latter for pronatory and supinatory rotation of the foot on a roughly longitudinal axis.

At heel strike, the foot is slightly inverted and the posterior lateral rim of the heel of the shoe first makes contact with the ground. It is at this stage in the walking cycle that shock absorption is most required within the foot and this is provided by the greater degree of mobility afforded to the small tarsal joints as the foot pronates. As weight is transferred progressively from the opposite foot, the hindfoot pronates at the subtalar joint to allow all the metatarsal heads to make contact with the ground and become fully weight-bearing. This movement is accompanied by some corresponding internal rotation of the tibia and talus. By the middle of the stance phase, the foot is fully loaded with the entire weight of the body.

As the foot progresses through the midstance phase, its function changes into that of a rigid lever to propel the body forwards. This involves supination of the foot with corresponding external rotation of the tibia—the heel leaves the ground and the final force at toe-off is concentrated on the plantar surfaces of the medial metatarsals and the hallux. This is the time of maximum loading of the forefoot and maximum stresses on the plantar soft tissues. It is during this period in the stance phase that mechanical defects, from wherever they originate, have the maxi-

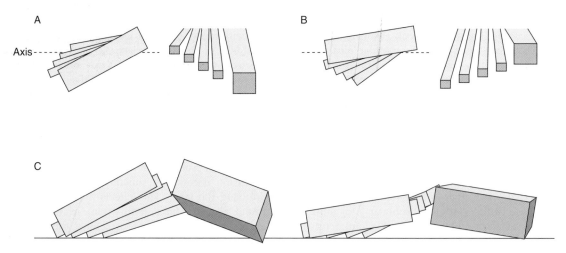

Figure 1.8 Frontal plane manifestations of a sagittal plane metatarsal motion. Positions of the metatarsals in (A) pronation twist; (B) supination twist. (C) How forefoot twist influences the position in pronation and supination of the posterior part of the foot. (From Hicks 1953, with permission.)

mum ill effects on the structure and function of the forefoot.

Variable factors affecting stance and gait

The normal variable factors which are of greatest clinical significance are shape, contour and mobility. These are interrelated and together determine the foot type, which is also related to the build of the body. All these factors have a bearing on the management of the patient.

Variations of shape

These are of importance in shoe fitting but they are also more indicative of the foot type than any other variable. There are three readily identifiable shapes: the short broad foot, the long narrow foot and the triangular foot. The short broad foot is subject to constriction from footwear of inadequate width and girth. The long narrow foot is more likely to be structurally unstable and is subject to impaction of the forefoot from footwear which is too short or which does not restrain the narrow foot from moving forward inside the shoe. The triangular foot has a broad forefoot and a narrow heel and is the most vulnerable of the three types.

Two further classifications exist related to the bisection lines of the forefoot and the calcaneus, namely the rectus foot and the adductus foot (Fig. 1.9). In a rectus foot shape, the forefoot bisection through the second metatarsal and the hindfoot bisection through the calcaneus are parallel to each other and the foot is straight. Because of this, if the foot suffers abnormal subtalar joint pronation, any forefoot deformity tends to develop in the sagittal plane, e.g. hallux rigidus or hallux limitus. An adductus foot shape is one in which the forefoot bisection is adducted relative to the hindfoot bisection and the metatarsals are angled towards the mid-sagittal plane. This foot shape tends to develop forefoot deformities in the transverse plane, e.g. hallux abductovalgus, if abnormal subtalar joint pronation occurs.

Variations of intrinsic mobility

Normal feet vary in their range of intrinsic mobility. The totality of movement within all the tarsal joints determines the degree to which the shape and contour of the feet change under the stress of weight-bearing. They may be relatively rigid, showing little or no change on weight-bearing, or relatively mobile, showing some lowering of the longitudinal arch and some

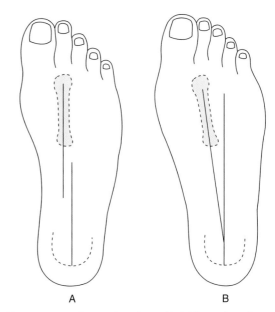

Figure 1.9   A: Rectus foot shape. B: Adductus foot shape.

consequential elongation while still remaining structurally stable. The former type has relatively little intrinsic capacity for shock absorption, while the latter has considerably more.

The term *hypermobility* indicates abnormal ranges of movement at joints. In the foot, on weight-bearing, this produces excessive pronation and flattening, significantly increasing its overall length. The breadth across the metatarsal heads may also be increased by splaying of the metatarsals. The term hypermobility is also applied to those metatarsal segments (specifically the first and fifth rays) where the range of movement at the proximal articulations is so marked as to affect the capacity of the metatarsal heads to accept their normal share of the weight-bearing load (see Ch. 5).

Variations in the metatarsal formula

It is difficult to gain agreement as to what constitutes the normal parabola of the metatarsal heads in the frontal plane, but there can be no doubt that variations do occur. Clinically, the most significant is the short first metatarsal, which gives the appearance of a short first toe. Like hypermobility, which may also be present, it may render the segment relatively incompetent for its essential weight-bearing function, causing some compensatory overloading of the adjacent metatarsal heads. The short first toe may be the cause of a mistaken measurement when footwear is being fitted and the

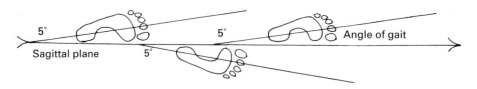

Figure 1.10 The angle of gait.

adjacent toe may suffer impaction from a short shoe. Shortness of the fifth or any other metatarsal may similarly overload its neighbour.

Variations in the angle of gait

The angle of gait is the deviation of the long axis of each foot from the sagittal plane (Fig 1.10). The norm is for the long axes of the feet to be nearly parallel or slightly out-toed. Marked in-toeing may arise from internal tibial or femoral torsion, from internal rotation of the hip joint, from bow legs or, in children, from active compensation for knock-knees. Marked out-toeing may arise from external tibial or femoral torsion, or knock-knees in adults. Whether or not these variations are significant clinically depends on their origins and on other variable factors such as age, weight and occupation.

REFERENCES

Elftmann H 1960 The transverse tarsal joint and its control. Clinical Orthopaedics 16: 41–45
Hicks J H 1953 The mechanics of the foot I. The joints. Journal of Anatomy 87: 345–357
Hicks J H 1954 The mechanics of the foot II. The joints. Journal of Anatomy 88: 25

Root M L, Orien W P, Weed J H 1977 Normal and abnormal function of the foot. Clinical biomechanics, vol II. Clinical Biomechanical Corporation, Los Angeles
Steindler A 1964 Kinesiology of the human body. Thomas, Springfield , Illinois

FURTHER READING

Close J R, Todd F N 1959 The phasic activity of the muscles of the lower extremity and the effect of tendon transfer. Journal of Bone and Joint Surgery 41(A): 189
Du Vries H L 1978 Surgery of the Foot, 4th edn. Mosby, St Louis
Jahss M H 1982 Disorders of the foot, vols 1 & 2. Saunders, Philadelphia
Jones F W 1943 Structure and function as seen in the foot. Ballière Tindall and Cox, London
Lake N C 1943 The foot, 3rd edn. Ballière Tindall and Cox, London
McMinn R 1982 Colour atlas of the foot and ankle. Wolfe, London

Mann R, Inman V F 1964 Phasic activity of the intrinsic muscles of the foot. Journal of Bone and Joint Surgery 46: 469
Morton D J 1935 The human foot. Columbia University Press, New York
Sgarlato T E 1981 Compendium of podiatric biomechanics. California College of Podiatric Medicine, San Francisco
Siebel M O 1989 Foot function – a programmed text. Williams and Wilkins, Baltimore
Vincent O T 1968 The mechanics of the foot. Chiropodist 23: 397–425
Williams M, Lissner H R 1977 Biomechanics of human motion. Saunders, Philadelphia

2

Examination and assessment

E. G. Anderson
J. A. Black

Keywords

Biomechanical examination
Case history
Circulatory assessment
Clinical laboratory tests
Clinical signs
Data Protection Act
Footwear patterns
Gait analysis
Motor assessment
Neurological assessment
Sensory assessment
X-rays

Establishing a diagnosis as a basis for treatment depends upon two sets of information, the *subjective symptoms* and the *objective signs*. Symptoms are those abnormal features of which the patient has personal experience. Signs are those detectable by a skilled observer with the help of various types of apparatus. The more information that can be made available from these sources, the more reliable the diagnosis is likely to be. Most of the foot disorders described in this book can be diagnosed by clinical examination, though some require laboratory or radiographic investigation as outlined in later pages.

For examination purposes, foot disorders can be conveniently subdivided into the superficial lesions of the skin and soft tissues, structural and functional disorders, and local manifestations of general or systemic disease. All three aspects need to be considered. Most of the superficial lesions are local symptoms of an underlying disorder and they cannot be treated effectively in isolation. However, it is practical to diagnose them separately since they need specific treatment over and above that required for the underlying fault.

The management of the foot problem cannot be divorced from that of any concurrent general or systemic disorder. Examination of the foot must include recognition of local signs and symptoms of more remote origins in order that fuller investigation may be instituted. This is particularly important when the foot disorder is the first presenting symptom of a more general pathology, as pes cavus may be in spina bifida, or as a swollen interphalangeal joint may be in rheumatoid arthritis. Depending on the findings, the patient may have to be referred for a full orthopaedic, circulatory, neurological, rheumatological or other general examination. In such circumstances, it is clearly impossible for the primary examination to explore all the possibilities of pathology remote from the foot. But the clinician must accept the responsibility to recognise and record clinical features of potential significance, to relate them to any local treatment that may be necessary, and to refer the patient for appropriate specialist examination with a summary of his reasons for doing so.

The foot is an integral part of the kinetic chain. It provides the musculoskeletal system with the mechanical interface between the ground and the lower limb, producing the leverage and propulsion necessary for walking and running whilst at the same time smoothing out the gross movements of locomotion, acting as an effective shock absorber and providing the subtle and delicate balance necessary to adjust to uneven terrain and changes in ground surface. It is important to realise that the leg and foot frequently mirror symptoms from one to the other, and each in turn can be the aetiological factor which results in symptoms experienced elsewhere in the kinetic chain. For example, anterior knee pain should not be diagnosed without a thorough examination of the foot, and conversely alterations in foot posture should not be considered without reference to the structural alignment of the legs, e.g. genu valgum or genu varum.

The lower limb must therefore undergo similar scrutiny so that the structural relationships between the foot and the lower limb can be appreciated. The position of the foot relative to the leg and the body planes must be ascertained, and also the ranges of motion of the hips, knees and the joints of the foot.

During the examination, all clinical observations, measurements and symptoms should be carefully noted in the patient's records. The method of referral to the clinician and all other relevant information, both medical and surgical, including possible drug therapy, must be similarly detailed. The practitioner must be meticulous in writing up case histories. Litigation alleging incompetence and negligence is ever increasing and no effort should be spared, irrespective of the contraints of time, to ensure that records are complete

and up to date. It is also worthy of note that as more records become stored on computer, all such data must be available for inspection under the Data Protection Act and the practitioner must be registered with the Data Protection Registrar. Individual comment relating to the patient should therefore always be of a professional nature.

Before commencing clinical examination, it is essential to put the patient at ease. Patients are frequently anxious, if not frightened, and consider the surgery a hostile environment, with the therapist an adversary. Whilst each consultation is just another in the day's work for the therapist, it is a major event for the patient. Reassurance and consideration are paramount. Simple things like a welcoming smile, ensuring the patient is comfortably seated, and not uncomfortably hot because no one has offered to take their coat, will ensure that clinical examination becomes a two-way exchange with information eagerly sought and willingly given. Time spent on this exercise, though sometimes abused, is never wasted, since it helps to quickly establish the relative significance of the complaint.

This exercise is of course even more important when children are the patients, and further reference is made to their particular requirements in Chapter 3.

CLINICAL EXAMINATION PROCEDURES

Before commencing any examination, there are two important features to be considered. These are the positioning and the exposure of the patient. When carrying out the initial examination with the patient seated, it is much more comfortable for the patient to be seated at a higher level than the examiner. This allows the patient to rest with a slightly flexed hip and knee, which is more comfortable than sitting with an extended knee.

Ideally, the whole limb being examined ought to be exposed, but in practice it is usually sufficient only to expose the leg from above the knee distally. The proximal parts of the limb can be examined in more detail if indicated. It is important to be able to see the knee and the patella, especially when the patient stands, and in order to do so, trouser legs have to be rolled up, not just pushed up. If they can't go up they have to come down. Both legs and feet should always be exposed and examined regardless of the complaint.

It is also helpful to the examiner to follow a set pattern of examination. This is good practice and helps to ensure that nothing is missed out. It is logical to proceed from the superficial (skin and soft tissues) to the deep structures (bones and joints) and thence from the local to the general.

Case history

Patients complain of symptoms. These may be local, e.g. pain, swelling, deformity or difficulty with footwear, or more general, such as abnormality of gait or symptoms related to other body systems. The purpose in taking a history is to find out as much as possible about these symptoms and to use the information, together with the clinical findings, first to determine the necessary investigations and then to arrive at a diagnosis. Then, and only then, can a treatment plan be formulated and a prognosis given. The symptoms of which the patient initially complains are the *presenting symptoms*, and it can be disconcerting to the patient if they are not examined first. They should always be given priority without prejudice to the coverage of other and possibly more important symptoms.

The salient features of symptoms are:

1. *Site and radiation of pain*: where is it, and does it go anywhere?
2. *Onset*: when, and the circumstances concerning it; gradual or sudden; relationship to an event, e.g. injury, sport, change of occupation or footwear.
3. *Nature*: severity and extent; is the pain sharp, dull, fiery, or just bearable discomfort?
4. *Influencing factors*: those that aggravate or relieve, e.g. exercise, rest, elevation. What is the duration of exercise tolerance? It is frequently the case that changes in body position provoke foot pain which then diminishes, or even disappears, with exercise, e.g. patients will often complain of pain when first rising from bed, the pain subsequently easing on mobility.
5. *Duration*: constant or intermittent?
6. *Relationship to general health*: e.g. are the symptoms related to any known health problem, such as diabetes mellitus, generalised arthropathy, circulatory or neurological deficiency, etc.?

To complete the history, it is worth enquiring as to the patient's past history and to social circumstances, particularly if the working environment is involved in their complaints.

Clinical signs

Skin

- Texture: coarse or fine, dull or shiny
- Colour: pallor, cyanosis, erythema, pigmentation, gangrene
- Temperature: cool, warm or distinctly hot (use the back of the hand and compare with the other limb)
- Humidity: dry, sweaty, areas of maceration
- Elasticity
- Hyperkeratosis (callosities)
- Hair: presence or absence, fine or coarse
- Integrity: fissures (heel or interdigital clefts), ulcers
- Dermatoses: eczema, psoriasis
- Surgical infections: AIDS may manifest with specific skin changes.

Nails

- Structure: ridged, cracked, thickened
- Extent: overgrown, onychogryphotic, stunted, ingrowing
- Subungual abnormality: swelling, pigmentation.

Swellings

- Tenderness: local, radiating
  Consistency: hard, firm, soft, fluctuant
- Adherence: to skin, to underlying soft tissue, to bone
- Transillumination
- Temperature.

Vascular status

Despite all the modern sophisticated methods of measuring blood flow, the basic clinical signs have stood the test of time and, in the overwhelming majority of cases, still provide both adequate and reliable information on the vascularity of the limb.

Skin colour and temperature. Whilst the relatively avascular foot may be pale and cool, the dysvascular foot, which may also be neuropathic, may be fiery red, especially at the extremities, sometimes tinged with a purplish suffusion.

Blanching of the tip of a toe with finger pressure will, in the former instance, result in a slow return of colour and, in the latter, in an excessively rapid flush of colour. Blanching also tends to occur on elevation, just as congestion does on prolonged dependency. Dependency may also result in cyanosis, more indicative of venous insufficiency.

The arterial pulses are palpated as shown in Figure 2.1. The dorsalis pedis is just lateral to the extensor hallucis tendon at the base of the first metatarsal; the anterior tibial is at the front of the ankle; and the posterior tibial is just behind and below the medial malleolus, with the foot slightly inverted. Pulses should be palpated with the middle three fingers, avoiding too much pressure, which might obliterate them. The thumb should never be used to feel for a pulse.

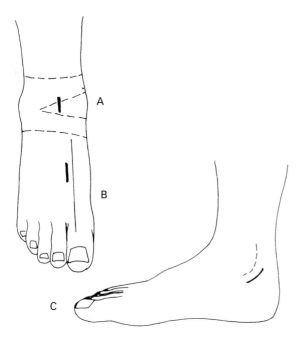

Figure 2.1   Arterial palpation points. A: Anterior tibial. B: Dorsalis pedis. C: Posterior tibial.

Comparing blood pressure in the arm with that at the ankles is another useful indicator of vascular flow. It is generally expressed as a ratio of ankle pressure/arm pressure. A ratio of 0.9 or less is indicative of a compromised circulation.

Oedema of the ankle and foot, when it is 'pitting', is a sign of more generalised cardiovascular insufficiency. Brawny oedema does not 'pit' and is usually due to lymphatic insufficiency.

Neurological status

The same principles apply to both the neurological and vascular examinations. Both the efferent (motor) and the afferent (sensory) systems must be examined.

Motor assessment. Muscle power is measured according to the Oxford (MRC) scale, as follows:

0—no muscle activity
1—muscle twitch without moving segment
2—segment moved with gravity eliminated
3—segment moved against gravity
4—segment moved against gravity and resistance
5—full power.

In practice, it is impossible to measure the power of every muscle, and so muscles are examined (mostly) in functioning groups. This is particularly true more proximally in the leg. In the lower leg and foot, the following should be tested:

- toe dorsiflexion (extension)—extensor hallucis longus and extensor digitorum longus
- toe plantarflexion (flexion)—flexor hallucis longus and flexor digitorum longus
- invertors—tibialis anterior and tibialis posterior; each of these can be tested separately by holding the foot in dorsiflexion and plantarflexion, respectively, when applying a resistance
- evertors—peroneal muscles
- ankle dorsiflexors—tibialis anterior, peroneus tertius together with the toe extensors
- ankle plantarflexors—calf muscles via the tendo Achilles. This group consists of two muscles: the soleus, whose origins are entirely within the lower leg; and the gastrocnemius, which has its origins on the distal femur. When spastic contraction is a problem, the origins of the contracture can be determined by testing ankle flexion with and without the knee bent; increased dorsiflexion on knee bending indicates the gastrocnemius as the tighter structure.

Sensory assessment. Sensation has several modalities of which touch, proprioception and pain appreciation are the most relevant to foot care, but temperature and vibration sense provide important information for the specialist. Accurate neurological testing is highly specialised and time-consuming, but it is important that the examiner can determine areas of gross sensory diminution or loss, and whether there has been any loss of position sense. The reflexes at the knee and ankle should be tested, as should the plantar (Babinski) responses.

A useful test of skin sensation can be obtained by the use of Semmes–Weinstein filaments. A single filament is pressed against the skin until it just begins to bend. If a sense of pressure is not felt with a filament of size 6.10 then there is significant sensory impairment. This method is particularly useful in the assessment of diabetic neuropathy.

Neurophysiologists are able to provide information on a nerve's conductive ability, and can perform electromyographic studies.

Other soft tissues

Tendons, ligaments, and fibro-fatty pads all require attention. It is necessary to note any local signs of tenderness along the structure, especially at points of attachment to bone, at localised swellings and at areas revealing crepitus on movement. Auscultation over tendons might also indicate a tenosynovitis. The plantar aponeurosis should be palpated for abnormal nodules and tenderness, especially at its insertion into the calcaneus. Tenderness on the medial border distal to the calcaneus may indicate a tear in its substance. The fibro-fatty subcutaneous tissue which forms the heel pad and the metatarsal pad should be examined to determine its integrity. It diminishes in thickness in the dysvascular and/or ageing foot, allowing bony prominences to be readily palpable subcutaneously. Lacking the shear absorbing capacity of the pads, the bony prominences are a potent source of pain in these people.

Some clinical signs are clearly of more importance than others and demand more urgent attention. Of these, the most important are signs of inflammation. Classically, they have been described as 'rubor, calor et dolor'—redness, warmth and pain. Inflammation does not necessarily mean infection—there can be many reasons for its presence—but certain features should be recorded:

- whether acute, subacute, or chronic
- if infective and localised, whether it is resolving or suppurating
- if infective and spreading, whether there is lymphangitis or lymphadenitis present; the former appears as longitudinal reddish streaks in the skin, and the latter as tender swellings at the site of the lymph nodes at the back of the knee and in the groin.

Any acute or subacute inflammatory lesion requires at least temporary priority in treatment over any associated deformity. Any spreading infection requires immediate reference for further investigation and treatment.

Local signs of systemic disease

The history and clinical signs elicited may point to the presence of systemic disease, and these of course require further referral. Reference should be made to subsequent chapters covering the respective systems, but the following text outlines signs and symptoms that should give rise to suspicion.

Circulatory. (See Ch. 24.)

- Arterial
  - intermittent claudication
  - rest pain
  - abnormal pulses
  - abnormal skin colour, texture or temperature

  - abnormal nails
  - incipient or established gangrene
- Venous
  - pain and swelling associated with thrombophlebitis or thrombosis, varicose eczema pigmentation, atrophie blanche
- Central
  - pitting oedema
  - breathlessness

Neurological. (See Ch. 27)

Almost every neurological symptom requires further investigation, but particularly:

- unexplained weakness
- ataxia
- spasticity
- absent or exaggerated reflexes
- any loss of sensory modality.

Other general conditions may necessitate referral for further investigation and treatment (see Chs 7, 25 and 26), e.g:

- obesity
- suspected diabetes mellitus
- gout
- rickets
- osteo- or rheumatoid arthritis
- generalised skin disorders.

Footwear

Footwear should also be examined during the patient's first visit and points of note recorded. The footwear should be checked for size, shape, style, suitability and indications of abnormal wear. Abnormal wear on the soles and heels often gives the best indication of the weight-bearing pathway during the gait cycle. It is not only the amount of wear but also the pattern which indicates the direction of causative forces: e.g. a circular pattern suggests a rotational element during gait. Inspection of the insole can also provide a valuable insight into the relative pressures occurring under the mid- and forefoot. Distortions of the uppers also give indications of abnormal frontal plane motion during gait. Points to note are:

- Heel wear
  a. Excessive wear at rear edge — calcaneal gait
  b. Excessive wear at front edge — broken shank, hyperpronated foot
  c. Excessive wear on lateral side — supinated foot due to, for example, pes cavus, painful first ray (postoperation)

d. Excessive wear on medial edge — hyperpronated foot
- Heel and sole wear
  a. Excessive on lateral side — supinated foot due to pes cavus; weakness of the evertor (peroneal) muscles
  b. Excessive on medial side — hyperpronated foot
  c. Lateral heel to medial sole — normal, but if excessive, leg may be externally rotated or forefoot abducted
  d. Lateral heel to lateral sole — leg may be internally rotated or the forefoot adducted
  e. Medial heel to medial sole — hyperpronated foot
- Sole wear
  a. Excessive across tread — pes cavus
  b. Excessive at tip — spasticity or foot drop
  c. Excessive under hallux — hallux rigidus
  d. Excessive under lateral side — metatarsus varus (adductus)
- Deformity of heel counters
  a. At back — heel 'bumps'
  b. Medial side — collapsed hyperpronated foot with valgus hindfoot
  c. Lateral side — supinated foot with varus hindfoot
- Deformity of the uppers
  Splay foot, hallux valgus, hammer toes, claw toes or the presence of other bony prominences.

Biomechanical examination

Joints

Assessment of the joints of the foot, their range and direction of motion, is crucial and no accurate diagnosis of the mechanics of the foot can be established without this information. Motion within their normal ranges should be pain-free and unrestricted. Features significant of joint pathology are pain on movement or limitation of movement (note any crepitus, subluxations or dislocations); deformity affecting either or both osseous components of the joint; tenderness on palpation indicating inflammation, suggestive of arthritis or sprain.

The *ankle joint* is a hinge joint and, irrespective of the position of the axis of motion, the only free movement permitted is that of plantarflexion and dorsiflexion. The range of motion may vary widely between individuals with 20–30° of dorsiflexion available in some cases, and between 30° and 50° of plantarflexion. The range of motion should be assessed with the knee extended and the subtalar joint in its neutral position.

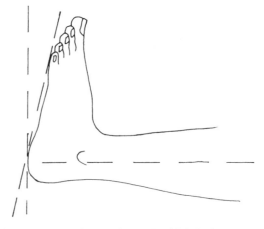

Figure 2.2 Dorsiflexion of the ankle. With the knee extended and the foot in neutral position, the angle between the long axis of the leg and the lateral border of the foot should be at least 10° less than a right angle. If dorsiflexion is limited, test the range again with the knee flexed.

It is possible to measure the angles between the long axis of the leg and the lateral border of the foot, in both plantarflexion and dorsiflexion, to determine the total range of motion. For normal function during walking, there should be at least 10° of dorsiflexion available (Fig. 2.2). Limitation of dorsiflexion may be caused by a tight gastrocnemius, determined by dorsiflexing the foot whilst the knee is fully extended, or by a tight soleus (if limitation persists with the knee flexed). Restriction may also occur as a result of anatomical variations or if there is joint damage.

Because it is easily observed, the ankle joint also provides a ready means of identifying rotational variations in the lower limb. With the patient supine, this may be done by measuring the positions of the malleoli relative to the frontal plane with an orthogauge (Fig. 2.3). The orthogauge is a rectangular sheet of rigid transparent plastic on which are marked the relevant angular and linear components for biomechanical examination.

The *subtalar joint* (talocalcaneal) provides the foot with triplane motion of inversion with adduction and plantarflexion, and eversion with abduction and dorsiflexion. In examining the subtalar joint, interest should concentrate on the total range of motion, its neutral position, and the amount of inversion and eversion from the neutral position. It is considered normal to have a range of inversion available that is twice that for eversion. Evaluation of the position of subtalar neutral can be assessed by palpation, by observation and by measurement, and all three methods must be used to establish the position accurately.

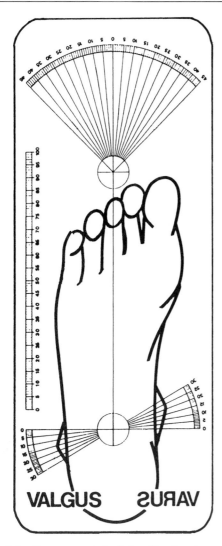

Figure 2.3 Measurement of rotational torsions by orthogauge. The patient lies supine, with the knee axis on the frontal plane and the foot at a right angle to the leg. The angle between a line through the tips of the malleoli and the frontal plane is measured by holding the orthogauge perpendicular to the leg.

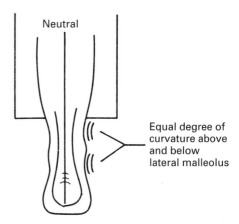

Figure 2.4 Visual observation of neutral subtalar position. Normally, the curves just above and below the lateral malleolus match each other. In calcaneal eversion, the lower curve is exaggerated; in calcaneal inversion, it is reduced.

The significance of the neutral position of the subtalar joint, or any other joint, is that from this position the foot will move maximally in a given direction. When applied to foot mechanics, the neutral position of the subtalar joint allows the practitioner to evaluate the relationship of the forefoot to the rearfoot and the foot to the leg.

Evaluation of the subtalar joint

By palpation. With the patient prone and the knee in full extension, the foot is dorsiflexed to 90° on the leg by applying pressure to the fourth and fifth rays, and the subtalar joint is inverted to its maximum. By palpating the joint about one thumb's breadth anterior to the distal margins of the medial and lateral malleoli, the lateral aspect of the head of the talus will be felt. This method is then repeated with the joint in maximum eversion, and the medial aspect of the talar head will be felt. When the head of the talus cannot be palpated on either the medial or lateral sides, the subtalar joint is in its neutral position.

By observation. It is possible to evaluate the neutral position by noting the curvatures just above the lateral malleolus and at the lateral aspect of the calcaneus. In neutral, these curves should match each other (Fig. 2.4). In eversion of the calcaneus, the curvature on the calcaneus is more exaggerated than that of the leg; with inversion, the curvature is reduced. The neutral position also approximates with the lowest point on the arc of movement of the plantar aspect of the heel.

By measurement (Fig. 2.5): a. With the patient prone to secure full muscular relaxation, and the foot extending beyond the leg rest, the leg is rotated to bring the back of the heel horizontal. The back of the heel and the lower third of the leg are marked with separate bisection lines.

b. The heel is swung into full inversion and into full eversion, care being taken to keep the foot perpendicular to the leg and to avoid any frontal plane movement in the ankle joint. At each extreme, the angles between the bisection lines are measured and added together to give the total range of movement.

Neutral position is at two-thirds from full inversion and one-third from full eversion, plus or minus 2°.

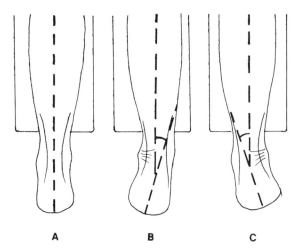

Figure 2.5 Assessment of neutral subtalar position. A: Bisection of back of leg and back of heel. B: Inversion angle (right foot). C: Eversion angle (right foot).

c. With the subtalar joint placed in its neutral position, the back of the heel is again bisected. The angle, if any, between this bisection and that of the leg denotes the degree of possible subtalar varus or valgus of the calcaneus. If there is no angulation, the calcaneus is vertical and the foot normal.

This method also indicates the degree of wedging or posting required in an orthotic appliance. Examples are given in Table 2.1.

Table 2.1 Sample measurements of the subtalar joint

Inversion angle	Eversion angle	Total range	Neutral position	Indications
21	9	30	20	Normal
27	6	33	22	5 varus
18	15	33	22	4 valgus

d. A convenient alternative method of measuring subtalar varus or valgus is by the use of an orthogauge. When applied with its centreline coinciding with the bisection line on the back of the leg and its transverse plane reference point on a level with the subtalar joint, degrees of subtalar varus or valgus are indicated by the calcaneal bisection line and can be measured by the protractor component of the orthogauge (Fig. 2.6).

The *midtarsal joint* is made up of the talonavicular and calcaneocuboid articulations, which for practical purposes can be considered to act as a single functional unit. Stability is provided by the calcaneocuboid articulation, whilst the talonavicular articulation provides mobility. Movements of the midtarsal joint are

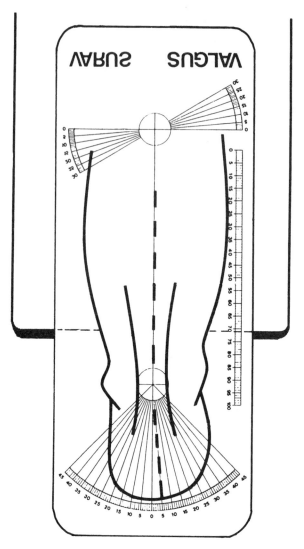

Figure 2.6 Measurement of subtalar varus or valgus by orthogauge. The centreline is placed over the bisection line marked on the leg. Degrees of subtalar varus or valgus are indicated by the calcaneal bisection line and can be measured by the protractor component.

dependent upon the shape of the articular surfaces and the restraint of the ligamentous structures. Of particular importance to the functioning of the midtarsal joint is the shape of the head of the talus. The talonavicular joint is similar anatomically to a ball and socket joint and the shape of the articular surface of the head of the talus largely dictates the amount of movement available.

Clinical examination should seek to determine the ability of the forefoot to adjust to the position of the hindfoot once the position of 'foot-flat' has been established during the gait cycle. It is therefore important that the range of movement should be assessed with the hindfoot in neutral, and also supinated and pronated. In the normal foot, when the subtalar joint is in its neutral position, the forefoot assumes a position where its plantar aspect is parallel to the transverse plane of the hindfoot. More motion is available during pronation of the hindfoot, and less motion when the subtalar joint is supinated. If, however, there are changes in the position of the axis of motion of the midtarsal joint, then the position of the forefoot relative to the hindfoot can also be changed. The forefoot may assume a position inverted or everted to the hindfoot; these abnormalities profoundly affect the normal mechanics of the foot and need to be evaluated (Fig. 2.7).

Pain on movement of the midtarsal joint with limitation of inversion may be suggestive of osteoarthrosis, rheumatoid arthritis or a tarsal synostosis.

The structure of the tarsometatarsal joints is such that it is difficult to isolate and evaluate their individual movements. It does, however, allow for clinical evaluation of the range of plantarflexion and dorsiflexion of the first and fifth rays, and whether such motion is excessive, or whether they are fixed in positions of dorsiflexion or plantarflexion relative to the transverse plane of the forefoot. Independent transverse motion of these units is practically non-existent, but it may be possible to quantify any abduction and adduction of the fifth and first rays, respectively.

The relationship of the forefoot to the hindfoot in the transverse plane is also quantifiable, and the practitioner can evaluate relative adduction or abduction by using a goniometer, an orthogauge or a tractograph.

The metatarsophalangeal joints should be assessed individually, then collectively. The range of motion of each should be noted, although only the first and fifth can be quantified. Any change in the integrity of the joints' surfaces, as in Freiberg's infraction, should be recorded. Test each of the joints for pain-free movement, noting any discrepancies in their motion. Note particularly any degree of hallux valgus, hallux limitus or rigidus, or hallux flexus; any possible subluxations or dislocations; and any toe deformities. The state of the metatarsophalangeal joints is critical to the diagnosis and prognosis of all forefoot disorders.

If this evaluation of the position and movements of the joints of the foot is carried out with precision, and the details noted, then an accurate assessment of function can be made, especially when it is coupled with other forms of investigation where initial examination has indicated potential pathology.

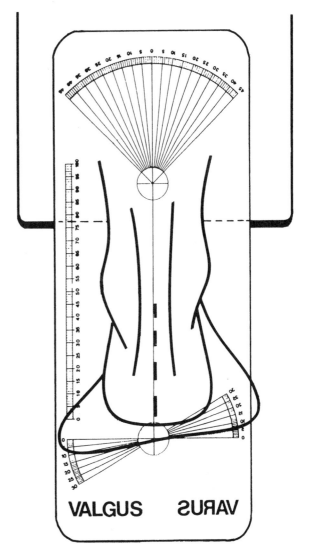

Figure 2.7 Evaluation of hindfoot/forefoot alignment by orthogauge. With the foot held in its neutral subtalar position, the orthogauge is placed with its centreline on the calcaneal bisection line. Degrees of forefoot varus or, by reversing the orthogauge, forefoot valgus are then evaluated by reference to the plantar aspect of the forefoot.

One must also be aware of the differences between individuals and whether there is generalised joint laxity (hypermobility) or hypomobility from joint stiffness. Both present problems for the clinician as it is virtually impossible to restrict generalised excessive movements within joints, and joints will not move beyond the limits imposed on them by their inherent anatomy. Where there is joint hypermobility, it is a recognised feature on X-ray that the articular surfaces are rounded and larger, and in hypomobility the articular surfaces tend to be smaller and more rectangular in shape, thereby restricting motion. Both conditions frequently result in pathology. The range of motion determined in the static examination may not equate with that utilised in gait.

Gait analysis

Analysis of the patient's gait is often necessary in order to develop a complete picture of the events taking place, particularly during the stance phase of gait. Gait analysis can be carried out both by visual observation of the patient walking and by other mechanical methods described later in this chapter. The two methods differ because the first observes the sequence of events from heel strike to toe-off, while the second examines the distribution of forces acting on the feet. It is helpful to use video equipment, but if this is not available then careful observation with the naked eye can reveal fundamental gait characteristics. Every person's gait pattern is specific to the individual, and it reflects not only leg length but the compensations which may be necessary relative to the anatomical positions of the feet and legs but not necessarily constant from step to step. A treadmill is also very useful since the visual parameters of the practitioner do not alter and cadence can be controlled at a constant rate. If no treadmill is available, a long well-lit corridor will usually suffice. It is important during this form of gait analysis to allow the patient a good 5 minutes' walking before beginning serious observation, because patients are usually very self-conscious about being observed. It is not possible to obtain reliable results from goniometers which are attached to the skin of the foot due to the relative motion between the skin and the underlying bone, and the small size of the bone.

The normal sequence of events which the clinician wishes to observe is as follows: prior to heel strike, the foot is supinated; it then pronates through to 'foot-flat' when the ground reaction forces reverse the rotation; the foot then supinates to become a rigid lever prior to take-off. Any alteration in these events necessitates further investigation. Abnormalities of a biomechanical nature are often only marginally abnormal, so that excessive pronation, early heel lift and other subtle changes require a trained eye to detect. It is frequently a help if more than one practitioner can observe the patient at the same time. After careful observation of the gait, it is then necessary to assess whether any apparent anomalies are of any functional significance and are related to the patient's symptoms. Many anatomical variations necessitate compensatory movements during walking which may not contribute to pathological symptoms.

FURTHER INVESTIGATIONS

Gait analysis

The clinical examination of gait has already been described. Here, those items of equipment which can add to the basic knowledge already acquired are mentioned. Many new sophisticated devices are now available, but for clinical use in the surgery simple tests can still provide most, if not all, of the information needed to treat patients. Devices are available for both the static and the dynamic evaluation of the foot in gait.

Static evaluation

1. The *plantarscope* shows how the plantar skin blanches under load; the pattern can be adjusted in some cases by the examiner to near normal by manipulating the foot and/or the leg of the patient. This can give a useful indication of the possible cause of the complaint (Fig. 2.8).

2. The *podometer* is a more elaborate form of the above device, combining measurement of the foot size

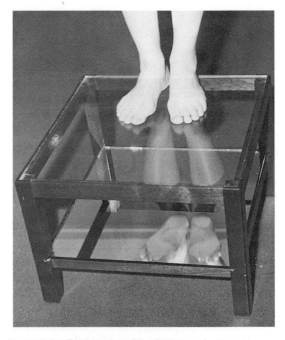

Figure 2.8   Examination of the feet on a plantarscope demonstrates weight distribution to the plantar surfaces.

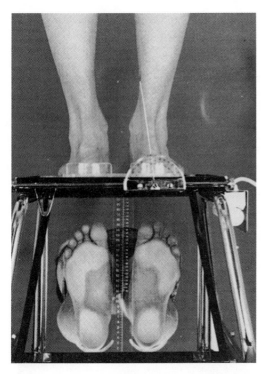

Figure 2.9 Examination of the feet on the podometer reveals foot size and calcaneal deviation, as well as the pattern of weight distribution.

Figure 2.10 The Harris & Beath mat provides mirror image prints of the pressure areas in standing or on walking.

and calcaneal deviation with the reflected image of the foot (Fig. 2.9).

3. The *pedobaroscope*. This device incorporates an internally illuminated sheet of plate glass, upon which is placed a plastic or, preferably, a card interface. The patient stands on this interface and a grey-scale image of the reflected light that is produced is assessed. The grey image is calibrated electronically and projected on a VDU screen as a colour image which can be photographed, stored on videotape, or printed out as hard copy. It has a very high resolution, recording the pressure under areas of the foot as small as 2 mm × 3 mm.

Dynamic evaluation

1. The simplest of these devices is to walk the patient over a black surface after dusting the feet with chalk. The resulting footprints will give a rough idea of high pressure areas, alignment of the foot and, if timed over a given distance, the cadence (in steps/minute).

2. The *Harris & Beath mat* is a rubber mat surfaced with tall ridges forming large squares, crossed by smaller ridges forming smaller squares, and even

smaller ridges forming even smaller squares. The mat is inked and covered with a sheet of paper over which the patient walks. Only the highest pressures record all three levels of ridge, these areas appearing darker. The print is, of course, a mirror image print which only shows the areas of maximum pressure during the stance phase of gait and is therefore not time-related. It can also be used for static prints, and is undoubtedly the most useful tool for everyday use in the clinic. Much helpful information can be gleaned from good prints (Fig. 2.10).

3. The *dynamic pedobarograph* is mainly a research tool and is a dynamic variant of the pedobaroscope. It works on the same principles but, like many other methods of measuring foot pressures and forces, if it is not used properly it may produce very attractive pictures which give quite erroneous information, e.g. in double foot strike. It is, however, reliable in that the results have been shown to be accurate and repeatable, and it has much the best resolution of any such apparatus. Single traces may not reflect the patient's normal gait pattern, and at least need to be taken for comparison.

4. The *Musgrave forceplate* system has been refined to produce a higher resolution, and is a mat of transducers placed on the floor, across which the patient walks. The Musgrave system, like many others, produces computer-generated pictorial results as well as a reading of the pressure between the foot and the

ground in kilograms per square centimetre (kg/cm^2). This enables foot pressures to be evaluated before and after treatment regimes (Figs 2.11 and 2.12).

5. The *E. Med* is a similar device of German origin, and produces an output not dissimilar to the Musgrave system, but of higher resolution. The apparatus is highly sophisticated and expensive; an insole version has also been developed, but is as yet of limited resolution.

6. The *electrodynagram* utilises pressure transducers applied directly to the skin and thus can be worn inside footwear. In theory, this is the ideal method to measure pressure, but of course it is subject to the effect of the specific footwear. The transducers are wired to a miniature recorder and the results are obtained via a computer. The repeatability of results using this method has been called into question by some centres, and the fact that there are transducers and wire leads under the foot may affect the gait pattern.

7. The *force plate* can also provide information about ground reaction forces in three directions, but the interpretation of these is complex and very much a matter for the researcher. A more useful clinical system is the *video vector*, utilising both a force plate and video recording of the patient walking. A computer provides a visible vector superimposed on the image of the walking patient on the screen.

8. *Videography* can be very helpful in that pictures can be replayed at leisure, as fast or as slow as one wishes, down to one frame at a time. This is a very instructive way of examining the foot disposition during gait. Like any of these dynamic systems, it does need space, not always readily available, and it is expensive. Video can be combined with use of the treadmill, which allows the patient to run at different speeds on different inclines, as well as to walk.

It is important to realise that most of these dynamic systems are sophisticated research tools. For the surgery, a Harris & Beath mat is probably the most

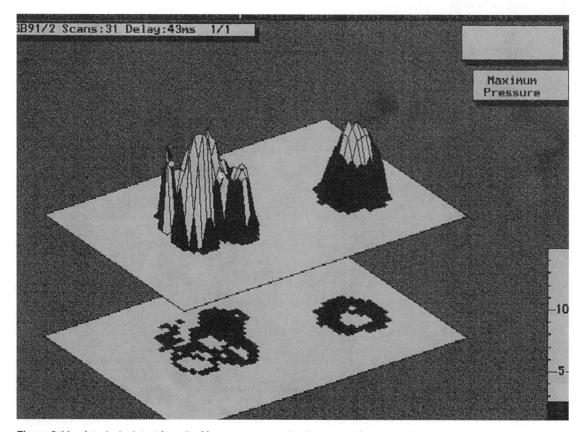

Figure 2.11   A typical printout from the Musgrave system showing areas of maximum load.

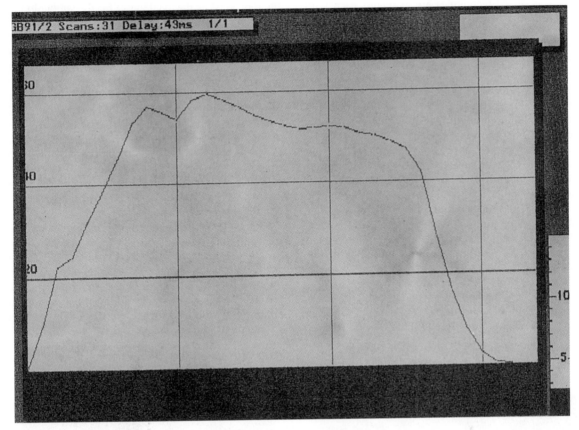

Figure 2.12 A visual representation of load from 'heel strike' to 'toe-off'.

useful single item. It can be used statically or dynamically, and takes up little space. It can be obtained as a kit in a box, complete with ink roller to spread the ink, and paper. It is important, too, to realise that static information must not be assumed to be an indication of what is occurring dynamically. The two modes are quite different, and if dynamic information is what is wanted, then data must be obtained in that form.

X-rays (see also Ch. 3)

Although many disorders of the foot can be safely diagnosed and treated without radiographic examination, some may need further investigation. This should, however, be supplementary to a thorough clinical examination. The main indications for radiographic examination of the foot are injury, deformity, swelling and pain which cannot be explained by clinical findings. These indications are not absolute: for example, the deformity of hallux valgus can be readily recognised on clinical examination; X-ray examination

would only be necessary if surgical treatment was being contemplated.

X-rays and safety

X-rays can be very helpful to the clinician, but they can also be dangerous. Strict precautions should always be enforced when X-rays are being taken, and they are ignored at some peril. Although modern X-ray machines produce little scatter of rays, and the intensity of X-rays is inversely proportional to the square of the distance from source, a lead apron should always be worn, or the clinician should retreat behind a screen. For small increases in distance away from the source, there are large decreases in X-ray intensity. Those involved with X-rays should also have their exposure to rays monitored regularly.

X-ray techniques

Plain radiographs are most commonly taken, but other

more specialised techniques are available, each with its particular indications.

Plain X-rays. Most radiological departments, if asked for X-rays of a foot, will provide non-weight-bearing anteroposterior (dorsoplantar) and oblique views. When suspecting diseased bone, or checking on a previously defined fracture, these may be adequate, but in general, assessment of foot structure ought to be made with standing views. Weight-bearing views are also useful when evaluating the mechanical status of the foot. Lateral weight-bearing radiographs enable the practitioner to determine the extent to which variations exist in the relationship between forefoot and hindfoot.

Standing anteroposterior and lateral views, together with an oblique view, will cover most eventualities, although the weight-bearing metatarsal profile view is helpful in determining the relative positions of the metatarsal heads and status of the sesamoids of the hallux. It is taken with the aid of a perspex stand which supports the feet in normal toe-out, with heels and toes both elevated by 30° (adjustable) wedges. Other plain films can be taken to show specific areas of the foot, such as the axial views for the subtaloid joint or the calcaneus. Most departments can now also provide 'microfocal' or 'macro' views, which present a much magnified view while still retaining a high resolution of bone structure (Figs 2.13A & B and 2.14 A & B).

Tomograms. These X-rays are taken with the purpose of finding out more about the three-dimensional characteristics of a lesion. The head of the X-ray tube swings in an arc as the X-ray plate moves below, allowing one spot to be kept in focus while the surrounding area remains blurred. By taking sequential exposures at, for example, 1 cm intervals through the lesion, a series of pictures can be obtained which will give an idea of the whole.

Contrast films. Normal cavities, e.g. joints, or abnormal ones and sinuses can be injected with radio-opaque dye to enable the position and shape of the cavity to be outlined either on plain films, or with tomograms. This is of use in determining the course of a sinus track, or arthrograms can outline soft tissue structures within the joint, e.g. the menisci in the knee.

Computerised axial tomography (CT scan). These are

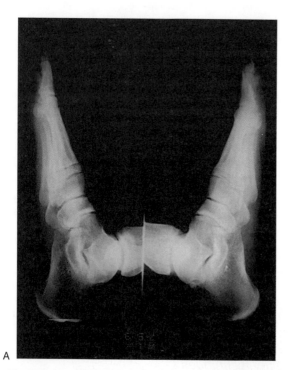

A

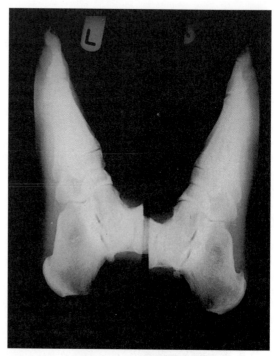

B

Figure 2.13 A: Weight-bearing lateral view of a normal foot. Note the smooth cyma line and the calcaneal inclination angle of 20°. B: Weight-bearing lateral view of forefoot valgus with a high angle of inclination of the calcaneus and interrupted cyma line.

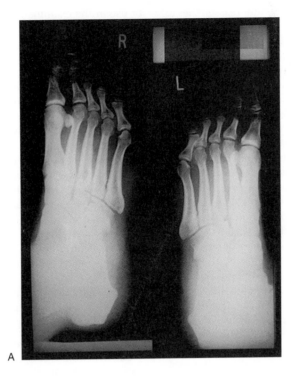

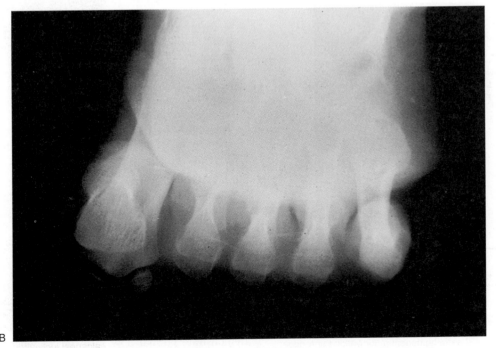

Figure 2.14 A: Non-weight-bearing oblique view. B: Weight-bearing metatarsal head profile.

simply tomograms which the computer reassembles to give a cross-sectional picture of the part being studied. They are still two-dimensional, but with a high resolution of structure. Unfortunately, the design of the scanner does not permit true weight-bearing scans of the foot to be carried out. To date, it has probably proved of most value in the foot in assessing fractures of the calcaneus and in determining the exact extent of tarsal coalitions.

Magnetic resonance imaging (MRI). This is a relatively new, non-invasive technique which is not strictly radiological. It involves exciting the structures of the cell nucleus with a magnetic field, and imaging the result. Longitudinal body cuts are then available in a three-dimensional format. It is of most use in determining the integrity of soft tissue structures, such as tendons and nerves, and in assessing the extent of soft tissue tumours (Fig. 2.15).

Ultrasound. This safe method of imaging is obtained by 'bouncing' ultrasonic waves through the tissues. It is a valuable aid in the visualisation of subcutaneous soft tissue structures such as tendons. It has the great advantage that tendon movement may be observed during the examination, and any abnormality of function as well as of structure may be identified. It is also

of use in the examination of the plantar fascia and of subcutaneous tumours.

Interpretation

Interpretation does need experience and skill, but there are some basic principles of interpretation common to all forms of radiological imaging which can help the novice. First, always look at the whole X-ray. You can usually tell the sex of the patient, if the name on the label is legible. Films show not only bone, but other soft tissue shadows, especially on CT scans, and they provide much valuable information. It should also be remembered that, in infants, the bones of the foot are represented by cartilaginous precursors, which may or may not contain centres of ossification, and thus the true 'shape' of the bone cannot be seen. In practice, clinical examination of the foot will suggest where the abnormality lies; nevertheless the whole film must be studied, as multiple abnormalities are not uncommon. More specifically, look for:

1. loss of continuity of bone cortex (e.g. fractures—but know where normal epiphyses and apophyses are to be found)
2. abnormal bone shape (e.g. developmental disorders or, more commonly, previous operations or old trauma)
3. alteration of relative position of bones (e.g. dislocations)
4. extra bones (e.g. accessory ossicles, extra digits or rays)
5. fusion of bones (e.g. congenital synostoses)
6. alteration in bone quality (or density), either local or general (e.g. disuse osteoporosis, periarticular porosis in rheumatoid disease)
7. expansions or outgrowths of bone (e.g. osteophytes, exostoses or tumours)
8. joint changes (e.g. osteo- or rheumatoid arthritis).

More than one of the above may be present; e.g. a fracture may have occurred through osteoporotic bone in a patient with a hallux valgus, where the hallux has a subungual exostosis.

Arterial pulse wave detection

The portable Doppler ultrasonic instrument may be used to detect the presence or absence of arterial flow in peripheral vessels in patients who, for example, have oedema preventing manual palpation of arteries. In some cases, the Doppler ultrasound technique will demonstrate normal flow in instances where pulses are palpable but appear diminished.

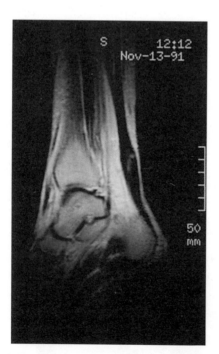

Figure 2.15 MRI showing degeneration within the tendo Achilles.

CLINICAL LABORATORY TESTS

Simple but useful tests can be carried out on body fluids and discharges, giving useful and sometimes essential information which may assist the clinician to reach a diagnosis or in planning appropriate treatment.

Urine

A midstream urine sample can be examined physically, biochemically and bacteriologically. Physical examination can determine volume, colour and specific gravity. The deposits may be examined microscopically for cells, casts and crystals, etc. (Fig. 2.16). Biochemical examination using Multistix (Ames) can determine specific gravity, pH and the presence of the following: proteins, glucose, ketones, bilirubin, blood, nitrites and urobilinogen. The bacteriological examination of urine using microscopes and culture techniques determines the morphology of infecting organisms and their sensitivity to antibiotics.

Blood

Haematological studies show the cell count and the morphology of the cells. The erythrocyte sedimentation rate (ESR) gives a non-specific indication of the presence of a disease process, such as infection. Biochemical examination for glucose, electrolytes, urates and many other more esoteric tests are readily available from the laboratory. Simple clinical testing which does not replace conventional laboratory methods includes the Dextrostix test for glucose. This is done using a drop of whole blood from a skin prick and should be carried out exactly according to the manufacturer's instructions. Bacteriological examination of blood is sometimes required if there is suspicion of systemic infection.

Discharge

Bacteriological examination of pus and other discharges from wounds is carried out for the purposes stated previously (Fig. 2.17). The importance of obtain-

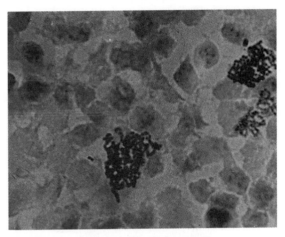

Figure 2.17   Pus from nail bed infected with *Staphylococcus aureus*. Gram film ($\times$ 100 objective).

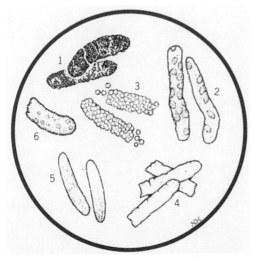

Figure 2.16   Urinary casts: 1, coarse granular casts; 2, epithelial cell casts; 3, red blood cell casts; 4, waxy casts; 5, hyaline casts; 6, casts with pus cells.

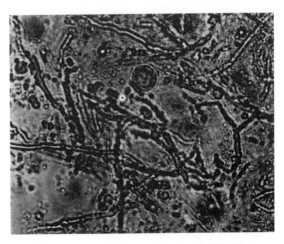

Figure 2.18   Tinea pedis: nail infected with *Trichiphyton rubrum*. KOH preparation ($\times$ 40 objective).

ing anaerobic cultures should not be overlooked, particularly with wounds of the feet which are not healing.

Skin and nail

Scrapings can be examined for confirmation of fungal infections and should be collected in the following manner.

Skin. Clean the area with 70% alcohol. Scrape the active edge of the lesion with a scalpel. Place the scales in a Petri dish. The roof of vesicles should be clipped off with appropriate tissue nippers.

Nail. After removing the thickness of the affected nail, scrapings should be taken from the advancing edge of the infection. Cotton wool swabs should not be used as the strands may resemble hyphae (Fig. 2.18).

FURTHER READING

Alexander I J 1990 The foot: examination and diagnosis. Churchill Livingstone, New York

Collee J G, Fraser A G, Duguid J P, Marmion B P (eds) 1989 Mackie & McCartney Practical medical microbiology, 13th edn (Microscopy and technical methods). Churchill Livingstone, Edinburgh

Gamble F O, Yale I 1975 Clinical foot roentgenology, 2nd edn. Krieger, New York

Hicks J H 1953 The mechanics of the foot 1. The joints. Journal of Anatomy 87: 345

Kapandji I A 1988 The physiology of the joints, 5th edn. Churchill Livingstone, Edinburgh

Ketwick J E 1982 Clinics in sports medicine. Saunders, Philadelphia

McRae R 1983 Clinical orthopaedic examination, 2nd edn. Churchill Livingstone, Edinburgh

Mann R A 1982 Biomechanics of running. Symposium on the foot and leg in running sports. Mosby, St Louis

Merriman L M, Tollafield D R 1995, Assessment of the lower limb. Churchill Livingstone, Edinburgh

Office practice of laboratory medicine 1987 Medical Clinics of North America 71(4)

Roche Scientific Services 1975 Urine under the microscope. Roche, Basle

Root M L, Orien W P, Weed J R 1977 Biomechanical examination of the foot. In: Clinical biomechanics, vol 1. Clinical Biomechanics Corporation, Los Angeles

Sgarlato T E 1978 Compendium of podiatric biomechanics. California College of Podiatric Medicine, San Francisco

Wright D G, Desai S M, Henderson W H 1964 Action of the subtalar and ankle joint complex during the stance phase of walking. Journal of Bone and Joint Surgery 46A

3

Radiological assessment for podiatrists

C. J. Fullerton

Keywords

Angular relationships on the dorsoplantar projection
Angular relationships on the lateral projection
Arthropathies
Bony mineralisation
Cyma line
Development of skeletal foot structure
Diabetic foot
Major axes of the foot
Radiographic charting
Radiographic interpretation
Radiographic projections
Sinus tarsi
Soft tissue examination
View of average foot
View of pronated foot

Diagnostic radiography is being utilised increasingly by podiatrists to improve the accuracy of diagnosis and the selection of appropriate treatment. Most diagnostic radiography is performed by a radiographer and interpreted by a radiologist, and therefore it is essential that precise guidance be given about the radiographic views required, the location of the suspected pathology, and a list of clinical symptoms and further details necessary to help the radiologist to arrive at a diagnosis. The standardised radiographic projections are performed to ensure radiographic images are diagnostically reliable. It is important that these procedures can be repeated with either the same patient or a succession of different patients to produce directly comparable images.

Some differences emerge in standardisation of views between podiatrists and radiographers, with podiatrists favouring views in a weight-bearing position. When taking a radiograph for charting purposes, it is necessary to take views of individual feet rather than both feet together. If both feet were viewed on the same exposure, divergence of X-rays would give a

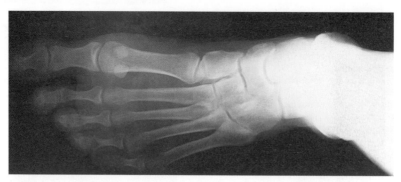

Figure 3.1 Dorsal plantar projection.

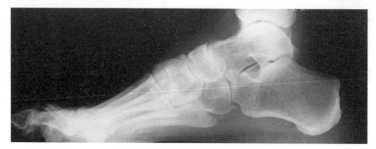

Figure 3.2 Lateral projection.

mildly distorted view. Finally, views should be taken in 'the angle and base of gait' position.

RADIOGRAPHIC PROJECTIONS

Dorsal plantar (D/P) projection

This is the most commonly taken projection of the foot which some radiographers refer to as the anterior/posterior (A/P) view. Wherever possible the D/P projection should be taken weight-bearing. It gives information concerning the phalanges, sesamoids, metatarsals, midtarsal bones and the distal aspect of the calcaneum and talus. The midtarsal joint, metatarsal–tarsal joints, metatarsophalangeal joints and interphalangeal joints can also be seen (Fig. 3.1).

Lateral projection

This projection shows the talus, calcaneum, navicular, medial cuneiform, cuboid, first metatarsal, great toe, medial sesamoid and most of the fifth metatarsal. The metatarsals and phalanges overlap to varying degrees. Any digit may be observed by elevating the part with a radiolucent object (Fig. 3.2).

Lateral oblique projection

This projection shows the phalanges, metatarsals, sesamoid bones and tarsal bones, with the cuboid being well defined. Any oblique projection of the foot shows the bones in a very distorted and magnified manner (Fig. 3.3). Podiatric indications for using this view include tarsal coalitions, abnormal bone shapes and exostoses.

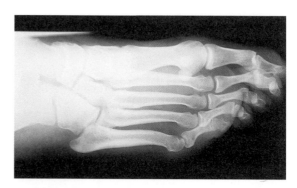

Figure 3.3 Lateral oblique projection.

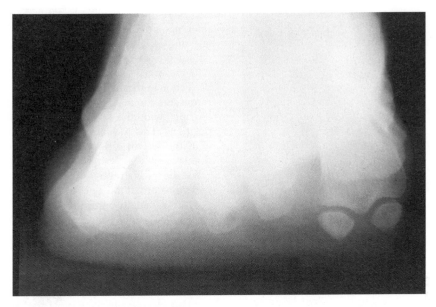

Figure 3.4 Axial sesamoid projection.

Axial sesamoid projection

This projection evaluates the sesamoid bones and their relationship with the metatarsal head plantarly (Fig. 3.4). It is used to evaluate the relative height of the metatarsal heads when determining if the metatarsal is plantarflexed.

Axial calcaneal projection

This projection is used to evaluate a fracture or an abnormally shaped calcaneum.

Mortice projection of ankle joint

This projection gives a clear outline of the joint space on both the medial and lateral aspects (Fig. 3.5).

Lateral projection of ankle joint

The trochlear surface of the talus is sharply outlined in this view (Fig. 3.6).

The above projections are the common radiographic views used in podiatric practice. If diagnostic information cannot be imaged on standard radiographic film, techniques such as bone scanning, computerised tomography and magnetic resonance imaging are alternatives.

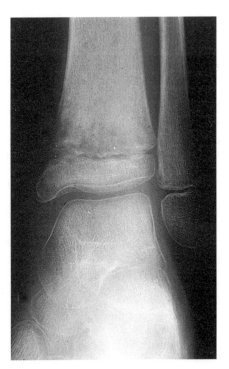

Figure 3.5 Mortice projection of ankle joint; osteomyelitis at the medial distal border of the tibia.

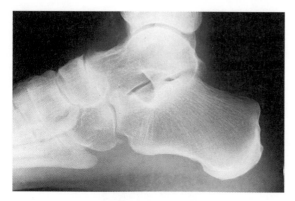

Figure 3.6 Lateral projection of ankle joint.

RADIOGRAPHIC CHARTING

Charting enables the clinician to enhance the written descriptive analysis and conclusion of the radiographic examination using reference points, lines, angles and relationships of osseous structures. This information is used to analyse pathology and positional relationships of osseous structures and to classify foot types. The information derived from this analysis can only be used as part of a general radiographic and clinical assessment of the foot, and not to impose rigid standards of normality or to initiate aggressive treatments. Noted that gross variations occurred in angular measurements of radiographs due to differences in technique between investigators.

Charting radiographs may be performed to aid diagnosis in aspects of traumatology, orthopaedics, paediatrics and podiatry. In podiatric practice, evaluation of hallux abducto valgus deformity and the determination of biomechanical foot types are the principal reasons for analysing radiographs using charting methods.

Information derived from charting is only reliable if the methods used are consistent and repeatable. Comparison of data from other studies must be regarded critically. Small variations in charting and radiographic technique can result in differing measurements for the same angle. In charting serial radiographs, one X-ray superimposed on top of the other is an easy method to determine if any changes in alignment have taken place.

There are numerous charting techniques available to podiatrists, some of which are of questionable value. Major errors can be caused by incorrect reference points and lines. This is due to attempting to bisect a three-dimensional osseous structure on a two-dimensional X-ray plate; thus care must be taken to determine exact reference points. Only the commoner reference lines and angles are described; further information can be obtained from a specialist radiology textbook.

There are several advantages of taking the X-ray projection in the angle and base of gait. This projection represents the average position of the foot in weight-bearing, with the bones in their relative functional positions. This technique allows the taking of X-rays with the feet in a position that can be easily reproduced.

As the radiograph forms an integral part of the patient record, it must not be defaced for charting purposes. It is usually appropriate to draw essential reference lines in fine pencil or to cover the radiograph with an acetate sheet and use markers to produce lines and angles.

Major axes (reference lines) of the foot on the dorsoplantar projection

Longitudinal axis of the rearfoot (Fig. 3.7)

If the posterior aspect of the calcaneum can be seen, a line should be drawn from the centre of the posterior aspect to a point at the anterodorso medial edge of the calcaneum and extended to the toes. If the posterior aspect cannot be seen and if the distal/lateral border of the calcaneus is straight, a line may be drawn parallel and medial for charting purposes. In most instances

LONG. AXIS

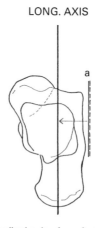

Figure 3.7 Longitudinal axis of rearfoot. This is a line drawn medial and parallel to line 'a' (a parallel line to the distolateral border of the calcaneus) for charting purposes. Gross irregularity of the distolateral calcaneal borderline will sometimes make the plotting of this reference axis somewhat difficult.

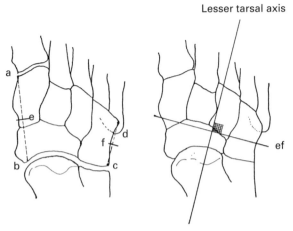

Figure 3.8 Longitudinal axis of the lesser tarsus. a: Medial/distal facet of the medial cuneiform; b: medial/proximal facet of the navicular; c: lateral/proximal facet of the cuboid; d: lateral/distal facet of the cuboid; e: bisection of line ab; f: bisection of line cd. The lesser tarsal axis is the line perpendicular to line ef.

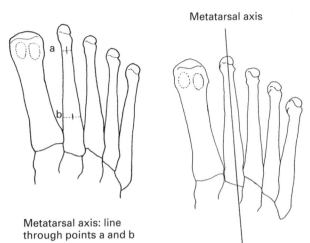

Figure 3.9 Longitudinal axis of the metatarsus. a: Bisection of the distal regular shaft of the second metatarsal; b: bisection of the proximal regular shaft of the second metatarsal.

the longitudinal axis of the rearfoot is roughly parallel to the longitudinal axis of the fourth metatarsal, although in many pathological instances this relationship does not hold true.

Longitudinal axis of the lesser tarsus (Fig. 3.8)

The longitudinal axis of the lesser tarsus, established by transecting the lesser tarsus, is useful when comparing the relationship of the lesser tarsus to both the position of the metatarsus and the position of the rearfoot.

Longitudinal axis of the metatarsus (Fig. 3.9)

The longitudinal axis of the metatarsus is the longitudinal bisection of the second metatarsal shaft.

Longitudinal axis of the digits

The longitudinal axis of the digits is the longitudinal bisection of the second proximal phalanx.

Angular relationships on the dorsoplantar projection

Talocalcaneal angle (Fig. 3.10)

The talocalcaneal angle is formed by a line bisecting the head and neck of the talus (collum tali axis), and

the longitudinal axis of the rearfoot. Normal range is approximately 17–21°. In pronation, the talocalcaneal angle will increase above 21°, and in supination it will decrease below 16°.

Approximately 75% of the head of the navicular should articulate with the talus in the normal stance. With pronation, the foot has moved in a lateral direction away from the talus, thus increasing the talocalcaneal angulation and causing the articulation between the talus and the navicular to be less than 75%.

The motion of pronation will also change the relationship between the longitudinal axis of the talus and the head of the first metatarsal. In normal stance, the axis of the talus should run through the centre of the first metatarsal head. When pronation occurs, it will run medial to the first metatarsal head. When supination occurs, it will project lateral to the first metatarsal head.

In the pronated talocalcaneal relationship, a notch or talocalcaneal gap will be revealed between the head of the talus and the distal portion of the calcaneus on the dorsoplantar film.

Cuboid abduction angle (Fig. 3.10)

The cuboid abduction angle is formed by a line representing the lateral aspect of the cuboid and the longitudinal axis of the rearfoot. Normal stance is 0–5°. When pronation involving the midtarsal joint occurs, the cuboid abduction angle tends to increase above 5°. With supination, the opposite occurs.

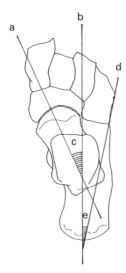

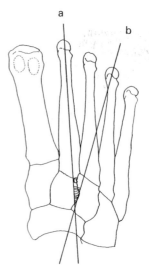

Figure 3.10 Talocalcaneal and cuboid abduction angles. a: Collum tali axis (i.e. bisection of the head and neck of the talus); b: longitudinal bisection of the rearfoot; c: talocalcaneal angle (average value 17–21°: with pronation the angle is above 21°, with supination the angle is less than 16°); d: lateral border of cuboid; e: cuboid abduction angle (this angle displays alteration in alignment of the midtarsal joint complex; the average value is 0–5°: with pronation the angle can be greater than 5°, and with supination the angle can be less than 0°).

Figure 3.11 Metatarsus adductus angle. a: Metatarsus axis; b: lesser tarsal axis; c: metatarsus adductus angle (average value is 8°, with a high normal of 12–14°; with a rectus metatarsus the angle is less than 12–14°, and with an adductus metatarsus the angle is greater than 12–14°). The metatarsus angle is normally adductory but is occasionally abductory in severe flat foot deformities or as a result of tarsometatarsal trauma.

Metatarsus adductus angle (Fig. 3.11)

The metatarsus adductus angle is formed by the intersection of the longitudinal axis of the metatarsus and the longitudinal axis of the lesser tarsus. The ideal angle is 16–18° and the angle is almost always adductory. If the angle is above 20°, this signifies that the adduction of the metatarsus will automatically make the medial aspect of the first metatarsal head more prominent and can contribute to hallux valgus deformity.

Intermetatarsal angle (Fig. 3.12)

This angle is also known as the metatarsus primus varus angle. It is formed by the intersection of the longitudinal axes of the first and second metatarsal shafts. The average angle is 8–10° and is an important consideration in determining the best procedure in cases of hallux valgus surgery. With an angle above 15° many podiatrists would consider that an osteotomy at the base of the metatarsal is preferable to an osteotomy at the distal end below the neck. Intermetatarsal angles which exceed 22° indicate that a first metatarsal medial cuneiform joint fusion or Lapidus procedure would be better.

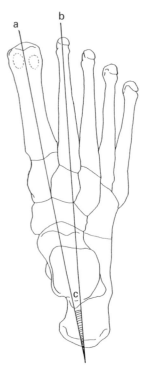

Figure 3.12 Intermetatarsus angle (metatarsus primus varus angle). a: First metatarsal axis; b: second metatarsal axis; c: first intermetatarsal angle. The average value of 'c' is 8°.

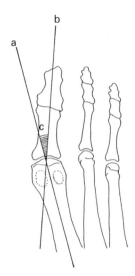

Figure 3.13 Hallux abductus angle. a: First metatarsal axis; b: hallux axis; c: hallux abductus angle. The average value of 'c' is 15–20°.

Hallux abductus angle (Fig. 3.13)

This angle is formed by the intersection of the longitudinal axis of the first metatarsal and the longitudinal axis of the proximal phalanx of the hallux. The average angle is 15°, and a value of 20° is considered to be abnormal.

Hallux interphalangeal angle

This angle is formed by the intersection of the longitudinal axis of the first proximal phalanx and the longitudinal axis of the distal phalanx. The average angle is 8–10°.

Tibial sesamoid position (Fig. 3.14)

The tibial sesamoid position is determined by the relative apposition of the tibial sesamoid to the first metatarsal axis.

Major axes (reference lines) of the foot on the lateral projection

Plane of support

The plane of support on the lateral projection is determined by connecting two points. The first is the most plantar aspect of the tuberosity of the calcaneus, and the second is the most plantar aspect of the head of the fifth metatarsal.

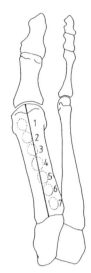

Figure 3.14 Tibial sesamoid position. This is determined by the relative position of the tibial sesamoid to the first metatarsal axis. Seven positions are identified: 1, tibial sesamoid lies medially clear of the first metatarsal axis; 2, tibial sesamoid laterally abuts the first metatarsal axis; 3, tibial sesamoid laterally overlaps the first metatarsal; 4, tibial sesamoid is bisected by the first metatarsal axis; 5, tibial sesamoid medially overlaps the first metatarsal axis; 6, tibial sesamoid medially abuts the first metatarsal axis; 7, tibial sesamoid lies laterally clear of the first metatarsal axis.

Calcaneal inclination axis (Fig. 3.15)

This is determined by connecting a point representing the most plantar aspect of the tuberosity of the calcaneus with the most distal plantar aspect of the calcaneus (at the calcaneal cuboid joint).

Collum tali axis (Fig. 3.16)

This is determined by the bisection of the head and neck (not the body) of the talus.

First metatarsal declination axis (Fig. 3.17)

Bisect the neck and the base end (not the base) of the shaft of the first metatarsal.

Angular relationships on the lateral projection

Calcaneal inclination angle (Fig. 3.15)

This angle is formed by the intersection of the plane of support and the calcaneal inclination axis. The normal

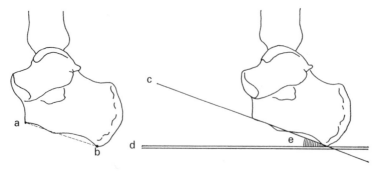

Figure 3.15 Calcaneal inclination axis and calcaneal inclination angle. a: Inferior limit, distal facet of the calcaneus; b: disto-inferior limit of the calcaneal tuberosity; c: calcaneal inclination axis; d: plane of support (line joining point b to inferior fifth head), e: calcaneal inclination angle. The average value of 'e' is between 18° and 22°. With pronation the angle can be decreased significantly; with supination the angle can be increased significantly.

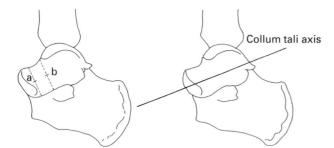

Figure 3.16 Collum tali axis (line through points a and b). The collum tali axis is a longitudinal bisector of the neck of the talus. Due to its variable shape, the radiographic plotting of the axis can be difficult. a: Bisector of the distal regular neck of the talus; b: bisector of the proximal regular neck of the talus.

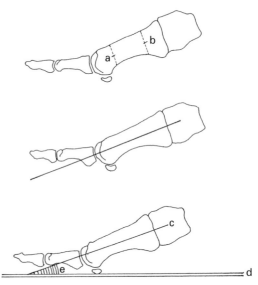

Figure 3.17 First metatarsal declination axis and first metatarsal declination angle. a: Bisector, distal regular shaft of first metatarsal; b: bisector, proximal regular shaft of first metatarsal; c: first metatarsal axis; d: plane of support; e: first metatarsal declination angle.

angle is between 15° and 30°. It is an index of relative arch height. In the pronated foot the angle can be decreased significantly.

Talar declination angle (Fig. 3.18)

This angle is formed by the intersection of the plane of support and the collum tali axis. The average value is around 21°. In the 'normal' foot, this axis will be collinear with the first metatarsal declination axis.

First metatarsal declination angle (Fig. 3.17)

Cyma line

The cyma line is another name for the midtarsal joint, or Chopart's joint. In the 'normal' foot, the talonavicular and calcaneocuboid portions of Chopart's joint should be in line with each other to form a continuous

S-shaped curve (Fig 3.19). In pronation, as the talus slides anteriorly, there will be an 'anterior break' in the cyma line.

Sinus tarsi

This is seen in the lateral projection of the foot. It appears as an oval area of decreased bone density, separating the posterior from the middle subtalar

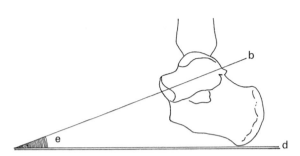

Figure 3.18 Talar declination angle. b: Collum tali axis; d: plane of support; e: talar declination. Normal value of 'e' is 21°. With pronation the angle is increased; with supination it is decreased.

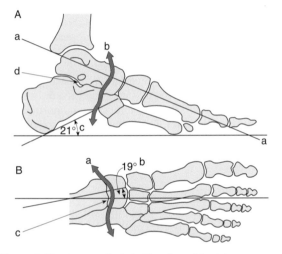

Figure 3.19 Average foot. A: Bisection of the talus passes through the shaft of the first metatarsal; the cyma line is an intact curve; angle of inclination of the calcaneus is normal; sinus tarsi is visible. B: Smooth uninterrupted midtarsal joint cyma line; talar deviation is 17–21°; the talonavicular joint is 75% congruent.

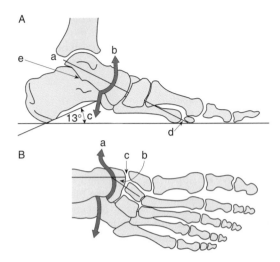

Figure 3.20 Pronated foot. A: Bisection of the talus passes below the shaft of the first metatarsal; anterior break in the cyma line; angle of inclination of the calcaneus is decreased; the talar declination line is increased; the sinus tarsi is obstructed. B: Broken midtarsal joint line; the talocalcaneal angle is greater than 21°; the talonavicular joint is less than

facets. In the normal foot, the sinus tarsi appears oval-shaped; in the pronated foot the sinus tarsi is obliterated (Fig. 3.20), and in the supinated foot it has a 'bullet-hole' appearance.

RADIOGRAPHIC INTERPRETATION

It is best to develop a constant approach towards radiographic analysis as this will reduce the possibility of missing major features or focusing on symptomatic sites alone. The approach recommended in this chapter is very similar to that suggested by Kaschak & Laine (1988), who suggested the mnemonic 'ABCDS' (Alignment, Bony mineralisation, Cartilage space, Distal to proximal, Soft tissue).

Distal to proximal

Due to the abundant information on a radiograph, it is easy to miss a small but important feature. On the D/P view, begin distally and read from medial to lateral. Moving through the levels from distal to proximal, note the soft tissue texture, bony mineralisation, bony alignment, cartilage space and trabecular pattern. Having the opposite foot for direct comparison is of vital importance when interpreting congenital deformities.

Soft tissue

This is often a neglected area of the examination. Soft tissue can yield a surprising amount of information about the systemic well-being of the patient. Where localised inflammation is present secondary to joint disease or infection, an increased localised density or fogging of the radiograph is noted. In diabetes mellitus, the tunica intima of the anterior and posterior tibial arteries are occasionally calcified and this can be detected on the radiograph. A generalised increase in brightness is noted with oedema.

An abrupt increase in brightness is noted as one moves distally to proximally on the proximal phalanges. This denotes the commencement of the plantar fat pad. Moving further proximal on the foot, there is an increased haziness on the radiograph denoting the increased bulk of soft tissue in the mid- and rearfoot.

Bony mineralisation

The assessment of bony mineralisation on a foot radiograph can prove to be extremely difficult. Localised demineralisation is easier to spot than the generalised case. The reason for this is that technical exposure factors can give the appearance of a pseudo-osteoporosis. A general guideline is to observe the blackness of the film in an area which contains no foot structure or soft tissue. A very black film background indicates overexposure which removes trabecular pattern detail, while a light grey background indicates underexposure, giving a false appearance of increased bone density.

On the D/P projection, the cortices appear smooth and white. These are best seen on the metatarsal bones, with the tarsal bones having cortices that are eggshell thin. The trabeculae lines are observed in the bases and heads of the metatarsals, the tarsal bones and the lateral view of the calcaneum. These lines denote lines of stress. The trabecular pattern and cortical appearance are good indicators of systemic health.

When observing the D/P projection, it is normal to see increased sclerosis (whiteness) in subchondral bone of the concave-shaped distal joint facets. This is particularly true in the metatarsophalangeal and talonavicular joints. Due to the difference in bone mass between the digital area and the midtarsal area, it is difficult for the radiographer to obtain a correct exposure for both areas. It is essential to communicate with the radiographer as to the location of the suspected foot pathology.

Alignment

One should not attempt to impose a rigid standard of normality concerning angular measurements between osseous structures. Instead, the measurements should be used in conjunction with the clinical examination and standard laboratory investigations to aid in the diagnosis. Abnormal alignments occur due to systemic disease, trauma, acquired deformity and foot imbalances.

Cartilage space

The joint space consists mainly of two smooth surfaces of articular cartilage with a thin space between them which is filled with synovial fluid. Articular cartilage does not show up on the radiograph and the joint space therefore appears unusually large. The joint space should be equidistant from the medial and lateral sides. The subchondral bone surface should be smooth and round.

Joint space narrowing will occur if all or part of the articular cartilage becomes eroded, as in arthropathy. Distension of the joint space will occur if a proliferative pannus forms between the joint surfaces in association with inflammatory joint disease. Diseases like acromegaly can cause a proliferation of the soft tissue, which includes articular cartilage, and therefore an apparent increase in the joint space.

The cartilage spaces are clearly seen in many joints, especially the interphalangeal and the metatarsophalangeal joints on the D/P projection. Some cartilage spaces overlap to give a confusing appearance. This occurs at the medial cuneiform/metatarsal joint and the cuneiform joints on the D/P view.

After developing a consistent approach towards reading the radiograph, it is important to study every individual bone in the foot to observe its normal and variant characteristics. This is important, as experience is required before one can determine abnormal bone shape.

Talus

On the D/P projection, only the head and neck of the talus is visible. Only 75% of the talar head articulates with the navicular. If the longitudinal axis of the neck and head of the talus is extended distally, it would pass through the first metatarsal head. In the pronated position, the axis would pass medial to the first metatarsal head. In the supinated position, the axis would pass lateral to the first metatarsal head. On the lateral projection, the convex trochlear surface of the talus is well visualised. The longitudinal axis of the neck and head of the talus, if extended distally, again passes through the metatarsal head. With pronation, the axis passes inferior to the first metatarsal head. With supination, the axis passes superiorly.

Calcaneum

On the D/P projection, only the anterior/lateral aspect of the calcaneum is observed. The rest of the calcaneum is hidden by the talus which is superimposed on it. With excessive pronation, the talocalcaneal notch is observed when the head of the talus is displaced medially on the calcaneum. On the lateral projection, the sinus tarsi is observed as an oval lucency situated within the talocalcaneal (subtalar) joint. The sustentaculum tali is identified as an increased density of a rectangular shape situated inferiorly to the sinus tarsi. The trabecular pattern is clearly observed, indicating lines of stress. In the centre of the calcaneum there is an area of sparse trabecular lines. The calcaneal inclination angle gives an indication of the height of the medial longitudinal arch.

Navicular

On the D/P projection, the navicular appears rectangular in shape. The medial aspect should not be excessively prominent.

Cuboid

On the D/P projection, the cuboid is an irregularly shaped bone. On the lateral projection, a sesamoid bone (os peroneum) is occasionally observed at the inferior border of the bone.

Midtarsal joint

The calcaneocuboid and the naviculocuneiform joints make up the midtarsal joint. Many authors state that an unbroken cyma line at the midtarsal joint indicates joint integrity here. A cyma line consist of two curves that are joined together to form a lazy S-type curve.

Cuneiforms

On the D/P projection, the medial cuneiform is clearly identified. The intermediate and lateral cuneiforms overlap each other and are not clearly outlined. On the lateral projection, the superior surfaces of the neck of the talus, navicular and medial cuneiform should form a straight line. With excessive pronation and the plantar displacement of the talar head and navicular, this causes a depression to occur at the naviculocuneiform joint, otherwise known as the naviculocuneiform fault.

First metatarsal

On the D/P projection, the first metatarsal has the thickest cortex of all five metatarsals. The medial aspect of the metatarsal head is frequently enlarged with occasional cystic degeneration. Confusion may arise over the appearance at the first metatarsocuneiform joint. This is due to an overlap of the joint surfaces. On the lateral projection, the rounded articular surface of the metatarsal head continues dorsally.

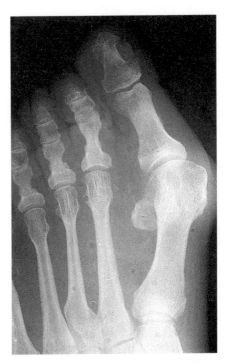

Figure 3.21 Rotation of proximal phalanx showing asymetrical borders of the phalanx.

Second to fifth metatarsals

On the lateral view, there is a great deal of overlap of the second, third and fourth metatarsals.

First proximal phalanx

On the D/P view, the curvature of the medial and lateral borders of the first proximal phalanx should be symmetrical. If there is increased curvature of the lateral border, this indicates rotation of the proximal phalanx such as that which may occur with a hallux valgus deformity (Fig. 3.21).

DEVELOPMENT OF SKELETAL FOOT STRUCTURE

At birth, all bone shapes are present in ossified or cartilaginous form. A radiograph of an infant foot shows only those skeletal elements which are ossified and not the cartilaginous portions. Gradually, the skeletal elements begin to ossify from primary centres of ossification. There is a predictable sequence of the appearance of these ossification nuclei in the developing foot. (See ossification timetable, Appendix 2)

At a later stage, secondary centres of ossification appear which are chiefly concerned with altering the shape or increasing the length of individual bones. An epiphysis is concerned with alteration in bone length and an apophysis is concerned with alteration in bone shape. The appearance of ossification centres can determine the (chronological) age of the child. It should be noted that the female skeleton reaches maturity 2 years earlier than the male skeleton.

Stages of foot development

At birth

The talus, calcaneum, metatarsal shafts and proximal phalanges are the only skeletal elements to be ossified at birth. The primary centre is present in 50% of the cuboid bone, with 90% being ossified at 6 months.

Six months to 2 years

The lateral cuneiform begins to ossify at 6 months. The medial cuneiform appears at 18–24 months. The secondary centre of ossification appears at the base of the first metatarsal and the bases of the proximal phalanges at approximately 2 years.

Two to 5 years

Between 2 and 3 years, the ossification centre of intermediate cuneiform appears. At 3 years, the primary ossification centre of the navicular appears. At this stage, the secondary centres appear at the bases of the intermediate and distal phalanges and the lesser metatarsal heads (Fig. 3.22).

Five to 12 years

During this phase, foot growth occurs in spasmodic episodes. The secondary ossification centre of the calcaneum appears at 8 years in females and 10–11 years in males (Fig. 3.23). The sesamoid bones appear at 9–11 years.

Twelve to 20 years

Final fusion of all epiphyseal areas as well as the calcaneal apophyses occurs during this period.

RADIOLOGICAL VARIATIONS OF THE FOOT

The growing tarsal and metatarsal bones are charac-

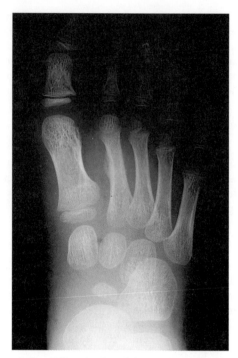

Figure 3.22 D/P projection of the right foot of a child of 3 years with suspected stress fracture of the second metatarsal shaft.

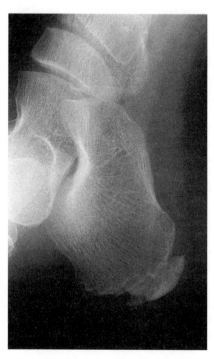

Figure 3.23 Lateral projection in a child of 9 years, showing secondary ossification centre of the calcaneum.

terised by numerous variations that may simulate pathological conditions. The podiatrist should be familiar with these normal anatomical variants in order not to misinterpret them as fractures, osteochondritis or bone disease.

Sesamoid and accessory or supernumerary bones

In the normal foot, there are two types of bones that remain unattached to the main body of any bone. These are the sesamoid and accessory bones.

Sesamoid bones

Sesamoid bones are located in tendons over bony prominences or where the tendon makes a change (angular) in course. The sesamoid is incorporated in the substance of the tendon and one surface of the sesamoid bone articulating with the adjacent bone. The sesamoid glides with the tendon.

Sesamoid bones are consistently located on the plantar surface, the most common being the two beneath the first metatarsal head. They develop from separate centres of ossification within the tendons of the flexor hallucis brevis. Occasionally an individual bone may be seen on radiograph as multipartite (several parts) or bipartite (two parts). Each part of a multipartite sesamoid bone is attached to its adjacent portion by fibro-cartilage and is developed from a separate centre of ossification (Fig. 3.24). The bipartite sesamoid bone consists of rounded ossifications and should not be confused with a fracture. Bipartite sesamoids are usually larger than the single sesamoid bones.

Less frequently, there are single sesamoids beneath the heads of the second, third and fourth metatarsals. Rarely, there are two beneath the fifth metatarsal head and on the plantar surface of the first interphalangeal joint. Infrequently, sesamoids are under all the metatarsal heads (Fig. 3.25). A sesamoid called the os peroneum is frequently found in the peroneus longus tendon as it turns under the cuboid to pass into the sole of the foot (Fig. 3.26).

Accessory bones of the foot

Accessory bones have been defined as inconstant, independent, well-defined bones in an otherwise normally developed foot (Trolle 1948). These supernumery centres of ossification occur in the foot more frequently than in any other part of the body, and far more often than in the hand. Their incidence varies from 18–30% in adults to 7% in children, excluding

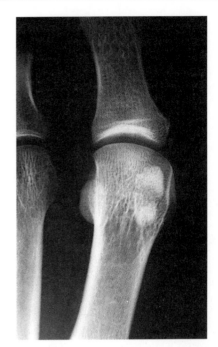

Figure 3.24   Projection of left foot showing bipartite tibial sesamoid.

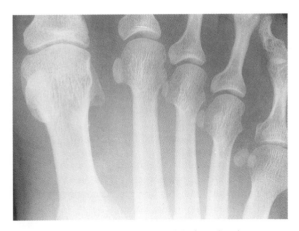

Figure 3.25   D/P projection of the right foot showing additional sesamoid bones.

those seen at and distal to the metatarsophalangeal joints (Shands & Wertz 1953).

Accessory bones are parts of prominences of the tarsal bones that are separated from the normal bone. Tendons or ligaments may attach to an accessory bone, but the latter do not slide with movement of the ten-

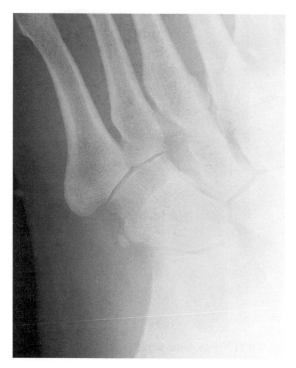

Figure 3.26 Lateral oblique projection showing an os peroneum beneath the cuboid.

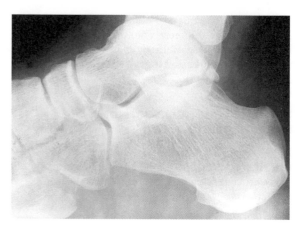

Figure 3.27 Lateral projection showing an os trigonum positioned posteriorly to the talus.

don. Accessory bones are considered to be secondary centres of ossification. They are usually asymptomatic and should be distinguished from fractures. The most common accessory bones in the foot are os trigonum and os tibiale externum.

Os tibiale externum. This is present as a separate bone in about 4–14% of normal feet (Lawson 1985). Three different types of accessory navicular have been described (Romanowski & Barrington 1991):

- *Type 1* is a sesamoid bone that lies in the tendon of tibialis posterior approximately 3 mm away from the navicular bone; this first type accounts for 30% of all accessory navicular bones.
- *Type 2* is united to the navicular by a synchondrosis and accounts for a further 70% of accessory navicular bones.
- *Type 3* is stated as being the end stage of type 2 accessory bone that has now completely fused with the parent navicular bone.

Shoe pressure on the accessory bone may also cause the formation of an inflamed adventitious bursa with local swelling and tenderness.

The accessory bone will be visible medially and proximal to the navicular bone. Its smooth and round-ed outline differentiates it from the irregular margin that characterises a fracture. In later adolescence, the accessory navicular may fuse with the body of the tarsal bone and present as an abnormally prominent and curved medial end of the navicular. This produces the same symptoms as the accessory navicular.

Os trigonum. The incidence of the os trigonum varies between 3 and 15% (Johnson et al 1984). On the posterior aspect of the talus there is a groove for the flexor hallucis longus tendon. The bony tubercle lateral to this tendon groove is usually larger than the medial one. Between 8 and 11 years of age, separate centres of ossification appear for the medial and lateral tubercles, and within a year they fuse with the main body of the talus. The lateral tubercle may remain separate as the os trigonum which is extremely variable in size and shape (Fig. 3.27).

A fused but large ossicle may become detached by sudden violence (Brodsky & Khalil 1987), particularly when union of the ossicle to the talus is by synchondrosis (cartilage joint). The absence of irregularity between the os trigonum and the main body of the talus distinguishes a synchondrosis from a fracture.

ARTHROPATHY

The diagnosis of a particular type of arthropathy cannot be made on the basis of X-ray alone. Initial assessment by a rheumatologist will involve clinical examination, laboratory analysis and plain film radiographic analysis.

Plain film radiographic analysis can aid diagnosis and determine the extent and severity of joint disease.

As in all radiographic evaluations, it is especially important to analyse the films in a logical fashion.

Initial review of a radiograph is best performed to detect general pathologic changes before committing oneself to a specific location or localised abnormality. This is accomplished by observing the soft tissue density, alignment of osseous structures, and finally assessing bone mineralisation.

Soft tissue swelling is denoted by the presence of soft tissue density on the film. This may be joint- or non-joint-related in cause. Increase in soft tissue density indicates a long-term inflammatory process indicative of various types of arthropathy.

Osseous malalignments and deformity of the foot are common with many forms of arthropathy and are not necessarily diagnostic. Although hallux valgus and digital deformities are common with rheumatoid arthritis, these deformities occur to varying degrees with other forms of arthropathy (Calabro 1966).

Periarticular osteoporosis is characteristic of rheumatoid arthritis. It is rarely noted in seronegative arthropathy. The interpretation of osteoporosis is subjective and only identifiable after 25–50% loss of mineral content. The diagnosis also depends on the film quality. Only after this general evaluation should each joint or cartilage space be visually examined for narrowing, erosions and distribution pattern of the disease.

Joint space narrowing is indicative of exacerbation of destruction of articular cartilage. Uniform joint space narrowing occurs with rheumatoid arthritis and seronegative arthropathy, whilst uneven joint space narrowing occurs with osteoarthritis. With gout, joint space narrowing does not occur until later in the disease process.

Marginal erosions appear 1–2 years following symptoms. Bone erosions are caused by inflamed synovial tissue, which demineralises the cartilage-free area of bone within the joint capsule at the metatarsophalangeal joint, or can occur at the posterior aspect of the calcaneum adjacent to the retrocalcaneal bursa. The erosions are characterised by their location, size and morphology.

Knowledge of the *distribution pattern* of disease outside the confines of the foot is essential to aid diagnosis. This is important when the disease pattern within the foot is similar to other forms of arthropathy. Using techniques suggested by Resnick (1981), *radiographic target areas* of the body are observed which aid the classification of arthropathy.

Proliferative bone production in the form of osteophytes and heel spurs. Inflammation at the ligamentous and capsular attachment to bone is termed 'enthesopathy'. This occurs with rheumatoid arthritis and seronegative arthropathy.

Radiology in rheumatoid arthritis (RA)

It takes, on average, 2 or 3 months before radiographic changes appear (Resnick & Niwayama 1981) and these are best seen in small joints of the hand and foot. The joints most frequently affected in the foot are the metatarsophalangeal joints, the fifth more often than the second, third or fourth, and the first less frequently than the second (Kumar & Madewell 1987).

Features of RA (Fig. 3.28)

1. Changes in soft tissue are best noted clinically. On X-ray it appears as fusiform swelling around affected joints. The swelling is symmetrical, unlike gout which is asymmetrical.

2. Initial joint space widening caused by synovial effusion. Later the joint space may be reduced uniformly due to cartilage destruction.

3. Osteoporosis at first tends to be juxta-articular (bone adjacent to joint) (Martel 1970).

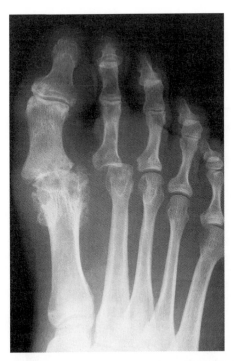

Figure 3.28   D/P projection showing rheumatoid arthritis with marginal erosions at the first metatarsal head and subluxation of the second metatarsal joint.

4. Erosions are first seen on the joint margin which then spread across the joint surface. Usually, these occur several years following the onset of joint symptoms (Brook & Corbett 1977). Patients receiving prolonged steroid therapy, either systemic or intra-articular, may develop gross articular destructive changes.

5. Subluxation may be observed, especially at the metatarsophalangeal joints.

Osteoarthritis (Fig. 3.29)

This is characterised by:
1. eccentric or uneven joint space narrowing
2. subchondral sclerosis of bone
3. osteophytic lipping at margin of joint
4. subchondral cystic formation.

Seronegative arthropathy

This group of arthropathies is characterised by less severe inflammation (Stiles et al 1988), no osteoporosis, osseous proliferation patterns (heel spurs) and asymmetry of articular changes. The radiographic

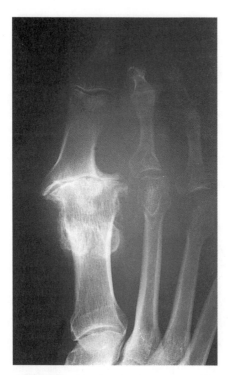

Figure 3.29   D/P projection showing osteoarthritis with gross osteophytic lipping.

changes are similar to rheumatoid arthritis but with an asymmetric pattern of distribution (Kumar & Madewell 1987).

Differentiating between the seronegative arthropathies can be difficult. Ankylosing spondylitis primarily affects the spine. Psoriatic arthropathy affects the spine and limbs, and Reiter's disease affects the lower limb (Resnick & Niwayama 1981).

Psoriatic arthropathy

The lesions which appear on a radiograph in psoriatic arthropathy are wide ranging and usually asymmetrical, and have the following characteristics:

1. There is consistent involvement of distal interphalangeal joints (Wright 1961).
2. The appearance of erosions on the articular surface is similar to those erosions seen in rheumatoid arthritis; the location of the erosions can differentiate between psoriatic and rheumatoid arthritis, since in the former the erosions appear primarily at the distal interphalangeal joint whereas in the latter they are located mainly at the metatarsophalangeal joint.
3. Deformities can range from mild to severe; severe deformities include arthritis mutilans, which is *mushrooming* or *pencil in a cup deformity* resulting from impaction of the distal end of one phalanx in the base of the next (Moll & Wright 1973).
4. There is reabsorption of ungual tufts.
5. Enthesopathy presents with the production of a heel spur which has a 'fluffy' appearance.

Ankylosing spondylitis

This arthropathy primarily affects the axial skeleton, with the first symptoms usually in the spinal column. The hip joint is commonly affected. Foot involvement occurs in only 15% of patients with this form of arthropathy. The disease has the following characteristics:

1. The sacroiliac joint is the primary target site with proximal migration up the spine as the disease progresses.
2. Enthesopathy is present, i.e. at the attachment of the tendo Achilles and the plantar fascia to the calcaneum (Hadler et al 1974).
3. Osteoporosis is slight.
4. Occasionally, bony ankylosis and bony proliferative changes of the metatarsophalangeal and interphalangeal joints of the hallux are seen.

Reiter's disease

The triad of arthritis, urethritis and conjunctivitis distinguishes Reiter's disease from other seronegative arthropathies. Heel involvement may occur as an initial symptom (Oloff 1988). Characteristics are as follows:

1. X-ray changes are not apparent except in chronic disease.
2. There is a proliferative heel spur with a 'fluffy' appearance.
3. Thickening of the tendo Achilles may be observed.
4. There is erosion of the posterior/superior aspect of the calcaneum; the degree of erosive changes is an indicator of the chronicity of the disease.

Gout (Fig. 3.30)

Modern drug therapy has significantly reduced the incidence of chronic erosive articular changes previously seen with gout. Erosions develop due to the deposition of sodium urate. The location of the erosion is mainly at the first metatarsophalangeal joint, followed by incidence at the first interphalangeal joint of the hallux and the medial cuneiform/metatarsal joint.

1. X-ray changes are not apparent except in cases of chronic disease.

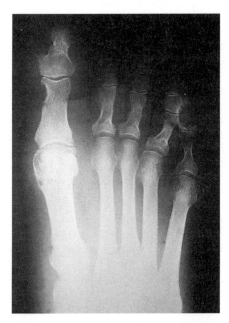

Figure 3.30 D/P projection of a foot with gout, showing 'punched out' erosion of the proximal phalanx and similar changes to the medial aspect of the metatarsal head. Note the osteoblastoma to the distal phalanx of the fifth toe.

2. There is absence of osteoporosis due to the inflammatory episodes being relatively brief in duration with little osteoclasis occurring.
3. Joint space narrowing is a relatively late manifestation. There is much bony destruction before articular cartilage loss supervenes.
4. Erosions are usually greater than 5 mm in diameter (Grahame & Scott 1970). Erosions appear near the joint margin and, as they enlarge, they tend to involve more of the cortex of the shaft rather than the articular surface.
5. Erosion of the bone is not apparent on radiograph until 2–3 years following the initial attack.

The diabetic foot

The aetiology of the osseous alterations manifested on plain X-ray film as a direct result of diabetes mellitus is not fully understood. However, it is accepted that two radiographic patterns of diabetic neuropathic osteoarthropathy (DNOAP) occur: one is the acute or early phase and the other is the chronic or late phase. The two are not separate pathologies but indicate the stage and severity of the neuropathic joint disease.

In one study, the tarsus and tarsometatarsal joints are affected in 54–60% of all cases, metatarsophalangeal joints in 30%, the ankle in 9–11%, and interphalangeal joints in about 5% in all neuropathic patients (Forgacs 1982). All patients with DNOAP will have had a peripheral neuropathy.

Acute or early phase

The acute phase is the atrophic form of DNOAP. Hyperglycaemia leads to deterioration of nerve impulses with an alteration in autonomic function, resulting in arteriovenous shunting with decreased blood flow to the distal soft tissues and increased blood flow to osseous structures (Edmonds et al 1985). High blood flow stimulates osteoclasis or bone reabsorption with softening of the bone which is liable to deform.

Radiographic features include osteoporosis, atrophy, destruction and disappearance of bone substance. Often this phase commences with osteoporosis of the metatarsals and phalanges, and usually the joint surfaces are spared, initially (Frykberg 1991). The cortical defects can often lead to severe osteolysis of metatarsal heads, leaving only the central shafts of the bones. Clinical features include soft tissue swelling, joint effusions and eventual subluxation. Sometimes this pattern of destruction may be confused with osteomyelitis.

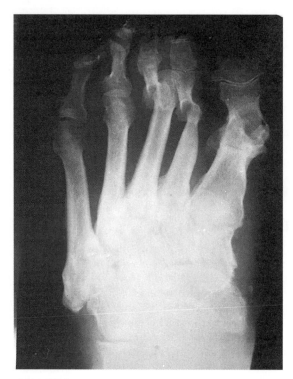

Figure 3.31 D/P projection showing diabetic neuropathic arthropathy.

Chronic or late phase (Charcot's joint)
(Fig. 3.31)

The chronic phase is the hypertrophic form of DNOAP, which is traditionally known as 'Charcot's joint'. The radiographic features include both reabsorption and sclerosis of joint surfaces with the production of large osteophytes. It is often described as 'osteoarthritis with a vengeance'.

This form of neuropathy is associated with gross neuropathic changes in ligament (Newman 1979). There is loss of normal protective reactions and relaxation of supporting structures within the foot leading to joint instability. With ligamentus laxity the joint surfaces fragment, leading to progressive destruction of joint surfaces and complete collapse of bone architecture. As healing takes place, there is gross proliferation of new bone at the joint margins.

Monckeberg's medial sclerosis

Medial calcification can occur in the posterior tibial and the dorsalis pedis arteries. On the radiograph it shows as a continuous pipe-like calcification on both the D/P and lateral projections.

Osteomyelitis

This represents a pyogenic infection of bone and/or bone marrow. A wide variety of microorganisms have been implicated in the disease, ranging from common infectious bacteria such as *Staphylococcus aureus* to less likely microorganisms including viruses and fungi (Roth & Pressman 1977).

The classification is as follows (Ingerman & Abrutyn 1986):

- direct extension osteomyelitis secondary to a focus of infection; usually the spread is from a skin ulceration which continues to the underlying bone
- osteomyelitis secondary to peripheral vascular disease; many of the patients in this category have diabetes mellitus (Mandel et al 1985)
- haematogenous osteomyelitis due to blood-borne bacteria which 'seed' in the metaphyseal end-arteries, e.g. metatarsal bone.

Overall, the various types account for 50%, 30% and 20% of osteomyelitic cases respectively.

Bone responds very slowly to inflammation and infection. Many of the radiographic signs of osteomyelitis do not show up on X-ray for 2 weeks after the start of bone infection (Ingerman & Abrutyn 1986). This delay is due to the fact that more than 50% of the bone matrix has to be removed before the radiographic change can be observed.

The earliest radiographic sign is soft tissue swelling. The other main radiographic signs of osteomyelitis include radiolucency, sclerosis, sequestration, involucrum, cloaca and subperiosteal calcification. Ingerman & Abrutyn (1986) stated that the sensitivity and specificity of routine X-rays are less than desirable. Bone scanning techniques have enhanced the clinician's ability to make an early diagnosis of osteomyelitis (Handmaker & Leonards 1976). The radiographic signs are interpreted as follows:

- *Radiolucency* nearly always presents as areas of decreased density.
- *Sclerosis* may represent bone repair, or the reverse, dead bone.
- *Sequestration* is a section of dead bone caused by pus eliminating the blood supply to the portion of bone; it can separate from the main body of bone and may be seen on X-ray.
- *Involucrum* is an area of new bone production — the accumulation of pus elevates the periosteum of the underlying bone and new bone is laid down on the inner surface of the periosteum.
- *Cloaca* is an area of decreased density at the

bone/periosteal junction; this area is an opening for discharging pus from the underlying bone.

Haematogenous osteomyelitis

This form of osteomyelitis tends to occur in children with clinical symptoms of soft tissue oedema, fever, chills and systemic toxicity, which is usually seen in the initial episode. In recurrent episodes, symptoms such as pain and drainage predominate, and systemic symptoms are usually absent. Due to the anatomical structure of growing bone, circulating bacterium can 'seed' in end-arteries of the metaphysis. The epiphyseal (growth) plate acts as a temporary barrier to infection spreading to the joint, but eventually infection breaks through the plate or may reach the joint via the periosteum.

Chronic osteomyelitis

Unless osteomyelitis is treated aggressively with antibiotics at an early stage, the condition can become chronic. There is a low grade infection with periodic discharge through sinus tracts to the skin surface. There are recurrent episodes where the condition can 'flare up' with increasing drainage and localised pain. The main radiographic features include areas of thickened sclerotic bone with irregular radiolucent areas and elevated periosteum. Soft tissue irregularities indicate sinus tracts from bone to the skin surface.

Osteochondroses

Brower (1983) defined osteochondrosis as a condition in which a primary or secondary ossification centre in the growing child undergoes aseptic necrosis with gradual reabsorption of dead bone and replacement by reparative osseous tissue. The bones of the foot affected by this disease process are the second or sometimes the third metatarsal epiphysis, the navicular and the sesamoid. A true ostechondritic process affecting the calcaneal apophysis is rare. It is recognised that a combination of trauma coupled with a significant reduction in vascular supply to the affected area may be implicated in the aetiology of this pathology. Diagnosis of the above conditions is made on the basis of clinical features, the age of the patient and the radiograph.

Freiberg's infraction (metatarsal head)

In the early phase of the disease, a rarefaction of the metaphysis, a relative sclerosis of the epiphysis and slight flattening of the metatarsal head are visible. Later there is widening of the articulating surface of the metatarsal head with flattening of the concave surface of the base of the proximal phalanx. There is thickening of the metatarsal shaft to the extent that the neck of the bone is obliterated. The joint space occasionally becomes wider.

Later, due to the irregular joint surfaces, secondary osteoarthritis occurs, with erosion of the articular cartilage and osteophytic proliferation at the joint margin taking place (Fig. 3.32).

Kohler's disease (navicular)

Kohler's disease is an ostechondritic condition of the navicular bone which occurs in males four to five times more frequently than in females at an average age of 3 years. The condition is quite rare (Dobas & Cachat 1978). The radiographic appearance shows a wafer-thin flattened navicular bone, with patchy areas of density and loss of trabecular pattern. A less common appearance shows a normally shaped navicular bone with a uniformly increased relative density compared to the other tarsal bones (Waugh 1958).

Sever's disease (calcaneum)

Scranton (Helal 1988) suggests that painful heels in children were often misinterpreted as avascular necrosis of the calcaneal apophysis or so-called Sever's disease. Scranton stated that true avascular necrosis of the calcaneal apophysis has never been documented.

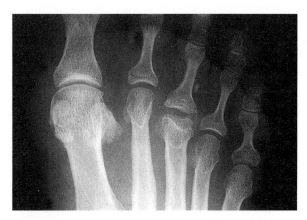

Figure 3.32 D/P projection showing secondary changes resulting from Freiberg's infraction of the third metatarsal head.

The ossification pattern of the calcaneal apophysis is highly variable, with unilateral differences on X-ray. An increased density of the calcaneal apophysis was recognised to represent the normal pattern of apophyseal ossification (Ferguson 1959). During development, flecks of calcification are first seen. Several centres may form, developing independently but coalescing to form the mature calcaneum.

REFERENCES

Brodsky A E, Khalil M A 1987 Talar compression syndrome. Foot and Ankle 7: 338–344

Brook A, Corbett M 1977 Radiographic changes in early rheumatoid disease. Ann Rheum Dis 36: 71

Brower A C 1983 The osteochondroses. Orthop Clin North Am 14(1): 99

Calabro J J 1966 A critical evaluation of the diagnostic features of the feet in rheumatoid arthritis. Ann Rheum Dis 25: 220

Dobas D C, Cachat P T 1978 Kohler's disease (a clinical study). Journal of the American Podiatry Association 68: 2

Edmonds M E, Clarke M B, Newton S, Barrett J 1985 Increased uptake of bone pharmaceutical in diabetic neuropathy. Q J Med 57: 843

Forgacs S 1982 Bones and joints in diabetes mellitus. Martinus Nijhoff Publishers, The Hague, p 94–109

Gould N 1982 Graphing the adult foot and ankle. Foot and Ankle 2(4): 213–219

Grahame R, Scott J T 1970 Clinical survey of 354 patients with gout. Ann Rheum Dis 29: 461

Green D, Weissman S D et al 1977 Roentgenologic analysis: angle of base of gait versus random positioning in relation to reducing X-ray exposure. Study performed at Pennsylvania College of Podiatric Medicine

Ferguson A, Gingrich R 1958 The normal and abnormal calcaneal apophysis and tarsal navicular. Clin Orthop 10: 87–95

Frykberg R G 1991 The high risk foot in diabetes mellitus.

Hadler N M, Franck W A, Bess N M et al 1974 Acute polyarticular gout. Am J Med 56: 715

Handmaker H, Leonards R 1976 The bone scan in inflammatory osseous disease. Semin Nucl Med 5: 95

Hlavav H F 1967 Differences in X-ray findings with varied positioning of the foot. Journal of the American Podiatry Assocation 57: 465

Ingerman M, Abrutyn E 1986 Osteomyelitis: a conceptual approach. Journal of the American Podiatric Medical Association 76: 9

Johnson R P, Collier B D, Carrera G 1984. The os trigonum syndrome: use of bone scan in the diagnosis. Journal of Trauma 24: 761–764

Kaschak T J, Laine W 1988 Clinics in Podiatric Medicine and Surgery 5(4): 798–804

Kumar R, Madewell J E 1987 Rheumatoid and seronegative arthropathies of the foot. Radiol Clin North Am 25: 1263

Lawson J P 1985 Symptomatic radiographic variants in extremities. Radiology 157: 625–631

Mandel G L, Douglas R G, Bennet J E 1985 Principles and practice of infectious diseases. John Wiley, New York

Martel W 1970 Acute and chronic arthritis of the foot. Semin Roentgenol 55: 391

Moll J M H, Wright V 1973 Psoriatic arthritis. Semin Arthritis Rheum 3: 55

Oloff L M 1988 Radiographic evaluation of inflammatory arthritis of the foot. Clinics in Podiatric Medicine and Surgery 5(4): 840

Resnick D, Niwayama G (eds) 1981 Diagnosis of bone and joint disorders. W.B. Saunders, Philadelphia

Romanowski C A J, Barrington N A 1991 The accessory ossicles of the foot. Foot 2: 61–70

Roth R D, Pressman M 1977 Clinical diagnosis of osteomyelitis. Journal of the American Podiatry Association 67: 10

Sgarlato T E 1965 The angle of gait. Journal of the American Podiatry Association 55: 645

Shands A R, Werts I J 1953 Foot problems in children. Surgical Clinics of North America 33: 1543–1566

Steele M W, Johnson K A, DeWitz M A, Ilstrup D M 1980 Radiographic measurements of the normal foot. Foot and Ankle, 1(3): 151–157

Stiles R G, Renick D, Sartoris D J 1988 Radiologic manifestations of arthritides involving the foot. Clinics in Podiatric Medicine and Surgery 5: 1

Talbott J H 1967 Gout, 3rd edn. Grune & Stratton, Philadelphia

Trolle D 1948 Accessory bones of the human foot. Munksgaard, Copenhagen

Waugh W 1958 The ossification and vascularization of the tarsal navicular and their relation to Kohler's disease. J Bone Joint Surg 40(B): 765

Wright V 1986 Psoriatic arthritis. In: Scott J T (ed) Copeman's textbook of the rheumatic diseases, 6th edn, vol 1. Churchill Livingstone, Edinburgh, p 775–786

FURTHER READING

Jahss M H 1982 Disorders of the foot. ch 6, p 116–139

Levy L A, Hetherington V J 1990 Principles and practice of podiatric medicine. Churchill Livingstone, Edinburgh

Scurran B L 1988 Clinics in podiatric medicine and surgery. Radiology of the Foot and Ankle 5(4)

Weissman S D 1983 Radiology of the foot. Williams and Wilkins, Baltimore

4

The growing foot

E. G. Anderson

Keywords

Accessory bones
Anatomical abnormalities
Cavus foot
Congenital abnormalities
Congenital talipes equinovarus
Coxa vara and coxa valga
Developmental conditions
Digital abnormalities
Extrinsic functional conditions
Flat foot
Genu varum and genu valgum
Intrinsic structural conditions
Malalignments
Normal growth and development
Polydactyly
Spina bifida
Structural deformities
Syndactyly
Talipes calcaneovalgus
Tarsal coalitions
Torsions
Trauma
Vertical talus

NORMAL GROWTH AND DEVELOPMENT

In the embryo, the limb buds appear at about the fourth week of intrauterine life, becoming segmented into proximal, intermediate and distal parts by the sixth week, and digitated by the seventh. By the ninth week, the thigh, leg and foot are recognisable entities. Ossification begins first in the larger bones of the leg and foot, extending gradually to the smaller bones. By the seventh month, the longitudinal arching of the skeleton of the foot is present. At birth, the skeletal framework is predominantly cartilage, but centres of ossification are present in the calcaneus, talus, cuboid, metatarsals and phalanges (see ossification timetable, Appendix 2). The infant's foot is thus highly malleable. This is important for two reasons. It allows some congenital deformities to be corrected more easily, but it also means that the feet may be deformed by premature or abnormal stresses of weight-bearing.

Abnormalities of intrauterine development of the foot will manifest themselves as congenital deformities. Some anomalies are characterised by failure of formation of parts, or extra parts, and must have their origin within the first few weeks of fetal development. Other deformities may be attributed to the abnormal intrauterine development of a basically normal foot. Little is known of the factors that control shape, form and size, other than that they are genetically determined but are capable of being modified by other influences. For example, the basic form of a bone is determined by the cellular tissue from which it is developed, but is then modified by pressures and stresses from surrounding tissues, such as developing muscles and the external environment. Deformities of the foot may be caused by imbalance of the action of muscles inserted into the developing foot. This is seen in extreme form when there is paralysis of muscle groups, as in spina bifida, but some deformities may be due to more subtle imbalance. Moreover, a foot deformity may itself contribute to abnormal development of muscles; thus it is uncertain whether the abnormal calf musculature found in children with talipes equinovarus is a cause or effect of the deformity.

At birth, the foot usually appears flat because of a fatty pad which is gradually absorbed as growth proceeds rapidly during the first year. Muscles are developed by the habit of kicking. The legs therefore should not be restricted by tight clothing, coverings or bed-clothes. At about 9–10 months of age the infant starts to crawl, and then learns to stand, at first with support and then unaided. Between 12 and 15 months the child begins to walk with assistance and gradually acquires proficiency with practice. Some children never crawl; they shuffle along on their bottoms and tend not to walk until they are nearer 2 years old. At first the stance is uncertain, with the feet widely spaced and variously abducted or adducted, while the gait is slow and deliberate. The processes of adopting an upright posture and learning to walk unaided depend upon the gradual development of neuromuscular pathways and coordination and should not be unduly or artificially stimulated, particularly in heavy babies, lest the immature foot be overloaded.

The child's foot is not a small-scale model of the adult foot. It is relatively shorter and wider, tapering towards the heel because the hindfoot is less fully developed than the forefoot (Fig. 4.1).

The shape of the foot is not finally determined until

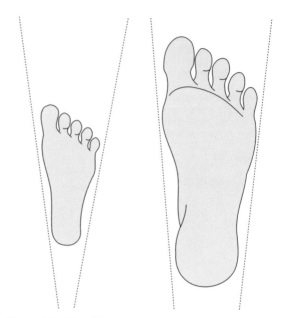

Figure 4.1 The different proportions of the immature and the mature foot.

growth ceases at about the 20th year; however, adult shoe size is usually reached by age 14. The growth rate of tissues is, in general, irregular, being very rapid in the first 2 or 3 years of life, slowing down at about 4 years of age, and spurting briefly at about 7 years. Thereafter, growth is retarded until puberty when the rate accelerates sharply, continuing into late adolescence. During this long growing period, footwear must be constantly adapted to current needs, being discarded when outgrown rather than when outworn. Maximum barefoot activity on suitable surfaces such as carpets, grass and sand should be encouraged as a means of stimulating muscle activity and development.

Most children are born with feet which, with normal growth and development, become both structurally stable and functionally efficient. They are subject thereafter only to the normal hazards of later life, e.g. infection, injury and disease. In some children, however, genetic and ontogenic abnormalities occur pre- and postnatally, giving rise to deformity and disability.

Those conditions present at birth are termed congenital disorders, while those that manifest later are developmental disorders. These defects can be considered intrinsic if they occur within the foot, and extrinsic if the effects on the foot are simply secondary to deformity elsewhere. The lower limbs, like other parts of the body, may also be affected by developmental defects occurring elsewhere, particularly those involving neuromuscular disturbances, such as spina bifida. The foot condition is then only part of a larger diagnostic and management problem. Foot disorders arising from systemic diseases are discussed in later chapters.

CONGENITAL ABNORMALITIES

These may arise from two sources: (i) adverse genetic factors, and (ii) adverse environmental factors acting on the developing fetus. Examples of the latter are drugs, e.g. thalidomide, and infections such as German measles. Some authorities believe that intrauterine pressure or abnormal fetal position may play a part in the development of some deformities. Most are probably multifactorial in origin. They vary widely in degree from mild to severe, and therapeutic measures likewise range from conservative mechanical correction to complex reconstructive surgery. They may require prolonged supervision, and with those conditions affecting the whole child, integrated care by several specialists is often required.

Full correction of some cases is not possible, and residual deformity remains as a chronic feature in adult life, requiring continuous supervision and management by means of special footwear, appliances and appropriate podiatric treatment.

Anatomical anomalies: excesses, deficiencies and fusions

Polydactyly (Fig. 4.2)

This term denotes the presence of additional digits on the hand or the foot. On the foot, two or more whole or rudimentary digits may develop from one metatarsal, or there may be complete supernumerary metatarsal segments. Depending on the nature and extent of the abnormality, selective amputation at an early age is indicated to ensure optimum function and to facilitate shoe fitting in childhood and adult life. As in any operation on the foot, it is important that the resulting scar is situated away from pressure areas.

Syndactyly

This term denotes total or partial fusion of neighbouring digits. There may be a congenital absence of one or more of the corresponding metatarsals. In its mildest forms, it appears as no more than the conjoined webbing of adjacent toes. It is very common in a partial form between the second and third toes. Surgery is rarely indicated as it is difficult to achieve a satisfactory result.

Accessory bones (Fig. 4.3)

The importance of recognising these accessory ossicles is to be able to distinguish them from fragments of bone resulting from injury. The commonest ones are:

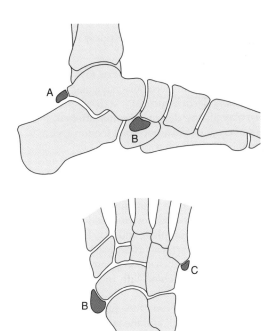

Figure 4.3 Accessory bones: os trigonum (A), accessory navicular (B), os vesalii (C).

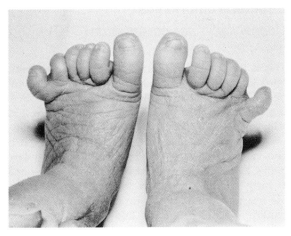

Figure 4.2 Polydactyly. The hands were similarly affected.

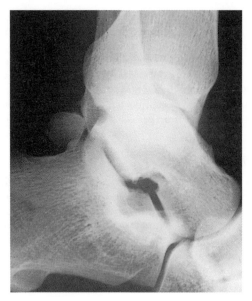

Figure 4.4 Os trigonum.

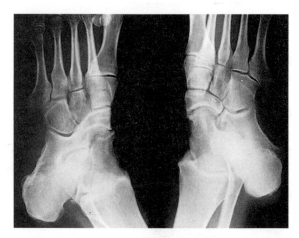

Figure 4.5 Calcaneonavicular bar.

- *os trigonum* — a vestigial bone which lies posterior to and sometimes attached to the talus (Fig. 4.4)
- *accessory navicular* — this lies medial to the medial end of the navicular, almost as an extension of it, and should be distinguished too from the sesamoid sometimes present in the tendon of the posterior tibial tendon
- *os vesalii* — this is much more rarely found at the base of the fifth metatarsal.

The os trigonum rarely gives rise to symptoms. Pain experienced over an accessory navicular may not simply be due to its presence, or just direct pressure upon it, but may also be due to abnormal stress applied to it by an overactive posterior tibial tendon trying to stop the foot hyperpronating.

Tarsal coalitions

In this condition there is an anomaly of ossification in which adjacent tarsal bones are fused together. Fusion may be partial or complete, and may be bony (synostosis) or cartilaginous (synchrondrosis).

The most common coalition occurs between the calcaneus and the navicular with union across the midtarsal joint (Fig. 4.5).

In a talocalcaneal coalition, fusion occurs between the sustentaculum tali and the talus.

Children with tarsal coalitions may never be aware they have them. On rare occasions they are responsible for acutely distressing painful symptoms, and

surgery is necessary for adequate relief. Between these two extremes are most children who have little trouble until they enter a growth spurt, when they develop the classical symptoms of the 'spastic flat foot'. This is a painful contraction of the peroneal muscles, and occurs as a protective mechanism. This results in a fixed everted abducted foot which resembles a flat foot, and from which it must be distinguished.

Diagnosis is not always easy. Examination reveals tender, taut and prominent peroneal tendons, and attempts to invert the foot will be painfully resisted. Specialised X-rays or a CT scan may be necessary to demonstrate the fusion.

Initial treatment consists of resting the foot, in a below-knee plaster of Paris cast if necessary, and reserving surgery for those with recurrent or intractable pain.

Structural deformities

Congenital talipes equinovarus (CTEV)
(Fig. 4.6)

This is the commonest form of structural deformity, often known simply as club foot. The foot is plantar-flexed and inverted, with the forefoot adducted. There is also an associated wasting of the calf muscles. The talus has been described as the hub of the deformity, with an abnormal neck directed both plantarwards and varus. Other structural anomalies are secondary to this. Two types are recognised: those which respond to early strapping in a corrected position, and those, the resistant talipes, which do not. This latter group require surgical treatment and this is performed between the ages of 3 and 6 months. The initial operation is one of elongation of the tendo Achilles and a

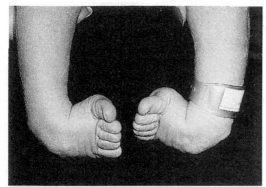

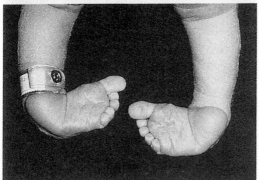

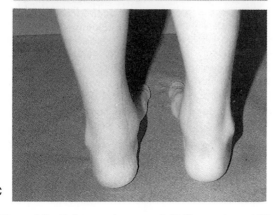

Figure 4.6 Talipes equinovarus. A, B: The newborn child. C: The same child, aged 6 years 3 months.

release of the right medial structures of the hindfoot to allow the foot to align as near normal as possible around the talus. Further surgery may be required at a later date if correction has been less than complete. Then, bony operations are required, either taking wedges from the calcaneus or fusing the peritalar joints. The fusing of hindfoot joints is always something to avoid if at all possible, as the consequences, especially in a growing foot, for the function of the forefoot are considerable. A club foot can cause much

trouble in adulthood, when pressures are maldistributed over the foot, often excessively along the outer border of the foot, producing painful callosities, and making provision of comfortable insoles and bespoke footwear essential.

Talipes calcaneovalgus

The 'opposite' condition to CTEV, this is considered by many to be a postural manifestation, and virtually always corrects with conservative manipulation and strapping. It is important, however, to recognise that this condition is associated in a few with congenital dislocation of the hip and deformity of the tibia.

Vertical talus

This is rather a rare deformity, known by several alternative names, such as 'rocker-bottom foot', and is primarily caused by a dislocation of the talonavicular joint. There are secondary structural effects which result in an equinus position of the calcaneus and a valgus dorsiflexed forefoot. Correction is surgical, and is aimed at reducing the dislocation of the talonavicular joint. The older the child, the more likely is bony correction or fusion to be necessary.

Metatarsus adductus

This condition is quite common in infants, and is found with a normal hindfoot. The great majority resolve spontaneously, but it is impossible to pick out the cases which will not. In these cases surgical release of tight medial structures can be carried out.

DEVELOPMENTAL CONDITIONS
Extrinsic structural conditions
Hip

Persisting femoral anteversion. This is one of the commonest 'variants' of normal (Fig. 4.7). The angle between the neck of the femur and the frontal plane is greatest at birth, and as the child develops and learns to walk, this angle decreases. The normal 'toe-out' attitude of the foot is the result, but in a not insignificant number of the population, this process is either arrested or never quite occurs, resulting in an in-toeing or 'hen-toed' gait. Whilst often quite an embarrassment to its owners, especially at a young age when they tend to trip over their feet, it is rarely the cause of symptoms, and needs no treatment.

Coxa vara and coxa valga (Fig. 4.8). The inclination of the neck of the femur to the shaft varies through the

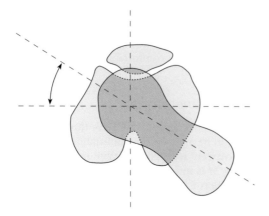

Figure 4.7 The femoral anteversion angle.

growing years, the normal angle in the adult being 125°. If less than this, the femoral shaft is abnormally adducted and the limbs are relatively shorter (coxa vara). If the angle is greater, the shaft is abducted and the limbs are relatively longer (coxa valga).

These deformities result in a malalignment of the femora, which must be compensated for at the knees to allow the individual to stand with the feet in a normal attitude. The consequence is a compensatory angular deformity of either genu valgum (due to coxa vara) or genu varum (due to coxa valga). They inevitably affect both gait and stance, especially if they are unilateral, as this tends to render the limb lengths unequal.

Knee—genu valgum and genu varum

Normal development of the child sees the varus bow legs of the infant straighten, and often 'overcorrect' into distinct valgus, or knock-knee, at about 6 years of age. The vast majority of these realign to the normal adult position of around 8° valgus. Persisting deformity in either direction is often associated with rotational deformity and always with altered posture of the feet. For example, genu valgum is associated with an abducted inverted foot on weight-bearing unless actively compensated, which often happens, resulting in the need for the forefoot to supinate. The converse of course applies with genu varum (Fig. 4.9). The treatment in severe cases is surgical realignment by means of osteotomy, but not infrequently the deformity is accepted and then the foot must be encouraged orthotically to adopt as normal a functioning posture as possible.

Torsions

These may occur as a result of abnormal joint alignment (as described above in relation to the hip) or to a built-in twist in the bones of the lower leg themselves. While internal torsions tend to be self-correcting, external torsions are not. The alignment of the legs is clearly reflected in the posture adopted by the feet, as for example in the in-turned leg. The natural adduction is compensated for by attempted abduction of the foot and its consequent pronation. With external torsions, however, the feet are still used in abduction, with a consequent hyperpronation and strain on the posterior tibial tendon. The alignment of the legs can be clearly seen by examining first the position of the patellae. A line projected forwards from the midpoint of the patella and at right angles to its transverse plane

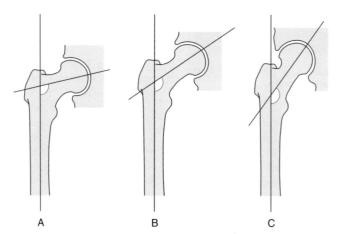

A   B   C

Figure 4.8 A: Coxa valga. B: Normal inclination angle between femoral neck and shaft—125° in adult. C: Coxa vara.

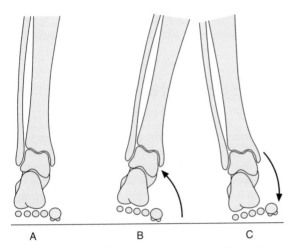

Figure 4.9 Genu valgum and genu varum. A: Normal alignment of the right leg and foot (from front). B: In genu valgum, the foot is everted as it bears weight and the forefoot supinates to the horizontal. C: In genu varum, the foot is inverted as it bears weight and the hindfoot pronates to bring the forefoot to the horizontal.

should normally intersect the foot between the second and third toes. Secondly, the line of the ankle joint axis, as visualised by projecting a line through the malleoli, can be compared with the patellar line. Whilst the latter indicates rotation at and above the knee, the former demonstrates the rotation of the whole leg, or when compared with the patellar line, that rotation due solely to the tibia.

Leg length discrepancy

It is important to realise two features about leg length. First, that up to 1 cm difference in true length is considered a normal variation. Secondly, that with normal clinical measuring techniques, leg length cannot be measured to an accuracy much greater than 1 cm. This discrepancy can be 'true' due to congenital underdevelopment, as a result of disease such as poliomyelitis, trauma and even surgical treatment. Apparent discrepancy exists where the limbs are actually the same length, but because of the alignment of one or other, are functionally different.

The effects of limb length discrepancy are either to cause a compensatory pelvic tilt and secondary spinal scoliosis, or to make the individual walk on his toes in order to effectively lengthen his leg. This latter response will in time result in an adaptive shortening of the tendo Achilles.

The importance of these conditions is that they impose abnormal stresses on the foot, particularly on

the talus in stance phase. These in turn may result in compensatory or adaptive changes in the function and structure of the foot with growth, and it is these which are important for the podiatrist.

Extrinsic functional conditions

These conditions affect function by virtue of an imbalance in the muscle control of the respective joints. Most of them are neurological diseases, although there are some primary muscular disorders to be considered.

The effects of the imbalance can be likened to a segmented flagpole supported in the upright position by guy ropes attached at different heights and directions. The loss of any one or more guy ropes will have a profound effect on both the stability and the shape of the pole. So it is with the leg and foot. The positions and functions of the foot are infinitely variable depending on exactly which muscle or muscle groups are inactive, partly active or even spastic or contracted. There is no virtue, therefore, in considering their effects in detail: it is more appropriate to highlight particular points of relevance.

Cerebral palsy (CP)

CP or brain injury results in an upper motor neurone type of paralysis of widely varying extent, from that which is indistinguishable to the untrained eye to the tragic spastic dysarthric who is unable to do anything for himself. CP can be found in different forms, most commonly as a spastic paralysis, but also as athetoid, ataxic or atonic. Surgery has little part to play in their treatment, and must be considered in relation to the child as a whole, and not just to a particular deformity. Inevitably this means that for the podiatrist, foot care may become the primary treatment. As with all of this group of conditions, however, there is great need for a team approach to management and integration of all modalities of therapy, so that the maximum benefit may be gained from each.

Spina bifida cystica

This is a congenital disorder where there has been a failure of fusion of the posterior spinal elements. It is only the severe cases that are easily recognised, but like CP, it can be found in all degrees from fatal to a minor bony deformity that exists unbeknown to the patient. The level in the spine at which the lesion occurs relates in some measure to the effects on the patient, but does not equate with their function. In high spinal lesions, total paralysis occurs and the foot is a malleable flaccid object. The problems arise in the foot in those with sacral lesions, where an imbalance primarily affects the muscles of the foot, resulting in deformity which can be very difficult to manage.

Hereditory sensory and motor neuropathy

Charcot–Marie–Tooth disease is a variety of this type of complaint.

Anterior poliomyelitis

As a result of the introduction of vaccination, the last major epidemic of poliomyelitis in the UK was 30 years ago and only isolated cases are now seen. The disorder is caused by an enterovirus which spreads from the bowel to invade the nervous system, particularly the anterior horn cells of the spinal cord. Its effects in the lower limb are seen in the muscles with weakness of inversion, eversion and plantarflexion of the ankle and also drop foot. Recovery from the disease is often incomplete and associated with contracture of muscles causing an equinovarus deformity, pes cavus or permanent foot drop. The resultant conditions may require surgical correction, but will demand considerable attention by the podiatrist due to the abnormal load-bearing of the foot and the need for special appliances and shoes.

Muscular dystrophies

These are probably primary muscle disorders, the best known of which is the progressive hereditary Duchenne type. This results in an increasing wasting of the muscles, with a life expectancy rarely exceeding 20 years.

Intrinsic structural conditions

Flat foot

This commonly used term can mean all things to all men. It is therefore necessary to define what is meant by flat foot. The arch of the foot can be made to disappear in two ways: the whole structure can simply collapse in a sagittal plane, or the foot can rotate so that the arch seems to disappear, i.e. the foot pronates (Fig. 4.10).

The collapsed foot is relatively uncommon and seems to be more prevalent in males. It gives rise to no symptoms other than anxiety to relatives who may notice that the foot is flat. Arch supports are of no benefit, and can be quite painful if used.

The hyperpronated foot is another matter altogether. Before considering the pathology to be primarily in the foot, the presence of more proximal causes must first be sought, as described above. Generalised joint hypermobility is sometimes associated with this condition, and renders it important to ensure that adequate treatment is undertaken as soon as the diagnosis is made. Treatment is with orthoses: in the pre-school child with a Salop ankle–foot orthosis, and in the older age groups with either a Yates–Helfet heel cup or simple Rose–Schwartz heel meniscus (Fig. 4.11). In each case the object is to maintain the foot in a neutral position while growth takes place.

The tendo Achilles is often noted to be shortened

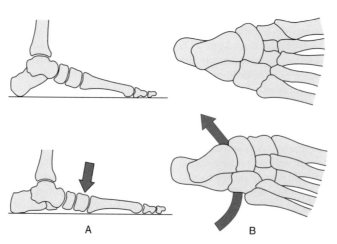

Figure 4.10   A: The collapsed foot. B: The pronated foot.

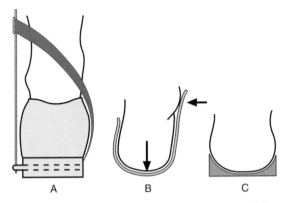

Figure 4.11 A: Salop ankle–foot orthosis. B: Yates–Helfet heel cup. C: Rose–Schwartz heel meniscus.

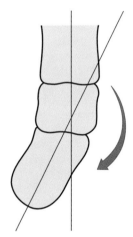

Figure 4.12 The turning moment on heel strike in the pronating foot.

also, but this is probably an adaptive shortening consequent upon the valgus attitude of the calcaneus produced by the hyperpronation. Only rarely does the tendon need lengthening.

If untreated, the hyperpronated foot may cease to be mobile and become fixed. Each step then produces a turning moment at the ankle on heel strike and increasing pain over the medial ligamentous structures as the body weight falls with the area of support of the calcaneus. Surgery may then be required (Fig. 4.12).

Cavus foot

The highly arched foot can also be considered as several different entities. The arch may simply be elevated in the sagittal plane as a result of muscle imbalance and this is associated with an increased inclination of the calcaneus. The presence of muscle imbalance suggests neurological disorder, and in many patients brisk reflexes in both upper and lower limbs would tend to confirm this and further suggest that the primary pathology may be intracerebral. In others, it is clearly a consequence of one of the extrinsic functional conditions described above.

Just as the flat foot could be produced by hyperpronation, so the cavus foot can be produced by excessive supination. The most frequently seen cause of this is where the first metatarsal is fixed in a plantarflexed position at the tarsometatarsal joint. This type of cavus foot is more likely to result in a fore- to hindfoot malalignment which, if the foot is unable to compensate, may require orthotic treatment.

The third type is simply called idiopathic, aetiology unknown, but there is more than a suggestion of a neurological element in many cases.

It is the neurological and idiopathic types of cavus foot which produce the greater problems in the long term. As the foot arches, the heel and the metatarsal heads become the primary weight-bearing areas, with a tendency for the first metatarsal head to take more than its fair share. Treatment is directed to straightening out secondarily clawed toes, the lesser toes by flexor to extensor (Girdlestone) tendon transfers, the hallux by a Robert Jones transfer of the long extensor into the metatarsal neck with fusion of the interphalangeal joint. The tight plantar structures can be released by stripping their origins from the calcaneus (Steindler). In older children where the deformity is more fixed, a wedge can be removed from the dorsum of the tarsus to straighten out the foot, or a chevron osteotomy performed to lower the forefoot. The management of the adult cavus foot is discussed in Chapter 5.

Malalignments

This term is used to denote an abnormal relationship between the transverse plane of the forefoot and the sagittal plane of the hindfoot. Normally this is about a right angle. It can be due to a primary hindfoot problem, or to one in the forefoot, but these do not necessarily give rise to symptoms unless the foot as a whole cannot compensate. Failure to compensate occurs in two particular situations: when the foot is overstressed, e.g. with severe athletic activity, or with increasing age, when the joints of the foot tend to stiffen. It is interesting to note that loss of joint mobility may also occur after prolonged immobilisation in a plaster cast, and this too can precipitate symptoms.

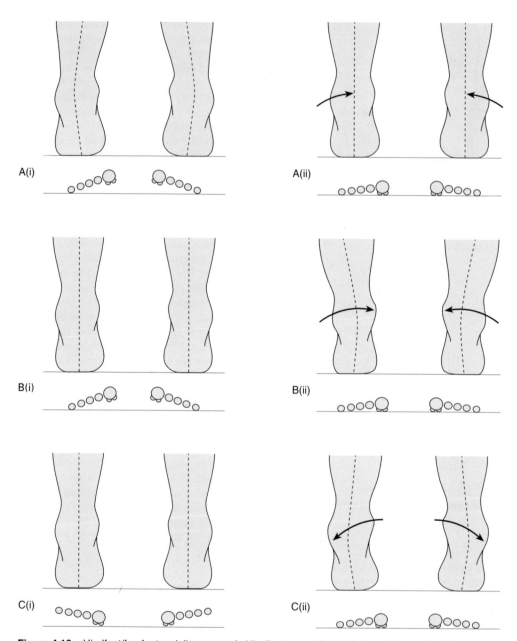

Figure 4.13 Hindfoot/forefoot malalignments. A: Hindfoot varus. (i) Hindfoot and forefoot both inverted. (ii) Usually compensated by pronation to the vertical to bring both plantar surfaces to the horizontal. B: Forefoot varus (supinated forefoot). (i) Forefoot only inverted. (ii) Usually compensated by pronation of hindfoot to bring plantar surface of forefoot to the horizontal. Alternatively compensated by hallux flexus. C: Forefoot valgus. (i) Forefoot everted. (ii) Usually compensated by supination of the foot to bring plantar surface of forefoot to the longitudinal.

Hindfoot varus (Fig. 4.13A). This situation arises, like persistent femoral anteversion, as a failure of development postnatally of an intrauterine position. The inversion of the hindfoot extends into the forefoot, and thus in order to bring the forefoot into a horizontal position, the foot has to pronate.

Forefoot varus, or supinated forefoot. Here the forefoot is inverted relative to the hindfoot, with the result that in order for the forefoot to come into the transverse plane at foot-flat during gait, the foot has to hyper-pronate, stressing the posterior tibial tendon, once it has utilised all the available midtarsal rotation. It has been suggested that the fixed plantarflexed first metatarsal is a compensatory mechanism too, but there is no more evidence for this than for it being a primary cause of the the valgus (pronated) forefoot (Fig. 4.13B).

Forefoot valgus, or pronated forefoot. With the forefoot everted relative to the hindfoot, compensation following saturation of midtarsal joint movement occurs by the foot supinating. As there is almost always much more inversion available at the subtalar joint than eversion, there is more compensation available for this particular malalignment (Fig. 4.13C).

Treatment is orthotic, aiming to control subtalar movement and compensating for (not correcting) the abnormal alignment.

Digital abnormalities

Children are frequently presented at an orthopaedic clinic with curly or otherwise slightly deformed toes. There are three elements to these deformities:

1. medial or lateral deviation from the midline of the digit
2. axial rotation
3. interphalangeal joint flexion.

Those present from birth frequently correct with growth. They are uninfluenced by strapping, although this may be an acceptable therapy to calm an anxious parent. If causing symptoms because of overlapping and rubbing in shoes, they are best treated with orthodigital splints. Surgery rarely has a place, but the curly overlapped fifth toe can be satisfactorily dealt with in this way. Claw toes can also be corrected by a flexor to extensor tendon transfer.

Juvenile hallux rigidus

Whilst not common, this condition causes much discomfort to its sufferers, who are usually teenage males. It is now thought that the aetiology is recurrent minor trauma, or a single incident which produces a chondral injury. The resulting pain and muscle spasm result in loss of extension at the metatarsophalangeal joint. The patient walks on the outer border of the foot to avoid the painful area. Rest in a cast is recommended first line treatment, with a proximal phalangeal osteotomy being reserved for those in whom symptoms persist.

Juvenile hallux valgus

As in many other foot problems, footwear has been universally blamed for the presence of this condition in teenagers. In almost all cases, a strong family history can be elicited. Footwear may aggravate an established tendency to valgus deformity, and may cause bunion formation by friction over the medial eminence of the metatarsal head, but does not cause hallux valgus. The valgus is often accompanied by a varus deformity of the first metatarsal. Up to 20° of valgus can be normal, but a useful guide to whether surgery is indicated is the position of the sesamoids on a profile X-ray: no subluxation, no operation. Surgery should not be carried out before the foot is skeletally mature, at about the age of 14. Until then, the position of the hallux can be controlled with an orthodigital splint.

Hallux varus

While this is an extremely uncommon condition in the UK, this is not the case elsewhere, e.g. in India. Commonly seen with metatarsus varus, it frequently corrects with growth. Occasionally surgery is necessary for the satisfactory fitting of footwear.

Sever's disease

Listed here for want of a better place, this condition was originally thought to be an osteochondritic lesion of the posterior calcaneus, associated with fragmenting apophyses. We now know that the X-ray appearances are normal, and believe that the condition is a traction apophysitis. It frequently responds to rest, but a cautionary warning must be given: forefoot malalignments may result in a varus or valgus calcaneus which may produce stress at the insertion of the tendo Achilles, and unless this primary problem is compensated, symptoms may not resolve, or may recur.

TRAUMA

Freiberg's infraction

This condition, once thought to belong to the osteochondritides, is now regarded as being the result of an osteochondral fracture. How this equates with its recognised incidence, mainly in girls around the age of 13 years, is difficult to explain. It may appear as an incidental finding in women with hallux valgus in the later years of life, with no recollection of ever having suffered symptoms. On the other hand, it can present as an acute arthritis of the second or third metatarsophalangeal joint with no X-ray signs being visible for several weeks. The metatarsal head flattens and occasionally produces prolific osteophytes and it is these which are more likely to cause symptoms. Treatment in the growing foot is variable, resting it when acutely painful, and relieving direct pressure on the metatarsal head by appropriate padding.

Fatigue fractures

These are most likely to occur in the athletic youngster, either in sport or in dance, and appear in the second and occasionally third metatarsal shafts. X-ray changes may not be visible until 3 weeks after the initial onset of symptoms. Treatment is rest in a plaster of Paris slipper cast. Very rarely, a fracture may occur towards the base of the fifth metatarsal (Jones fracture). It can be difficult to heal, but this may be due to the continuation of the precipitating forces, as would happen with a supinated forefoot, and thus the foot should always be examined closely for evidence of such abnormality.

THE RATIONALE OF TREATMENT

The first requirement is of course to make a diagnosis, and to this end it must be re-emphasised that the foot is at one end of a kinetic chain, and therefore responsive to variations in normal anatomy and pathological disorders above it. Before deciding that the foot is the primary seat of pathology, careful examination of the whole limb is required, and in a child this is particularly relevant. Identification, or even suspicion, of disorders more proximal requires referral to an orthopaedic surgeon for evaluation.

Once these problems have been dealt with, or not, whichever is the case, attention can be turned to the foot. Surgery may or may not have been carried out in the meantime, and an understanding surgeon will always keep in mind what the orthotist and podiatrist can contribute, and tailor her surgery accordingly. This is surgico-orthotic integration and is a very important concept in the treatment not only of children, but of all patients. Conversely, the orthotist and the podiatrist must have some idea of what they can do to help the surgeon make the most of surgery. It is two-way teamwork.

The general requirement is to have a plantargrade, painless, mobile foot. Developmental structural deformities such as juvenile hallux valgus are best not operated on until after skeletal maturity, and conservative management with orthodigital orthoses is preferred until that time is reached. In this case pre-operative care is in the hands of the podiatrist. Similarly, where a forefoot malalignment is diagnosed, and where operation has no place, short- or long-term care may be required. Postoperatively, the podiatrist can offer much help in the treatment of residual symptoms and deformity.

FURTHER READING

Anderson E G 1990 Fatigue fractures of the foot. Injury 21: 275–279
Fixsen J, Lloyd-Roberts G 1988 The foot in childhood. Churchill Livingstone, Edinburgh
Gould J S 1988 The foot book. Williams and Wilkins, Baltimore

Hessinger R N 1987 The pediatric lower extremity. Orthopedic Clinics of North America 18: 4
Jahss M H 1982 Disorders of the foot, vols 1 & 2. Saunders, Philadelphia

5

Disorders of the adult foot

G. C. Rendall
C. E. Thomson
P. M. Boyd

Keywords

Ankle equinus
Digital deformities
Digital malfunctions
Forefoot equinus
Forefoot valgus
Forefoot varus
Hallux abducto valgus
Hallux flexus
Hallux rigidus
Heel conditions
Ligamentous laxity
Morton's neuroma
Osteochondritis
Pes cavus
Plantarflexed first ray
Rearfoot valgus
Rearfoot varus
Subtalar pronation

The foot is a sophisticated, durable example of engineering, capable of withstanding many millions of contacts over a lifetime. Its function is highly variable and it is programmed to adopt the most mechanically appropriate position for the activity. When instability, overuse, trauma or other external or internal problems arise, the foot has a large number of protective mechanisms to limit and repair damage and restore maximal mobility in the shortest possible time. The highly developed nature of the foot indicates its evolutionary importance. Unfortunately, the foot is often forgotten about or neglected, covered with shoes which are often vested with more importance than the foot which is hidden and viewed as a rather unattractive appendage. Only when there are problems do feet arouse interest. In gait, the foot cannot be considered an appendage. It is the first point of contact: the stability and progression of the body in walking are highly dependent on the interaction of the foot with the ground below it and the lower limb above. Not surprisingly, in such a highly stressed and complicated system, things may go wrong. Problems often emerge from poor foot mechanics, but may also be developmental or idiopathic in origin, or related to a systemic pathology. The most damaging conditions often arise from a combination of underlying problems, such as a mechanically unsound neuropathic foot or a foot distorted by rheumatoid arthritis. The main focus of this chapter is on problems which can be related to mechanics, although a number of other problems are also discussed.

PRONATION AND SUPINATION

Pronation and supination occur at the subtalar joint. They are triplanar movements across all three body planes. Pronation describes movement of the foot in the direction of eversion, dorsiflexion and abduction, while supination moves the foot in the opposite direction, that of inversion, plantarflexion and adduction. These are normal movements provided they occur at the appropriate times during the gait cycle and to the correct magnitude (see Ch. 1).

The subtalar joint and the ankle joint comprise the link between the leg and the foot. These joints act together as a universal joint, able to move, and absorb movement, in all three cardinal body planes. The ankle joint has primarily sagittal plane motion, permitting the foot to plantarflex and dorsiflex on the leg and, in midstance phase, permitting the leg to pivot forward over the loaded foot. The subtalar joint is often described as a *torque translator* as it permits frontal plane forces in the foot (e.g. calcaneal eversion) to be absorbed as transverse plane rotation in the leg (e.g. internal rotation). Its relationship with those joints immediately distal (i.e. talonavicular and calcaneocuboid) is the key to the foot's ability to be, at different times, both a flexible mobile adapter for the early part of the midstance phase and a rigid lever for propulsion. This enables the foot to adapt to variations in walking surfaces and body posture, and to absorb shock, thereby lessening the impact between the foot and ground during the contact phase of gait. It is these same motions that allow the subtalar joint to compensate for deformities in the foot and lower limb.

The ability to compensate enables the individual to function with a plantargrade foot in what appears to be a smooth and efficient manner. Motion used to compensate for deformity may limit that available for

normal locomotion and disrupt the normal timing of pronation and supination during the gait cycle. This abnormal compensatory pronation and supination may give rise to secondary deformity and associated symptoms.

FLAT FOOT—PES PLANUS

Flat foot is an umbrella term for a range of conditions which tend to lower the medial longitudinal arch. Subtalar pronation which occurs as compensation for structural abnormalities tends to destabilise the midtarsal joint and medial column, thereby creating a functional flattening of the arch. The vast majority of feet described as flat are functional flat feet which respond to treatment with functional orthoses.

Intrinsic effects of subtalar pronation

As pronation occurs, normally in the contact and early midstance phases, the talus plantarflexes and adducts and the calcaneus everts. Most of the frontal plane motion is therefore transmitted to the forefoot through the calcaneus, whilst most of the sagittal and transverse plane motions are transmitted through the talus.

Eversion of the rearfoot with pronation twists the medial side of the foot against the ground. Medial ground reaction forces push up on the medial side of the forefoot, supinating it about the longitudinal axis of the metatarsophalangeal joint and dorsiflexing the first ray. The longitudinal axis lies very close to the transverse and sagittal planes so that most of its supinatory motion is inversion (i.e. frontal plane). This 'unlocking' of the longitudinal axis can be seen as forefoot inversion. Hicks (1952) suggested a further means of inverting the forefoot by serial dorsiflexion of adjacent metatarsals. By dorsiflexing the first more than the second, the second more than the third, etc., the forefoot would function as if inverted (see Ch. 1).

Adduction and plantarflexion of the talus with subtalar joint pronation effect a change in the range and direction of metatarsophalangeal joint motion. The subtalar joint consists of four bones which form two joints: the talus articulates with the navicular on the medial side and the calcaneus articulates with the cuboid on the lateral side. Each of these two joints, the calcaneocuboid and the talonavicular, has a separate axis of motion. For motion to be maximised these axes must be parallel. When the subtalar joint is in the neutral position the two axes are angulated away from each other. Movement of the two joints therefore occurs in different directions, so that they create tension in shared ligaments and jamming in contiguous bones, and thus they restrict each other's range of motion. This effect is exaggerated when the subtalar joint is supinated, rendering the metatarsophalangeal joint very inflexible in the normal propulsive phase (Elftmann 1960). Adduction and plantarflexion of the talus lowers the axes of motion of the talonavicular and calcaneocuboid joints and increases their parallelism (Fig. 5.1). This effects an increase in the total range of motion available at the oblique axis of the metatarsophalangeal joint. Lowering the axis of motion of the metatarsophalangeal joint also has the effect of raising the inclination of the plane of motion of the joint, so that more of its motion occurs in the sagittal plane. To summarise, pronation of the subtalar joint increases the total range of motion and particularly the amount of dorsiflexion available to the forefoot around the oblique axis of the metatarsophalangeal joint. Subtalar joint pronation can therefore be said to unlock the oblique axis of the metatarsophalangeal joint.

Plantarflexion of the talus also reduces the congruence of the talonavicular joint, destabilising it, so that the range of motion is increased medially. Winson et al (1994) have shown that most medial column motion (approx 75%) occurs at the talonavicular joint. Destabilising the navicular increases the motion and reduces the axial stability of the first ray. Subtalar joint pronation also flattens the line of action of the peroneus longus muscle across the plantar arch (Root et al 1977). This reduces the plantarflexion function of the muscle, further destabilising the first ray so that it is readily dorsiflexed when subjected to sagittal plane ground reaction force.

Increased ranges of motion enhance adaptability, and thus are useful to the foot in the contact and early midstance phases. When pronation occurs late in the gait cycle, or to such an extent that the foot cannot recover, hypermobility renders the forefoot incapable of normal function. Reaction forces produce misalignment of the joints of the forefoot and midtarsus. Typical results of these misalignments are structural foot deformities such as hallux abductovalgus, hallux rigidus, lesser toe deformities and flat foot. These abnormal reaction forces can also be transmitted to the rearfoot and leg, causing problems outwith the foot.

Extrinsic effects of subtalar pronation

Abnormal subtalar joint pronation may occur out of phase or to excess, the effect being to create instability and misalignment of the lower limb. It is widely accepted that, particularly under conditions of high usage such as in athletics, it can produce injury outwith the foot. Research into this is minimal, so that relationships between pronation and lower limb symptoms are somewhat conjectural. Clinical observation indicates that treating abnormal pronation with functional orthoses often reduces symptoms in a wide range of lower limb problems, such as anterior knee pain syndrome, posterior and anterior shin splints and Achilles tendinitis. Dannanberg (1993) reported a number cases of intransigent low back pain improving after provision of foot orthoses. What follows is a brief

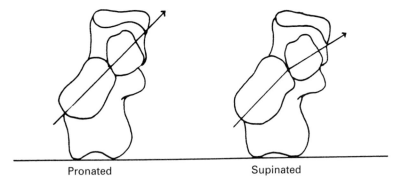

Pronated   Supinated

Figure 5.1 The oblique axis has two components: the calcaneocuboid axis and the talonavicular axis. During subtalar pronation, these become parallel, acting as one to increase midtarsal mobility. In the supinated foot, they diverge and oppose each other, leading to restriction of movement.

outline of basic pronatory theory and its relationship to the remainder of the lower limb.

Basic pronatory theory suggests that the talar trochlea is held firmly between the tibia and fibula at the ankle joint. In the weight-bearing limb, movements of the calcaneus are transferred via the talus to the tibia and fibula. This can be seen with normal pronation and supination of the subtalar joint during walking. As the calcaneus everts during pronation in the contact phase of the gait cycle, the talus adducts and plantarflexes causing internal rotation of the tibia and fibula. At the same time the loaded knee is forced into flexion. As the knee flexes, the medial condyle of the femur rolls more quickly than the lateral, so that transverse plane (internal) rotation of the tibia precedes that of the femur. In this way tibial rotation assists the normal shock-absorbing mechanism of the lower limb. As the cycle progresses, the opposite motion occurs. The pelvis rotates externally on the weight-bearing limb, which gradually follows it as the centre of mass and the limb move over the top of the foot. The foot is twisted laterally but this is resisted by ground reaction forces through the transverse plane. This assists subtalar supination, helping to turn the foot into a firm propulsive lever.

Where there is an underlying abnormality, or instability, pronation may become exaggerated or prolonged. As with normal compensatory motion the action is referred through the talus to the rest of the lower limb. Excessive subtalar pronation exaggerates internal rotation of the tibia. Late pronation may reverse the direction of the slowly externally rotating limb, causing the tibia briefly to rotate internally in late midstance against an externally rotating femur.

Abnormal pronatory patterns disrupt the timing of recovery to supination for propulsion. The tibia may lag behind the externally rotating pelvis and femur, introducing a damaging torque within the knee joint. The knee may now be unstable and vulnerable to the stresses produced by propulsion, so that the genicular ligaments and muscles come under strain. If the limb as a whole remains internally rotated, this may result in impaired function being referred into the trunk. One reason for this may be an inability to use the medial column appropriately to assist fluent transition from midstance to propulsion. Elevation of the hypermobile first ray prevents movement of the metatarsal phalangeal joint (see section on 'hallux rigidus/limitus', p. 91), so that there is distal resistance to the smooth forward progression of the centre of mass. This momentarily reverses the direction of movement of the hip and lower spine in early propulsion from extension and lordosis to flexion and straightening.

Whilst the change is small, it is repeated many times. Dannanberg (1993) suggests that this sagittal plane blockade may occur 2500 times per limb per day in a normal subject. He associates it with lower back pain, suggesting that it may be a repetitive strain injury of the muscles which support the lower spine and the sacroiliac joint. In highly active individuals the number and frequency of repetitions are higher, as are the forces. It is estimated that the average long-distance runner may make 2 million foot strikes per year, and in elite marathon runners this could be doubled. Contact and propulsive forces in these athletes may be 2.5 times the body weight. In such cases very small abnormalities can create significant problems.

Structural causes of abnormal subtalar pronation

The classification of structural abnormalities is dependent on variables such as the cardinal body plane in which the deformity is found, the type of compensation necessary to cope with the abnormality, the intrinsic or extrinsic structural abnormality and the timing during the gait cycle of the compensatory mechanisms. This last category is significant as it determines the amount of damage that can be inflicted on the foot or lower limb. An abnormality, such as forefoot varus, that requires abnormal compensatory pronation late in the gait cycle, when the foot is in propulsion, will tend to be more damaging than one such as rearfoot varus, which requires a greater amount of pronation but at the correct time of the gait cycle, contact and early midstance phase. The instability of the foot produced by abnormal compensatory pronation at a late stage in the cycle makes it vulnerable to the greater ground reaction forces experienced during propulsion. Secondary deformity and pain associated with hyperkeratotic lesions are usually the result. In contrast, where increased pronation occurs at the early phase of the gait cycle, the foot may recover into supination prior to propulsion, thereby minimising abnormal function. The common structural abnormalities are described below and listed in Table 5.1.

Structural abnormalities

In determining abnormalities, the foot is generally referenced to subtalar neutral with the midtarsal joint locked in maximal pronation and the ankle approximating 90°. This can be done in a weight-bearing or non-weight-bearing position for the rearfoot, but should be restricted to a non-weight-bearing position for forefoot analysis. There is considerable debate over

Table 5.1   Classification of functional abnormalities

Name	Definition and functional implications
Frontal plane	
Coxa vara	Increased angulation of the femoral shaft and neck; tends to precede development of tibial valgum
Coxa valga	Decreased angulation of the femoral shaft and neck; tends to precede development of tibial varum
Tibial varum/genu varum	Angulation of the tibia relative to the supporting surface, in which the distal end of the tibia is directed toward the midline of the body; tends to produce rearfoot varus
Tibial valgum/genu valgum	Angulation of the tibia relative to the supporting surface, in which the distal end of the tibia is directed away from the midline of the body; tends to produce forefoot supinatus
Rearfoot/hindfoot varus	Inversion of the heel relative to the supporting surface when the STJ is in neutral and the patient is in their normal angle and base of gait. Where sufficient motion is available, compensatory pronation of the STJ occurs
Rearfoot/hindfoot valgus	Eversion of the heel relative to the supporting surface when the STJ is neutral and the patient is in their normal angle and base of gait. Where sufficient motion is available, compensatory supination of the MTJ (longitudinal axis) usually occurs, producing forefoot supinatus
Subtalar varus	Inversion of the calcaneus relative to the tibia when the STJ is neutral; tends to produce rearfoot varus
Forefoot varus	Inversion of the forefoot relative to the rearfoot when the STJ is neutral and the MTJ is locked in both axes. Where sufficient motion is available, compensatory pronation of the STJ usually occurs (see also forefoot supinatus)
Forefoot valgus	Eversion of the forefoot relative to the rearfoot when the STJ is neutral and the MTJ is locked in both axes. Where sufficient motion is available, compensatory supination of the MTJ (longitudinal axis), and also the STJ, usually occurs
Sagittal plane	
Flexion contractures of the hip and knee are common in patients with neural pathology and are important functionally, in that they tend to preclude normal muscle alignment and function	
Flexion of the knees	Often associated with tight hamstrings and may lead to gastrocnemius equinus
Genu recurvatum	Hyperextension of the knee may produce or be a result of ankle equinus
Ankle equinus	Limitation of ankle dorsiflexion to less than 10°. Pronatory compensation occurs in the STJ and MTJ (oblique axis). Alternatively, early heel lift and rapid, late abduction of the hip may be seen
Ankle calcaneus	Excessive ankle dorsiflexion: leads to prolonged heel loading and a propulsive gait
Forefoot equinus	Plantarflexion of the forefoot relative to the hindfoot will tend to be compensated at the ankle joint. Using ankle dorsiflexion to enable heel contact often creates functional equinus of the ankle
Plantarflexed first ray	Creates an everted forefoot to hindfoot relationship (i.e. forefoot valgus). When hypermobile, compensatory dorsiflexion of the first ray occurs
Elevated first ray	Tends to produce restriction of first MTPJ motion
Transverse plane	
Internal torsion/rotation of the hip, femur or tibia	Produce lateral forefoot loading in propulsion, and therefore late STJ pronation
External torsion/rotation of the hip, femur or tibia	Produces medial forefoot loading in propulsion and therefore late supination of the MTJ (longitudinal axis). May lead to development of forefoot supinatus
Forefoot adductus	Fixed adduction of the forefoot relative to the rearfoot destabilises the intrinsic musculature and leads to toe deformities
Miscellaneous factors	
Forefoot supinatus	Fixed supination of the longitudinal axis as a result of chronic calcaneal eversion in stance and gait. Functionally indistinguishable from forefoot varus
Limb length differential	Leads to pelvic tilt and asymmetrical gait. Classically, pronation occurs in the longer limb and supination and ankle plantarflexion in the shorter (see also Ch. 10)
High activity levels	Will tend to lead to higher stress on joints and higher ranges of motion. Propulsive pronation can be a major source of problems in such cases (see also Ch. 10)

MTPJ—metatarsophalangeal joint; MTJ—midtarsal joint; STJ—subtalar joint.

the validity of foot measurement (Menz 1995). Briefly, non-weight-bearing measurement of the rearfoot involves maximally inverting and everting the foot and then calculating the neutral position to be two-thirds of the total range from the position of maximal supination (Root et al 1977). This method has been shown to be a broad generalisation but it is not an accurate way of determining subtalar neutral for all cases (Kidd 1991). The relationship of the calcaneum to the supporting surface can be seen with the subject standing on a flat surface, then taking a few steps on the spot, thus restoring a normal angle and base of stance. The tibia is then externally rotated until the talonavicular joint is congruous. This can be identified by palpation or by visually identifying a position in which the concavities below each malleolus are equal (in reality the position at which the experienced eye thinks it looks best). Reliability studies indicate that there is poor inter-rater but reasonable intra-rater reliability in measurements of subtalar neutral position. This demonstrates that examiners' perceptions of what constitutes subtalar neutral vary, and thus measurement of subtalar neutral position is a debatable concept. Podiatrists are not alone in persisting with the use of questionable methods of clinical measurement. Hayes (1992) showed that informing physical therapists of the fundamental unreliability of their measurement method in no way eroded their confidence in that measurement. Indeed, in Hayes' study, the group who had been informed of this basic unreliability had significantly more confidence than the group who had not. It is likely that, in all branches of medicine, practitioners persist in using fundamentally unreliable diagnostic practices. Other than denial of evidence and an inherent reluctance to change, there are probably three main reasons for this:

1. whilst recognising the flaws, experienced practitioners have sufficient critical skills to view these measurements within the context of a complete picture in formulating a diagnosis
2. nothing better or more practical is available
3. therapy based on such examinations works, so why change a winning formula?

These ideas are being questioned and tested through research but it is important that this is not viewed negatively. The purpose of research is to build information, not to strip confidence. New technology and the development of a worthwhile body of research into foot function mean that the last decade has provided a considerable growth in understanding. It is possible that practitioners' faith in their overall clinical judgement and skills will be vindicated by future research, and therefore the following section is submitted with a small note of caution but in an atmosphere of growing understanding. It categorises foot types principally by site and plane of deformity.

Rearfoot (hindfoot) varus (Fig. 5.2)

With the ankle at 90° and the subtalar joint in the neutral position, the calcaneus is inverted relative to a flat supporting surface. The rearfoot is intrinsically unstable, being supported entirely on the medial weight-bearing tubercle. It requires the forefoot to be plantargrade to achieve stable equilibrium. Compensation is a simple matter of the rearfoot following the forefoot until it is flat on the ground. In rearfoot varus, the foot presenting to the ground in an inverted position must evert to become flat (plantargrade). The forefoot has no eversion available to it as it locks in maximal eversion parallel to the rearfoot when the subtalar joint is in neutral. Eversion must, therefore, come from subtalar pronation. The foot needs only to pronate until such time as it is flat, and in rearfoot varus this should coincide with calcaneal vertical. This compensatory pronation occurs in the midstance phase. Pronation is therefore excessive but at the correct time. The effect is that there will be delayed recovery from pronation and medial structures are likely to be stressed. Delayed recovery from pronation means that the foot is ill-prepared for propulsion. The knee may be slow to externally rotate and the first ray remains hypermobile, so being elevated by ground reaction forces.

The associated deformities and symptoms include hallux valgus and rigidus, tibial strain syndromes, Achilles tendinitis, plantar fasciitis and shearing stress lesions of the heel and forefoot. Subclassification is by level of compensation. Compensated rearfoot varus indicates the ability to pronate until the calcaneus is vertical. Partially compensated rearfoot varus pronates to the end of the range but remains inverted, and uncompensated rearfoot varus would be indicative of a very rigid foot unable to provide any compensation at all. Loading patterns vary considerably between these subtypes, moving medially with the degree of available compensation. In compensated rearfoot varus the plantar surface may show hyperkeratotic lesions under the second, third and fourth metatarsal heads and along the medial borders of the heel and the hallux. If there is no pronatory compensation, lesions are likely to develop at the base and the head of the fifth metatarsal and possibly externally on the fifth toe. A further possibility is that active compensation may occur to stabilise the forefoot and bring the medial

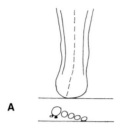

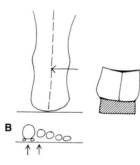

Figure 5.2 Hindfoot varus: 'chronic foot strain'. Relative positions of hindfoot and metatarsal heads of right foot at rest (A) and under load (B), from rear.
A: Calcaneus inverted: moderate to high arch, tending to be rigid; foot also inverted, possibly mildly adducted.

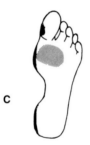

B: Lateral border overloaded unless hindfoot pronates to vertical; symptoms of postural fatigue in foot, leg and lower back; possible retrocalcaneal bursitis from heel movement. Shoes worn from lateral heel to medial sole; bulging of medial heel counter. (Arrows below line indicate abnormal pressures; arrow above line indicates movement.)

C: Plantar callosities possible at medial heel, second, third and fourth metatarsal heads and medial side of hallux.

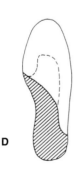

D and E: Management options.
1. Supporting padding and strapping if foot strain symptoms are acute or severe.
2. Palliative valgus insole with medial heel wedge; metatarsal cushioning if required.
3. Functional orthosis with medial hindfoot posting to stabilise inversion.

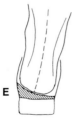

aspect into ground contact. In such cases, a plantar-flexed first ray or hallux may be seen concurrent with rearfoot varus, though it is difficult to attribute cause and effect with any certainty.

Forefoot varus (Fig. 5.3)

With the subtalar joint in neutral and the midtarsal joint locked in maximal pronation, the forefoot is inverted relative to the rearfoot. Forefoot varus creates a major problem for the foot because of the duration of its effect. The foot becomes plantargrade by excessive pronation of the subtalar joint. This means that the calcaneum will be everted, generally to the extent of the varus problem. The forefoot is inverted, and therefore the rearfoot is required to maintain this everted position throughout the midstance phase. Normally, as the heel lifts, the plantar fascia tightens and the first metatarsal plantarflexes to hold the forefoot on the ground against an inverting rearfoot. In forefoot varus, pronation may have destabilised the first ray to such an extent that the Hicks' windlass cannot function. The forefoot loses its means of stabilising the rearfoot in propulsion and the subtalar joint may remain pronated throughout the propulsive phase. In such cases, the adducted and plantarflexed talus and the elevated first ray will tend to become fixed by ligamentous contracture. Subjects with forefoot varus may exhibit all pronation-associated symptoms in the foot and leg, but midtarsal strain is a particularly common occurrence. The midtarsus becomes enlarged and osteoarthrosis often develops. The hallux may be held firmly plantarflexed, either in a bid to stabilise the forefoot or as a result of the excessive elevation of the first ray. The inevitable result of such a position is hallux rigidus or flexus.

This overloads the interphalangeal joint, which becomes hyperextended. Alternatively, and particularly if the first (alone) or all the metatarsals are adducted, the hallux may become laterally subluxated at the metatarsophalangeal joint, progressing to hallux abductovalgus. Impaction and constriction of the lesser toes, secondary to pronation and elongation of the foot, are likely to cause medial deviation and clawing of these toes. This process is aggravated by the tension of the long flexor tendons becoming more oblique as the rearfoot tilts into pronation, and the metatarsophalangeal articulations of these toes are deviated from their normally straight alignments. The hypermobility of the first metatarsal entails substantial overloading of the second, third and fourth metatarsal heads, with the consequent formation of heloma and callosities at these sites and probably another under the interphalangeal joint of the hallux.

In uncompensated forefoot varus, the lower limb is highly unstable in propulsion as it pivots around the lateral column of the weight-bearing foot. In order to overcome this instability as the forefoot load increases, the leg may externally rotate sharply so that the foot abducts abruptly towards the end of the midstance phase. This abductory twist reduces the evertory moments around the joints of the foot as weight is transferred to the opposite limb. Heloma and callosities are likely to develop over the fifth metatarsal head. The pronatory loads are so high in forefoot varus that an uncompensated form is rare unless accompanied by more general foot deformity such as ankle calcaneus (calcaneovarus). This type of foot tends to obviate normal gait, producing a short step with a high proportion of the gait cycle spent in double support and a short or absent propulsive phase (see Ch. 11).

Ankle equinus (Fig. 5.4)

Ankle equinus is a limitation of ankle movement in which dorsiflexion is restricted to less than 10°. It can be due to bony malformation of the ankle mortice, congenital shortness of triceps surae muscles, acquired triceps surae muscle shortness due to footwear, or as part of general ligamentous laxity. External torsion of the tibia or external rotation of the limb will also lead to inadequate sagittal plane motion at the ankle joint.

Dorsiflexion is required in the second half of the midstance phase as the centre of mass passes over the fulcrum that the ankle joint provides throughout midstance and as load in the forefoot increases. It permits the tibia to rotate over the top of the loaded foot prior to heel lift. This acts both to smooth the passage of the centre of load, by minimising its vertical displacement, and to preload the posterior muscle group in preparation for propulsion. When ankle equinus is present, the foot and lower limb compensate either by adapting the gait or by using other joints to achieve the range of motion required. Some of the common compensations are: shortening the length of the stride; keeping the knee slightly flexed through the gait cycle, thereby releasing a tense gastrocnemius muscle; raising the heel prematurely at heel lift, which produces a bouncy or springy gait; late pronation at the subtalar joint, unlocking the midtarsal joint to allow some dorsiflexion of the forefoot at that joint; and, finally, an abductory twist of the foot prior to heel lift.

By far the most problematic of these compensatory mechanisms is late pronation. Pronation of the subtalar joint occurs as a result of high loads on the forefoot being transmitted backward through the foot. During the pre-propulsive period of the stance phase, the sub-

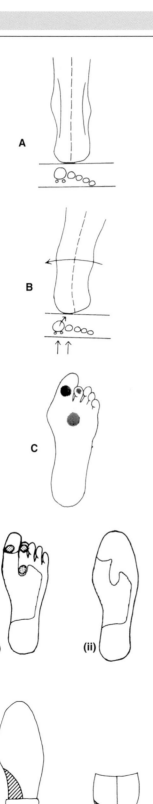

Figure 5.3 Forefoot varus. Relative positions of hindfoot and metatarsal heads of right foot at rest (A) and under load (B), from rear.
A: Forefoot inverted on hindfoot; possibly also mildly adducted.

B: Marked compensatory pronation of hindfoot to enable forefoot to become horizontal; resultant hypermobility of forefoot; first metatarsal segment hypermobile and elevated; second metatarsal overloaded; hallux plantarflexed. Shoes worn from medial heel to medial sole; possible broken shank; bulging on medial side of uppers. (Arrows below line indicate abnormal pressures; arrow above line indicates movement.)

C: Variable symptoms of foot strain—flattening and elongation of medial arch, possible hallux flexus, probable hallux abductovalgus. Possible plantar fasciitis or heel spur syndrome. Plantar lesions under second metatarsal head and interphalangeal joint of hallux.

D and E: Management options.
1. Valgus and shaft padding to support medial border and to relieve overloading of second metatarsal head and interphalangeal joint.
2. Symptomatic treatment for forefoot lesions and pain in heel.
3. Palliative valgus and shaft insole.
4. Functional orthosis with medial forefoot posting.
5. Half Thomas heel and medial flare if shoe distortion severe.

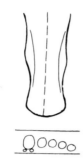

A

Figure 5.4 Ankle equinus, short or tight tendo Achilles group. Relative positions of hindfoot and metatarsal heads of right foot at rest (A) and under load (B), from rear.
A: Limitation of dorsiflexion at ankle; foot usually well arched, tending to be rigid but may be flexible.

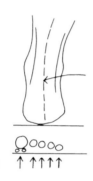

B

B: Compensatory pronation at subtalar joint to permit further dorsiflexion at midtarsal joint. Forefoot relatively elevated, supinated and hypermobile. Springy gait as heel lifts off prematurely .(Arrows below line indicate abnormal pressures; arrow above line indicates movement.)

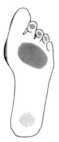

C

C: Possible symptoms of foot strain, plantar fasciitis or calcaneal spur. Secondary forefoot conditions may include metatarsalgia, hallux abductovalgus and clawed toes with associated dorsal and apical lesions. Midtarsal joint subluxation.

D: Management options, depending on cause.
1. Stretching for tight posterior muscle group.
2. If insufficient, raise heels to compensate for ankle equinus, or insert heel lifts in shoes; or consider tendon lengthening.
3. Palliative valgus and metatarsal insole if foot strain symptoms severe.
4. Symptomatic treatment for possible plantar fasciitis or calcaneal spur.
5. Symptomatic treatment for secondary forefoot lesions.
6. Functional orthosis if indicated.

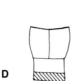

D

talar joint will normally be supinating from a position of maximum pronation at approximately midstance (i.e. as the malleoli pass each other). In equinus, large dorsiflexion moments unable to be absorbed by rotating the ankle joint cause the subtalar joint to buckle into pronation. The subtalar joint, with an average axis only 16° from the sagittal plane, has very little dorsiflexion available (Manter 1941). Pronating the subtalar joint has the effect of unlocking the oblique axis of the midtarsal joint and increasing the proportion of its triplane movement which occurs in the sagittal plane. As the leg rotates forward, the fulcrum around which it pivots is shifted forward from the ankle joint to the midtarsal joint. This can affect foot stability as it enters the propulsive phase, and Root et al (1977) suggest that ankle equinus is the most difficult functional problem encountered by the podiatrist. As the heel lifts, midfoot structures are strong only when the subtalar joint is supinated. Pronation tends to make the forefoot hypermobile. High medial forefoot loads immediately before heel lift cause the talus to plantarflex and the first ray to dorsiflex, so that the medial longitudinal arch undergoes substantial flattening. Laterally, the cuboid is forced into dorsiflexion on the calcaneus and the fifth metatarsal dorsiflexes on the cuboid. This means that, even in fairly mild equinus, the lateral side can have a convex (rocker-bottom) appearance immediately before heel lift. As the heel lifts, the forefoot is unstable and is unlikely to have sufficient time or power to restore a normal position in the propulsive phase. Loss of plantarflexion of the medial column makes this even less likely. The foot often remains fully pronated throughout the propulsive phase, or alternatively may oscillate rapidly as supinators (e.g. tibialis posterior) attempt to restore stability before the toe-off phase. The effect is to produce high shearing forces on the forefoot and high torque forces within the foot and the rest of the lower limb. This very late compensatory pronation can lead to subluxation of tarsal and metatarsal joints, causing severe damage to the foot, and a rigid rocker-bottom foot with tarsal arthritis is a possible result. Where equinus occurs concurrently with the insensitive foot, high forefoot pressures and midtarsal torque can render the foot inviable.

Lack of pronatory compensation also carries problems. Early heel lift produces a rapid shift of load to the forefoot, resulting in a vertical shift in the centre of mass. This carries high energy costs, equivalent to constantly going up and down stairs. In extreme cases, such as spastic gait where large, erratic triplane movements of the centre of mass may occur, energy output may be several times greater than that of normal sub-

jects. Early heel lift also increases the duration of forefoot loading and this is likely to increase the severity of forefoot lesions. A rare alternative compensation is for the subject to hyperextend the knee in order to advance the centre of mass over the foot. In the experience of the authors, functional (as opposed to passive) hyperextension has been limited to patients with lower motor neurone (flaccid) paralysis of the lower limb.

Ankle equinus, in addition to being one of the most damaging of foot deformities, is also one of the most over-diagnosed. In one podiatry report, 96.5% of new patients were diagnosed as having clinical equinus; this may have arisen from the practice of testing ankle dorsiflexion passively and non-weight-bearing. This leads to the situation where an examiner attempts, with the power of his hand and a very short lever (the length of the foot), to overcome residual tension in the triceps surae, whilst simultaneously holding the subtalar joint in neutral and measuring the angle of the lateral border to the tibia with a goniometer, a feat requiring both considerable force and legerdemain. Alternative approaches, such as paralysing the tibial nerve with local anaesthetic, have been suggested but these are also passive, non-weight-bearing and subjective. An alternative objective method in which high peak ankle torque ratios are analysed (comparing peak internal ankle torques before and after tibial block) indicates the likelihood of contracture as a source of equinus. The integrated analysis system, involving two Kistler forceplates, a three-dimensional motion analysis system and the Biodex dynamometer, is probably beyond the needs or budgets of clinicians.

A more clinically viable approach is to view the patient standing. With the subject in angle and base of stance, place the subtalar joint in neutral with the patient standing 60 cm from, and facing, a wall. Dorsiflex the big toe to maintain subtalar neutral and have the subject lean forward towards the wall keeping knees straight and heels on the ground. Measure the angle of the fibula relative to the ground. The external moments created by the centre of mass rotating around the ankle and ground reaction forces resisting its rotation will be very much closer to those created in gait and so more able to overcome any latency in the triceps surae, which provide the main internal force. Using this method, the clinician has a clearer reference point (the ground) against which to measure the angle of the tibia and a free hand with which to hold the goniometer. If equinus is present, measure again with the subject flexing the knees. This releases the gastrocnemius so that, if there is still less than 10° of dorsiflexion, the gastrocnemius is not responsible for the deficit. Next, test the subject sitting with knees flexed. If the end of the range of motion is springy, it is likely that soft tissue, probably the soleus, is responsible. If the end of range is hard and inflexible then it may be an osseous equinus. The diagnosis of source impacts on the choice of therapy.

Tightness of the gastrocnemius dictates stretching exercises with knees straight. One format which may be used is known as the CRAC (**C**ontract, **R**elax, **A**ntagonist, **C**ontract) technique, in which the subject stretches, then contracts by standing on tiptoe, then passively stretches and finally actively stretches by contraction of the antagonist. Contraction of the antagonist is thought to create deeper stretch in the agonist and has been shown to increase significantly the effects of stretching. Those with soleus equinus should follow a similar routine but with the knees bent. Therapists should observe subjects in the clinic performing the exercise and repeat this observation on review. Written instructions aid compliance (see Ch. 6). Patients who subluxate the lateral column during these stretches should not continue the programme. This will be clearly visible in the clinic as a marked convexity of the lateral column and perhaps by dorsal creasing at the base of the fifth metatarsal.

These patients, those who do not respond to stretching and those with osseous equinus should be provided with heel raises or advised to wear a shoe with a raised heel. This plantarflexes the foot in midstance, permitting a larger range of dorsiflexion in the pre-propulsive phase. Research is required to vindicate this apparently common-sense approach.

Forefoot valgus

Forefoot valgus is eversion of the forefoot relative to the rearfoot when the subtalar joint is in the neutral position and the midtarsal joint is locked in maximal pronation. It may be a true valgus of the whole forefoot caused by an everted position of the midtarsal joint, or a result of the plantarflexed first ray creating an impression of forefoot evertus. Functionally, there is little difference between them: in a mobile foot, ground reaction compels the first ray to elevate and the forefoot to invert around the longitudinal axis. This creates a forefoot that is plantargrade in early propulsion but not locked. The locking mechanism is eversion of the heel until such time as external lateral moments, created by ground reaction forces, around the forefoot are equalled by internal medial moments, created by the supinators, around the rearfoot.

In this case the rearfoot has to supinate excessively in propulsion to create equilibrium. If first ray and midtarsal motion are insufficient to compensate for the level of valgus deviation, inversion is found by supinating the subtalar joint. Subtalar supination is required in early midstance as the forefoot is loaded. This strains lateral ligaments and peroneals and is more problematic than the mobile variant. Lesions tend to be located diffusely over the middle three metatarsal heads in mobile forefoot valgus, but as compressional foci over the first and fifth in the rigid form, particularly when the first ray is plantarflexed. Dorsal lesions on the fifth are a very common finding in both types, probably as a result of friction from shoes associated with the excessive frontal rotation. Treatment is by propping the lateral side of the foot either with a plantar metatarsal pad (PMP) to include the second to the fifth metatarsal heads, or with a forefoot post higher on the lateral side by the extent of the deformity.

Ligmentous laxity

This describes a body phenomenon which can be classed as within the normal range from being a very mild form of laxity manifesting as increased flexibility of the fingers and toes, to being extremely lax where there is marked hyperextension of elbows, knees, toes and fingers. The position of the lower jaw can also be a sign of ligamentous laxity; it may appear to protrude further than the upper jaw and often the teeth are irregular and the fitting of braces is required.

Part of the picture in ligamentous laxity is a relative tightness of the triceps surae muscle group. This produces an ankle equinus that is usually compensated for by abnormal pronation at the subtalar joint with consequent unlocking of the midtarsal joint, particularly in females. Males tend to compensate with an early heel lift. With severe ligamentous laxity, the looseness of the ligaments can cause the foot to roll into excessive pronation, and the tightness of the triceps surae group perpetuates this situation.

Other effects of ligamentous laxity are to exaggerate movements, particularly those of pronation. In an otherwise structurally sound foot, it is possible to find excessive pronation with eversion of the calcaneus simply because ligamentous structures are too elastic to maintain the normal arch configuration. Similarly, lax ligaments will exaggerate compensatory pronation for structural abnormality, giving marked features of abnormal pronation.

Rearfoot valgus (congenital pes plano valgus) (Fig. 5.5)

Rearfoot valgus has been described as *normal flat foot*,

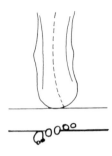

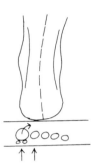

A

Figure 5.5 Pes planovalgus: hindfoot valgus, 'congenital flat foot'. Relative positions of hindfoot and metatarsal heads of right foot at rest (A) and under load (B), from rear.
A: Calcaneus everted; low convex medial arch; prominent medial malleolus; tarsus usually rigid; forefoot abducted on hindfoot and everted.

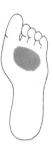

B

B: Fixed eversion of hindfoot; bowing of tendo Achilles (Helbing's sign); forefoot supinated to horizontal; first metatarsal hypermobile, elevated and inverted. 'Flat-footed' abducted angle of gait; shoes worn down at lateral heel and medial sole; shank flattened, possibly broken. (Arrows below line indicate abnormal pressures; arrow above line indicates movement.)

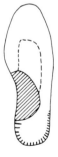

C

C: Variable plantar lesions, depending on state of metatarsophalangeal joints; possibly diffuse callus; deformity may be asymptomatic or present symptoms of tarsal arthritis.

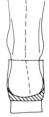

D

D and E: Management options.
1. Accommodative insole with heel cupped for fixed calcaneal eversion; resilient valgus support if symptomatic; additional metatarsal cushioning if necessary.
2. If foot mobile, valgus flange also.
3. Symptomatic treatment for forefoot lesions.
4. Wedge-soled shoes suitable, but not rigid shanks.

E

since it is defined as flat foot without pronation or exceptional dysfunction. This condition was formerly thought to be an important and frequent cause of flat foot, but current thinking postulates that it is a relatively rare cause, and that most cases of flat foot are the result of abnormal subtalar pronation. Rearfoot valgus may originate in the subtalar joint but is more often associated with genu valgum. The tibia is usually splayed and the calcaneum tends to retain a position of eversion relative to the ground. The forefoot becomes plantargrade by inverting/supinating at the longitudinal axis of the midtarsal joint, so that development of a supinatus deformity is not uncommon. It is often associated with ligamentous laxity and obesity, and where this is the case, knee pain and medial ankle instability are common sequelae. There may be also a problem with late pronation, particularly in the presence of supinatus. Foot problems vary, but substantial skin lesions are not necessarily found. Foot strain, as well as pain and instability in the knees, hips and lower back, may cause persistent problems which do not have straightforward solutions. Similarly, lax ligaments will exaggerate compensatory pronation for structural abnormality, giving marked features of abnormal pronation. Management options are discussed in Figure 5.5.

Other forms of flat foot

Arthritic flat foot is seen occasionally in advanced rheumatoid arthritis; the foot is held in eversion and abduction as a consequence of the disease process in the tarsal joints. *Traumatic flat foot* may follow fractures of the ankle or calcaneus. These are chronic deformities which require accommodation in appropriately modified footwear, together with supporting orthoses to relieve symptoms and to prevent further deformation of the foot on weight-bearing.

Paralytic flat foot may occur following injury or disease affecting the posterior tibial nerve, leading to paralysis of the invertor and flexor muscles and resulting in a flaccid flat foot. *Spastic flat foot* is due to spasm of the peroneal muscles which hold the foot in an everted and abducted posture, usually because of some painful focus in the tarsal joints. This is usually identified as a tarsal synostosis (see Ch. 4).

Foot drop, in which dorsiflexion capacity is lost following poliomyelitis and paralysis of the anterior tibial nerve, is another flaccid condition requiring differentiation by examination and history. *Congenital vertical talus* is a rare extreme flat foot condition in which the obliquity of the talus to the calcaneus and forefoot is such that the talus is driven vertically between the talus and fore-

foot. There is usually subluxation of the subtalar joint and often aplastic talus (see Ch. 4).

Profound sensory neuropathy, which may be seen in diabetes or leprosy, can lead to chronic disintegration of the midfoot. In such cases of tarsal disintegration, there is total collapse of the medial longitudinal arch and a complete loss of foot structure. The talus tends to 'fall off' the front of the calcaneus, creating a highly unstable, rocker-bottom foot, in which the forefoot is dysfunctional and the weight is taken predominantly on the heel (see Chs 4 and 28).

Management of subtalar joint abnormalities

Since the underlying defects are of a permanent character, more durable measures are required in the longer term. These must both accommodate the primary deformity and control the secondary symptoms. This necessitates the design of functional or accommodative orthoses, together with any necessary footwear modifications. Bearing in mind the different sources of the primary abnormal pronation, the following procedures may be indicated.

Rearfoot varus (Fig. 5.2)

a. Medial heel wedging or cupping to stabilise the inverted position of the rearfoot and to prevent abnormal pronation on weight-bearing
b. Valgus support to the medial border of the foot but without elevating the first metatarsal
c. Metatarsal padding to relieve possible plantar lesions and symptoms of metatarsalgia
d. Functional orthotic with medial rearfoot posting
e. Footwear with broad-based heels of average height.

Forefoot varus (Fig. 5.3)

a. Medial forefoot wedging to prevent abnormal pronation
b. Valgus support to the medial border of the foot
c. Shaft padding to the first metatarsal and proximal phalanx of the hallux
d. Metatarsal padding with a U-shaped cavity to relieve overloading of the second metatarsal head
e. Functional orthotic with medial forefoot posting
f. In severe long-standing cases, an extended heel (a half Thomas heel) and a medial flare
g. Symptomatic treatment of forefoot lesions.

Ankle equinus (Fig. 5.4)

The treatment varies with the cause. In the bony form or congenital shortage of the triceps surae muscle group, heel lifts can be inserted into the shoes or a higher-heeled shoe can be worn. Where the deforming effects of equinus have been long-term and foot realignment is necessary, a functional orthotic device can be prescribed, in combination with the heel lifts.

In acquired ankle equinus, first line management is to stretch out the triceps surae muscle group with a daily muscle stretching regime, after which a functional orthotic can be issued to realign the foot if necessary. If prolonged pronation has been the mode of compensation used for the condition, functional orthoses will help to keep the muscle group stretched.

Ligamentous laxity

The treatment is to stretch the triceps surae muscle group with a suitable daily stretching and maintenance regime. Functional orthoses with high medial posting will control the abnormal pronation, allowing the foot to function from its ideal position, and will help to sustain the muscle stretch.

Surgery

Patients with these conditions which result in pes planus deformity may obtain adequate relief from the use of orthotic devices. However, the clinician should not be misled into believing that pes planovalgus is a benign condition, as the instability present in this foot type may lead to other problems such as hallux valgus and hammer toes.

Surgical intervention should be considered in adult patients with symptomatic deformity which fails to respond to conservative measures and in children with gross deformity and/or instability. Adults will usually undergo arthrodesing procedures, while younger patients may obtain good results with reconstructive measures prior to osseous adaptation. Many patients undergoing surgical repair of the deformity will also require Achilles tendon lengthening or gastrocnemius recession.

PES CAVUS—THE HIGHLY ARCHED FOOT

Pes cavus is an umbrella term which describes a foot with a high arch. The term does not imply a cause and encompasses highly arched feet no matter what the aetiology and pathology.

In two-thirds of cases, some underlying neurological condition is responsible for the foot deformity, and in the remainder, some intrinsic structural defect is responsible. It is important to determine the cause, as pes cavus may be the only presenting feature of an underlying neurological condition which requires to be identified so that the appropriate management can be undertaken and the prognosis determined. Tests which may help identify the cause include nerve conduction, electromyography, somatosensory tests and muscle biopsy.

Neurological causes of pes cavus include Charcot–Marie–Tooth disease or peroneal muscular atrophy, spinocerebellar degeneration, spina bifida, poliomyelitis, cerebral palsy, polyneuritis, muscle dysplasia, trauma and arthrogryposis (see Ch. 27).

The causative mechanisms are unknown, although several theories have been suggested, such as muscle imbalances with either weakness or overactivity of extrinsic or intrinsic muscles, contracture of the plantar fascia and tight plantar ligaments. The more severe forms of pes cavus tend to be neurological and progressive in nature, leading to rigidity and marked deformity. Problems arise from instability in gait to pain from plantar callosities and heloma, and difficulty in obtaining well-fitting shoes.

Management may require surgery to produce stability and gain optimum function combined with podiatric care for chronic residual deformity with associated pressure lesions. Appropriate orthotic therapy and footwear modifications will produce the best long-term management (Fig. 5.6).

Non-neurological pes cavus appears to be an anomaly in development which has given rise to this high-arched structure. Certain mechanisms have been identified as being responsible for the appearance of the foot and these can vary in severity, from a very mild form with little or no interference to mobility, to severe pes cavus and its associated problems.

Forefoot valgus

This is a structural abnormality where the plantar aspect of the forefoot is everted in relation to the plantar aspect of the hindfoot, when the subtalar joint is referenced to its neutral position and the midtarsal joint is maximally pronated (Fig. 5.6). The range of motion of the first ray is normal.

The compensation for this deformity is to allow inversion of the forefoot so that it becomes parallel with the ground. This usually occurs at the longitudinal axis of the midtarsal joint which supinates. The highly arched appearance of this foot when non-

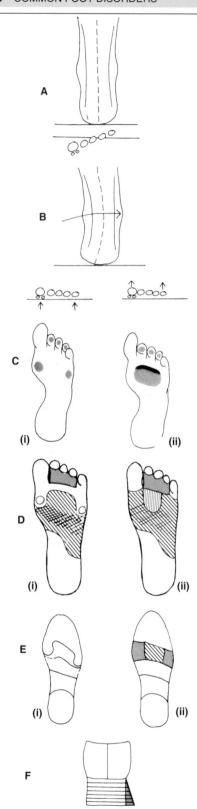

Figure 5.6 Pes cavus: forefoot valgus, plantarflexed first ray, hindfoot varus. Relative positions of hindfoot and metatarsal heads of right foot at rest (A) and under load (B), seen from the rear.
A: High arch, mobile or rigid; forefoot everted on hindfoot; first ray plantarflexed, possibly fifth also; both commonly relatively fixed, but mobile in some cases. Tight plantar fascia, possibly some metatarsus adductus.

B: Postural instability from compensatory inversion of hindfoot; possibly chronic ankle sprain. Forefoot lesions variable, depending on behaviour under load of first and fifth rays. (Arrows below line indicate abnormal pressures; arrows above line indicate movement.)

C: (i) If both first and fifth rays fixed, plantar helomata under both metatarsal heads, probably severe, often vascular. (ii) If both first and fifth rays hypermobile and elevating, diffuse callosity under middle metatarsal heads, usually heavy. A combination of such lesions is possible. Liability to ulceration in neuropathic states. Clawing of middle toes with apical and dorsal lesions.

D: First stage management. (i) Double-winged metatarsal padding extended posteriorly to load medial border. Alternatively, metatarsal padding only on foot with tarsal platforms in shoes. Orthodigital splints for toes. (ii) If metatarsophalangeal joints mobile, padding as above; if fixed, plantar cover extended posteriorly to lateral border with cavity (-ies) for 2, 3 and/or 4 as required. Maximum metatarsal bar effect required. Orthodigital splints for toes.

E: Long-term management. (i) Insole with tarsal platform extended to metatarsals 2, 3 and 4; metatarsal bar effect accentuated. Orthodigital splints for toes. (ii) Insole as above if metatarsophalangeal joints mobile; if fixed, plantar cushion for middle metatarsal heads with tarsal platform extended anteriorly into shafts under first and fifth. Maximum metatarsal bar effect required. Orthodigital splints for toes.

F: Buttressed heel if required to maintain lateral postural stability.

weight-bearing changes as the arch flattens substantially on loading. This is sometimes termed mobile pes cavus.

When the forefoot valgus deformity is too large to be compensated for by the midtarsal joint, it occurs at the subtalar joint which supinates to allow the forefoot to become parallel with the ground. In stance, the foot has a supinated appearance, with a high arch and a heel position which is varus; the lower limb is externally rotated. The foot, being a rigid structure which lacks adaptability, thus gives rise to lateral ankle instability. The metatarsals become plantarflexed and the proximal phalanges dorsiflex. This causes a tension on the long flexor tendons which plantarflex the intermediate and distal phalanges, giving rise to claw toes which may develop as flexion contractures and perpetuate the features of pes cavus.

Plantarflexed first ray deformity

This deformity is defined as a structural abnormality where the first ray has a greater range of plantarflexion than dorsiflexion (Fig. 5.7). This is determined by placing the subtalar joint in the neutral position, maximally pronating the midtarsal joint and putting the first ray through its full range of motion. Normally the first ray will be able to dorsiflex above the transverse plane of the lesser metatarsals to the same extent as it can plantarflex below, about 1 cm.

The plantarflexed first ray has a greater range of

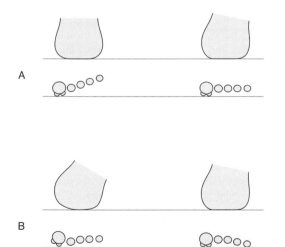

Figure 5.7 A, B: Uncompensated and compensated forms of forefoot valgus and plantarflexed first ray. Skin lesions develop under the first metatarsophalangeal joint (MPJ) in forefoot valgus, and under the first and fifth MPJs in a plantarflexed first ray deformity.

plantarflexion than dorsiflexion, and in severe cases dorsiflexion is so reduced that the first metatarsal cannot dorsiflex to the level of the lesser metatarsals.

The foot with a plantarflexed deformity looks similar to that with a forefoot valgus, and compensation mechanisms are also similar. Initially, midtarsal joint supination is utilised to allow the first metatarsal head to dorsiflex to a transverse plane in line with the other metatarsals. Where the plantarflexion deformity is large, or where the range of motion in the first ray or midtarsal joint is small, as with advancing age, the subtalar joint must now compensate by supinating. This causes inversion of the heel, which increases the mechanical advantage of peroneus longus as it plantarflexes the first ray. Eventually, the peroneus longus muscle increases this plantarflexed position of the first ray, which requires more subtalar joint supination. This is a progressive deformity and gives rise to the pes cavus appearance. Lateral instability with callosities on the plantar surface of the first and fifth metatarsal heads is common.

Rearfoot varus

This deformity can be identified by examining the position of the calcaneus when in the neutral calcaneal stance position. The calcaneus will be inverted in relation to the weight-bearing surface. There will be a moderate to high arch depending on the degree of varus. Normally this deformity is compensated for by the subtalar joint pronating until the calcaneus becomes vertical. In situations where there is insufficient subtalar joint motion to allow the calcaneus to become vertical to the supporting surface, it will remain inverted to a greater or lesser degree and the subtalar joint will be maximally pronated. In this situation there is often active plantarflexion of the first ray to allow ground contact by the medial side of the sole of the foot. This accentuates the height of the arch, and the plantarflexed metatarsals cause triggering of the hallux and clawing of the lesser digits. Often there are plantar lesions under the first and fifth metatarsal heads.

Forefoot equinus

This is a congenital deformity where all the metatarsals are abnormally plantarflexed, and the effect is to give a highly arched appearance. The deformity may occur at the tarsometatarsal joints or at the midtarsal joint. In either case, the metatarsals have an acute downward angle. Because of this angle of declination, the proximal phalanges of the toes rotate to the dorsal surface of the metatarsal heads in acute dorsiflexion, which gives rise to retracted or claw toe deformities.

Forefoot equinus is first compensated at the ankle joint taking away valuable motion, allowing the heel to contact the ground in stance. Subsequent compensation is with subtalar joint pronation, which releases motion at the oblique axis of the midtarsal joint, leading to subluxation of this joint and instability of the forefoot in propulsion.

Ankle equinus

A supination deformity of the foot with increased arch height and forefoot overloading can occur where there is severe limitation of ankle dorsiflexion. This limitation can be caused by congenital shortness of the triceps surae or bony limitation of the ankle which prevents the heel from contacting the ground during stance. The muscles that supinate the subtalar joint are mainly resisted by the ground reaction forces on the lateral side of the foot, but when the heel does not contact the ground, this pronatory effect by ground reaction is lost and the foot supinates abnormally.

Clinical features

The foot is characterised by a high medial longitudinal arch with the forefoot plantarflexed in relation to the hindfoot. The hindfoot may be plantarflexed, neutral or dorsiflexed in relation to the tibia, but the arch is always high. Sometimes there is a lateral arch and usually there are trigger, retracted or claw toes.

Standing lateral radiographs are useful when evaluating the extent of the cavus deformity, and gait analysis will help in assessing stability and function. The deformity may be fixed and rigid or there may be considerable reduction in its height on weight-bearing. This will depend on the cause of the deformity; it is more likely to be fixed when plantar ligaments are in contracture, and there is more likely to be a varus deformity of the heel with contracted ligaments where there is supination of the subtalar joint.

With a varus heel, there is more likelihood of postural instability; the varus deformity usually denotes subtalar joint supination, which means lack of pronation, locked midtarsal joints, external tibial rotation and poor shock-absorbing capacity of the foot and lower limb. This can give rise to foot and lower limb fatigue and pain in the knee, hip and lower back. If there is an underlying neurological condition then walking becomes even more difficult and the individual has to cope with falls and ankle sprains as well.

It is the high arch configuration and retracted toes that usually give rise to most discomfort in the foot of the adolescent and adult. The exposed metatarsal heads pinned down by the claw toes become liable to excessive pressure. There is reduced resilience in the arch and the overall load-bearing area is reduced, particularly where there is a heightened lateral arch. The fibro-fatty padding is forced anterior to the weight-bearing area and its cushioning properties are lost. The toes no longer function effectively in propulsion as only the apices have ground contact and there is increased leverage on the metatarsal heads. In the case of forefoot valgus and plantarflexed first ray, the first metatarsal head is the initial part of the forefoot to bear weight in midstance. This weight is prolonged and as the midtarsal joint supinates, the fifth metatarsal head undergoes increased loading and heloma and callosities develop on these two sites. Over time they may become fibrous and contain neurovascular elements, giving rise to severe pain and disability.

In the mobile foot which flattens under load and where there is laxity of ligaments, shearing stresses may cause diffuse callosities over the second, third and fourth metatarsal heads. Plantar fasciitis and heel pain are common complications.

Triggering of the hallux and retraction and clawing of the lesser digits give rise to pressure areas on the toes from the shoe. The hallux may have a bursa and/or a callosity on the interphalangeal joint and the fifth toe may be retracted and varus, giving rise to a pressure lesion on the proximal interphalangeal joint; clawing of the toes leads to apical lesions.

Where the cause of the pes cavus is neurological, there is the added possible complication of impaired sensation and reduced blood supply. The deformed foot, having lost its sensory stimulation of pain, may unknowingly be severely overloaded, and in tissues already devitalised this increased pressure may cause ulceration and infection. The first and fifth metatarsal heads are most susceptible to excess pressure and develop thick callosities which may mask underlying necrosis and infection. Necrosis of bony tissue may encompass joint cavities, and infection may spread to the deeper tissues. These perforating ulcers will depend on the extent of the neurological deficit.

Management (Fig. 5.6)

Management of the condition needs to be directed towards three distinct areas:

1. the fatigue and discomfort of the lower limb and foot

2. the specific pain related to pressure lesions
3. the difficulty in obtaining well-fitting shoes.

The fatigue and discomfort of the lower limb and foot are due to their instability and lack of shock-absorbing capacity. The reduced weight-bearing area of the foot adds to this problem. The postural instability must be addressed by controlling the forefoot deformities which cause the supinatory compensation at the subtalar joint. This supination prevents the natural adaptive effects of the foot and shock-absorbing mechanisms, and increases the risk of falling and ankle sprains. By controlling these forefoot deformities with functional orthoses and forefoot lateral posting, the supination and varus heel can be reduced, restoring some of the adaptive properties of the foot. It may also restore some shock absorption and relieve the knee and hip of lateral stress.

Supporting the varus heel with medial heel wedging on an orthosis stabilises the contact phase of gait, thus giving the heel a broader platform. In the case of uncompensated rearfoot varus, it reduces subtalar joint pronation to more normal amounts. Forefoot and ankle equinus require heel raises or shoes with an appropriate heel height to reduce the need for subtalar joint compensation.

Increasing the load-bearing area of the foot not only improves the stability of the foot but reduces some of the most concentrated areas of pressure. Functional or palliative devices, particularly where there is a lateral arch on the foot, can incorporate medial and lateral arch domes to form a tarsal cradle which improves the weight distribution and lateral stability. Filler pads can also be incorporated to improve conformity of the orthosis to the foot.

Specific pain related to pressure lesions is sometimes the most disabling symptom. Reduction of heloma and callosities, and the debridement and treatment of ulcers (see Ch. 9), are of prime importance in restoring comfort and reducing the risk of infection. Short-term adhesive padding in the form of plantar covers winged to the first and fifth metatarsal heads and short return appointments made for the patient will improve the lesions until more long-term orthoses can be manufactured. Digital padding may also be needed to relieve the pressure lesions on the toes. These may come in the form of short-term felt pads (Ch. 9) and long-term moulded splints (Ch. 14).

Footwear is an area where the patient faces a dilemma. Whenever possible, the patient will want to wear normal shoes with some degree of fashionable appearance. Fitting highly arched feet into normal footwear is often the start of pressure lesions, particularly if there are also clawed or retracted toes. If there is inadequate depth in the toe box of the shoe, extra pressure will be exerted on the toes. The lack of shock absorption in the foot and the varus attitude of the heel soon distort the shoe, breaking down the heel counter and giving rise to lateral instability.

At the present time, trainers are widely accepted and provide a solution for many patients. The shock-absorbing sole and soft uppers allow the patient to function comfortably without having to resort to surgical footwear. There are other options too. Reasonably priced hand-made shoes and boots in soft leather and suede are now available, and shoes made with broader, deeper toe boxes in stretch material are also available from retail stores. Adaptations to improve stability come in the form of heel extensions into the lateral arch, and reinforced heel counters are also possible from hospital orthotic laboratories. Where deformity is extreme, the surgical boot-maker can make customised boots and shoes to fit these deformed feet.

HEEL PAIN

POSTERIOR HEEL PAIN

Superficial bursitis (syn: Haglund's bumps, pump bumps, heel bumps, winter heel, calcaneal (retrocalcaneal) exostosis) (Fig. 5.8)

This is an adventitious bursa found superficial to the insertion of the Achilles' tendon. It is a common condition seen mainly in young (adolescent) females; it is not a condition which is seen in later life.

Clinical features

Pain is located in the posterior aspect of the heel and is often associated with a particular pair of shoes. The patient may report seasonal fluctuations, the problem being more prevalent in the winter months and often associated with recurrent chilblains.

On examination, tenderness may be elicited directly over the calcaneum at the insertion of the tendo Achilles, situated just lateral to the midline of the heel and coinciding with the upper edge of the back of the heel of the shoe.

Aetiology

The cause is bursitis of an adventitious (acquired) bursa over a posterior bony prominence of the calca-

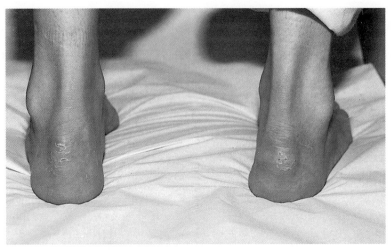

Figure 5.8 Superficial bursitis (Haglund's bumps).

neum. Some individuals are predisposed because of an increased pitch of the superior posterior surface of the calcaneum. The bursa is a result of pressure from footwear and is commonly found with compensated rearfoot varus because of compensatory frontal plane motion of the calcaneum.

Treatment

Conservative. Initially, this should be advice regarding more appropriate accommodative footwear. Padding is used, such as fleecy web to reduce shearing stress or foam to cushion and oval cavity pads fabricated from semi-compressed felt to redistribute pressure. These can be applied to either the foot or the shoe.

Footwear modifications can be carried out, the most straightforward being the removal of the heel stiffening overlying the bump; thermoplastic heel cups with 'doughnut pads' in closed cell rubber, or foam heel linings on the heel counter are alternatives.

Surgery. Operations are performed only rarely. One option is to shave off the bony prominence but this is difficult because of the site of attachment of the Achilles' tendon. Radically, a closing wedge osteotomy alters the posterior profile of the calcaneum but requires a 3-month recovery period.

Retrocalcaneal bursitis

Anatomy

This is inflammation of an anatomical bursa located between the posterior angle of the calcaneum and the Achilles' tendon near its insertion. It is a horseshoe-shaped structure, about 2 cm in length, 1 cm wide and 0.5 cm in depth (Frey et al 1992). It lies over the postero-superior aspect of the calcaneum and is bi-concave anteriorly, lying against the Achilles adipose pad, and posteriorly it lies against the tendon. The bursa has a synovial lining filled with a highly viscous fluid.

Clinical features

Pain is located to the posterior aspect of the heel and is exacerbated by dorsiflexion of the foot, e.g. walking upstairs. On examination, pain is less well located, and the bursa is usually palpable anterior (deep) to the tendon. There may be soft tissue bulging (bi-lobed) at both sides of the tendon and pain on dorsiflexion of the foot which compresses the bursa between tendon and bone (Fig. 5.9).

Differential diagnosis

- Achilles tendinitis
- Prodrome for rheumatoid arthritis or seronegative arthritis.

Further investigations

- Lateral X-rays for evidence of erosions
- Injection of radio-opaque dye (bursography).

On X-ray examination, prominence of the superior portion of the calcaneal tuberosity may be seen in

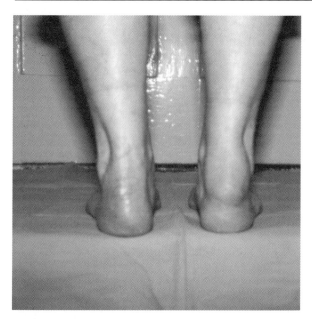

Figure 5.9 Unilateral retrocalcaneal bursitis.

association with superficial bursitis. It is often found with inflammatory arthropathies such as rheumatoid disease and seronegative arthropathies, and in these instances there may also be erosions at the upper end of the Achilles' tendon insertion.

Pathology

With inflammation of the deep retrocalcaneal bursa, the bursal walls become thickened and oedematous.

Treatment

This involves aspiration of the bursa and injection of a corticosteroid with a local anaesthetic. Identify the cause, e.g. attention to footwear. The patient may benefit from the application of a heel raise in the shoe.

Achilles tendinitis (paratendinitis)

This is the most common peritendinitis of the tendons of the foot and is an over-use syndrome affecting the Achilles' tendon near its point of insertion. Athletes, joggers, runners and other sports people are most commonly affected (see Ch. 11).

Clinical features

Initially, pain is experienced first thing in morning or after activity. If unresolved, symptoms may progress

to unrelenting pain. On examination, there is usually unilateral fusiform swelling in the lower third of the Achilles' tendon (about 2 cm from insertion). The tendon is hot and inflamed, and pain is elicited on active plantarflexion of the foot and when standing on tiptoes.

Differential diagnosis

- Deep (retrocalcaneal) bursa
- Seronegative arthritis.

Aetiology

It is an over-use injury but may be aggravated by a high heel tab on running shoes as well as improper training.

A suggested classification is:

1. Non-insertional—just proximal to the tendon insertion. Most instances are peritendinitis with inflammation limited to the peritendon or it may be peritendinitis with tendinosis, i.e. degeneration of the tendon. On palpation it will feel thickened and nodular and may predispose to a tear or rupture. The blood supply to the tendon, 2–6 cm proximal to its insertion, is at its least viable and this may be related to the cause of non-insertional tendinitis. (Rupture also tends to occur in this region).

2. Insertional. This involves the tendon/bone interface and is associated with a Haglund's deformity (deformity in which bone is seen to extend excessively above the upper pitch line). The bony prominence associated with chronic inflammation of the retrocalcaneal bursa will mechanically abrade and chemically erode the Achilles tendon at its insertion and may develop a retrocalcaneal spur.

Further investigations

- Soft tissue X-ray
- Tenogram.

Treatment

Steroid injections are contraindicated because of the danger of intramuscular injection and therefore rupture of the tendon. Underlying biomechanical deformities must be corrected and it is necessary to rest from sporting activity. Attention should be paid to the to footwear, in particular a heel counter which acts as an irritant. Physical therapies such as the use of ice and strapping in the acute stages, and ultrasound and contrast footbaths to reduce inflammation (see Ch. 15) are common treatments. A heel raise to rest the tendo Achilles is often useful but more chronic conditions may require a plaster cast. After the injury has resolved, a rehabilitation programme for the muscles and tendons should be encouraged, e.g. an intensive regime of stretching and exercises (see Ch. 11).

HEEL PAIN SYNDROME

This is often referred to as plantar fasciitis and is a generic term to cover a group of conditions of similar origin: plantar fasciitis, subcalcaneal pain, heel spur syndrome and painful heel syndrome.

Anatomy of the plantar fascia and heel pad

The plantar fascia is non-elastic material consisting mainly of collagen, with only occasional elastic fibres. It is arranged into three longitudinal divisions, each covering one of the superficial layers of intrinsic muscles of the sole and giving partial origin to it. The central portion, sometimes referred to as the plantar aponeurosis (Mitchell et al 1991), is thicker and stronger than the others and is important in maintaining the longitudinal arch of the foot.

The plantar aponeurosis is triangular in shape and attached proximally, by dense fibrous tissue, to the medial plantar calcaneal tuberosity where it is narrowest and thickest. Fibres of the plantar fascia are continuous with those of the Achilles' tendon. From this point, the plantar aponeurosis fans out distally, becoming broader and thinner and dividing into five bands over the respective metatarsals. The distal attachment of the central portion inserts through the longitudinal septa into the proximal phalanges of each toe.

These also divide into superficial and deep layers proximal to the metatarsophalangeal joints. The superficial layers become attached to the dermis of the ball of the foot, anchoring the skin and providing support from shearing forces. The deep layer of each band splits into medial and lateral septa, which surround the sheaths of the flexor tendons of the toes and adjacent ligaments and insert dorsally into the periosteum at the base of the proximal phalanges. Through these deep connections to the proximal phalanges, the plantar fascia tightens as the toes are extended (Hicks' windlass).

Normally, the heel pad is about 18 mm thick without load, being thicker in males than females (Prichasuk 1994). The superficial subcutaneous layer of the fatty pad consists of septa with equal amounts of collagen and elastic tissue, and is separated from a deeper subcutaneous layer by another layer of septa. The deep layer is thicker, lying above the calcaneus and containing wider septa with more elastic tissue (Buschmann et al 1995).

The clinical picture

Medial plantar heel pain is a common condition occurring at any time of life, although studies indicate that the age group 40–60 years is most frequently affected. Males and females are equally affected and bilateral presentation occurs in about 10–20% of cases.

Presenting symptoms are distinct. Onset of pain is usually gradual, appearing for no apparent reason and without history of trauma. Pain on weight-bearing is described as sharp, usually worse first thing in the morning, gradually subsiding, then recurring after rest and at the end of the working day. Pain after sleep and rest may be explained by increased effusion at the site of the lesion, this oedema placing pressure upon local nerve endings (Whiting 1974). An alternative explanation is contraction of the relaxed plantar fascia during sleep which is then suddenly stretched on weight-bearing (Wapner & Sharkey 1991).

On examination

The exact site of tenderness is located by applying tension to the plantar fascia, dorsiflexing the great toe (Hicks' windlass) and then running the thumb from distal to proximal along the medial aspect of the central portion (plantar aponeurosis) towards the calcaneum. While carrying out this test, the examiner should simultaneously concentrate on the patient's facial expression. A grimace elicited from firm pressure over the point of origin of the plantar fascia at the medial plantar tubercle of the calcaneum is diagnostic of the condition.

Heel pain with a mechanical origin
Aetiology

Three main factors are implicated as the cause of mechanical heel pain.

Abnormal subtalar joint pronation (pes planus). Although frequently cited as a cause of heel pain, the relationship between excessive subtalar joint pronation and heel pain has yet to be substantiated by clinical research. Prichasuk & Subhadrabandhu (1994) suggest an association between pes planus and heel pain, comparing the calcaneal pitch of patients with symptoms against a control group. Hicks (1954) described the windlass effect of the plantar fascia in maintaining the arch of the foot. As the metatarsophalangeal joints extend, the non-elastic fascia draws the calcaneum forward. This occurs during the latter stage of the stance phase, when pronation is prolonged and elongation of the foot increases the tension on the attachment of the plantar fascia.

Plantar heel pain does not occur exclusively in low-arched, pronating foot types; it may also be associated with pes cavus. In pes cavus, symptoms are likely to be due to contracture of the plantar fascia compounded by compressional forces on the heel through lack of shock absorption.

Heel pad thickness. The pad of fat under the heel acts as a firm cushion to ground reaction forces. Increased compressibility of the fatty pad is also considered to be an important aetiological factor in plantar heel pain (Snook & Chrisman 1972). Prichasuk (1994) reported that the elasticity of the heel pad decreases with age and its resistance to compression is reduced in patients with heel pain. Howells (1994) pointed out that heel pad thickness must be considered relative to foot size, and recommended the use of a 'heel pad index'.

Buschmann et al (1995) noted, in comparing normal and atrophic heel pads, that the latter (as occurs with senescence, peripheral neuropathies and various collagen vascular diseases) results in septal hypertrophy and fragmentation of elastic fibres but that there is no significant difference in the percentage of collagen to elastic tissue. They also observed that the adipocytes were smaller in atrophic heels compared to normal heels. These changes in the make-up of the fatty pads are thought by Buschmann et al to cause loss of resilience.

Obesity. Obesity is a consistent finding in relation to the development of this condition and numerous studies have substantiated this fact. Most authors agree that the incidence of obesity occurring in association with plantar heel pain is of the order 30–50% (Hill & Cutting 1989). Heavy body weight accounts for additional load on the foot with increased elongation and tension on the origin of the plantar fascia exacerbating the influence of biomechanical factors and compressibility of the heel pad.

Pathology

Entheses, the point of ligamentous attachments to bone, have a characteristic structural appearance. The fibres become more compact, then cartilaginous and calcified, before merging with the periosteum at a *cement* line (Whiting 1974). It is widely accepted that

mechanical tensile stress applied to the plantar fascia produces injury to the enthesis which results in a localised inflammatory response (enthesitis). The trauma which initiates the enthesitis may tear away small fragments of subperiosteal bone into which some of the fibres are inserted, and the subsequent bone healing represents the process by which calcaneal spurs form (traction spurs) (Whiting 1974).

Ultrasound and radioisotope bone scans support the inflammatory theory (Williams et al 1987, Wall et al 1993) but Snook & Chrisman (1972) point out that painful symptoms are not replicated by stretching the plantar fascia. Graham (1983) has demonstrated stress concentration at the origin of plantar pain and proposes that the spurs represent a reaction of fatigue fracture rather than a traction spur as was commonly believed.

Heel pain as a result of inflammatory joint disease (seronegative spondarthritides)

Aetiology

Early literature considered plantar heel pain to be a symptom of gonorrhoea. It is now established that enthesitis at the point of insertion of the Achilles tendon and origin of the plantar fascia is a familiar finding of seronegative spondarthritides, specifically ankylosing spondylitis, psoriatic arthritis and Reiter's syndrome. The latter is presumably the cause of confusion with gonorrhoea, as Reiter's syndrome can be sexually transmitted and there is the possibility of coincidental disease. Rheumatoid arthritis is also responsible but to a lesser extent.

The term 'talalgia' (heel pain) was coined by Gerster (1980) as a label for this dual source of pain emanating from both the above sites. He remarked on the high concordance (91%) between severe talalgia and HLA-B27 (human leucocyte antigen B27) and the frequency of radiological sacroiliitis (64%). Furthermore, Gerster was able to point out that severe talalgia is more common in Reiter's syndrome and psoriatic spondylitis than in ankylosing spondylitis. Gerster & Piccinin (1984), in a prospective study, aimed to determine the prevalence of heel enthesopathy in juvenile onset seronegative spondylarthropathy. This study indicated a high presentation (27%) of severe talalgia with juvenile onset spondylarthropathy. Heels were the most common site of enthesopathic lesions in children with seronegative enthesopathy and arthritis. Patients presenting with heel pain and involvement of other joints, especially the sacroiliac, raise the possibility of spondarthropathy, particularly if the patient is a young male. A thorough clinical history is required and, if necessary, referral to a rheumatologist for further investigation (see Ch. 26).

Heel spurs

In the early days of X-rays, calcaneal spurs were presumed to be the source of pain, acting as a foreign body impinging on the surrounding soft tissue. The significance of plantar spurs is not clear; they appear to be common in the general population, increasing in frequency with age (10–16% of the over-50s; Banadda et al 1992), and have no direct relationship to heel pain (Williams et al 1987). Resnick et al (1977) showed in a control group that 16% had plantar spurs, 11% had posterior spurs and 4% had both. Closer scrutiny of the size of heel spurs, rather than just their presence, reveals that, when symptomatic (Fig. 5.10), they are larger than controls (Wainwright et al 1995). In general, heel spurs are considered a normal variant and an insignificant finding when they are small and well-defined with smooth, regular cortical contours.

In relation to seronegative arthritis, inflammation develops in many localised sites in the body, particularly at entheses (i.e. points of union between fascia, tendons or ligaments and bones). Enthesopathy is characterised by local infiltration of lymphocytes and local inflammation, leading subsequently to fibrosis and calcification. During the active phase of these diseases, spurs are more prominent, but during remission, bone undergoes a phase of repair reflecting the disease process. Unlike the normal heel spurs described above, those seen in association with seronegative spondarthropathies can be described as pathological. In comparison, they are large, the cortical margins are ill-defined and irregular in outline, and they are commonly described as 'fluffy' or 'fuzzy' in appearance (Fig. 5.11).

Box 5.1　Case study: heel spurs

Figure 5.12A shows a radiograph of a young Asian male presenting with plantar and posterior heel pain (he also complained of pain in the hip). On examination there was gross swelling of the posterior aspect of the calcaneum at the insertion of the Achilles tendon, which was extremely tender. X-rays demonstrated posterior and plantar heel irregularities. Further investigation revealed a raised erythrocyte sedimentation rate (ESR) and ankylosing spondylitis was later confirmed; sacroiliac enthesopathy was revealed to be the cause of the hip pain. Subsequent X-rays were taken during remission and revealed remodelling of the calcaneum (Fig. 5.12B).

Other causes of plantar heel pain

Subcalcaneal bursitis

Plantar heel pain has been related to a subcalcaneal bursitis (policeman's heel), although there is little evidence of such a bursa, congenital or acquired. A few papers make cursory reference to it, apparently out of historical obligation rather than factual evidence, but Lapidus & Guidoff (1965) stated that a bursa does not exist in this site. It seems likely that the inflammatory

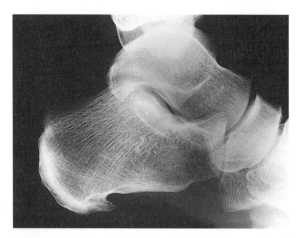

Figure 5.10　Lateral radiograph of a large symptomatic heel spur.

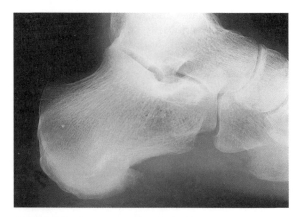

Figure 5.11　Lateral radiograph of a large, irregular and painful plantar heel spur in a patient with psoriatic arthritis.

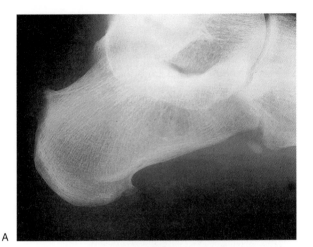

A

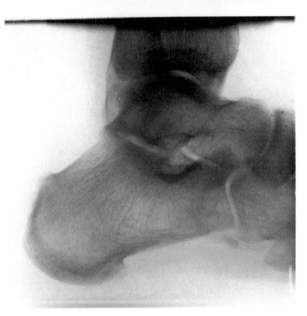

B

Figure 5.12 A: Lateral radiograph of plantar and posterior heel spurs. This patient was later diagnosed as having ankylosing spondylitis. B: Subsequent radiograph taken during remission shows remodelling of the calcaneum and reduction of the spurs.

symptoms associated with medial plantar heel pain have been confused with the presence of an inflamed bursa.

Nerve entrapment

Entrapment of the medial calcaneal nerve (Beito et al 1989) or first branch of the lateral plantar nerve to abductor digiti minimi (Schon et al 1993) has been identified as the cause of recalcitrant heel pain which is medially located and associated with a sharp (electric) shooting pain, often radiating up the leg. Chronic fibrosis of this nerve is alleged to be due to over pronation resulting in repetitive microtrauma to the medial aspect of the heel. Treatment may involve surgical removal of the nerve.

Radiculopathy of first spinal nerve

This is proximal compression of the nerve, leading to referred pain in the distribution area of the medial plantar nerve (Schon et al 1993).

Treatment of heel pain

The treatment is much the same regardless of the aetiology. In the sedentary individual, this condition is often self-limiting. Wolgin et al (1994) noted that 82% of patients had complete recovery after the application of a variety of conservative measures, with an average time to resolution of symptoms of 5–7 months. Those patients who do not respond to conservative measures present a challenge to podiatric treatment. The natural course of events is that the problem resolves with or without treatment and, generally, palliative measures are sufficient in helping the patient through the painful stages. The condition lasts for about 6 months to 1 year, and occasionally 2 years, but this is the exception rather than the rule. In order to alleviate discomfort during the painful phase, a range of therapies aimed at reducing either mechanical stress or inflammation is available.

Padding and orthotics

Treatment by this method is essentially palliative. Padding includes the use of simple heel cushions fabricated from sponge or pads shaped like a 'doughnut' to deflect pressure from the painful site. Commercially available shoe inserts are useful and may provide valuable shock absorption. Valgus pads can be used either alone or in combination with cushioning and medial heel wedges or menisci (such as cobra pads) to limit hindfoot eversion.

Reduction of the tensile stress on the fascial attachments to the calcaneum will relieve some of the pain. A reinforced figure-of-eight strapping (see Ch. 12), which inverts the calcaneus and increases its angle of inclination, is helpful in the short term. The calcaneum may be tilted upward at its anterior end by a felt bar fitted into the shoe. A tarsal platform (filler pad) acts similarly by elevating the cuboid. Combined with sponge heel cushions, these forms of padding offer alternative methods of short-term treatment while an orthotic is being constructed and specific forms of treatment are undertaken. The combined valgus filler insole (tarsal cradle) relieves part of the tensile stress on the calcaneal attachments. The provision of such appliances should be thought of as an adjunct to more active forms of treatment rather than as a complete treatment in itself.

Spread of the compressible heel pad can be contained by heel cups or an orthotic with a deep heel seat providing cushioning to the calcaneum (Snook & Chrisman 1972). Wapner & Sharkey (1991) and recommend stretching the Achilles tendon by the use of night splints and exercises, respectively. Non-steroidal anti-inflammatory drugs (NSAIDs) prescribed by a physician are also suggested as an adjunct to the aforementioned therapies. Furey (1975) stated that obese patients responded least well to treatment and so attention to weight loss is an important component of treatment.

Ultrasound

Ultrahigh frequency sound diathermy (ultrasound) enables the practitioner to direct a localised beam of energy onto the area, thereby producing a number of effects, which include an increase in temperature (see Ch. 15). There is some debate surrounding the efficacy of ultrasound therapy. Crawford & Snaith (1996) have demonstrated that therapeutic ultrasound at a dosage of 0.5 W/cm, 3Mz pulsed 1:4, applied for 8 minutes twice weekly for 4 weeks, is no more effective than placebo in the treatment of plantar heel pain.

Hydrocortisone

If the above measures fail, the next possible line of treatment is an injection of hydrocortisone (e.g. 1 ml Depo-Medrone) directed from the plantar aspect into the point of maximum tenderness. As this is a painful injection, requiring a large calibre needle (e.g. 23 gauge) to penetrate the thick plantar skin, a posterior tibial nerve block prior to heel injection allows more satisfactory access. Multiple heel injection may produce calcified deposits in the calcaneal fatty pad (Fig. 5.13).

Surgical management

Most of the literature advocating surgical treatment emanates from the USA. These involve plantar fasciotomy at its origin, often with resection of the bony spur or Steindler's release (the stripping of soft tissue from its attachment to the calcaneum), but there is little reference to the consequences on foot function when deprived of the windlass mechanism (Daly et al 1992). Sometimes the severance of the nerve to abductor hallucis is advocated.

Plantar fibromatosis

Dupytren's contracture of the palmar fascia. This is a condition of contracture of the palmar fascia affecting 1–3% of the population and resulting in a flexion deformity of the fourth and fifth fingers. It has a specific geographical distribution, being more common in northern Europe. There is a strong genetic association (dominant inheritance) and there is an association with other diseases such as diabetes, alcoholism and particularly epilepsy.

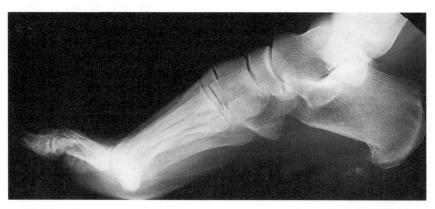

Figure 5.13 Calcified deposits in the calcaneal pad of fat following multiple heel injections with corticosteroid. (With permission from A. Wilson, The London Foot Hospital.)

Plantar fibroma is less common than Dupytren's and less problematic; contraction is not a feature in the foot as it is in the hand. Males are much more frequently affected and it presents in the older population most frequently in the fifth and sixth decades.

Clinical features

Patients may complain of a painful lump or a swelling but just as often it is asymptomatic. The fibromata may be single or multiple, unilateral or bilateral. They are seen in the medial longitudinal arch or just proximal to the metatarsophalangeal joints. On examination, there are subcutaneous, fibrous, nodular swellings which are firm and fluctuant on palpation.

Treatment

Usually none is required. If pain is experienced then an injection of hydrocortisone can be successful in reducing the size of lesions. Occasionally surgery is indicated, but fibromata often recur.

Tarsal tunnel syndrome

This is an uncommon entrapment neuropathy involving the posterior tibial nerve as it passes around and below the medial malleolus between the tibia and the flexor retinaculum. It is analogous to carpal tunnel syndrome in the hand.

Clinical features

The patient experiences burning pain and paraesthesia in the sole of the foot and in the toes, corresponding to the distribution of the tibial nerve. Symptoms can be worse at night and relief is achieved by hanging the foot out of the bed or walking around the room (Lam 1967). Percussion over the site of entrapment will reproduce symptoms in the distribution of the nerve (positive Tinel's sign), as will sustained digital pressure (Lam 1967). In chronic cases, sensory loss may be evident, as well as motor changes resulting in weakness of the intrinsic muscles.

Aetiology

The tibial nerve becomes tethered within a restricted fibro-osseous tunnel formed by the flexor retinaculum of the ankle and the medial malleolus (Cimino 1990). It is seen in association with rheumatoid arthritis due to compression of the nerve with synovitis of the tibialis posterior tendon. Pressure on the nerve results in a decrease in its ability to transmit impulses. Surgical decompression of the nerve may expedite a rapid recovery.

DISORDERS OF THE FOREFOOT

HALLUX RIGIDUS

Hallux rigidus and hallux limitus are conditions in which dorsiflexion of the hallux at the first metatarsophalangeal joint is restricted. It is generally accepted that around 60° of dorsiflexion is required for normal gait, although reliable indicators of normal motion at the first metatarsophalangeal joint are difficult to obtain.

Biomechanics

There is a popular perception of the big toe having an important role in gait, but its precise function is poorly recognised. The first toe must dorsiflex on the metatarsal during the propulsive phase of gait in order that the centre of mass can pass forward from the loaded foot to the opposite foot. The pivot for this action comprises the metatarsal heads and during this period they are often described as the anterior rocker. This action triggers Hicks' (1954) windlass mechanism causing metatarsal plantarflexion which is essential to create forefoot stability. The windlass (see Ch. 1) is dependent on retention of an angle of dorsiflexion at the metatarsophalangeal joint. During propulsion, the heel lifts and the first toe is subjected to an upward ground reaction force. This creates tension in the plantar fascia so that the heel and toe are pulled towards each other. As the toe is pulled by the fascia, it presses on the metatarsal head, forcing the metatarsal to plantarflex by sliding over the sesamoids. The greater the angle of dorsiflexion at the metatarsophalangeal joint, the bigger the turning force applied to the metatarsal.

Shereff et al (1986), using cadavers, described a mean normal range of sagittal plane motion at the first metatarsophalangeal joint of 111° (+/− 11.5°). In normal barefoot subjects the first metatarsal could attain an angle of over 90° to the horizontal at toe-off (Fig. 5.14). Most of this rotation would occur around a toe which is flat to the ground. The point at which the metatarsal head leaves the ground is the point at which the metatarsal angle relative to the ground exceeds the available dorsiflexion at the metatarsophalangeal joint. At this point the anterior rocker shifts forward from the metatarsal heads to the interpha-

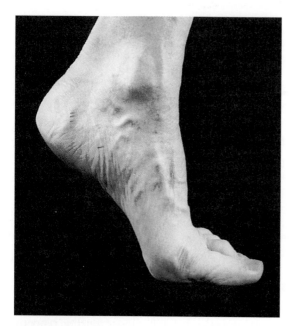

Figure 5.14 Normal range of dorsiflexion of the first metatarsophalangeal joint.

langeal joints. The centre of rotation of the first metatarsophalangeal joint is retained within the metatarsal head, and for most of the range of motion (below 40° of dorsiflexion) the proximal phalanx slides over its distal surface. In extremes of dorsiflexion, the articular surfaces become compressed (Shereff et al 1986). In cadavers with hallux rigidus these authors reported marked early jamming of the first metatarsophalangeal joint. It is possible to create this jamming effect in feet with a full range of first metatarsophalangeal joint motion. If the dorsiflexion angle at the first metatarsophalangeal joint is lost, then the tension created in the plantar fascia by dorsiflexing the toe and raising the heel compresses, rather than plantarflexes, the first metatarsal. This can be demonstrated by first plantarflexing the metatarsal and dorsiflexing the toe, and then maximally dorsiflexing the metatarsal and dorsiflexing the toe.

Dorsiflexion at the metatarsophalangeal joint will be reduced substantially by the inability to plantarflex the metatarsal. The reduced ability to rotate the joint about its axis means that a smaller proportion of the movement that does occur is a result of glide between the joint surfaces. Instead, the end of range of motion, now achieved within the functional range, moves the pivot point distal to the metatarsal head and the last few degrees of motion are achieved by closing the joint space. The dorsal surface of the metatarsal head is then compressed against the adjacent portion of the hallux and this creates a jamming of the joint.

In gait this jamming may occur quite early in the propulsive phase, inhibiting the smooth forward progression of the centre of mass over the top of the weight-bearing foot (Dannenberg 1993). To enable the subject to continue to pivot over the foot, the pivot point must move forward from the metatarsophalangeal joint to the interphalangeal joint. Normally this is a transient shift and it occurs at a time when most of the body weight is being taken by the other foot. Where dorsiflexion of the hallux is limited the metatarsal head lifts earlier, so that the anterior rocker may be the first metatarsophalangeal joint for a substantial portion of the gait cycle. It is during this small part of the gait cycle that the features of hallux rigidus are developed.

Pathology

As the heel rises, the upper margin of the convex metatarsal head impinges with considerable force against the dorsal rim of the concavity at the base of the proximal phalanx. Constant repetition of this process of compressive and shearing stresses induces a subacute arthritis, with eventual erosion of the articular cartilage, narrowing of the joint space, increased density of subarticular bone and proliferation of osteophytes on the dorsolateral margins of either or both of the two bones, often referred to as dorsal lipping (Fig. 5.15). The joint becomes enlarged, stiff and painful to move, until such time as immobility renders it pain-free. The interphalangeal joint hyperextends, subluxated by propulsive ground reaction forces, and the fatty pad below the toe is compressed dorsally around the toenail, often producing symptoms of ingrowing toenail.

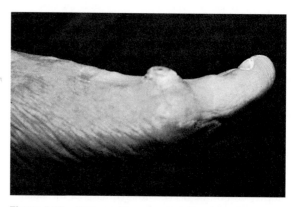

Figure 5.15 Hallux rigidus, showing dorsal exostosis.

Functional effects are primarily the result of losing the Hicks' windlass mechanism. Dorsiflexion of the toe is essential if the metatarsal is to plantarflex. Plantarflexion, which occurs mostly at the talonavicular joint (Winson et al 1994), enables the medial longitudinal arch to be raised and the propulsive forefoot to be stabilised against an inverting heel. Reaction forces stiffen the raised medial column by osseous compression (Dannanberg 1993). Failure of plantarflexion of the first ray precludes restoration of the medial longitudinal arch and reduces stability. The inability to dorsiflex the toe means that the first ray cannot plantarflex and therefore the metatarsal does not bear load during the propulsive phase. This produces medial instability until such time as the interphalangeal joint becomes loaded later in propulsion. At this time, the tread line, usually the first interphalangeal joint and the second and fifth metatarsal heads, will be oblique to the line of progression and will encourage late and possibly excessive supination. These points along the tread line are frequently overloaded and therefore develop callosities. The resultant high pressure on the distal phalanx is likely to cause hyperextension of the interphalangeal joint. Nail problems may develop as a result of back pressure from the shoe on the hyperextended toe, but are more usually the result of the pulp being distorted by plantar pressure and forced around the nail.

In later stages movement becomes gradually more restricted because of osteophytic formations and the degeneration of the articular cartilages (Fig. 5.16). Pain may then become less severe and, ultimately, may cease altogether as all movement is lost, but pain from the secondary features such as plantar heloma may be considerable. The oblique thrust of weight-bearing stresses through the foot consequent upon its inversion and adduction may also cause some compression and deformity of the lesser toes, with associated dorsal and interdigital lesions.

Aetiology

The most critical aetiological factor is hypermobility of the first metatarsal on weight-bearing. This may be a localised hypermobility of the first ray or part of a general hypermobility of the foot caused by persistent abnormal pronation of the hindfoot. Elevation of the metatarsal head which occurs under load for either of these reasons disrupts the normal function of the joint. In the earlier stages this impaired function may be completely pain-free, and passive first metatarsophalangeal joint motion may be normal. This is termed functional hallux limitus, indicating that the limitation

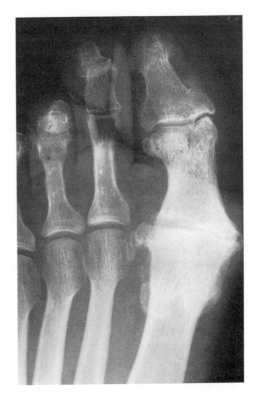

Figure 5.16 Hallux rigidus: X-ray showing joint changes.

only occurs with gait as a secondary effect of abnormal pronation or elevation of the first ray. At this stage normal joint function can often be restored by judicious use of orthoses. It is also possible that pain may exist without obvious joint damage. In such circumstances it has been suggested that protective spasm of the flexor hallucis brevis may hold the toe relatively immobile. Impaction through constant stubbing in the toe box was long held to be the primary cause of hallux rigidus. It has fallen from favour but should not be disregarded as a causal factor, particularly in cases where the subject's occupation or hobbies predispose them to such trauma (e.g. kicking a ball). Feet which elongate excessively may be liable to both impaction and functional limitus, and thus show an increased propensity for developing limitation.

Trauma may also be a causal factor, particularly when it leads to osteochondral pathology such as osteochondritis dissecans. In such cases a subchondral fragment may become displaced and disrupt the integrity of the articular surface. Osteochondritis of the talar dome can be classified in a way that can usefully be applied to other weight-bearing joints. It is suggested that the fragment may:

1. settle and resume its position, in which case damage will be minimal
2. settle in a slightly offset position
3. become fully displaced and float within the joint space
4. settle into the hollow in such an orientation that union is impossible, acting as dead tissue to preclude satisfactory healing.

In types '1' and '2' there is likely to be some cartilage damage and irregularity of the articular surface, so that slowly developing pathology is probable. Types '3' and '4' predispose to substantial articular remodelling with the fragment acting as an irritant and, in type '4', as an obstruction to healing. The joint will tend to remodel, eventually filling in the pit left by the fragment but becoming flattened.

Management

Management of hallux rigidus has been developed by experience, anecdote and rule of thumb. There follows a general description of short- and long-term management options, with the author's preference indicated. Conservative management of the adult deformity is directed to three objectives, namely to relieve pain, to maintain maximum pain-free movement and to compensate for the disturbance of normal weight-bearing.

In the many cases where relief of pain is the first consideration, immobilisation of the joint by padding and strapping is indicated in the short term. It can quickly be effective, provided the design of the padding and the application of the strapping are correctly matched to the needs of the individual case. An essential preliminary is to ascertain the most tolerable position of the joint and to design the padding accordingly. When pain is acute, a shaft pad under the joint gives immobilisation, particularly if combined with immobilising strapping, extending from the hallux and incorporating the metatarsal area. When pain is less acute or receding, some gentle movement of the joint can be tolerated and a plantar metatarsal pad with a single wing applied to the first metatarsal head and held in place by a half metatarsal strapping (see Ch. 12) may help. In some cases it is necessary to protect a painful dorsal exostosis with an oval cavity pad, or the plantar aspect of the interphalangeal joint with a cavity pad shaped to the full size of the toe to transfer pressure from the joint to the full length of the proximal phalanx. Added depth in the shoes is essential, and upper insertions, slit releases or balloon patches may achieve this (see Ch. 14).

In addition to such local measures, the hypermobili-ty must be restrained as much as possible. Normally this arises from abnormal subtalar pronation and must be controlled. Medial heel wedges or a cobra pad where a medial meniscus is extended distally to lie under the navicular in the form of a 'D' pad can be used with the initial short-term padding. A metatarsal pad extending from the second to the fifth metatarsal, in which the first is encouraged to plantarflex, should be used where the limitus is primarily a result of a dorsiflexed first ray. Heat therapy applied between re-application of the preferred dressing at weekly intervals may also be beneficial in relieving pain.

All the foregoing measures are short-term and are useful when the patient must be kept ambulant. They need to be used discriminately to ensure the earliest possible relief from pain. Easy fitting, but stiff-soled, shoes are imperative at this stage, as is the abandonment of any footwear likely to cause impaction of the hallux. Attention must be given to any plantar or digital lesions.

When pain has subsided, manual traction and circumduction of the hallux may be instituted. These manipulations should be preceded by heat therapy and the patient should be encouraged to repeat the movements daily. Adhesive dressings should be discontinued in favour of durable orthoses, incorporating such protective padding previously found to have been effective (Fig. 5.17). Hallux shields in latex or silicone may be necessary to shield the area of the joint, particularly if there are prominent exostoses.

For long-term conservative management, reliance must be placed mainly on patient-specific orthoses. These should meet three criteria: to stabilise the foot by controlling abnormal pronation or supination, to encourage stable pain-free movement in the joint, and to protect overloaded areas of the plantar surface. Dannenberg (1993) describes an excellent orthosis (the kinetic wedge) for encouraging dorsiflexion of the first metatarsophalangeal joint. The kinetic wedge consists of an antipronatory orthotic with a biaxial forefoot addition. The key difference between this and a simple plantar metatarsal pad covering metatarsals two to five is that in the kinetic wedge the metatarsal head sits in a pocket and the distal part of the addition actively dorsiflexes the toe. This maintains an angle of dorsiflexion at the metatarsophalangeal joint, so reducing the risk of jamming at this joint, (i.e. functional hallux limitus). Where there is virtually no pain-free movement, a rigid splint may be provided to stiffen the medial side of the foot, particularly across the metatarsophalangeal joint. Many materials have been used for this, including steel, aluminium and graphites. The author uses 4 mm thickness suborthelene, running

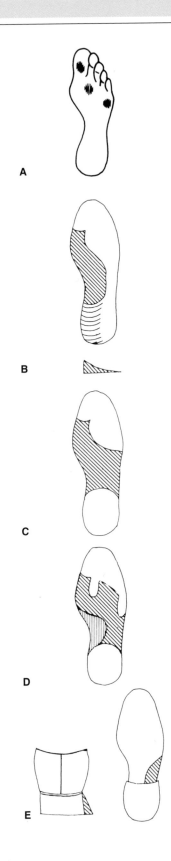

Figure 5.17 Hallux rigidus.
A: Typical distribution of plantar lesions.

B: Medial heel wedging with valgus and shaft padding to control pronation, stabilise elevated first metatarsal, and minimise movement in first metatarsophalangeal joint.

C: Tarsal platform and shaft padding to stabilise compensatory supination and minimise overloading and strain of lateral border and ankle. Metatarsal bar element may be added if required to aid rocker action and to reduce supination of forefoot.

D: Combination of tarsal platform, valgus, shaft and shaped metatarsal padding to balance foot mediolaterally and to protect second and fifth metatarsal heads and interphalangeal joint of hallux from overloading. Metatarsal bar element and/or heel wedges added as necessary.

E: Flared heel and/or reverse Thomas heel if lateral ankle instability present.

it along the line of the first metatarsal from just below the navicular to the front of the retaining insole. Where this fails and the patient is compliant, an external rocker can be applied to the shoe to permit a pain-free early propulsive phase.

Surgical treatment

If severe degenerative changes are not evident, it may be possible to salvage the joint. Cheilectomy may remove osteophytic hypertrophy, but will not relax the periarticular tissues sufficiently to alter the long-term prognosis. A modified Watermann or Austin procedure (see Ch. 21), which shortens the first metatarsal, will assist in relieving joint tension. Plantarflexion of the capital fragment may be performed simultaneously to offset the functional loss of weight-bearing length.

If the joint is deemed non-functional, then arthroplasty with either a hemi- or total joint implant may be used. Adequate resection of bone is necessary to ensure that the implant is not subjected to the excessive tension which was present prior to surgery. A structural metatarsus primus elevatus may also lead to hallux limitus, and is best managed by plantarflexory osteotomy of the first metatarsal.

HALLUX ABDUCTOVALGUS

Hallux abductovalgus (HAV) is a complex deformity of the medial column involving abduction and external rotation of the first toe, and adduction and internal rotation of the first metatarsal (referenced to the midline of the body). The displacement of the hallux occurs at the metatarsophalangeal joint, whilst the metatarsal is displaced largely at the metatarsal/medial cuneiform joint. Deformity is said to exist when abduction of the hallux on the metatarsal is greater than 10–12°.

Prevalence

Population estimates are difficult, as incidence increases with age and cultural features such as shoe styles. In Sim Fook & Hodgson's (1958) study, 33% of all shoe wearers had hallux valgus. Shine (1965) found HAV in 48% of women and 16% of men who had worn shoes for 60 years or more. It is more common in women than men, with 90% of all surgical cases being female (Hardy & Clapham 1952), although no such gender-related difference has been observed in children or adolescents (Johnston 1956). Both the degree and the frequency of HAV increase with age, though this may

be misleading. Shine found a linear increase in mean angle and incidence with years of shoe wear rather than with age.

Biomechanics/pathomechanics

Abnormal subtalar pronation is generally accepted in the podiatric community as the dominant cause of hallux abductovalgus, although it is likely that this is most damaging when accompanied by constrictive footwear, heavy weight-bearing and/or adductus of the first ray.

Pronation of the subtalar joint reduces the vertical/sagittal effect of peroneus longus, so that the first metatarsal is displaced more readily by sagittal plane ground reaction forces. It also lowers and increases the parallelism of the neutrally divergent, calcaneocuboid and talonavicular joint axes. This increases movement of the forefoot on the rearfoot, particularly in the sagittal plane (Elftmann 1960). Plantarflexion and adduction of the talus also reduces the congruency, and therefore stability, of the talonavicular joint where most first ray movement occurs (Winson et al 1994). The combined effect is of an unstable first ray unable to provide the required resistance to ground reaction forces in gait. These dorsiflex and invert the first ray on its axis, which runs approximately parallel to the transverse plane and at 45° to the frontal and sagittal planes. The first ray has greater dorsiflexion in hallux valgus but it is likely that inversion is the more active element in causing hallux abduction. Hardy & Clapham (1952) showed a highly significant correlation between first toe rotation and hallux valgus angle, with a mean angle twice as high when associated with toe rotation. In the normal foot the main (transverse) axis of motion of the first metatarsophalangeal joint runs through the first metatarsal head and lies parallel to the frontal and transverse planes. This means that the motion from this axis will be purely in the sagittal plane (i.e. dorsiflexion and plantarflexion). Inversion of the first ray rotates the transverse axis of motion of the first metatarsophalangeal joint out of the transverse plane, so that sagittal plane ground reaction force on the toe effects transverse plane deviation. This means that the normal dorsiflexion seen in the propulsive phase is accompanied by abduction.

Abduction occurring with propulsive phase dorsiflexion angulates the toe to the line of progression, so that reaction forces are more medial than normal. Any eversion occurring at this time will increase the abductory effect due to increased displacement of the metatarsal (Root et al 1977). Once this process of displacement has been initiated, the musculature and tensile structures that surround the toe perpetuate and worsen it.

Snijders et al (1986) describe a mechanical model in which, by displacing the flexor musculature laterally, the flexors create an abductory moment (midline of body as reference), referred to as 'bow-stringing'. This and the other plantarflexing mechanisms, principally the plantar fascia through Hicks' windlass, will tend to both fix and exacerbate the deformity of the toe and impart deforming forces to the metatarsal. With the toe abducted and tension in the fascia, the backward force of the toe pushes the metatarsal head not only plantarly but also medially. The more laterally displaced the toe, the more medial will be the force on the metatarsal. These deformities, hallux abductovalgus and metatarsus primus adductus, are entirely reciprocal, so that it is no surprise that Hardy & Clapham (1952) noted a correlation between them which grew stronger with increasing hallux valgus angle (greater than 25°). If pronation occurs or an abducted foot position is maintained during the propulsive phase, tibiotalar internal rotation, resisted by abductory ground reaction force applied through the first toe, will also tend to produce lateral deviation. In this case the deviation occurs in the vertical axis of the metatarsophalangeal joint. This axis normally has only minimal transverse plane motion available. Subjected to repeated abduction, medial ligaments stretch, increasing available abduction. Eventually the first metatarsophalangeal joint may subluxate medially, producing the hallux abductus deformity.

The term hallux valgus is a universally accepted misnomer, in that the primary deformity is transverse plane deviation (abductus) rather than frontal plane (valgus). The term hallux abductovalgus is more correct as there is usually evertory frontal plane rotation (valgus) in the toe. Root et al (1977) provide a rationale for this. During late midstance and propulsion, flexor hallucis longus and brevis fix the hallux to resist sagittal plane reaction forces. Fixation of the hallux by the flexors also maintains its position in the frontal plane so that it cannot invert with the unstable metatarsal. This establishes an evertory torque at the metatarsophalangeal joint, which rotates the toe relative to the metatarsal, creating the frontal plane (valgus) component of the deformity.

Aetiology

Several aetiological factors predispose to hallux abductovalgus:

- heredity
- shoes
- gender
- pronation of the foot
- rheumatoid arthritis
- miscellaneous factors
  - neurogenic imbalance of the foot
  - excessively long first ray
  - excessive rounding of the first metatarsal head
  - forefoot adductus
  - pronation of the first metatarsal
  - muscle imbalance and ligamentous laxity
  - obesity
  - trauma
  - amputation of the second toe.

Of these aetiological factors, the authors consider the first five to be of the greatest significance, and these are the areas which will be considered in some detail.

Heredity

Around 60% show a family history. This is significantly more than in controls but the very high prevalence of hallux abductovalgus and possible heightened awareness among those sufferers make such statistics vulnerable to scrutiny. To date, no accepted genetic trait has been identified for hallux abductovalgus, but it is possible that some other predisposing factors (e.g. forefoot adductus or ligamentous laxity) may be passed genetically or that familial behaviour patterns (e.g. relating to footwear) may predispose subjects. Heredity is therefore generally accepted as a possible causative factor.

Shoes

Causation has traditionally been attributed to narrow footwear and this belief persists in the mind of the public. A number of studies lend weight to the argument that footwear is a major cause. Barnicott & Hardy (1955) compared a predominantly shoe-wearing European population with a predominantly barefoot African population in Nigeria. Europeans had a significantly higher hallux valgus angle than Africans. Gender comparisons showed that female Europeans had significantly higher hallux valgus angles than male Europeans and this was not the case in the African population. The authors suggested that the reason for this was constrictive footwear. It has been suggested that by wearing very broad shoes, the abduction angle of the hallux could be reduced over a period.

Other comparative studies between shod and unshod populations in St Helena (Shine 1965) and

Hong Kong (Sim Fook & Hodgson 1958) agree that there is a markedly higher prevalence of hallux abductovalgus in shod populations. In the latter case the ratio was 17:1. While there is clear evidence to implicate footwear as a major causative agent, in all studies substantial hallux valgus deformity has been found in subjects who have never worn shoes, albeit less frequently than in those who have. A number of other factors must be considered, the most import of which is foot function.

Gender

All studies show a clear increase in hallux abductovalgus in women who wear shoes compared to other groups. Hardy & Clapham (1952) quoted that 85% of those seeking surgery are female. Barnicott & Hardy (1959) supported this, showing a mean hallux valgus angle significantly greater in European women than in men (mean difference 4.1°) in a predominantly young sample (mean age below 25 years). That this difference is not seen in adolescents or in non-shoe wearers feeds the general assumption that women's fashion shoes are the exciting primary factor. Current preferences for broader less sexually definitive footwear may make or break this association.

Pronation of the foot

It is generally accepted that pronation of the foot is a deforming factor in the development of hallux valgus, and Hardy & Clapham (1952) showed a highly significant correlation between them. The precise reason why this should be so is still based largely on conjecture. The most widely accepted rationales for functional aetiology are presented in the preceding section on biomechanics/pathomechanics of hallux abductovalgus.

Rheumatoid arthritis

Rheumatoid arthritis (see Ch. 26) is a painful inflammatory polyarthropathy in which small joints are most often affected. Ulnar deviation in the hand and fibular drift in the feet are very common and hallux abductovalgus often develops. It may be extreme (often greater than 90°) and is often associated with considerable pain. The pathology is somewhat different to that generally found in HAV, in that rheumatoid arthritis causes osteoporosis and whittling of bone ends. Joint surfaces may therefore be considerably reduced in area, and the joints may be unstable and

subject to very high pressures. Intrinsic muscle power is often diminished. Muscles waste and the small joints become unstable, particularly in the sagittal and transverse planes. Total lateral dislocation of metatarsophalangeal joints is a possibility, and plantar bursae form and painful callosities are a frequent finding.

Clinical features

In an established case the clinical features include:

1. Abduction and valgus deviation of the hallux, adduction of the first metatarsal and lateral subluxation of the metatarsophalangeal joint. In extreme cases the joint may become dislocated. The hallux impinges on the second toe which it may override or, more frequently, underlie. The second toe often develops into a hammer toe which may also eventually become dislocated at the metatarsophalangeal joint.

2. The central toes are usually abducted and clawed, while the fifth toe may be displaced medially and underlie the fourth. Their respective metatarsophalangeal joints may become subluxated, or even dislocated in some instances. Metatarsalgia is usually present and sometimes severe.

3. Secondary osteoarthrosis of the first metatarsophalangeal joint is a common feature, with peripheral osteophytic proliferation which may limit dorsiflexion of the hallux.

4. Numerous secondary lesions occur where the skin and soft tissues are subjected to trauma. These include bursitis over the medial prominence of the metatarsal head; plantar heloma and callosities; dorsal, apical and interdigital helomata on the toes; and deformities and other conditions of the nails.

The basic deformity ranges in degree from slight to very severe and the symptoms are highly variable. Pain in and around the joint may be experienced, probably from ligamentous strain or muscular spasm consequent upon the disordered function. In many cases the deformity itself is painless, having gradually developed from childhood. In some cases the secondary osteoarthrosis may give rise to considerable pain. Symptoms may also result from ischaemia or neuritis in vessels and nerves as they are stretched around the medial eminence. The chief sources of pain are the superficial lesions, particularly bursitis, digital and plantar heloma and callosities.

Pathology

Authorities differ as to the precise mechanisms by which the deformity becomes established, but the sequence of pathological processes may be summarised as follows:

1. The first toe becomes displaced laterally.
2. Due to reaction from the forces on the first toe and first metatarsal instability, the first ray is displaced medially. As a result of the transverse plane angle created at the first metatarsophalangeal joint, the hallux is no longer stable and is pulled laterally by the transverse head of the adductor hallucis. The abductor hallucis is working at a mechanical disadvantage because of the pronation of the foot and is unable to balance the pull of the adductor sufficiently to prevent the initial angulation at the metatarsophalangeal joint becoming increased. This deformation is further exacerbated by the tension on the long extensor and flexor tendons across the joint, the so-called 'bowstring' effect.
3. The capsule and collateral ligaments of the joint adapt to the deformation, the medial ligament stretching and the lateral one shortening. Weight-bearing stresses force the metatarsal head medially and its sesamoidal ridge overrides the medial sesamoid, becoming gradually eroded. The sesamoids appear to be laterally displaced on X-ray, but the main movement has been that of the first metatarsal head medially as the metatarsal becomes progressively more adducted.
4. Osseous changes occur in response to the altered function of the joint. Osteophytic proliferation from constant irritation may accentuate the medial prominence. Additional bone may be laid down on the dorsolateral aspect of the metatarsal head to maintain an articulation with the base of the hallux. A similar adaptation may occur at the lateral plantar aspect to maintain articulation with the sesamoids. Persistence of the elevated position of the first metatarsal imposes a limitation of dorsiflexion on the hallux, so that a degree of hallux limitus is also present.
5. As the deformity progresses, the second toe tends to be displaced dorsally by the abduction of the hallux, developing a hammer-toe deformity, possibly with subluxation or even dislocation of its metatarsophalangeal joint. The third and fourth toes may become clawed and retracted, and the fifth metatarsophalangeal joint becomes deformed, the fifth toe becoming adducted and the metatarsal abducted as splaying of the metatarsals occurs. In extreme cases, the hallux becomes completely dislocated and may lie at right angles to its metatarsal.
6. The skin and soft tissues overlying bony prominences are subjected to abnormal shearing and compressive stresses, which cause various superficial lesions. A bursitis (*bunion*) is a common occurrence over the medial prominence of the metatarsal head and this is often the chief source of pain, particularly if it should become infected. Even without infection, recurrent bursitis can be very troublesome. In addition to the painful swelling, a sinus may form from which the bursal contents exude to the surface and periodically dry up into a hard corneous plug. A fistula may develop from the bursa into the joint, provoking copious discharge of synovial fluid and exacerbating the risks of infection. A bursitis may also develop over the lateral aspect of the fifth metatarsal head (*Tailor's bunion*), although this condition may occur independently. Dorsal, interdigital and apical heloma result from deformities of the lesser toes; the dorsal lesions sometimes develop into bursitis. The overloading of the metatarsal heads, which results from the disturbance of normal forefoot function, causes the formation of plantar heloma and callosities, notably under the second and third metatarsal heads. Complications may include metatarsalgia, as well as involution, onychophosis and onychocryptosis affecting the nail of the hallux.

Surgical treatment

According to Giannestras (1973), over 80 types of surgical procedure for hallux abductovalgus have been described. Many of these techniques are now obsolete and others are personalised modifications of standard techniques. Three types of approaches are now commonly used (Fig. 5.18):

1. osteotomy—to correct metatarsus primus adductus
2. arthroplasty—removal of part of the joint leaving an intact, if altered, joint
3. arthrodesis—fusion of the joint.

The main criterion for selection of procedure appears to be age. Osteotomies of the metatarsal are used in young patients with mild to moderate hallux abductovalgus. Keller's arthroplasties (resection of the proximal portion of the proximal phalanx) are used for mild to severe hallux abductovalgus in older patients. Arthrodesis is used mainly in more severe cases and more commonly in the younger age group.

Two other approaches worthy of mention are the bunionectomy and the McBride procedure. Bunionectomy is a minimum trauma procedure used mainly on elderly patients to remove a painful medial prominence. The McBride procedure involves transferring the abductor hallucis tendon from the phalanx to the metatarsal in order to discourage adduction of the metatarsal. This is used in children and adolescents. In

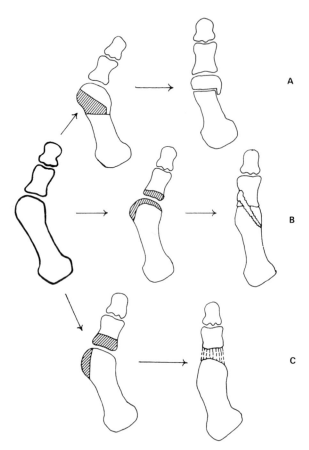

A

B

C

Figure 5.18 Main operations for hallux abductovalgus. A: Osteotomy of the first metatarsal. B: Arthrodesis of the first metatarsophalangeal joint. C: Keller's arthroplasty.

such cases the underlying cause of the deformity should always be sought and, where appropriate, a regime including functional orthoses instituted (see also Ch. 21).

HALLUX FLEXUS

This term describes the abnormal position of the hallux, which is plantarflexed from the first metatarsophalangeal joint. The deformity is usually mobile, but may become fixed.

In the great majority of cases it is only of significance as a secondary feature of one or other of the following syndromes: forefoot varus, a hypermobile or short first metatarsal, or a congenital metatarsus primus elevatus. In all such cases, the plantarflexion of the hallux occurs as a functional compensation to improve the stability and functional capacity of the forefoot in the

presence of an unstable and relatively incompetent first metatarsal. The plantarflexion is initiated by the flexor muscles of the hallux, but secondary contractures in the joint capsule from persistence of the abnormal attitude result in some limitation of dorsiflexion, even at rest. Eventually, pathological changes in the joint similar to those in hallux limitus may ensue, further limiting dorsiflexion and consolidating the flexion deformity. The effect is to disturb the normal pattern of weight-bearing by overloading the interphalangeal joint and the second metatarsal head, with the probable result of painful lesions developing at these sites.

Hallux flexus may also develop temporarily in response to painful stimuli from the region of the plantar surface of the first and second metatarsal heads, e.g. from a verruca. The diagnosis and cure in these cases is usually obvious. Occasionally, hallux flexus may be the result of either direct or indirect trauma, e.g. paralysis of the extensor muscles of the hallux resulting from damage to the anterior tibial nerve.

The treatment of the deformity and its effect depend on the identification of the primary syndrome and the application of appropriate measures designed to balance the foot posture with foot orthoses, which will also protect overloaded areas of the plantar surface (see also the section on 'hallux rigidus' and Fig. 5.17).

METATARSALGIA

Metatarsalgia is a general term denoting pain in the metatarsophalangeal area and it is symptomatic of many different conditions. Metatarsalgia may be considered as functional and non-functional in origin.

Functional metatarsalgia

Functional metatarsalgia denotes pain caused by abnormal mechanical stresses resulting from disordered function of the foot. The differential diagnosis and management of functional metatarsalgia depend on the underlying condition. Its association with pes planovalgus, pes cavus and hallux abductovalgus has already been mentioned, but it may also be symptomatic of other metatarsophalangeal abnormalities.

Metatarsophalangeal abnormalities

In stance, the five metatarsal heads lie in the same transverse plane on weight-bearing and share the load equally, except that the first takes a double load through its two sesamoids. The middle three metatarsals are firmly articulated at their bases and have only a very limited range of dorsoplantar movement at their heads, for the purpose of shock absorption and adaptation to the surface. The first and fifth, however, have the capacity for movement in all three planes, and this enables them, in locomotion, to adjust to varying attitudes of the forefoot to the ground and to varying and uneven surfaces.

Apart from the previously mentioned effects on the metatarsophalangeal area of hindfoot deformities and hallux abductovalgus, the position and functioning of the middle three metatarsal heads are usually disturbed only by malposition and malfunction of their respective digits, e.g. when they are pinned down by digital retraction or subluxation. The first and fifth metatarsals, on the other hand, may in some cases be either hypermobile or dorsiflexed relative to the others. In each case they are elevated excessively under load, are incompetent as weight-bearing members and thereby overload their neighbours. In other cases they may be relatively plantarflexed and held in that position by tight fascial bands so that they themselves are overloaded, forming an actual 'transverse metatarsal arch', which is pathological. Such disturbances of normal weight-bearing are reflected in the pattern of hyperkeratotic lesions seen on the plantar surface.

Mediolateral stability of the metatarsophalangeal area is provided, passively, by the transverse metatarsal ligaments and actively by the transverse head of the adductor hallucis, which, together, restrain the natural spread of the metatarsals under load. When the foot as a whole is hypermobile, as with persistent abnormal pronation, and also hallux abductovalgus, these structures are often unable to prevent the metatarsals splaying apart because the adductor hallucis no longer has a stable anchorage at its medial insertion. The splaying is most marked in the case of the first and fifth metatarsals, as they are less firmly articulated at their bases than the others. This not only increases the width of the forefoot, it also initiates or increases the tendency to abduction of their metatarsals. Both hallux abductovalgus and digitus quintus varus deformities are thereby precipitated or worsened. The splaying of the metatarsals, together with the hypermobility of the foot, causes shearing stresses on the first and fifth metatarsal heads from contact with the sides of the footwear, with resultant bursal formation at these sites.

The plantar tissues of the forefoot undergo compression, shearing and tensile stresses in the normal course of standing and walking. The excessive stresses which provoke the pain responses comprised under the term metatarsalgia may be produced in various ways.

Abnormal compression. This occurs from undue rigidity of the foot (as in rigid pes cavus, ankle equinus and forefoot equinus); from fixation of one or more metatarsals or metatarsophalangeal joints, such as may occur from impaction and constriction of the toes or fixed plantarflexion of the first and fifth rays; from fixed retraction or clawing of the toes; or from subluxation or dislocation of any of the metatarsophalangeal joints. In hallux abductovalgus, the second toe may become hammered and the metatarsophalangeal joint subluxated or dislocated. Persistent abnormal compression of the plantar tissues may result in contusion and inflammation of the soft tissues and in nucleated plantar keratoses.

Abnormal shearing stress. Abnormal shearing may occur from hypermobility of the whole foot, from hypermobility of the first and fifth rays and also from forward movement of the foot in an ill-fitting shoe. This results in inflammation of the plantar tissues, diffuse plantar keratosis and possibly bursal formation beneath and anterior to the metatarsal heads.

Abnormal compression and shearing may occur concurrently in the same foot, as in a hypermobile foot with a subluxated hammer toe. Evidence of both types of stress is presented in the form of a diffuse plantar callosity with a nucleus under the fixed metatarsal head.

Abnormal tensile stress. This results from the splaying of the metatarsals, and the resultant strain on the transverse ligaments and muscles, with the intrinsic muscle fatigue, contributes to the pain of metatarsalgia.

Other causes. Other contributory factors include excessive weight-bearing (obesity, pregnancy, occupational factors) and unsuitable footwear (short and narrow shoes which impede toe function, incorrect heel-to-ball fitting, soles too thin to give adequate protection). Local ischaemia, however caused, may also be a factor. Atrophy or displacement of the plantar fibro-fatty pads under the metatarsal heads, with consequent loss of shock absorption, is seen in rheumatoid arthritis and in old age.

Persistent traumatisation of the plantar tissues induces fibrosis in the dermis as a functional adaptation, often accompanied by some corresponding diminution of adipose tissue. Fibrosis is clinically manifest as a toughening or induration of the integument into deep folds or craters underlying plantar helomata and callosities. After enucleation of the epidermal lesions, the structural deformations in the dermis are clearly observable as fixed corrugations or pits in the otherwise uniform texture of the plantar skin. Their shape and size are indicative of the types of abnormal stresses which have caused them and are significant diagnostically. If the abnormal stresses are not adequately controlled, such dermal deformations provide ready-made sites for continuing hyperkeratotic activity and add significantly to the chronicity of plantar lesions. The papillae at the crests or margins of these irregularities are often hypertrophied, the neurovascular elements within them providing a further source of pain. In addition to whatever mechanical therapy is indicated, the use of astringents, caustics, exfoliants or emollients may be required for the local dermal fibrosis.

Management

The successful management of metatarsalgia, as is the case with other conditions, depends on identifying the causes and eliminating or mitigating their ill-effects. In cases where metatarsalgia is a symptom of forefoot rather than hindfoot malfunction, the main consideration must be to ensure maximum function of the lesser toes and their metatarsophalangeal joints. Retraction and clawing of the toes, which impair their normal function and restrict their respective metatarsal heads, need to be corrected as far as possible by orthodigital splints which straighten the toes, improve their alignment with their metatarsals and promote better toe function. When necessary, metatarsal padding should be used, with or without a metatarsal brace (Fig. 5.19). The same design is also effective as a palliative measure when no improvement in digital function can be expected.

Passive and active exercises should be instituted to stretch the toes and improve range of movement of the metatarsophalangeal joints. Re-education of the intrinsic muscles may be assisted by the use of Faradic footbaths, which also relieve the metatarsalgia (see Ch. 15).

Various types of metatarsal padding are illustrated in Chapter 12. Palliative metatarsal cushioning is indicated in cases of atrophy or displacement of the plantar fibro-fatty pads. In the majority of cases, symptoms are relieved completely by attention to the underlying foot fault and to shoe fitting problems.

When metatarsalgia is due to prominence of a single metatarsal head and symptoms are unrelieved by conservative measures, metatarsal osteotomy may be helpful (see Ch. 21). The cut is made obliquely through the neck of the metatarsal, allowing the head to find a new position in the same plane as the adjacent metatarsal. Some transfer lesions are to be expected, although these tend not to be as severe as the original ones.

Non-functional metatarsalgia

Morton's neuroma (Morton's metatarsalgia, plantar digital neuritis)

Morton's neuroma is a common, intermittent, neural-

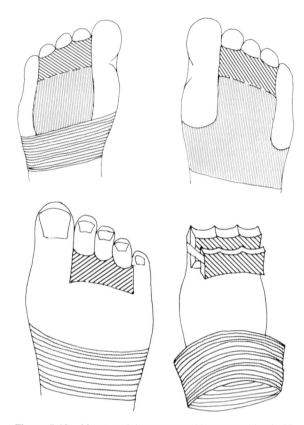

Figure 5.19 Metatarsalgia: metatarsal brace combined with orthodigital splints.

gia affecting the web spaces of the toes, typically the third. The source of pain is a pathological change to the plantar digital nerve as it divides to supply the adjacent sides of the toes.

A wide variety of synonyms is attributed to this condition, there being a distinct lack of consistency in nomenclature within the literature. The condition is eponymous with Thomas G. Morton, and neuroma and metatarsalgia are probably the more widely used terms, neither of which is accurate. The lesion affecting the nerve is not proliferative or inflammatory, and therefore neuroma and neuritis are misnomers, as is the term metatarsalgia, which implies pain in the metatarsals when, in fact, it occurs distal to the metatarsals, often involving the digits. In the past, metatarsalgia has been the predominant term but more recent literature favours neuroma. Thomas et al (1989) have proposed Morton's digital neuralgia as a suitable option and this would be more appropriate. Adding yet another name to a long list risks perpetuating the confusion and so the readily identifiable

Morton's neuroma is the term of choice throughout this chapter.

Anatomy of the plantar digital nerves. The lateral and medial plantar nerves, branches of the tibial nerve, give rise to the plantar digital nerves. The former supplies both sides of the fifth toe and lateral fourth, whilst the medial side of the fourth toe is innervated by the medial plantar nerve, which also supplies both sides of the first, second and third digits. The literature refers to a communicating branch of the lateral plantar nerve anastomosing with the medial plantar nerve to supply the third interdigital space (Fig. 5.20).

The metatarsal heads are separated by bursae which are superior to the transverse plantar ligament; the neurovascular bundles lie deep to this ligament and between the metatarsophalangeal joints.

Clinical features. The mean age of presentation is between 45 and 50 and, overwhelmingly, females are affected by this condition. Both feet may be affected equally but bilateral presentation is relatively uncom-mon, as is the occurrence of more than one lesion in the same foot.

The complaint is that of a severe, sharp, sometimes lancinating pain (often likened to a hot needle) which occurs suddenly while walking. At onset, the patient must stop to remove their shoe (usually found to be constrictive) and relief of pain can be aided by massaging the foot or manipulating the toes. In the worst cases, pain becomes debilitating and patients are apprehensive about walking. Incipient cases describe milder symptoms of burning or tingling sensations.

The third web space is most frequently involved followed by the second; only rarely do symptoms occur in the first or fourth web spaces. On examination, the foot will appear normal, although on rare occasions an intermetatarsal swelling may be evident. The exact site of tenderness is located to a point between and just anterior to the heads of the two adjacent metatarsals. This area should be palpated from the plantar surface using the thumb to apply upward and backward pressure on the affected web space, which elicits focal tenderness and which can be exacerbated by simultaneously compressing the foot laterally.

Lateral compression of the metatarsal heads may be accompanied by a palpable, painful Mulder's click (Mulder 1951) as the neuroma is expressed from between the metatarsal heads. Painless clicks are also commonplace and easily demonstrable on compression of asymptomatic feet. Sometimes a firm mass is noticeable in the web space.

In describing the distribution of pain, Nissen (1951) stated that, in his study of 27 feet, pain was felt in both the plantar region and the toe. In nine, pain was confined to the tip of the toe, and in only four was pain confined to the plantar aspect. Few other authors detail the extent of digital involvement but it is generally accepted that the toes are often involved. Variably, there is an associated hypoaesthesia or paraesthesia in the toes.

Sensation should be tested using firm but careful pressure with a sharp instrument, comparing sensory perception in all the interdigital spaces. On the whole, testing sensation in the toes, particularly of the older population, is unsatisfactory. In the rare instance of unambiguous loss of sensation in the interdigital space, this should be considered as strong supportive evidence of a positive diagnosis.

One further clinical test may be of value in carefully chosen patients. This involves the injection of a small quantity of a local anaesthetic such as lignocaine. The anaesthetic solution should be introduced accurately at the level of the metatarsophalangeal joints and deposited beneath the transverse metatarsal ligament.

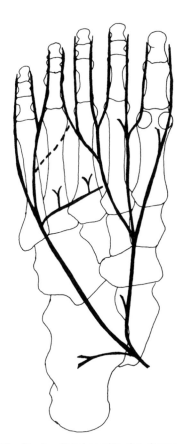

Figure 5.20   Plantar digital neuritis: the plantar nerves.

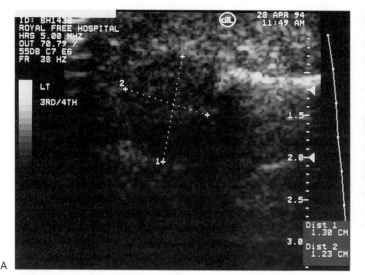
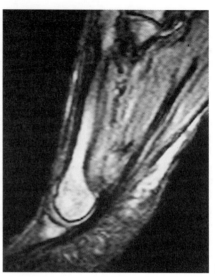

Figure 5.21   A: Ultrasound scan of intermetatarsal space, three-quarters of which reveals a large neuroma. B: MRI of the same site, which fails to identify the neuroma. (With permission from A. Wilson, The London Foot Hospital.)

This is advocated not as a treatment but as an aid to diagnosis, the premise being that, for a positive diagnosis, the local anaesthetic will temporarily ameliorate symptoms immediately after the injection. This test will not necessarily rule out other soft tissue lesions in the area but it may be useful in excluding bone or joint pathology.

Diagnosis of Morton's neuroma is dependent on thorough history-taking, accruing as many of the above signs and symptoms as are present in order to arrive at a definitive diagnosis. More objective methods have been sought; Guiloff et al (1984) reported on a prospective study using sensory conduction tests to confirm diagnosis. This proved to be of limited value.

Modern imaging techniques may improve detection of neuroma (Fig. 5.21). Ultrasound scanning has been shown to be successful in positively identifying neuroma in the plantar digital nerve (Redd et al 1989, Pollak et al 1992, Williams 1993). Typical sonographic appearance is that of a hypo-echoic mass (varying in density from the surrounding tissue), orientated parallel to the long axis of the metatarsals. Neuroma require to be a minimum of 5 mm in diameter in order to be detected in this manner. Neither the equipment nor the specialist knowledge for ultrasound scanning is readily available, although access to such simple and low cost techniques may result in fewer faulty diagnoses, forestalling the need for investigative operations.

Magnetic resonance imaging (MRI) (Sartoris et al 1989, Unger et al 1992, Resch et al 1994) and computed

tomography (CT) (Turan et al 1991) have both been shown to be helpful in observing neuroma but are rather elaborate and expensive means of investigating this condition as results merely confirm the clinical findings.

Aetiology. The precise nature of this common affliction has become an enigma, with much literature devoted to the various hypotheses. Four main arguments are considered here.

Anatomical factors: double origin of nerve. Regarding the frequency of involvement of the third web space, Betts (1940) hypothesised that this may be due to the peculiarity of this nerve, being derived from both the medial and plantar nerves. This nerve is therefore larger than the other plantar digital nerves and may be more susceptible to trauma. In addition, Betts stated that the two nerves forming the fourth plantar digital nerve both pass across the muscle belly of flexor digitorum brevis, so that dorsiflexion of the toes during walking subjects the nerve to further stretching due to the contraction of this muscle. The work of Betts is supported by McElvenny (1943) and Bickel & Dockerty (1947), but it fails to explain the occurrence of lesions in the other web spaces. The double origin theory has been disputed by Levitsky et al (1993), who found, in a study of 71 cadaveric feet, communication between the medial and lateral plantar nerves in only 19 (26.8%) specimens.

Furthermore, nerves formed by the anastomosis of the medial and lateral plantar nerves in the third web space were not thicker than those of single origin. The argument of these researchers is weakened, as their study was based on cadavers with no known history of symptoms. Levitsky et al (1993) do suggest an alternative anatomical explanation, showing that the intermetatarsal head distance in web spaces two and three were significantly smaller than those in spaces one and four.

Ischaemic theory. In examining postsurgical specimens histologically, Nissen (1948) concluded that, as many of the plantar digital arteries showed severe degenerative changes, including disruption of the arterial wall, thrombosis and incomplete recanalisation, the changes in the nerve were ischaemic in nature. Also, as the common symptoms were of pain occurring after walking a specific distance and persisting as a severe ache for a number of minutes after rest, this bore the stamp of ischaemia (Nissen 1951). Nissen (1948) was unable to provide a reason why the digital vessels to the third web space should be prone to degeneration but proposed that: 'The most likely factor would seem to be repeated minor trauma to the digital artery from pressure transmitted through the sole'. Graham & Johnston (1957) also found ischaemic changes in the plantar digital arteries. Making comparisons between 50 cadaveric specimens of varying ages, they found that although these nerves were normal, arteriolar degeneration was a constant feature in the adult foot. They concluded that this may combine with multiple trauma to bring about pathological changes to neural tissue. Since then, other authors have utilised control groups with specimens obtained from cadavers or amputated limbs and have also demonstrated changes in the plantar digital artery (Meachim & Abberton 1971, Bossley & Cairney 1981, Ringertz & Unander-Scharin 1950).

Bursa theory. Mulder (1951) postulated the role of the 'intermetatarsal' bursa, following an earlier theory, but without being able to substantiate his theory. Some years later, Shephard (1975) produced evidence from a study which suggested that the primary cause may be due to inflammation of the intermetatarsophalangeal bursa, commenting on the adherence of the bursa to the nerve at operation. Some years later, Bossley & Cairney (1981) produced one of the more illuminating pieces of work in recent years as to the possible cause of Morton's neuroma.

Using cadaveric feet, they injected radio-opaque dye into the bursae between the metatarsals. They demonstrated that in the second and third web spaces, the bursa extended beyond the level of the transverse metatarsal ligament and beyond the joint. They also showed that distal to this ligament the bursa wall was

in close approximation to the neurovascular bundle. In the fourth web space, the bursa did not extend as far as the ligament or the joint. This was described as an intermetatarsal bursa, unlike its counterparts which were labelled intermetatarsophalangeal bursae. This helps to explain the paucity of symptoms in the most lateral web spaces. Unfortunately, their study makes no mention of the bursa in the first web space.

Ensuring that the solution was confined to the bursa, Bossley & Cairney (1981) went on to inject steroid into the intermetatarsophalangeal bursa in patients with symptoms. This proved successful in relieving symptoms in all patients, albeit only temporarily in most. They concluded that, on lateral compression, the bursitis is squeezed between the metatarsal heads and irritates the plantar digital nerve, resulting in the pathological changes of secondary fibrosis, a view which was propounded by Mulder some 20 years earlier. They do not elucidate the cause of the bursitis.

Mechanical theory. Some of the above studies made only casual observation of the foot type involved: Graham (1983), laxity of the transverse arch; Nissen (1951), anterior flatfoot; Mulder (1951), splayed metatarsals. None of the studies reviewed goes further than these brief comments and it is regrettable that there is no recorded data pertaining to foot type.

The majority of feet affected tend to be flat, broad, pronating type feet, but not exclusively so. The above studies commenting on the structural abnormalities seem to indicate such foot types. Excessive subtalar joint pronation, which occurs as compensation for forefoot or rearfoot varus, renders the forefoot hypermobile, leading to shearing stress between bone and bursae and causing irritation and subsequent fibrosis of the plantar digital nerve.

Synopsis of aetiology. As none of the above provides a definitive explanation, it is conceivable that the actual cause of Morton's neuroma is not a single factor but a combination of all or some of the above, with anatomical peculiarity, ischaemia, bursa and mechanical theories all playing a role in the aetiological process. Predominantly, this is a condition of females, suggesting an important relationship to footwear, and it is well recognised that if footwear tends to be constrictive, relief of symptoms is achieved upon removal of shoes.

Hypermobility of the forefoot, due mainly to abnormal subtalar joint pronation and compounded by lateral compression from constricting footwear, creates shearing stress and friction on the intermetatarsophalangeal bursa, establishing an inflammatory process. The increased fluid within this bursa produces pressure in the restricted confines of the second and third web spaces. The bursa becomes extruded and impinges on the neurovascular bundle, leading to an entrapment type neuropathy.

Pathohistology. During surgery, neuroma are observed as a fusiform swelling of the nerve which is white and glistening (Fig. 5.22), firm and nodular on palpation (Graham & Johnston 1957). Bickel & Dockerty (1947) demonstrated that neuroma occur in three different sites along the plantar nerve: proximal to, distal to, or at the bifurcation of the digital branch. It should be noted that swellings have been observed in control material and, paradoxically, symptomatic nerves have appeared normal during surgery but resection has provided relief of symptoms.

McElvenny (1943) described the swelling as tumours, labelling them as neurofibromata or angioneuromata. This implicates proliferation of nerve tissue and therefore neoplasm. Winkler et al (1948) could find no evidence of proliferation, concluding that the deposition of hyaline and collagenous material was essentially degenerative in nature, trauma being the most probable cause. Other descriptions available include sclerosing neuroma, endoneural vascular fibrosis and perineural fibrosis.

Meachim & Abberton (1971) provided a comprehensive and objective account of the pathological changes,

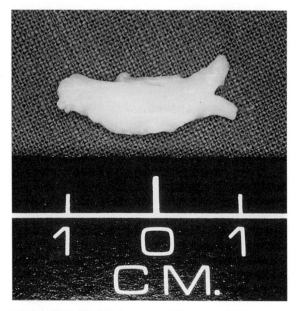

Figure 5.22 Resected neuroma. (Reproduced with permission from G. Hooper, Princess Margaret Rose Orthopaedic Hospital.)

the value in this study being their comparison with a control group. They concluded that the histological findings in Morton's neuroma are not specific; they represent degeneration and reactive changes. They stated that the swelling found in the plantar digital nerve was best described as a 'fibrous nodule', formed by myxofibrosis among fat lobules, fibrous septa and nerve. The nodule envelops and separates nerve bundles, showing a variable amount of segmental degeneration, and usually extends to tendon sheath or bursal lining. The plantar digital artery lies in or near the nodule. Guiloff et al (1984) commented on the marked local thickening of the affected nerve, which was usually adherent to the bursa. This is in keeping with the views of Bossley & Cairney (1981), who also commented on the fibrinoid necrosis of the bursa wall.

The pathological changes to the plantar digital nerve consistent with Morton's neuroma are:

1. variable loss of myelinated fibres
2. excessive collagen deposition in the endoneurium
3. fibrosis of endoneurial blood vessels (endarteritis)
4. fibrosis that is often continuous with the intermetatarsal bursa.

These changes are degenerative and consistent with other forms of nerve entrapment (Gauthier 1979, Lassman 1979).

Management

Conservative. Palliative treatment of this condition is difficult and only likely to be successful when the presenting symptoms are mild. Given that constriction due to footwear is a consistent finding and is likely to be an important aetiological factor, the first line approach to treatment should be to persuade the patient to alter the style of footwear, which alone can provide relief. This can be complemented with forefoot padding or insoles. However, to provide padding in the existing constrictive footwear is likely to exacerbate rather than resolve the problem. If footwear can be changed to allow prescription of palliative orthoses, then redistributive or cushioning padding should be tried and, if successful, converted into an insole.

Other measures include a 'half-boiled egg' pad or metatarsal dome, the function of which is to spread the affected metatarsals, relieving compression from the plantar digital nerve or metatarsophalangeal bursa. Accuracy of application is all-important and is probably best applied on a dynamic leather board template. The apex of the 'egg' should be placed between and just proximal to the affected metatarsal heads.

If the patient presents with an underlying biomechanical anomaly then orthotic control should be attempted (Gaynor et al 1989). Failure of orthotic intervention may be due to the fact that hypermobility creates a permanent nerve pathology, which persists in spite of restoration of function.

Hydrocortisone. Failing these measures, an injection of hydrocortisone is the second line consideration. One millilitre of hydrocortisone, such as a depot preparation of prednisolone, and 1 ml of lignocaine in combination injected into the painful site (as previously indicated) offers symptomatic treatment and some relief of symptoms in the short term, from a few days to, at best, a few months, and occasionally pain reduction is satisfactory. Greenfield et al (1984) obtained complete relief in 30% of patients after a series of injections (average 3.8 injections), and temporary relief in 50%. After 2 years, 17 of 18 patients remained asymptomatic, while 41% had slight discomfort. Gaynor et al (1989) were less successful with cortisone and suggest that, so poor is the outcome of conservative management of Morton's neuroma, the initial treatment should be surgical, thus echoing the sentiments of Jones (1887) a century previously:

Nothing short of an operation is satisfactory . . . operative measures are so safe and simple and other measures so prolonged and troublesome that most patients do not hesitate which course to accept.

Mann & Reynolds (1983) reported that, although patients obtained some relief from conservative management (change of footwear, padding and steroids), the majority (70–80%) were sufficiently symptomatic to elect to have surgery.

Surgical. In the past, when symptoms were so severe, patients were apparently willing to undergo radical operations, including resection of the metatarsal head and toe, as advocated by Jones. In 1940, Betts refined the surgical approach by describing resection of the nerve through a plantar incision.

The plantar incision allows ready access to and a complete view of the nerve. The nerve is exposed through a longitudinal incision of about 3–4 cm between the affected metatarsal heads. The incision is deepened and the nerve located to where it crosses the transverse plantar ligament. The nerve is then traced proximally and the whole nerve and sometimes the vascular bundle are removed. A recent report testifies that the plantar incision is still favoured by British orthopaedic surgeons today (Prior 1995).

The dorsal approach has the twin advantages of avoiding a painful weight-bearing scar, which can be problematic, and allowing for quicker weight-bearing after surgery (see Ch. 20). For these reasons it is the preferred procedure of surgeons in America, presumably for litigation purposes. The incision begins at the

web space and is continued proximally to the level of the metatarsal head. The disadvantage of the dorsal approach is that the neuroma lies deep to the transverse plantar ligament, necessitating division (Mann 1978). This was once thought to be detrimental, leading to splaying of the metatarsals. Addante et al (1986) advocated division of the transverse plantar ligament in all instances, reporting the success of a 'web splitting' approach, originally described by McElvenny (1943).

This incision begins at the metatarsal head, extending between the toes to the plantar skin. The nerve is severed as far proximal as possible and under tension, allowing the stump to retract into the space proximal to the metatarsal heads. The obvious benefit of this procedure is the unobtrusive scar postoperatively. Studies indicate a satisfactory outcome of surgical management in about 80% of cases (Mann & Reynolds 1983, Schroven & Geutjens 1995).

It is generally recognised that recurrence of symptoms is due to the formation of a terminal stump which results from neural regeneration. To avoid terminal nerve stumps, it is advocated that the nerve should be resected sufficiently proximal to the transverse plantar ligament (Johnston et al 1988, Amis et al 1992, Young & Lindsey 1993).

Alternative surgical methods. As reported by Dellon (1992), no other compression neuropathy is treated by complete resection of the affected nerve. The reason that this particular nerve is dealt with in such a manner is probably because the subsequent hypoaesthesia is fairly inconsequential. Although the majority (68%) of interdigital spaces are left permanently numb, Mann & Reynolds (1983) maintain that some patients retain normal sensation. Recovery of sensation must be due to infiltration of surrounding nerves. Nonetheless, trends in surgical approaches seem to be moving away from amputation of the nerve and less aggressive options are being discussed.

Neurolysis involves releasing the nerve from intramuscular fibrosis and fascial slips crossing the nerve. Good results from this technique are reported by Gauthier (1979), Price & Miller (1992) and Dellon (1992). Gauthier, the innovator of this procedure, reported an 83% success rate in his substantial sample size of some 206 patients (304 neuroma). The advantages of this particular method are that sensation is retained and there is no risk of a resultant terminal nerve stump. Percutaneous electrocoagulation has been described by Finney et al (1989), and Barrett & Pinetti (1994) have pioneered the use of endoscopes to decompress the neuroma or entrapped nerve. Angel (1995, personal communication) found success in relocating the nerve dorsal to the transverse plantar ligament without need for resection. If trends continue, complete amputation of the affected nerve in Morton's neuroma might one day be resigned to the archives, but at present it remains the mainstay of treatment for Morton's neuroma.

Fracture of the metatarsals

Stress fracture (fatigue fracture). Stress fractures occur in normal bones subjected to normal forces occurring for a prolonged or repeated period. These forces are insufficient to cause an acute fracture. Classically, the patient was an army recruit, the stress fracture being induced by strenuous military training or route marching (march fracture). This is a good demonstration of the need for adaptive changes in both soft tissues and bony structures (Davis' law and Woolf's law). Stress fractures of the metatarsals can also be seen in highly trained athletes through overuse. In sedentary individuals the cause is usually related to unaccustomed activity.

It has been reported that metatarsal fractures are the most common stress fracture to occur in the lower limb, accounting for 35% (Wilson & Katz 1969). Stress fractures of the metatarsals most frequently involve the second and third, these being the longest and the narrowest. The first metatarsal accounts for 7–8%, and the fourth and fifth for 3% (Levy 1978). Males and females are equally affected, fractures occurring at any age, although rarely before adolescence. Bilateral presentation is rare.

Clinical features. The patient presents with a recent history of dull aching pain in the forefoot, experienced on prolonged weight-bearing and exacerbated by walking. Pain is not severe initially and disappears with rest; if the activity is continued, the pain intensifies. Thorough history-taking is important, often relating to a recent history of some unusual, moderately strenuous activity such as running or dancing.

On examination there will be local tenderness located to one or more metatarsals. Dorsal swelling is a diagnostic feature and will appear 3–10 days after injury, located to the second or third metatarsal. Swelling is accompanied by erythema and should be differentiated from cellulitis.

Radiographs. Dorsoplantar X-rays are the most valuable and initially may appear normal. In the absence of immediate radiological evidence, a stress fracture should be presumed when there is a clear cut clinical history. Radiographic evidence does not always appear until 3 weeks after injury when endosteal and periosteal bone callous becomes evident (Fig. 5.23).

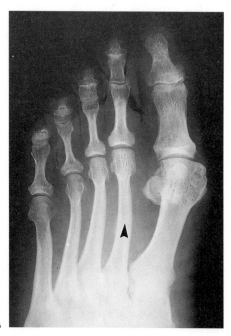
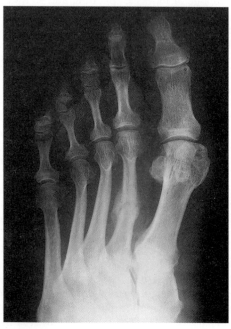

A

B

Figure 5.23   A: Hairline crack in the second metatarsal. B: Same foot 6 weeks after immobilisation in a plaster cast. Bone callus formation denotes good union.

Radioisotope bone scans (scintigraphs) utilising technetium phosphate ^{99m}Tc, (half-life 6 hours) detect metabolic bone changes within 24 hours.

Insufficiency fracture. Insufficiency fractures are defined as a particular type of stress fracture that occurs in abnormal bone under normal stress (Berquist & Johnson 1989). The elderly are prone to insufficiency fractures of the metatarsals as a result of generalised or localised osteoporosis. The latter occasionally present secondary to first ray surgery through disuse atrophy by enforced immobilisation and the altered distribution of forces within the foot (Battey 1980) (Fig. 5.24). Similarly, patients on systemic steroid therapy are also susceptible to this type of fracture.

Traumatic fracture. Resulting from direct injury, the most likely site of fracture is in the neck of the metatarsal, which is narrower and weaker than the shaft. This is usually a complete fracture, except in children when incomplete (greenstick) fractures may occur.

Treatment. Depending on circumstances, palliation such as protective padding, appropriate footwear and advice to rest can suffice. In the young, fit individual, the normal course of events is that the fracture will heal without immobilisation. Sports people should be reassured and refrain from activity for 3–8 weeks. External immobilisation in the form of a below-knee walking plaster cast is advisable for pain relief and quick recovery. Healing is confirmed by periosteal callous formation on follow-up X-rays, 6–8 weeks later.

Box 5.2   Case study: metatarsal fracture

A male, 29 years of age, presented with persistent pain and swelling in the left forefoot of approximately 14 weeks' duration (Fig. 5.23). The problem began after the patient jumped from a bus when there was an audible crack. The patient was concerned about the severity and chronicity of the condition. On examination, the dorsum of the left forefoot was inflamed, swollen and extremely tender. A fracture was diagnosed and X-rays requested. Dorsoplantar films (see also Ch. 3) demonstrated a slight hairline crack in the neck of the second metatarsal. Treatment was to apply a below-knee walking plaster which was left in place for 6 weeks. Follow-up X-rays confirmed bony union with significant callous formation.

Osteochondritis—Freiberg's infraction
(Freiberg's disease)

Osteochondritis of the second metatarsal, Freiberg's infraction, is a common, crushing-type osteochondritis (juvenilis) leading to avascular necrosis (osteonecrosis) of the metatarsals. The second metatarsal is most commonly involved (68%), then the third (27%), but rarely the fourth or fifth (Gauthier & Elbaz 1978). Both feet are equally affected and the condition is most prevalent in adolescence (most commonly ages 12–14 years), affecting females more than males. Despite being considered a condition of teenagers, it may occur at any age and its occurrence in later life is recognised (Hay & Smith 1992). Presentation in the adult foot is more likely to be due to premature osteoarthritis of the metatarsophalangeal joint.

Clinical features. The patient presents with pain in the region of the involved metatarsal head and painful limitation of metatarsophalangeal joint movement, particularly extension, which may elicit crepitus. Patients may additionally have difficulty standing on tiptoe when tested. Palpation of the dorsal surface of the metatarsal head, with the toe flexed, will reveal a distinctive diagnostic bony ridge and can be accompanied by diffuse soft tissue swelling.

Aetiology. Freiberg (1914) noticed skin callus under

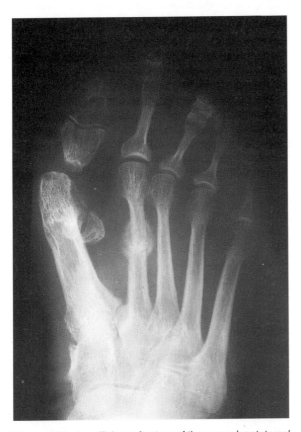

Figure 5.24 Insufficiency fracture of the second metatarsal following Keller's arthroplasty of the first metatarsophalangeal joint.

the second metatarsal head, and presumed that a long second metatarsal might predispose to trauma resulting in this disorder. Since then it has been reported as the result of some incident to the epiphyseal plate, namely an interruption of the blood supply to the epiphyseal bone, such as occlusion of a small end artery possibly related to trauma. The metatarsal head receives its blood supply from radial arteries that penetrate the bone medially and laterally and unite to form a central arterial network. Branches from this network supply the subchondral bone. Congenital anomalies in the blood supply or damage to the vessels may place the metatarsal head at risk.

Excessive pressure on the second metatarsal head, leading to microfractures, has not been substantiated by recent foot pressure assessments (Stanley et al 1990). They proposed that the length of the metatarsal was the most important factor, demonstrating that the second was the longest metatarsal in 85% of feet in their study. Correspondingly, a short first metatarsal may also be significant in overloading the second metatarsal head.

Pathology. An interference with the blood supply results in avascular necrosis of the subchondral bone which becomes more dense. Initially there are no radiographic changes, until the head of the metatarsal head collapses (Fig. 5.25). When this does occur, there is increased density of bone (osteosclerosis), with expansion of the metatarsal head and neck. There then follows a reparative process, with formation of bone callus which is subsequently converted to normal bone. Later, there is flattening of the articular surface and expansion of the metatarsal head, and, although initially preserved, eventually there is loss of joint space and osteophytosis which may fragment, resulting in loose bodies in and around the joint. There may also be cortical thickening (hypertrophy) of the metatarsal shaft.

Smillie (1957) summarised the pathological changes into five stages:

1. fissure fracture
2. bone absorption
3. bone absorption with sinking of central portion
4. loose body separation
5. flattening deformity and arthrosis of the second metatarsophalangeal joint.

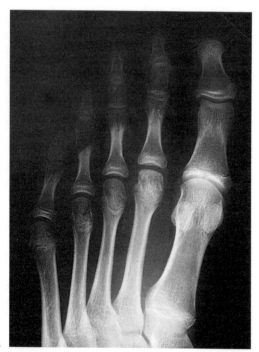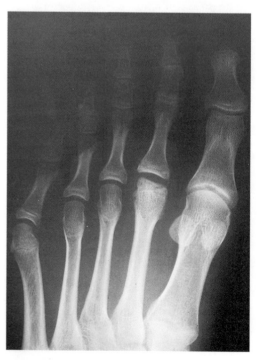

A   B

Figure 5.25 A: Freiberg's infraction—radiographs of the foot on initial presentation appear normal. B: Radiographs taken 6 months later; these demonstrate collapse of the metatarsal head and a positive diagnosis of Freiberg's infraction.

Treatment. Initially, conservative measures involve local redistributive padding, and insoles incorporating metatarsal bars may provide benefit. Adaptations to footwear, namely rocker soles may be advantageous, but are difficult to implement in the younger patient. Local injections of hydrocortisone offer symptomatic treatment, providing only some short-term relief.

Surgery. If the above measures prove to be unsuccessful then a variety of surgical techniques are available, dictated by the severity of symptoms and the age of the patient. Gauthier's procedure is performed on the basis that mainly the dorsal articular surface of the second metatarsal head is damaged and the plantar portion preserved. A wedge of bone (base 5 mm) is removed from the neck of the metatarsal and the head reflected backwards as a dorsireflexory osteotomy (Tollafield 1993). Smith et al (1991) describe excellent results produced by shortening the metatarsal. In the older patient, where degenerative changes are the cause of discomfort, a proximal hemiphalangectomy is more appropriate.

Hallux sesamoids

Adult hallux sesamoids have dorsal cartilaginous facets articulating with the metatarsal head. The joint capsule encloses the superior articular margin of each sesamoid, while fibres of the flexor hallucis brevis tendon invest its rough, non-articular surface. The sesamoids are separated from each other by the flexor hallucis longus tendon on its way to insertion into the distal phalanx. The hallux sesamoids are situated at a point of maximum pressure and they serve to elevate the metatarsal head and protect it and the long flexor tendon.

Developmental variations. Sesamoids may have one, two or more centres of ossification. This results in partition of the sesamoids and they may be bi-, tri-, quadri- or multi-partite. According to Inge & Ferguson (1933), tibial partite sesamoids occur in about 10% of the population, and partition is unilateral 75% of the time. The tibial sesamoid is usually the larger. Partite sesamoids are much larger than their normal counterpart and their parts are well corticated all round.

Symptomatic sesamoids. Partite sesamoids themselves can be the source of pain. Sesamoid injuries are more frequently seen in pes cavus type feet with a rigid plantarflexed first ray.

Causes of pain in the sesamoids

Fracture. True fracture of the sesamoids is rare and is more likely to be stress-related. Tibial sesamoids are more frequently affected.

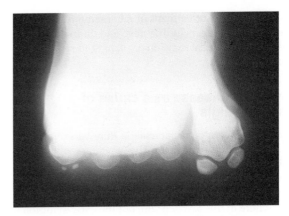

Figure 5.26 Tangential (skyline) view of the hallux sesamoid bones. This X-ray also demonstrates sesamoid bones at the fifth metatarsophalangeal joint.

Clinical features are those of pain on walking, particularly during the propulsive phase, and swelling localised to the metatarsal head. Anterior/posterior and axial (skyline) views are required for a positive diagnosis (Fig. 5.26). Close scrutiny of the X-ray film is required to differentiate fractures from partite sesamoids.

Fractures are mainly of the tibial sesamoid. A fractured sesamoid is not corticated at its fracture line and is only slightly longer than its normal neighbours, and as large. A bipartite sesamoid is usually larger than a single sesamoid and partite segments are usually oval with smooth concave/convex opposing edges, whereas fractures exhibit an irregular, serrated line of division with interruption of the peripheral cortex and exaggerated separation of segments. The partition lines are usually transverse, as opposed to oblique or longitudinal. The following are also worth consideration: an unusual position, multiplicity of fragments, absence of similar findings on opposite side and, lastly, bone callus on subsequent films.

Chondromalacia of the sesamoid (sesamoiditis). In the foot, chondromalacia exclusively involves the tibial sesamoid (usually bipartite) and is the result of repetitive mechanical stress. Pain is located to the medial sesamoid, occurring only on weight-bearing.

Osteochondritis (Treve's disease). Avascular necrosis of the sesamoids is uncommon. It is characterised by irregularity of the trabecular pattern, giving a stippled appearance on X-ray. Its cause may be related to a crush fracture.

Arthritis. The sesamoids may undergo degenerative changes and can become eroded with rheumatoid arthritis.

Treatment. The treatment of all sesamoid injuries is much the same, including rest and immobilisation. Sometimes surgical excision or planing to reduce their bulk is required.

Systemic disease as a cause of metatarsalgia

Systemic causes of metatarsalgia may be exemplified in rheumatoid arthritis. The metatarsophalangeal joints are affected in 90% of patients with this disease and are often the first site of onset. The features of the established rheumatoid foot are discussed at length elsewhere in this text (Ch. 26), but the early symptoms have relevance at this point as an important differential diagnosis from the aforementioned functional and non-functional causes.

The incidences of initial hand and foot involvement are approximately equal (15.7% versus 14.7% respectively). Radiologically, erosive changes most commonly appear first in the feet. The first site of erosions is found at the fifth metatarsal, followed by the third, fourth, second, and then the first, the daylight sign (Fig. 5.27). In rheumatoid disease, the response to pressure is the formation of bursae over the prominent metatarsal heads, offering intrinsic protection. A familiar picture is that of individual bursae overlying each of the metatarsal heads. These become extremely tender and in chronic conditions may be prone to ulceration (Fig. 5.28). Treatment is palliative, aimed at restoring the natural upholstery by the use of cushioning materials. Forefoot arthroplasties such as Fowler's

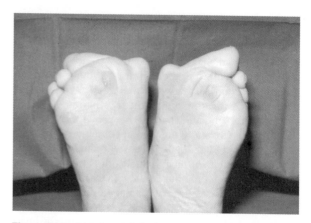

Figure 5.28   Metatarsalgia in rheumatoid disease, with characteristic prominent, painful metatarsal heads.

or Kates Kessel and Kay procedures are justified when pain is unremitting or when ulceration is recurrent despite attempts at palliation (see Ch. 26).

Other systemic diseases giving rise to pain in the metatarsophalangeal area in adults are gout (primarily the first metatarsophalangeal joint) and those diseases leading to neuropathic changes in the foot (see Ch. 25).

DIGITAL MALFUNCTIONS AND DEFORMITIES

Retracted toes

In this condition, the toes are drawn back into a dorsiflexed position and are less effective in locomotion. They are subjected to shoe pressure on the dorsum of the interphalangeal joints with resultant dorsal lesions. The condition may be one aspect of the ankle equinus, with limitation of dorsiflexion of the foot, tightness of the tendo Achilles group of muscles, relative inefficiency of the tibialis anterior, and overaction of the digital extensors in assisting dorsiflexion of the foot. This is termed extensor substitution.

The primary condition needs correction or accommodation, as previously described. Additionally, exercises may be indicated to improve the muscle imbalance. Orthodigital splints are effective in improving the alignment and function of the toes, and protecting their dorsal surfaces from shoe pressure. Surgical correction is discussed in Chapter 20.

Claw toes

In this condition, the interphalangeal joints are flexed and the toes are drawn into a claw-like position. They

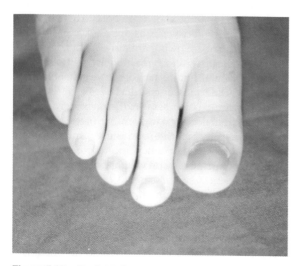

Figure 5.27   Daylight sign: metatarsophalangeal joint synovitis.

are usually extended at the metatarsophalangeal joints and may suffer from greatly increased pressure on their apices and on the dorsum of their proximal interphalangeal joints. These areas are commonly the sites of painful and persistent apical and dorsal helomata and/or bursitis.

In some cases, the deformity is merely the end result of persistent impaction and constriction from ill-fitting footwear. More commonly it is symptomatic of various alternative aetiologies.

In abnormal pronation of the foot, the tibialis posterior and the long digital flexors may overact to maintain stability. In so doing, the long flexors overpower the interossei and lumbricales, thus buckling and clawing the toes. This process is termed flexor stabilisation.

In pes cavus of neurological origin, notably Charcot–Marie–Tooth disease, wasting of the intrinsic muscles, which normally keep the toes straight, results in imbalanced flexor/extensor activity which contracts the toes into the typical clawed toe deformity. In other cases of pes cavus, where there is no neurological involvement, the forefoot is both adducted and plantarflexed at the midtarsal or tarsometatarsal joints. The toes are correspondingly abducted and dorsiflexed at their articulations with the metatarsals. Their lumbricales and interossei are mechanically at a disadvantage, and the action of the long flexors and extensors on the terminal phalanges is consequently unrestrained. Without the moderating influence of the lumbricales and interossei on the interphalangeal joints, the toes are contracted into the clawed position.

Overaction of the long flexors may also occur to compensate for weakness of the tendo Achilles group in locomotion—flexor substitution.

In upper motor neurone lesions, clawing of the toes occurs from spasmodic contraction of the long and short digital flexors. This phenomenon may also be seen in rheumatoid arthritis, as a result of the inflammatory process in the interphalangeal joints.

Clawing of the toes entails progressive subluxation of the metatarsophalangeal joints, so that the metatarsal heads are more firmly held in contact with the ground and thereby overloaded in locomotion. This deformation of the metatarsal segments is clearly seen in clawing of the hallux. The first metatarsal is plantarflexed, the proximal phalanx extended and the distal phalanx flexed. This deformity is sometimes incorrectly called hallux flexus, but that term should be confined to flexion deformity of the whole toe, and not just the terminal phalanx as in this case. Plantar hyperkeratosis develops under the first metatarsal head and possibly under the distal phalanx, and a dorsal lesion may

appear over the interphalangeal joint. The latter may develop into a bursitis and an underlying exostosis. The lesser toes may be subjected to similar lesions on their dorsal surfaces and/or their apices. Ulceration and infection may supervene at any of these sites.

Management

The conservative management of claw toes is directed to the treatment of their associated lesions and to protective padding. For the middle toes, orthodigital splints provide the most effective means of protection. For the first and fifth toes, individual shields in silicone or latex rubber are generally more satisfactory. Surgery is indicated if the deformities of the toes are too marked and well established to be controlled adequately by conservative means. Arthrodesis of the interphalangeal joints of the lesser toes may be carried out, and for the hallux, transfer of the tendon of extensor hallucis longus to the neck of the first metatarsal (Chs 20 and 21).

Hammer toe

This is essentially a plantarflexion deformity of the proximal interphalangeal joint, the distal interphalangeal joint remaining normal or possibly dorsiflexed. It may occur in any of the three middle toes, the second being the most commonly affected. The proximal phalanx is extended and the deformity therefore exposes the proximal interphalangeal joint to dorsal pressure and friction, and the apex of the toe to concentrated pressure as it bears weight. The abnormal joint positions become more or less fixed by adaptive contractures of the surrounding capsule and tendons, depending on how long the deformity has persisted. In most early cases, it is possible to correct the deformity with the use of corrective padding and manipulation, which may have to be applied for a prolonged period. Ankylosis of the proximal interphalangeal joint may occur in long-standing cases.

The deformity is caused in various ways. It may be concomitant with a short first metatarsal segment, the abnormally short hallux exposing the second toe—and possibly the third—to impaction from footwear fitted too short because the unusual digital formula has been overlooked. The second toe is commonly deformed by pressure from an abducted hallux, which may more or less override the intermediate and distal phalanges. The fourth toe often becomes hammered because the fifth toe underrides it, elevating its proximal phalanx and causing shoe pressure on the dorsum of the proximal interphalangeal joint. The immediate cause of deviation of the fifth toe is pressure from the lateral side of the shoe, which may be too narrow or pointed, but hallux valgus and splaying of the metatarsals are the main factors, coupled with the abduction of the forefoot where this occurs in pes valgus.

Where all three of the middle toes are affected, the primary cause may lie in failure of the lumbricales to keep the toes straight in locomotion, thus allowing the proximal phalanges to be excessively dorsiflexed on their respective metatarsal heads. The digital flexors then act more powerfully on the intermediate and distal phalanges, flexing them into deformity ('flexor stabilisation').

The chief effect of these deformities is to cause painful and persistent digital helomata. Inflammation of adventitious bursae also commonly occurs on the dorsal sites, particularly on the second and fourth toes, occasionally becoming secondarily infected. Ulceration may occur at the apices, especially where the nutrition of the tissues is impaired by circulatory, neurological or metabolic deficiencies. Painful nail conditions may also arise from persistent trauma to the distal phalanges.

Management

Conservative management is directed to correction of deformities by splinting and manipulation, where correction is still possible, or to provide maximum protection of both dorsal and apical pressure points in chronic cases. Padding to deflect pressure may be necessary to bring a particular lesion under control, but the maximum degree of protection or correction can be ensured only by controlling the position and alignment of all three toes simultaneously. This ensures that correction or protection of one toe is not obtained at the cost of displacement of the others.

Surgery is indicated if conservative treatment does not resolve the problem of recurrent pressure lesions other than by its long-term application. An arthrodesis of the proximal interphalangeal joint may be performed, correcting any flexion deformity (Fig. 5.29). It may be necessary to divide the capsule and the tendon at the metatarsophalangeal joint to correct dorsiflexion of the proximal phalanx. In older patients, an alternative is to remove the proximal half of the proximal phalanx of the affected toe, making it slightly floppy and able to take up a position where there is no pressure upon it (Ch. 20).

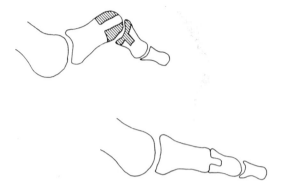

Figure 5.29 Arthrodesis for hammer toe.

Mallet toe

This is an abnormal plantarflexion of the distal phalanx only, most commonly of the second or third toes. It may be the cause of persistent apical lesions but can also be symptom free. It is amenable to the same treatment as hammer toes by means of orthodigital splints. If pressure on the apex is insufficiently relieved by the use of deflective padding it may be straightened by arthrodesis of the terminal interphalangeal joint. Partial amputation, although less acceptable aesthetically, is an effective alternative.

Digitus quintus varus

This common deformity of the fifth toe is often congenital (see Ch. 4), but if it appears in adulthood it is most commonly acquired. As with hallux abductovalgus, the persistent moulding effect of pointed footwear is a relevant factor, but the abduction of the forefoot secondary to pes planovalgus is probably more important. The toe is not only abducted but axially rotated and flexed, indicating an oblique pull on the phalanges by the flexor tendons due to the abduction of the forefoot on the hindfoot.

The deformity is the immediate cause of painful pressure lesions dorsally, interdigitally and distally, which can be best relieved by the latex or silicone rubber shields designed to provide optimum correction and protection. The abnormal pronation leading to the abduction of the forefoot must also be adequately controlled and any footwear faults eliminated as far as possible. Surgery may be indicated (Ch. 20).

REFERENCES

Addante J B, Peicott P S, Wong K Y, Brooks D L 1986 Interdigital neuromas: results of surgical excision of 152 neuromas. Journal of the American Podiatic Medical Association 76(9): 493–495

Amis J A, Siverhus S W, Liwnicz B H 1992 An anatomic basis for recurrence after Morton's neuroma excision. Foot and Ankle 13(3): 153–156

Banadda B, Gona G, Vaz R, Ndlovu D 1992 Calcaneal spurs in a black African population, Foot and Ankle 13(6): 352–354

Barnicott N A, Hardy R H 1955 The position of the hallux in West Africans. Journal of Anatomy 89: 355–361

Barrett S L, Pignetti T T 1994 Endoscopic decompression for intermetatarsal nerve entrapment – the EDIN technique: preliminary study with cadaveric specimens; early clinical results. 33(5): 503–508

Battey M A 1980 The lesser metatarsal stress fracture as a complication of the Keller's procedure. Journal of the American Podiatry Association 4(70): 182–186

Beito S B, Krych S M, Harkless L B 1989 Recalcitrant heel pain: traumatic fibrosis versus heel neuroma. Journal of the American Podiatric Medical Association 79(7): 336–339

Berquist T H, Johnson K A 1989 Trauma. In: Berquist T H (ed) Radiology of the foot and ankle. Raven Press, New York, ch 3, p 197

Betts L O 1940 Morton's metatarsalgia: neuritis of the fourth digital nerve. Medical Journal of Australia 1: 514–515

Bickel W H, Dockerty M B 1947 Plantar neuromas, Morton's toe. Surg. Gynecol. Obstet., 84: 111–116

Bossley C J, Cairney P C 1981 The intermetatarso-phalangeal bursa – its significance in Morton's metatarsalgia. Journal of Bone and Joint Surgery 62B(2): 184–187

Buschmann W R, Jahss M H, Kummer F, Dessai P, Gee R, Ricci J 1995 Histology and histomorphometric analysis of the normal and atrophic heel fat pad. Foot and Ankle 16(5): 254–258

Cimino W R 1990 Tarsal tunnel syndrome: review of the literature. Foot and Ankle 11(1): 47–51

Crawford F, Snaith M 1996 How effective is therapeutic ultrasound in the treatment of heel pain? Annals of the Rheumatic Diseases 55

Daly P J, Kitaoko H B, Chao E Y S 1992 Plantar fasciotomy for intractable plantar fasciitis: clinical results and biomechanical evaluation. Foot and Ankle 13: 188–195

Dananberg H J 1993a Gait style as an etiology to chronic postural pain, part I. Functional hallux limitus. Journal of the American Podiatric Medical Association 83(8)

Dananberg H J 1993b Gait style as an etiology to chronic postural pain, part II. Postural compensatory process. Journal of the American Podiatric Medical Association 83(11)

Dellon L A 1992 Treatment of Morton's neuroma as a nerve compression. The role for neurolysis. Journal of the American Podiatric Medical Association 82: 399–402

Elftmann H 1960 The transverse tarsal joint and its control. Clinical Orthopaedics 16: 41–45

Finney W, Wiener S N, Catanzariti F 1989 Treatment of Morton's neuroma using percutaneous electrocoagulation.

Journal of the American Podiatric Medical Association 79(12): 615–618

Frey C et al 1992 The retrocalcaneal bursa: anatomy and bursography. Foot and Ankle 13(4): 203–207

Furey J G 1975 Plantar fasciitis: the painful heel syndrome. Journal of Bone and Joint Surgery 57A: 672–673

Gauthier G 1979 Thomas Morton disease: a nerve entrapment syndrome. Clinical Orthopaedics 142: 90–93

Gauthier G, Elbaz R 1978 Freiberg's infraction: a subchondral bone fatigue fracture, a new surgical technique. Clinicial Orthopaedics and Related Research 142: 93–95

Gaynor R, Hake D, Spinner S M, Tomczak R L 1989 A comparative analysis of conservative versus surgical treatment of Morton's neuroma. Journal of the American Podiatric Medical Association 79(1): 27–30

Gerster J C 1980 Plantar fasciitis and Achilles tendinitis among 150 cases of seronegative spondarthritis. Rheum and Rehab 19: 218–222

Gerster J C, Paccinin 1984 Enthesopathy of the heels in juvenile onset sero-negative B27 positive spondylo-arthropathy. J. Rheum 12(2): 310–314

Giannestras N J 1973 Foot disorders – medical and surgical management, 2nd edn. Lea and Febiger, Philadelphia

Graham C E 1983 Painful heel syndrome: rationale of diagnosis and treatment. Foot and Ankle 3(5): 261–267

Graham W D, Johnston C R 1957 Plantar digital neuroma. Lancet 7: 470–471

Greenfield J, Rea J, Ilfield F 1984 Morton's interdigital neuroma: indications for treatment for local injection versus surgery. Clinical Orthopaedics 185: 142–144

Guiloff R J, Scadding J W, Klenerman L 1984 Morton's metatarsalgia: clinical, electrophysical and histological observations. Journal of Bone and Joint Surgery 66B: 586–591

Hardy R H, Clapham J C R 1952 Hallux valgus – predisposing anatomical causes. Lancet 1180–1183

Hay S M, Smith T W D 1992 Freiberg's disease: an unusual presentation at the age of 50 years. Foot 2: 176–178

Hayes K W 1992 The effect of awareness of measurement error on physical therapists' confidence in their decisions. Physical Therapy 72(7): 515–561

Hicks J H 1953 The mechanics of the foot, 1. The joints. Journal of Anatomy 87: 345

Hicks J H 1954 The mechanics of the foot, 2. The plantar aponeurosis and the arch. Journal of Anatomy 88: 25–31

Hill J J, Cutting P J 1989 Heel pain and body weight. Foot and Ankle 9(6): 254–256

Howells R J 1994 Plantar heel pain. Journal of Bone and Joint Surgery 74(B): 850

Inge G, Ferguson A 1933 Surgery of the sesamoid bones of the great toe. Archives of Surgery 27: 466–489

Johnson J E, Johnson K A, Unni K K 1988 Persistent pain after excision of an interdigital neuroma. Journal of Bone and Joint Surgery 70A(5): 651–657

Johnston O 1956 Further studies of the inheritance of hand and foot anomalies. Clinical Orthopaedics 8: 146–160

Jones R 1887 Plantar neuralgia. Liverpool Medico-Chirurgical Journal, January

Kidd R 1991 An examination of the validation of some of the more questionable cornerstones of modern chiropodial diagnosis. Journal of British Podiatric Medicine, September: 172–173

Lam S J S 1967 Tarsal tunnel syndrome. Journal of Bone and Joint Surgery 49B(1): 87–97

Lapidus PW, Guidoff F P 1965 Painful heel: report of 323 patients with 364 painful heels. Clinical Orthopaedics 39: 178–186

Lassman G 1979 Morton's toe: clinical, light and electron microscopic investigations in 133 cases. Clinical Orthopaedics 142: 73–83

Levitsky K A, Alman B A, Jevsevar D S, Morehead J 1993 Digital nerves of the foot: anatomic variations and implications regarding the pathogenesis of interdigital neuroma. Foot and Ankle 14(4): 208–230

Levy J M 1978 Stress fractures of the first metatarsal. AJR 130: 679–681

McElvenney R T 1943 The etiology and surgical treatment of intractable pain about the fourth metatarsophalangeal joint (Morton's toe). Journal of Bone and Joint Surgery 25B(3): 675–679

Mann R 1978 Diseases of the nerves of the foot. In: Mann R (ed) DuVries surgery of the foot, 4th edn. Mosby, St Louis, p 463–468

Mann R, Reynolds J 1983 Interdigital neuroma: a critical analysis. Foot and Ankle 3: 238–243

Manter J T 1941 Movements of the subtalar and transverse tarsal joints. Anatomical Record 80: 4

Meachim G, Abberton M J 1971 Histological findings in Morton's metatarsalgia. Journal of Pathology 103: 209–217

Menz H B 1995 Clinical hindfoot measurement: a critical review of the literature. Foot 5: 57–64

Mitchell I R, Meyer C, Krueger W A 1991 Deep fascia of the foot: anatomical and clinical considerations. Journal of the American Podiatric Medical Association 81(7): 373–378

Mulder J D 1951 The causative mechanism in Morton's metatarsalgia. Journal of Bone and Joint Surgery 33B(1): 94–95

Nissen K I 1948 Plantar digital neuritis: Morton's metatarsalgia. Journal of Bone and Joint Surgery 30B: 84–94

Nissen K I 1951 The etiology of Morton's metatarsalgia. Journal of Bone and Joint Surgery 33B(2): 293–294

Pollak R A, Bellacosa R A, Dornbluth N C, Strash W W, Devall J M 1992 Sonographic analysis of Morton's neuroma. Journal of Foot Surgery 31(6): 534–537

Price B A, Miller G 1992 Internal neurolysis. Journal of Foot Surgery 31(3): 250–259

Prichasuk S 1994 The heel pad in plantar heel pain. Journal of Bone and Joint Surgery 76B(1): 140–142

Prichasuk S, Subhadrabandhu 1994 The relationship of pes planus and calcaneal spur to plantar heel pain. Clinical Orthopaedics and Related Research 306: 192–196

Prior T D 1995 British orthopaedic foot surgery society: review of the thirteenth annual scientific meeting. Journal of Bone and Joint Surgery 7(1): 19

Redd R A, Peters V J, Emery S F, Branch H M, Rifkin M D 1989 Morton's neuroma: songraphic evaluation. Radiology 171: 415–417

Resch S, Stenstrom A, Jonsson A, Jonsson K 1994 The diagnostic efficacy of magnetic resonance imaging and ultrasonography in Morton's neuroma: a radiological–surgical correlation. Foot and Ankle 15(2): 88–92

Resnick D, Feingold M L, Curd J, Niwayama G, Goergen T D 1977 Calcaneal abnormalities in articular disorders. Radiology 125: 355–366

Ringertz N, Unander-Scharin L 1950 Morton's disease – a clinical and patho-anatomical study. Acta Orthop Scand 19: 327

Root M L, Orien W P, Weed J H 1977 Normal and abnormal function of the foot. Clinical biomechanics, vol II. Clinical Biomechanics Corporation, Los Angeles

Sartoris D J, Brozinsky S, Resnick D 1989 Magnetic resonance Images. Journal of Foot Surgery 28(1): 78–82

Schon L, Glennon T, Baxter D 1993 Heel pain syndrome: electrodiagnostic support for nerve entrapment. Foot and Ankle 14(3): 129–135

Schroven I, Geutjens G 1995 Results of excision of the interdigital nerve in the treatment of Morton's metatarsalgia. Foot 5: 196–198

Shephard E 1975 Intermetatarsophalangeal bursitis in the causation of Morton's metatarsalgia. Journal of Bone and Joint Surgery 57B(1): 115–116

Shereff M J, Bejjani F J, Kummer F J 1986 Kinematics of the first metatarsophalangeal joint. Journal of Bone and Joint Surgery 68A(3)

Shine I 1965 Incidence of hallux valgus in a partially shoe wearing community. British Medical Journal 5461: 1648–1650

Sim Fook L, Hodgson A R 1958 A comparison of foot forms among non-shoe and shoe wearing Chinese populations. Journal of Bone and Joint Surgery 40: 1058–1052

Smillie I S 1957 Freiberg's infraction (Kohler's second disease). Journal of Bone and Joint Surgery 39B: 580

Smith T W D, Stanley D, Rowley D I 1991 Treatment of Freiberg's disease: a new operative technique. Journal of Bone and Joint Surgery 73B: 129–130

Snijders C J, Snijders J G N, Philippens M M G M 1986 Biomechanics of hallux valgus and spread foot. Foot and Ankle 7(1)

Snook G A, Chrisman O D 1972 The management of subcalcaneal pain. Clinical Orthopaedics 82: 163–168

Stanley D, Betts R P, Rowley D I, Smith T W D 1990 Assessment of the etiologic factors in the development of Freiberg's disease. Journal of Foot Surgery 29(5): 444–447

Thomas N, Nissen K I, Helal B 1989 Disorders of the lesser rays. In: Helal, Wilson (eds) The foot. Churchill Livingstone, Edinburgh, p 493–499

Tollafield D R 1993 Freiberg's infraction: surgical management by osteotomy; a forgotten technique? British Journal of Podiatric Medicine and Surgery 5(2):

Turan I, Lindgren U, Sahlstedt T 1991 Computed tomography for diagnosis of Morton's neuroma. Journal of Foot Surgery 30(3): 244–245

Unger H R, Mattoso P Q, Drusen M J, Neumann C H 1992 Gadopentetate-enhanced magnetic resonance imaging with fat saturation in the evaluation of Morton's neuroma. Journal of Foot Surgery 31(3): 245

Wainwright A M, Kelly A J, Winson I G 1995 Calcaneal spurs and plantar fasciitis. Foot 5(3): 123–126

Wall J R, Harkness M A, Crawford A 1993 Ultrasound diagnosis of plantar fasciitis. Foot and Ankle 14(8): 465–469

Wapner K L, Sharkey P F 1991 The use of night splints for treatment of recalcitrant plantar fasciitis. Foot and Ankle 12: 135–137

Whiting M F 1974 Pain in the plantar fascia and associated tissues. Chiropodist, September, 275–295

Williams R 1993 The foot: a joint approach. From the report

of a seminar at the Royal Society of Medicine by C E Thomson. Journal of British Podiatric Medicine 48(9): 151–152

Williams P L, Smibert J G, Cox R, Mitchell R, Klenerman L 1987 Imaging study of the painful heel syndrome. Foot and Ankle 17: 345–349

Wilson E S, Katz F N 1969 Stress fractures: an analysis of 250 consecutive cases. Radiology 92: 481–486

Winkler H, Feltner J B, Kimmelstiel P 1948 Morton's metatarsalgia. Journal of Bone and Joint Surgery 30A(2): 496–500

Winson I G, Lundberg A, Bylund C 1994 The pattern of motion of the longitudinal arch of the foot. Foot 4(3): 151–154

Wolgin et al 1994 Conservative treatment of plantar heel pain: long term follow-up. Foot and Ankle 15(3): 97–102

Young G, Lindsey J 1993 Etiology of symptomatic recurrent interdigital neuromas. Journal of American Podiatric Medical Association 83(5): 255–258

6

Patient education

G. Dunlop

Keywords

Communication
Compliance
Health education
Health promotion
Memory
Patient education
Teaching methods

The specific goal of patient education is to teach patients about their illness, and about their health, in order that they can become more involved in the decisions that are made concerning their own care. Teaching patients is not new to patient care and has been practised throughout the latter part of this century by medical carers with varying degrees of success and failure. However, recent developments in patient care have established a need for medical carers to adopt good patient education practice into their daily, routine patient care and to be effective in the use of patient education techniques. Recent changes in attitude towards the overall approach to patient care, such as the introduction of the Patient's Charter, have established the principle that patients must be better informed as a means of ensuring equity in patient care. As an example, the Patient's Charter, which was published in 1991, promises that all patients who use the National Health Service in Scotland are given 'accurate, relevant and understandable explanations' and that they 'will be involved so far as is practical in making decisions about their own care, and wherever possible given choices'.

Other developments that have contributed to a change in attitude to patient care are the introduction of health promotion, particularly in the Western world, which is set to improve health for individual nations by making people more aware of how to maintain a healthy lifestyle; as well as the move to encourage health professionals to consider psychosocial issues associated with illness when caring for an individual patient. Providing the patient with knowledge about her condition is simply an approach to patient care that recognises the patient as an active participant in the caring process and not merely a passive recipient who is expected to conform with little or no understanding.

Medical carers should now consider the patient as part of the health care team, as someone who can contribute to the development of her own care and help to make decisions on how the care may be conducted. Patient empowerment is advocated by the World Health Organization (WHO 1978) as being a basic human right of every individual in matters concerning their health and welfare. Patients must be well informed so that they can adopt good health practice in relation to their own lifestyle and within the context of their own social demands. Informing patients about their health and illness is merely a means to establishing good patient relationship, and goes some way to maintaining patient compliance (Sarafino 1990, Sheridan & Radmacher 1992).

An explanation of the purpose of patient education is perhaps necessary, as the term is often used synonymously with health education or with health promotion. There are, however, distinct differences between these three terms even though they are interlinked:

1. Health promotion aims at achieving equal opportunities for all members of society, both for those who are well and for those who are sick, in order that they may achieve their fullest health potential (WHO 1978). Health promotion is a means of preventing disease and seeks to improve the health status of the individual, and of communities as a whole, by making people more aware of how they may improve their health or prevent disease. British government legislation, such as the White Papers in 1989 and 1991 on health care, advocate the use of health promotion initiatives in the care of all patients.

2. Health education also aims at preventing disease and illness, but is a method of achieving health promotion. Teaching members of the public about healthy lifestyles and potential risk factors is one of the ways of promoting health for members of society and is probably most familiar to the public in the form of advertising campaigns or distribution of leaflets.

3. Patient education is also concerned with prevention but is aimed specifically at individuals who are receiving health care. The education, therefore, is more likely to be concerned with the issues surrounding the patient's condition and is generally conducted between a health professional and the patient. The purpose of patient education is to provide the patient with information about her condition in order that she may become more actively involved in the care and maintenance of her own health.

HOW IS PATIENT EDUCATION PRACTISED?

Patient education, therefore, involves more than giving patients advice about their condition(s) or giving instructions about the treatment programme. Common practice in educating patients would be to give patients detailed information on matters dealing with the cause of their complaint; the development of the condition; the therapeutic options available to treat the condition; prevention; how the condition may be aggravated or encouraged to recur; the likely outcome; short- and long-term effects on lifestyle; and self-monitoring of the condition. Therefore patient education must be patient-specific, being tailor-made for each individual patient in order to establish relevant information for each individual. Just as each patient receives individual consultation in order to establish her own special health care needs, each patient must be given personal education to sustain those health care needs. Patient education, must therefore be integrated into each patient consultation and thus become as normal a process as examining a patient or as planning a care programme. Medical carers should aim for a patient consultation that encourages patient interaction, and an environment for patients to discuss their concerns and anxieties, which are just as relevant to the health complaint as are the signs and symptoms. Medical carers should seek to develop a caring environment that is patient-centred, encouraging patients to ask questions about their condition, and responding by giving patients information that is useful and helpful to their needs (Webb 1994). However, what is equally important is that the patient is able to understand the information given, is able to remember the information and is confident enough to use it to care for her own health and illness. Information given to patients should be such that it will help them understand the care of the condition, enabling them to have more control in maintaining their own health care. If patients are more knowledgeable about their care then they can become more involved in the decisions that are made concerning the treatment of their condition (see Box 6.1). Consideration should be given to the fact that the patient has a very large part to play when treating the condition, and in many instances, the treatment will only progress as far as the patient wishes.

Box 6.1 Case study 1: self-monitoring by the patient after avulsion and phenolisation of the nails

The healing process after the avulsion and phenolisation of nails requires close monitoring, much of which can be carried out by the patient, who can be taught to change the dressings as well as how to assess the healing process. A female patient of 49 years of age, who was to have the nails of the hallux of both toes avulsed, was informed that she would be expected to be involved in the postoperative care, which was to consist of changing the dressings and checking the appearance of the area. The patient was in agreement with the proposed arrangement and problems were were identified which would prevent the patient from doing so. Prior to the procedure, the patient was given written instructions as well as information concerning the arrangements she should make.

Pre-nail surgery advice sheet
On the day of your appointment for nail surgery:

* *Bring a slipper or sandal to wear after the procedure which will allow room for dressings which may be bulky when applied to your toe.*
* *Make transport arrangements for your return home. You will be able to walk after the operation but you should rest the foot as much as possible. If possible, arrange for a lift, as you are strongly advised not to drive until the effects of the local anaesthetic have worn off at the site of the procedure, which will be about 1 hour.*
* *If you are under 16 years of age a responsible adult must be in attendance.*
* *The operation will have a duration of approximately 15 minutes, but you should expect the appointment to last at least 1 hour.*
* *You will be required to attend for the postoperative care of the wound at the same clinic.*

After the procedure was completed an advice sheet was given to the patient explaining what should be expected.

Advice to patients following nail surgery
* *Do not walk for long distances.*
* *Avoid driving while the toe is numb and for up to 12 hours while the systemic effects of the anaesthetic continue.*
* *As the effects of the anaesthetic wear off, you may become aware of some throbbing sensations in the toe which has been treated. If this becomes uncomfortable you should take the painkiller you would take normally for a headache.*
* *Try to be off your feet as much as possible for the first 24 hours after the operation. If you have to work during this time, light duties while off your feet should be arranged.*
* *If you notice blood seeping through the dressing DO NOT remove the dressing but apply a further dressing and keep your foot elevated.*
* *Keep the dressing dry until you have it redressed at the clinic.*
* *Your toe will be seen at regular intervals until it has healed, which usually takes about 4–6 weeks.*
* *In the unlikely event of persistent bleeding or if you are in discomfort, contact the following number (number given).*

The patient was then informed that the dressing would be removed in 1 week's time by the podiatrist. The patient left the clinic with the copy of the postoperative advice sheet, an appointment for 1 week later and a dressing pack for the toe containing enough sterile gauze, tubular gauze and hypoallergenic tape for home use should the dressing fall off accidentally.
     On return the patient was asked to discuss her postoperative experience. The dressing was removed by soaking the foot in a tepid saline footbath lined with a plastic liner to reduce cross-contamination. At this point it was explained to the patient that she would be expected to attend to her toe twice before her next appointment in 2 weeks' time. By giving the footbath in the clinic, the patient was able to appreciate the temperature of the footbath and the fact that the water must cover the toe, as well as understanding the relevance of lining the footbath to reduce cross-contamination.
     The area was then dried and a replacement dressing was applied. The patient was taught how to apply the gauze without touching the wound and how to apply the tubular gauze using the fingers if she did not wish to purchase an applicator. The patient was then alerted to any signs which might suggest that bacteria had infected the toe, i.e. pain, dark-coloured stain on the dressing and a strong unpleasant odour. The patient was given an advice sheet on dressing procedures, which was accompanied by an explanation, and was encouraged to discuss with the podiatrist the contents of the list. An adequate supply of dressings was given, as well as a contact telephone number in case of problems.
     The patient was given a list of instructions which again were accompanied by an explanation, and she was encouraged to discuss the contents of the list with the podiatrist. A supply of dressings was given.

Dressing procedures advice sheet
* *While bathing or taking a shower keep the dressing dry.*
* *Remove the soiled dressings as directed by bathing your foot in warm water with 25 g salt dissolved in it, as demonstrated.*
* *Keep your foot immersed in the salt solution for about 10 minutes.*

Box 6.1 (cont'd)

- *Dry the foot with a clean towel, dabbing the wound with the gauze supplied.*
- *Open the dressing pack and place the dressing on the toe, taking care not to touch the side of the dressing that will come into contact with the wound.*
- *Cover the dressing with the tubular gauze, as demonstrated, and secure with the tape provided.*
- *Redress your toe once a week unless instructed otherwise.*
- *If you have any problems or queries do not hesitate to contact the following number (number given)*

The patient left the clinic with:
- the dressing procedures advice sheet
- a return appointment for 2 weeks later
- a dressing pack (enough for two dressings)
- a contact number.

This format of postoperative care was continued for the subsequent visit, 2 weeks later, and again for the visit scheduled 1 month later.

The female patient experienced a successful and quick recovery, being discharged 7 weeks after the procedure was carried out, and she needed to attend the clinic only four times. Obviously not all cases will follow the plan of management exactly, as bacterial infections may develop and/or the patient may not comply with the home care. Examples can be given where patients have had bacterial infection and have alerted the podiatrist to the abnormal signs and symptoms, thus allowing the pathology to be diagnosed and controlled. To date, out of 50 patients, four have developed a postoperative bacterial infection; of those four, only one patient has required systemic antibiotics.

All patients were questioned about the experiences of changing their dressings at home. The patients accepted the responsibility, but to varying levels, and the outcome suggests that good patient education improves the postoperative care. The experience also taught the patients to care for their own open wounds.

WHAT IS THE VALUE OF PATIENT EDUCATION?

Aside from political and current trends in patient care, consideration should be given to the benefits for the individual patient and for the health carer when effective patient education is practised. Patient education has an important part to play in the individual care of a patient, as a means of sustaining the effects of a treatment plan and as a means of promoting preventative care (Tolsma 1993). Patients are likely to be more compliant with the treatment and the advice given to them by their health carer if they are given detailed information (Sarafino 1990, Hilton 1992). Effective patient education has shown that not only has the health of the patient improved, but that patients in general have tended to appreciate the information they have been given about their condition and have responded by becoming more compliant and cooperative with the care programme. Various studies have shown that the more patients understand about their health problem(s) and about the consequences of the treatment, the more they are likely to adhere to the care plan (Ley 1988). Teaching patients about the care of their own health and welfare will allow for the prevention of additional ailments or for the recurrence of conditions. Encouraging patients to share in the treatment of their own condi-

tion(s) is a means of improving therapeutic efficacy and of relieving symptoms.

Effective patient education has also improved the relationship between the patient and the medical carer. Patients have reported a greater satisfaction with the care they had received, as they felt their needs had been identified and dealt with, and reported an increase in confidence in the relationship with their carer (DiMatteo et al 1979, Stiles et al 1979). Patients were more satisfied with the overall care they received from the health carer when they were given informative knowledge about their condition and were more likely to complete the course of therapy (Stiles et al 1979, Howard et al 1987, Ley 1988, Hilton 1992).

PATIENT EDUCATION IN PODIATRY

Teaching patients about their foot problems is not a new concept in podiatric care, although practitioners in past years have often referred to the practice of educating patients as foot health education rather than patient education. Kemp & Winkler (1983), in their extensive study on the needs of podiatric expertise in the UK, highlighted the necessity to give patients better information on the requirements of well-fitting footwear. These authors concluded that, because so many foot problems were associated with ill-fitting footwear, patient teaching in this area would contribute to a considerable reduction in disabling foot problems. Cole & Stiles (1983) discussed in detail the role of the podiatrist as a foot-health educator, giving examples of how podiatrists could practise such an approach. Edwards & Jackson (1986), recognised that a great number of chiropodists of the time were involved in foot-health education in some form or another but were unaware of what teaching material was available, created an index of foot-health material. This information was received with great approval and gratitude by the profession. Bradshaw (1990) discussed the merits of using a custom-designed foot care leaflet to teach patients suffering from diabetes how to avoid the development of foot ulcers. He gave an account of how such a leaflet may be designed and produced in order that other practitioners may learn from his experience.

THE HEALTH PROFESSIONAL'S ROLE AS A PATIENT EDUCATOR

It would seem, therefore, that podiatrists have recognised the value of informing patients about their foot health as an important aspect of patient care. There is also evidence to suggest that podiatrists are now accepting the principle of adopting patient education, as recent studies carried out by Valente & Nelson (1995) and Wormald (1995) both promote the importance of patient education as an integral part of caring for patients suffering from diabetes mellitus. These authors state the case for podiatrists to become more involved in patient teaching as a means of preventing problems in the lower limb that are associated with patients' lack of knowledge about their illness. Nevertheless, what has also become evident is that podiatrists, although aware of the benefits of teaching patients, do not teach all of their patients all of the time (Dunlop 1994). Podiatrists are similar to other health care professionals in this respect; as Ley (1988) concluded, many health carers do not give their patients clear informative information about their condition nor do they attempt to educate their patients in any form.

Health care professionals are in the advantageous position of being able to teach their patients about the care of their condition(s) and, as a consequence, about their health. However, many health care professionals have been dubious about the benefits of educating patients and feel that it is a time-consuming business that makes very little difference to the outcome of a patient's care, despite copious evidence to suggest the contrary. Health care professionals would seem to be discouraged about the benefits of patient education, as many unsuccessful attempts to educate patients have been reported. Some have reported that patients have been unable to understand medical terminology or that patients were over-anxious and had problems remembering what they had been told (McKinlay 1975). Others suggest that non-compliance is due to patients misunderstanding or misinterpreting information (Segall & Roberts 1980). A breakdown in communication between the health care professional and the patient would certainly seem to be a common feature leading to patient non-compliance. However, Ley (1988) suggested that health carers are themselves often non-compliant in their commitment to patient care. Very often health carers do not fulfil their role as health providers and fall short in their use of good communication skills and effective patient education.

Consideration should be given to the fact that the patient is not the only party involved in the communication process. Several studies have looked at the effectiveness of the health professional in educating their patients and have concluded that the reason for patient non-compliance does not lie totally with the patient; health professionals also have some shortcomings.

This apparent lack of patient teaching in podiatry is most probably due to the fact that podiatrists, like many other health professionals, are not aware of the most effective methods of teaching patients (Dunlop 1994) and are unaware of how these can be integrated into daily practice. Undergraduate training has given little attention to the subject of educating patients. Powrie (1992) concluded that the levels and depths of study in health education varied enormously throughout the recognised teaching institutions. Although the relevance of patient education is understood, for many podiatrists the practical application of the process remains a mystery.

EFFECTIVE TEACHING METHODS FOR EDUCATING PATIENTS

Successful patient education must comprise two components:

- helping patients to remember what they have been taught
- encouraging patients to change their behaviour, to use what they have learned.

Helping the patient to remember

Teaching patients about their own foot health will only be effective if the patient is able to remember

---

Box 6.2 Case study 2: fitting a heel post

A male patient, aged 29, was prescribed a functional orthosis with a 15° heel post to treat his knee pain when running. The aim of the therapy was explained to the patient, as well as his part in monitoring the progress of the treatment and cooperating with the treatment recommendations. The device and its fitting into the shoe were demonstrated to the patient, after which he walked for a short distance in the clinic. Following this, there was a discussion of the issues concerning the treatment, and in particular those signs and symptoms the patient might experience when wearing the device as detailed on the advice sheet.

Advice sheet for wearing orthoses
At first the orthoses may feel uncomfortable but the following guidelines will help you to become accustomed to them:

● *Wear the orthoses for short periods, starting with an hour a day and increasing the time by an hour if this is comfortable. If the orthoses remain uncomfortable or become painful, wear them only for short periods and not at all if you cannot tolerate them.*
● *At the time of your next appointment in 2 weeks it should be possible to wear them for the better part of the working day.*
● *You may experience discomfort in your legs or back during the first few days as your muscles are adapting. If this pain or discomfort continues beyond the first few days, stop wearing the orthoses and report the symptoms at your next appointment.*

The patient left the clinic with:

● the instruction sheet on how to wear the device
● a return appointment for 2 weeks later
● a contact telephone number.

On his return visit the patient felt confident discussing the signs and symptoms with the practitioner and it was decided to make an adjustment to the device which improved its function.

The teaching methods used in this instance consisted of a demonstration carried out by the practitioner to the patient and between the patient and the practitioner, and a discussion between the patient and the practitioner. Written instructions with reinforcement by repetition were chosen to improve the patient's understanding, in addition to offering the patient ownership of the treatment plan.

---

of presenting information to the adult learner that have enhanced memory, and some of these methods have been identified as being equally effective in teaching patients (Box 6.2).

Amount of information

As the ageing process develops, the efficiency of the adult memory reduces. There are many reasons as to why this occurs; some are due to the physiological changes of the ageing body and others due to a change in the ability of the adult to process and recall information (Perlmutter & Hall 1992, Aitkinson et al 1993). It has been well documented that the average adult can recall no more than between seven and nine pieces of information at any one time (Rogers 1977). Medical studies have demonstrated that patients remembered less than half of 10 pieces of information (Joyce et al 1969). Podiatrists can help their patients by presenting only small amounts of information at any one time. Other methods, such as repeating information, may be useful in assisting memory recall. The podiatrist may repeat the information for the patients, or the patient themselves may be requested to repeat the information. Both methods have been successful in enhancing memory recall (Bertakis 1977, Ley 1988).

Podiatrists must also be aware that a high number of patients receiving podiatry care will have a medical history which itself may have an effect on the patient's ability to recall detail, and may in addition create anxiety and worry that will affect information retrieval. Podiatrists should therefore be aware of the limitations of their patients' ability to remember large amounts of informative detail and be prepared to use methods that will reduce the burden on the adult memory. For many of these patients written information will be of great benefit (see Box 6.3).

Written information

Written information should be used to enhance memory and not used to present new information. Miller & Shanks (1986) identified that written information was most useful when the carer had initially discussed the issues with the patient, and then followed the discussion with written information. Written information used on its own would seem to have little value. Written information must be clear, legible and readable. Again, a patient's medical history must be taken into consideration, with attention to those conditions that will affect eyesight, such as diabetes, rheumatoid arthritis and cataracts. Consideration should be given to the size of the writing, which should be large

what she has learned. In this respect, it is clearly relevant that the main recipients of podiatry patient education will be adults. Even if the patient is a child, the education will often be presented to the parent or to the guardian. Therefore, by adopting certain teaching techniques that are favourable to improving adult memory, podiatrists can achieve effective patient education. Adult educationalists have identified methods

> **Box 6.3** Case study 3: home therapy for anhidrosis and epidermal fissures
>
> A male patient, 79 years of age, presented with a heel problem of anhidrosis and epidermal fissures of many months' duration. The patient was given a clear and concise explanation as to why the skin was cracking and how the regular use of an emollient could stop or control the cracking of the skin, thus reducing the possibility of bleeding and the entry of bacterial infection. It was decided to use a simple aqueous cream, obtainable at retail outlets, which was easy to purchase and above all not expensive. Selecting this home therapy and ensuring the patient understood the rationale made it more likely that the treatment would be effective. The cream was applied to the foot at the end of the treatment and the patient was asked to observe how much cream was used and how best to apply it. The name of the cream was written down for the patient, together with a few short details on how the cream should be applied. It was agreed that the condition should be reviewed in 4 weeks unless there was any deterioration in the meantime.
> The patient was given:
> - hand written instructions
> - an appointment for 4 weeks later.
>
> On the patient's return, the condition of the foot had improved. Although the skin was still dry, there was no evidence of fissuring. The patient was congratulated on his success in treating the fissures and some discussion followed on how the dry skin condition could be further improved. The patient admitted that he did not use the cream every day as recommended. The patient feedback was useful as the patient agreed on the next stage of management, which was to use the cream regularly as well as checking the skin for any sign of recurrence of fissuring. It was also agreed that although the patient may forget to use the cream occasionally, the important issue was to prevent the recurrence of the fissures. With this information and his previous experience of the condition, the patient would be able to control any recurrence; he was discharged.

enough for the patient to be able to read easily. Podiatrists should also be aware that, even in the healthiest individual, vision will become reduced as ageing progresses. Vision is reported to be at its best at the age of 18, and from then on it declines gradually with time (Cross 1981, Perlmutter & Hall 1992).

At the beginning or at the end

The adult will best recall information that has been presented at the beginning or at the end of a process. In other words, adult patients will remember the first few pieces of information they are given and the last few pieces. The reason for this pattern of recall is best explained by Atkinson et al (1993), who theorised that information that is presented first, primacy, will enter the short-term memory and will be easily processed into the long-term memory as there is little else in the short-term memory to interrupt or confuse that information. Similarly, the information that is presented last is easily stored into the long-term memory as there is no information following on that will create a confusion. Within the process of the patient consultation, podiatrists should be aware of the best time to present information that has to be remembered by the patient. Common practice by podiatrists is to give patients instructions during the treatment process when, by all accounts, there is a lot of activity going on (Dunlop 1994), and when, unfortunately, they are least likely to recall it.

Changing the patient's behaviour

It is common practice for a podiatrist to request that patients carry out part of their treatment plan by themselves in their own environment. In doing so, the podiatrist is requesting patients to change their behaviour by adding some activity to their lifestyle, e.g. daily use of an antifungal agent, or by taking something out of their lifestyle, e.g. a fashionable pair of shoes that are harmful to healthy foot function. Various approaches to educating patients have been identified as being successful in encouraging patients to use what they have been taught and make some changes to their lifestyle. It is, however, unrealistic to assume that using such methods will assure total patient compliance to every care plan, but what is evident is that there are a variety of methods that have been successful in changing patients' behaviour.

Communication skills

Medical studies have shown that patients respond more favourably to those medical practitioners who adopt a caring attitude and are willing to listen to what the patient has to say. When patients were asked about their relationships with their doctors, it was found that they were more likely to return to the same doctor and to adhere to the care plan if they felt that the doctor cared about them as individuals, if the doctor took time to listen and explain to them, and if the doctor was accessible when needed (DiMatteo et al 1979). Although this study was based on relationships between doctors and their patients, components of the study can easily be related to podiatry practice. The patients were predominantly adult and ambulatory, and their illnesses included diabetes mellitus, heart disease, arthritis and musculoskeletal problems. The overall outcome of the study concluded that patients in general are sensitive and responsive to the interaction they have with their medical carer.

Patient contracting

Patients are actively more compliant with the instructions given to them about their health care when they are involved in the decision-making process (DiMatteo et al 1979, Stiles et al 1979, Becker & Maiman 1990, Sarafino 1990). Negotiating with the patient and coming to an agreement on the treatment plan, i.e. forming a contract with the patient, have been shown to be useful methods for encouraging patients to change her behaviour (Leslie & Schuster 1991). Forming a contract with a patient is based on the principle that patient and carer will together set down in a written contract what is achievable to the patient in maintaining her own care. The advantage is that the patient can share in the responsibility and will have the opportunity to agree or disagree with the plan. It is fair to say that contracting with patients has not been successful in all instances; the reasons for its failure have been the setting of unrealistic goals, which were difficult for the patients to adhere to, and a lack of consideration of the patients' social surroundings (Morgan & Littell 1988).

HOW AND WHAT SHOULD PODIATRISTS TEACH PATIENTS?

Patient education may be adopted into all aspects of podiatric care: podiatric conditions that are minor and easily prevented, e.g. interdigital hyperhidrotic fissures, and also those conditions that are limb-threatening, e.g. arterial disease. Podiatrists have a wealth of knowledge about the conditions associated with foot problems, as well as specialised knowledge concerning the care and maintenance of foot health. This wealth of knowledge will well equip podiatrists to educate their patients about all aspects of foot care. However, the difficulty has been knowing how to include patient education in a care programme. How might this be done?

Common in podiatry practice is the patient suffering from rheumatoid arthritis who seeks pain relief for a combination of foot problems which are the result of osseous deformity and/or vascular and sensory impairment. Podiatrists, with their specialist skills, will attempt to reduce the foot pain using palliative techniques, therefore allowing the patient to be more mobile and pain-free. However, in caring for such a patient, the podiatrist must also give attention to the additional needs that are a consequence of the illness. For many patients suffering from rheumatoid arthritis, controlling their pain is not the only problem. Other problems include dealing with their disabilities and coping with their loss of independence. These patients often feel that they do not have the capabilities to cope with their rheumatoid arthritis, not because of any physical disability but because they themselves as individuals lack the confidence or the knowledge to help them cope (Taal et al 1993). Using patient education in the podiatric care of the patient suffering from rheumatoid arthritis can help the patient to understand how she herself can improve her foot pain and can become active in coping with her illness rather than depending on the next podiatry appointment—in short, allowing the patient more control in coping with her illness.

CONSULTATION WITH PATIENT EDUCATION

As with any other consultation, the patient's problems and diagnosis are established. The podiatrist will begin to teach the patient about his condition with a clear explanation of how the condition is related to the foot problems. A treatment plan is formulated; however, in forming the treatment plan the patient is fully consulted in the decision-making process and is given an explanation about the treatment choices that are available. Here the patient must be well informed in order to understand the consequences of the therapies and the role he has to play in maintaining the therapeutic efficacy.

At this stage of the consultation, the patient's contribution will be valuable in order to establish how the treatment will best be conducted within his social surroundings and physical limitations. This is where agreement and understanding from both parties is required to plan a course of management that will be acceptable and manageable for the patient. Following on, the patient has to be taught how he himself can cope with his foot problems within his own environment, instead of being dependent on the next visit to the podiatrist. The benefit here is once again allowing patients more control and independence, and there are also benefits to be gained from patients using medical services only when necessary, as stated by Davis et al (1994):

The patient must have sufficient knowledge about the disease and its pathology to identify when to apply and modify treatment methods and when consultation with medical and health professionals is necessary.

Patients must be given clear information that they are able to remember. This process may seem very time-consuming but that need not be the case. Within the average 20-minute consultation, the podiatrist has a one-to-one relationship with the patient which is the perfect environment in which to establish a patient's personal needs. Although friendly conversation is a useful means of building rapport, some of the conversation can allow the patient to address his needs, which will equally produce a good patient relationship. Much of the general explanation can be given to the patient while treatment is being carried out, instead of having long moments of silence. To reinforce the pertinent details, a verbal summary can be given at the end of the consultation, accompanied by written information. Demonstration may be given to the patient during the treatment when there is time, e.g. applying medica-

ments or exercising, but demonstrations must be used with verbal explanation followed by written detail. At the beginning of the next consultation, some time should be given to assess the patient's progress.

Review of how the patient has coped with the responsibility for her own care will again involve patient interaction and effective communication skills. The purpose of the review process is to evaluate the progress of the patient's condition. One of three things may be required in the review of the patient's case: setting new targets for the patient as the previous ones were unachievable; repetition or readjustment of the educational programme as the patient has misunderstood or has forgotten; or, ideally, reinforcing the benefits and merits for the patient who has been successful in achieving her goals and has maintained efficacy in the care of her condition.

REFERENCES

Aitkinson R L, Aitkinson R C, Smith E E, Bem J 1993 Introduction to psychology, 11th edn. Harcourt Brace Jovanich, Florida

Becker M H, Maiman L A 1980 Strategies for enhancing patient compliance. Journal of Community Health 6(2): 113–135

Bertakis K D 1977 The communication of information from physician to patient: a method for increasing patient retention and satisfaction. Journal of Family Practice 5(2): 217–222

Bradshaw T 1990 The concept, development, anatomy and physiology of a footcare leaflet for people at risk of developing diabetic foot ulceration. Chiropodist 45(2): 30–32

Brandberg Y, Berenmar M, Bolund C, Michelson H, Mansson-Brahme E, Ringborg U, Sjoden P 1994 Information to patients with malignant melanoma: a randomised study. Patient Education and Counselling 23: 97–105

Carter W B, McKenna M, Martin M, Andersen E M 1989 Health education: special issues for older adults. Patient Education and Counselling 13: 117–131

Cole R, Stiles C S 1983 The chiropodist and health education. Chiropodist 38(6): 206–210

Cross P 1981 Adults as learners. Jossey Bass

Davis P, Busch A, Lowe J C, Taniguchi J, Djkowich B 1994 Evaluation of a rheumatoid arthritis patient education program: impact on knowledge and self-efficacy. Patient Education and Counselling 24: 55–61

DiMatteo R M, Prince L M, Taranta A 1979 Patients' perception of physicians' behaviour: determinants of patient commitment to the therapeutic relationship. Journal of Community Health 4(4): 280–290

Dunlop G M 1994 Approach to the use of patient education in the care of podiatry patients. Unpublished thesis, University of Glasgow Department of Adult and Continuing Education

Edwards L M D, Jackson F V P 1986 Health education resources. Chiropodist 41(4): 135–137

Ewles L, Simnett I 1985 Promoting health: a practical guide to health education. John Wiley, Chichester

Hilton S 1992 Does patient education work? British Journal of Hospital Medicine 47(6): 438–441

HMSO 1989a Working for patients in the health service: caring for the 1990s. HMSO, London

HMSO 1989b Caring for people: community care in the next decade and beyond caring for the 1990s. HMSO, London

HMSO 1991 The health of the nation: a consultative document for health in England. HMSO, London

Howard J E, Davies J L, Roghmann K J 1987 Respiratory teaching of patients: how effective is it? Journal of Advanced Nursing 12: 207–214

Joyce C R B, Caple G, Mason M, Reynolds E, Matthews J A 1969 Quantitative study of doctor–patient communication. Quarterly Journal of Medicine XXXVIII(150): 183–194

Kemp J, Winkler J T 1983 Problems afoot: needs and efficiency in footcare. Disabled Living Foundation, Milton Keynes

Kemper D W, Lorig K, Mettler M 1993 The effectiveness of medical self-care interventions: a focus of self-initiated responses to symptoms. Patient Education and Counselling 21: 29–39

Leslie M, Schuster P A 1991 The effect of contingency contracting on adherence and knowledge of exercise regimens. Patient Education and Counselling 18: 231–241

Ley P 1988 Communicating with patients: improving communication, satisfaction and compliance. Chapman and Hall, London

McKinlay J B 1975 Who is really ignorant – physician or patient? Journal of Health and Social Behaviour 16: 3–11

Miller G, Shanks, C 1986 Patient education: comparative effectiveness by means of presentation. Journal of Family Practice 22(2): 178–181

Morgan B S, Littel D H 1988 A closer look at teaching and contingency contracting with type II diabetes. Patient Education and Counselling 12: 145–158

Permutter, Hall 1992 Adult development and ageing, 2nd edn. Wiley, Chichester

Rogers J 1977 Teaching adults, 2nd edn. Open University Press

Sarafino E P 1990 Health psychology: biopsychosocial interaction. John Wiley, Chichester

Segall A, Roberts L W 1980 A comparative analysis of physician estimates and levels of medical knowledge among patients. Sociology of Health and Illness

Sheridan C L, Radmacher S A 1992 Health psychology. Challenging the biomedical model. John Wiley, Chichester

Stiles W B, Putnam M D, Wolf M H, James S A 1979 Interaction exchange: structure and patient satisfaction with the medical interviews. Medical Care XVii(6): 667–679

Taal E, Johannes J R, Erwin R S, Oene W 1993 Health status, adherence with health recommendations, self-efficacy and social support in patients with rheumatoid arthritis. Patient Education and Counselling 20: 63–76

Tolsma D D 1993 Patient education objectives in healthy people 2000: policy and research issues. Patient Education and Counselling 22: 7–14

Valente L A, Nelson M S 1995 Patient education for diabetic patients: an integral part of quality care. Journal of the American Podiatric Medical Association 85(3): 177–179

Verhaak P F M, van Busschbach J T 1988 Patient education in general practice. Patient Education and Counselling 11: 119–129

Webb P (ed) 1994 Health promotion and patient education: a professional's guide. Chapman and Hall, London

Wormald T 1995 Lower limb amputation in the diabetic: causation and prevention – the role of the podiatrists. Journal of British Podiatric Medicine 50(5): 63–67

7

Affections of the skin and subcutaneous tissues

M. F. Whiting

Keywords

Bacterial paronychia
Bullous disorders
Bursae
Bursitis
Cellulitis
Deficiency states
Disorders of sweating
Eczema and dermatitis
Erythema pernio
Erythrasma
Fibrosis
Ganglion
Heloma durum
Heloma miliare
Heloma molle
Hyperkeratosis
Infection
Intertrigo
Juvenile plantar dermatosis
Lichen planus
Lymphadenitis
Lymphangitis
Mechanical stress factors
Psoriasis
Purpura
Pustular psoriasis
Reiter's disease
Staphylococcal infections
Streptococcal infections
Synovial sacs
Talon noire
Tinea pedis
Trophic ulceration
Tumours
Ulceration
Urticaria
Verrucae

The environment in which the foot functions predisposes to a range of disorders which arise from, or are related to, one or more of the special conditions which apply to the shod foot. Mechanical damage arises from interaction with the shoe or ground, and the role of the foot in weight-bearing and transmission results in the need for a high level of adaptation to meet demands placed upon the tissues of the foot. The enclosed, warm and humid environment of the shoe is conducive to the development of extensive microbial flora, which, combined with the possibility of mechanical abrasion, increases the risk of infection. These same environmental factors create conditions in which increased sweating easily takes place, with water retention in the skin due to non-evaporation associated with occlusion.

The foot is supplied by blood vessels which are located at the most distant periphery of the circulatory system and which are therefore more prone to damage from pathological processes and gravitational effects. Metabolic and neurological disease are both likely to involve the foot at some stage. The skin of the foot may also be affected by skin disease occurring elsewhere in the body, and this has implications for it, often associated with the physical environment in which the foot is required to function.

As a result of the interaction of these factors, the skin and subcutaneous tissues of the foot are prone to a range of disorders, some of them specific to the foot. It is possible to classify them into five groups:

1. *Conditions arising from mechanical stress.* Of these, the most common are heloma (corns), callosities (tyloma), bursitis and a range of complications which arise from them. Because of their frequency and potential to produce chronic disability, these conditions are discussed in some detail.

2. *Conditions arising from infection.* Bacterial infections of the foot mainly occur as complications of traumatic lesions or are associated with circulatory, neurological or metabolic disease and will be mentioned in these sections. Verrucae (warts) are caused by the human papilloma virus (HPV) and are a common viral infection affecting the skin of the foot. Tinea pedis (athlete's foot) is a common mycotic infection and is caused by a number of pathogenic fungi. Each of these common infections is discussed separately.

3. *Disorders of the sweat glands.* Hyperhidrosis and anhidrosis are relatively frequent states of altered levels of activity of the sweat glands and have potential clinical significance.

4. *Deficiency states.* These arise from circulatory, neurological and metabolic disorders. Atherosclerosis affecting the arteries of the leg places the foot at risk of ischaemic ulceration and gangrene. Diabetes mellitus,

as a result of both disordered metabolism and its associated macro- and microangiopathy, is prone to give rise to complications in the foot. Vasomotor dystrophy and vasospastic disorders which give rise to erythema pernio, Raynaud's disease, vascular spasm and trophic ulceration are included. The gravitational effects giving rise to varicose veins and varicose ulcers are considered in relation to the tissues of the foot.

5. *Dermatological conditions.* These affect the skin of the foot as part of their overall manifestation and require management by the dermatologist. They are not considered here in detail.

CONDITIONS ARISING FROM MECHANICAL STRESSES

The mechanical stresses to which the skin and subcutaneous tissues of the foot are subjected are classified as *compressional, tensile, shearing* and *torsional* (Fig. 7.1). Understanding the way in which these stresses arise in the foot, during movement and when standing, is necessary in order to design an effective programme of treatment.

Compressional stress arises from two convergent forces acting in opposite directions, e.g. the plantar tissues of the heel and forefoot undergo compression between superimposed body weight and the resistance of the ground beneath. Less obviously, the interdigital surfaces of the toes are compressed when the toes and forefoot are subjected to compression in the front of a tightly fitting shoe.

Tensile stress results in the stretching of tissues. It occurs when a force is applied in a single plane but is divergent, acting in the opposite direction, e.g. the plantar ligaments and fascia are subjected to tensile stress on weight-bearing. Tensile stress is applied to the skin when the soft tissues are compressed under the heel and forefoot and the skin is stretched laterally during weight-bearing.

Shearing stress arises when forces act in different planes and in opposite directions. Shearing occurs commonly in the tissues of the feet because of movements of the bony structures within the foot, relative to the soft tissues, and when there is movement between the foot and shoe during walking. It is potentially damaging to the other tissues of the foot when one layer is forced violently over another.

Torsional stress is shearing combined with rotation. It occurs within the plantar tissues when the foot makes any pivoting motion.

Each of these mechanical stresses is normally well tolerated by the tissues of the foot but may give rise to pathological changes if the toleration threshold of the

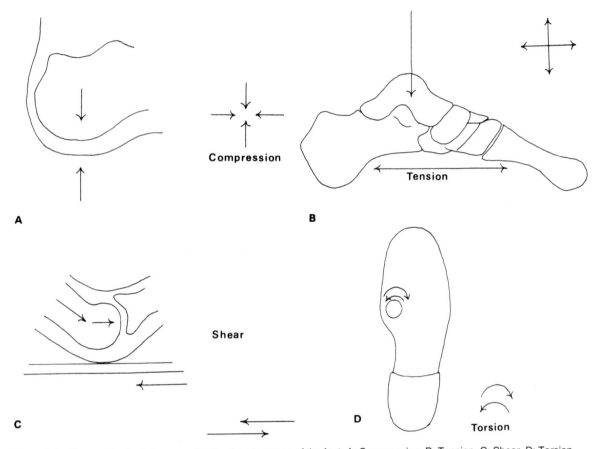

Figure 7.1   The mechanical stresses affecting the structures of the feet. A: Compression. B: Tension. C: Shear. D: Torsion.

affected tissue is exceeded. The strength of tissues may be reduced in pathological states and give rise to a reduced threshold of tolerance such that damage is more easily produced; for example, normal skin is strongly resistant to splitting from tensile stress (fissures), but skin which has been weakened by sweat retention and maceration, or is anhidrotic, splits easily.

When the tolerance of skin and subcutaneous tissue to mechanical stress has been exceeded, each produces its own characteristic response. However, the mechanics of the foot are complex, and mechanical effects are usually combined into complex stresses which, if severe enough, may result in tissue trauma and injury. Sustained mild injury to the skin and soft tissues of the foot may give rise to heloma, callosities, bursitis, blisters and small ulcerations. The nature of the lesion which is produced reflects the types of mechanical stress giving rise to it and the response potential of the affected tissues. Analysis of the mechanical cause of a lesion indicates the approach to remedial action which is likely to be most effective.

Hyperkeratosis

This is the name given to a state of thickening of the keratinised layers of the skin. It occurs in a wide range of skin disorders but in the foot is most commonly seen in the form of callus, which is a discreet area of thickened skin, or in heloma, which are small areas of callus containing a deep centre or nucleus of parakeratotic cells that press into the underlying dermis to cause pain.

The normal physiological process of keratinisation (or cornification), which maintains the stratum corneum as a horny protective covering, becomes stimulated to overactivity under the influence of intermittent compression. The resultant hypertrophy of the stratum corneum is thought to be the product of accelerated proliferation of epidermal cells, stimulated by reactive hyperaemia, a stronger cohesion of the surface cells and a decreased rate of desquamation. This response is termed hyperkeratosis and it is a normal protective response of the skin, as seen, for example, in the hands of manual labourers. Any asymptomatic area of such physiological callus on the foot has a protective function and does not require to be removed. Hyperkeratosis becomes pathological only when it is so thick that it causes painful symptoms and significant deformation to the normal papillary stratification of the skin. Hyperkeratosis may also result from congenital, hormonal, occupational and infective factors, but in the present context only traumatic hyperkeratosis is considered.

Hyperkeratotic lesions

The size, shape, thickness and density of an area of traumatic hyperkeratosis are indicative of the stresses responsible for its development. A callus (callosity or tyloma) is a diffuse area of relatively even thickness. An heloma is an area of callus which is complicated by a deep central mass of cornified cells, called a nucleus, which presses into the underlying dermis. The nucleus is usually an inverted cone but may vary in shape and size according to the location and the prevailing mechanical stresses.

Corns (Latin *cornu*: a horn) or helomata (Greek *helos*: a stone wedge) are classified as hard (heloma durum), soft (heloma molle), vascular (heloma vasculare) and neurovascular (heloma neurovasculare).

Heloma durum (Fig. 7.2). These occur, typically, on the dorsum of the interphalangeal joints of the toes, on their apices and on the plantar surface of the foot beneath the metatarsal heads. Less frequently, they arise on the plantar medial aspect of the interphalangeal joint of the hallux. They also occur interdigitally, beneath a nail (subungual heloma), or in the nail sulcus (onychophosis).

Heloma durum is always indicative of concentrated, intermittent pressure affecting the lesion site, often as a result of deformity or dysfunction of the foot or the toes. On the plantar surfaces and the apices of the toes, pressure arises from the interaction of body weight, footwear and ground resistance. At other sites, pressure is generated between the weight-bearing foot and footwear, or between adjacent toes due to the constraining effect of tight shoes. The nuclei lie underneath a margin of surrounding callus (Fig. 7.3).

Treatment involves the removal of overlying callus by minute dissection with a scalpel, followed by the excision of the nucleus by partial or whole section. This can be achieved, podiatrically, without breaching the dermo-epidermal junction, although a small amount of bleeding can be regarded as acceptable if the thorough removal of an established, irregular nucleus is undertaken in a single procedure. Keratolytic medication is

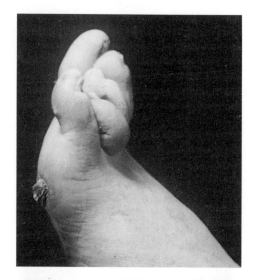

A

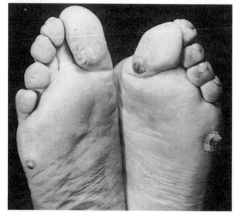

B

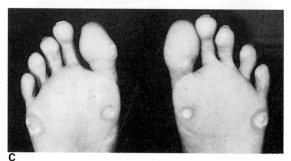

C

Figure 7.2 A, B, C: Plantar helomata.

sometimes used if it is not possible to remove the whole of the nucleus (see Ch. 12) as part of a longer term treatment strategy.

Protective padding, designed to deflect pressure from the site of the lesion, should be applied to protect the area postoperatively. In the longer term, the

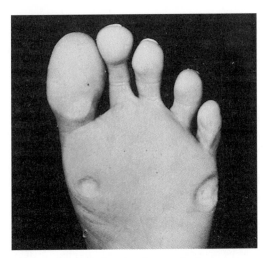

Figure 7.3   Plantar helomata after enucleation.

causative mechanical factors should be identified and a management scheme developed to correct function or accommodate fixed deformity. Frequently, it is possible to design and fabricate an orthotic device which affords long-term protection and possibly correction. In most instances, shoe advice is necessary and orthotic treatment should be delayed until there is compliance with footwear advice (see Ch. 14).

Complete cure is possible but critically depends upon the cooperation of the patient, who should be prepared to follow footwear advice and use orthotics which have been prescribed to correct underlying mechanical dysfunction.

Heloma molle. These occur only interdigitally, commonly in the fourth cleft but also in the other interdigital spaces. There is usually no nucleus. A typical lesion is either wholly or partially ring-shaped with a central area of atrophy in which the skin is extremely thin, appearing almost denuded of normal stratum corneum. This general shape and appearance is determined by the moulding of the intervening skin between the opposing bony prominences of the interphalangeal joints. In the fourth web, however, the lesion usually arises between the lateral aspect of the base of the proximal phalanx of the fourth toe and the medial aspect of the proximal interphalangeal joint of the fifth toe. Extreme deformity or dislocation of the fifth or fourth toe may cause exceptions to this common pattern. Characteristically, there is maceration of the ring-shaped hyperkeratosis. This is due to the retention of sweat, which the close proximity of the toes does not allow to evaporate.

The treatment is the careful removal of the rubbery hyperkeratosis with a scalpel, followed by the application of medication to dry the skin. Advice to keep the interdigital spaces dry by careful towelling and powdering after bathing may be sufficient. Alternatively, the application of a suitable alcohol-based solution once or twice daily may provide sufficient astringency to prevent the recurrence of the symptoms of maceration. Relief of interdigital pressure is essential and may be achieved with a soft silicone interdigital orthotic. Advice concerning footwear, aimed at achieving reduction in interdigital pressure, should be given.

Vascular and neurovascular heloma. Small blood vessels and nerve endings arising from the dermis become caught up in the region of the dermo-epidermal junction at the nucleus of an heloma which has become complicated by secondary injury. In such instances, the dermo-epidermal junction is grossly disrupted and the dermal papillary structure is deformed by long-standing or repeated injury, e.g. to a coterminus chilblain, inexpert self-treatment with a razor blade or otherwise incompetent treatment. Hypertrophic dermal papillae project around the periphery of the lesion and often within the nucleus itself. These appear as an irregular pattern of capillary loops between a number of small concentrations of dense stratum corneum (micronuclei). Interspersed between these abnormal structures are white, grey or discoloured yellow specks and lines, which arise from dense connective tissue containing nerve endings and dilated small blood vessels. Dermal elements disorganised in this way and pinched by hyperkeratotic skin give rise to intense pain and discomfort. Capillary haemorrhage is likely to result from unskilful operating, repeated attempts at which progressively worsen the deformation of the skin strata.

Treatment is complicated by the difficulty of enucleating multiple small nuclei and the presence of nerve endings and blood vessels which give rise to pain and bleeding during operative treatment. Skilful enucleation is possible in some instances, and infiltrated local anaesthesia with a 1% solution of plain lignocaine enables the reduction of overlying callus and a significant proportion of the nuclear elements, provided that bleeding can be controlled. The application of escharotic medication, such as silver nitrate or the reducing agent pyrogallol, in suitable strengths is effective but requires several treatments before the micronuclei are removed. Pyrogallol has the advantage of being analgesic, and thus facilitates further operative reduction without the need for local anaesthetic infiltration for subsequent treatments. Pyrogallic acid should not be applied to broken skin because of the risks of absorption into the bloodstream and its systemic effects. Pyrogallol should not be used on more than three successive occasions, because at therapeutic concentrations it is cumulative in effect and can produce a sudden tissue breakdown which can be difficult to resolve. Salicylic acid is not used, because the maceration and 'fogging' effect on the epidermis which it produces prevents discrimination between nuclei and connective tissue elements. Once the complications of the lesion have been reduced, treatment continues as for hard corns. Electrosurgery, using recently developed apparatus, shows promising results (Ch. 12).

Heloma miliare (seed corns). Unlike other heloma, these are not produced solely by mechanical injury, although they occur most frequently under the weight-bearing aspect of the foot. They are localised areas of parakeratotic stratum corneum cells, closely resembling the nucleus of heloma durum without any surrounding callus. In common with the nucleus of heloma durum, it can be shown histologically that the granular layer of the epidermis is absent immediately beneath the funnel-shaped cone of parakeratotic cells which form the lesion. Apart from the retention of cell nuclei in these stratum corneum cells, they are not otherwise remarkable. Histochemically, they do not contain significantly increased amounts of cholesterol, as has been suggested by some. Although usually found in relation to areas of increased pressure, they also occur on apparently non-weight-bearing sites and are more common in dry skin conditions, such as anhidrosis.

The treatment is by the removal of symptom-producing lesions by partial or whole section using a scalpel. The majority of lesions produce no symptoms and do not require treatment. However, the regular application of an emollient will improve the hydration of the skin, and improvement in the texture of the skin is often associated with a reduction in the number of focal hyperkeratotic plugs. In more severe cases, the regular application of a keratoplastic topical medicine such as 10% urea will assist treatment.

Complications of hyperkeratotic lesions

If the pressure which gives rise to heloma becomes particularly intense, or if the intermittent pattern is replaced by continuous compression due, for example, to the fixation of a deformity or intense pressure from ill-fitting footwear, then the soft tissue under the lesion may break down and become necrotic. Due to the tough nature of the overlying hyperkeratosis, the inflammation and exudation which is often associated with such necrosis is contained. Exudate subsequently macerates the overlying hyperkeratotic skin, which becomes weakened, allowing a route for colonisation by pathogens. Infection of the skin may follow and, depending upon the colonising organism and state of the host defences, this either remains localised or spreads into the surrounding tissue (cellulitis).

Infection. Infection is a constant hazard because of the foot's confinement in a warm, humid environment. Such infections usually remain localised and resolve rapidly once treated locally with drainage and antiseptic dressings. In the foot, due to the potential for a reduced blood supply, the possibility of a spreading cellulitis, particularly if there is debility, should be considered. Stringent pre- and postoperative antiseptic procedures are always necessary in the practice of podiatry. Even minor infections of the skin of the foot should be speedily and effectively treated. A detailed account of the procedures to be followed is given in the section on bacterial infection (see also Chs 9 and 16).

Ulceration. Ulceration arises from the loss of continuity of the skin surface due to necrosis of skin cells. It is commonly associated with the following causative factors:

1. continuous trauma (in the foot, this is frequently compression)
2. loss or degeneration of subjacent adipose tissue
3. poor peripheral circulation, which results in trophic changes
4. neuropathy from any cause (diabetes is the most frequent).

An ulcer may exude clear uncontaminated tissue fluid or a purulent discharge, which indicates secondary infection (Fig. 7.4).

Ulceration associated with hyperkeratotic lesions usually heals well following the careful removal of the hyperkeratotic mass and deflection of pressure away from the affected site with appropriate padding. The ulcer is cleaned by irrigation with sterile saline and dressed with a sterile environmental dressing under which cell regeneration can take place rapidly. If there is cellulitis and evidence of spreading infection, then treatment with a suitable antibiotic is necessary.

Perforating ulcer. This form of deep ulceration may penetrate underlying structures such as joints or tendon sheaths; in this way, infection may be spread into deeper structures, even to the extent of entering bone (osteomyelitis). Ulceration which perforates into subjacent structures is consequently a serious complication of plantar hyperkeratosis and requires urgent treatment, possibly with simultaneous administration of antibiotics by mouth. This type of ulceration usually

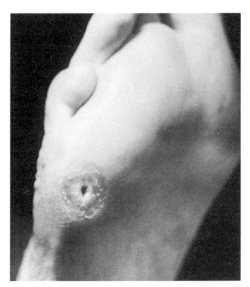

Figure 7.4 Perforation ulcer under the fifth metatarsal head. The sinus at the centre of the lesion may penetrate to the underlying metatarsal head and the metatarsophalangeal joint.

occurs underneath the metatarsophalangeal joints, particularly the first and fifth, although any may be affected.

In addition to the causative mechanical component, which is typically continuous pressure due to fixation or disordered function of the affected metatarsophalangeal joint, there is frequently coexistent neuropathy. This may be due to any neurological disorders, but most commonly will be found in association with diabetes. Neuropathy leads to reduced or absent pain sensation and consequently minor injury is not sensed, nor is subsequent infection, so that the first manifestation noted by the patient is a discharge which may be profuse or slight and which has a characteristic musty odour. Alternatively, no outward signs may be present and on reduction of a plantar callus a necrotic area is found, leading to a deep sinus which penetrates into the foot, possibly into the joint cavity. If only a small amount of clear discharge is present, there is no infection, while the copious discharge of pus is indicative of acute septic arthritis.

Following the complete removal of overlying hyperkeratosis, the cavity is drained and carefully cleaned by irrigation with sterile saline. The ulceration is dressed with a sterile dressing which may contain an antiseptic such as chlorhexidine. In some instances it is necessary to pack the cavity gently with a sterile tulle dressing to maintain adequate drainage. It may be nec-

essary to repeat the cleaning and debridement of the ulcer site and continue treatment with antiseptics until healing from the base of the ulcer takes place (see Ch. 9). Antibiotics by mouth may also be necessary. The maximum possible relief of weight-bearing should be provided by means of padding or a well-designed orthotic device. A metatarsal bar placed across the sole of the shoe to provide a rocking action may assist in preventing further damage. Reduction of body weight may also be indicated if this is thought to be a factor in increasing mechanical damage to the sole of the foot. If no local cause can be established for the ulceration, further investigation, directed at determining potential neuropathy, circulatory deficit or metabolic disease, should be undertaken.

Fibrosis (Fig. 7.5). Fibrosis (an increase of fibrous tissue) occurs in the dermal and subdermal tissues, most commonly on the plantar aspect of the foot, as a response to long-standing mechanical stress and injury. It arises from repeated damage and chronicity of low grade inflammation with delayed healing, which results in the accumulation of scar tissue in the dermis. Subcutaneous fascia is often depleted with a consequent reduction in protective shock absorption locally. The surrounding soft tissues tend to become adapted to the presence of the lesion, thus creating a 'crater' which may rapidly fill with hyperkeratotic skin unless the mechanical damage is prevented.

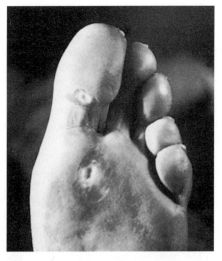

Figure 7.5 Long-standing plantar helomata after enucleation. Their appearance resembles that of the perforating ulcer in Figure 6.4, but these cavities have bases and sides of tough fibrous tissue which tend to perpetuate their recurrence.

Fibrosis is commonly implicated in the chronicity of many hyperkeratotic lesions.

Treatment depends on the repeated removal of overlying hyperkeratosis and effective deflection of pressure and shearing stress. Carefully designed and fitted orthotics, associated with appropriate footwear advice, with good compliance on the part of the patient, are essential, if progress is to be made in treating these resistant lesions. The use of escharotic caustic substances, such as pyrogallol and silver nitrate, assist in the reduction of both overlying hyperkeratosis and connective tissue elements in the dermis. Vitamin therapy, e.g. the use of fat-soluble vitamins A and E, either alone or with pyrogallol, is effective in some instances. It is likely that fat-soluble vitamins have a role to play in stimulating the activity of dermal cells, in particular the fibroblasts. Combined with effective mechanical therapy and regular reduction of the hyperkeratosis, the use of these topical medicines can be highly effective. Electrosurgery can also be employed in the management of such conditions (Ch. 12).

Synovial sacs. These small sacs containing synovial fluid are cavities created in the tissues by persistent shearing stress. Skin and subcutaneous tissue are subjected to chronic exposure and low grade shearing stress, resulting in the development of semi-organised synovial structures in the connective tissue of the dermis. Such tissue damage occurs as a rupture just below the dermo-epidermal junction, often beneath heloma durum or deep callus at a site of intermittent pressure and shearing stress. Small superficial bursae formed in this way fill with synovial fluid which may exude on enucleation. Elimination of the incomplete bursae can be achieved by employing appropriate astringent topical medication, such as silver nitrate, or by electrosurgical removal. Protective padding, aimed at reducing the effects of shear, is necessary to avoid recurrence. Such synovial structures occurring at a deeper level may form a sinus which communicates to the surface or with the underlying joint to form a fistula. The structure may become consolidated and fibrotic, to create a chronic adventitious bursa with recurrent episodes of bursitis.

Dermal protrusions. Dermal protrusions are small herniations of the dermis beyond the level of the dermo-epidermal junction. Two common examples are those which occur at the apex of a lesser toe and those in association with plantar heloma. The apex or pulp of a toe, most commonly the fifth as it underlies the fourth, may be affected by constant compression and pinching. This results in deformation and hypertrophy of the dermal papillae, which protrude from the dermis like a small coxcomb. The epidermal covering is very thin and there may be fissuring of the surface and discolouration from extravasation of blood from the hypertrophic papillae.

In the case of long-standing plantar heloma beneath the metatarsal heads, excessive reduction by operating or exfoliation may denude the epidermal layer to such an extent that the underlying dermal elements protrude into the enucleated area, simulating a vascular corn. In both cases, the excessive compression responsible for the dermal protrusions must be relieved before topical medication with astringents can have any effect in reducing the hypertrophic dermal papillae.

Furrowing. Furrowing is seen in plantar callus when it becomes pinched into a deep trough. This may occur between adjacent metatarsal heads, as in a splayed foot which has been constricted in narrow footwear, or immediately anterior to the metatarsophalangeal joints, as seen in mobile pes cavus. The margins of the furrow are often highly vascular and may contain fibrotic elements associated with enlarged hypertrophic dermal papillae. Like other cutaneous deformations, furrows are indicative of the causative mechanical stresses, which effective treatment will aim to moderate.

Fissures. Fissures are splits in the epidermis resulting from a loss of elasticity in the skin or alteration of its texture and strength due to changes in hydration. They occur interdigitally when the skin is macerated, and around the heel when the skin is excessively dry. Careful drying and astringent medication are required interdigitally for fissures associated with maceration, while, in contrast, the regular application of emollients is indicated for dry heel fissures. The edges of heel fissures may be heavily calloused and need to be reduced operatively before medication is administered. Weight-relieving padding will help to reduce the compression of the plantar heel tissues and consequently the tensile stress exerted on the epidermis as the skin bulges on weight-bearing.

Principles of treatment

All mechanically induced hyperkeratotic lesions and their associated complications require a comprehensive regime of treatment, involving operative, medicinal and mechanical aspects of therapy. The objective is to restore the skin and subcutaneous tissues as nearly as possible to normal and to eliminate or mitigate the stresses responsible for the condition. This objective is usually attainable, provided a programme of treatment is planned and conducted over an adequate period of time. Treatment which is merely episodic and temporarily palliative is usually ineffectual and tends to become endlessly repetitive, which is unsatisfactory to both the patient and the practitioner.

The enucleation of heloma and the reduction of callosities can be achieved succesfully, painlessly and without bleeding provided that the correct scalpel is chosen and a careful operating technique is employed. The maintenance of firm skin tension is essential to a safe technique.

An important element in treatment is the relief of abnormal mechanical stresses which produce hyperkeratosis. For plantar lesions, this entails the identification and correction of underlying structural and functional defects (Ch. 5). Dorsal lesions and those on the lateral aspect of the foot require careful identification of the mechanical stresses occurring between the foot and its covering footwear. Mechanical protection is achieved with properly designed digital padding. Initially, this may be adhesive, but subsequently should be detachable. The range of devices available includes corrective and protective orthodigital splints for the intermediate toes, shields for the hallux and fifth toe, and interdigital wedges. These may be fabricated from a variety of materials which are described in Chapters 12 and 14. When combined with suitable footwear and given satisfactory compliance on the part of the patient, such measures provide good clinical results.

Bursae

Bursae occur both naturally (anatomically) and adventitiously (developing in response to external stimuli, usually superficial) in the subcutaneous tissues. They are small connective tissue sacs which become organised and lined with synovial cells secreting synovial fluid. Anatomical bursae are found at sites where there is a functional need to reduce both friction and shearing. They facilitate smoothness of movement at points of potential resistance to free movement. Adventitious bursae can develop beneath heloma, and at sites where the soft tissues are subjected to excessive shearing stresses, as in hallux abductovalgus (Fig. 7.6). Sites in the foot where bursae are liable to become inflamed due to mechanical trauma are:

- on the medial aspect of the first metatarsal in hallux abductovalgus
- on the posterior aspect of the heel, either superficially between the skin and the tendo Achilles, or retrocalcaneally between the calcaneus and the insertion of the tendo Achilles
- under the plantar aspect of the calcaneus
- over the lateral aspect of the cuboid in talipes equinovarus

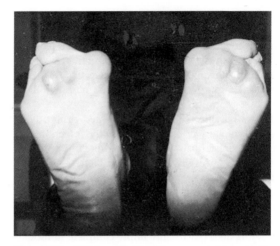

Figure 7.6   Plantar callus and fibrous nodules under the middle metatarsal heads, indicating overloading secondary to hallux abductovalgus deformity.

- under an heloma on the dorsum of an interphalangeal joint.

Inflamed bursae arise as a result of either trauma or infection.

Traumatic bursitis. This is caused by undue shearing stress at any one of the sites mentioned, and there is frequently pain and swelling. If there is continued irritation and injury, the condition may become chronic, with further distension due to the accumulation of fluid within the bursal sac. Synovial fluid may track either towards the surface, through a sinus, or inwards to the joint through a fistula. Both channels may develop, allowing synovial fluid from a joint to discharge onto the surface.

Infective bursitis. This may be established by spread of infection via a sinus or through the cavity left after enucleation of helomata. The resulting inflammation frequently extends over a considerable area. It may resolve if the infecting organism is not virulent, but otherwise suppuration and further spread of the infection into the surrounding connective tissues may ensue.

Treatment of bursitis

Traumatic bursitis. In acute cases where there is no sinus, the most effective treatment is to rest the area and reduce the hyperaemic phase of the inflammatory process by the use of cooling lotions, such as in a wet compress, or by the application of cold in an appropriate form. Once the acute episode has subsided, the reabsorption of the excess synovial fluid within the bursal sac may be increased by the application of heat and rubefacients. When bursitis occurs beneath an heloma, reduction of the hyperkeratosis often exposes a sinus. The sinus should be cleaned and then closed, if possible, by means of astringents (see Ch. 12). Any potential trauma to the area must be eliminated by protective padding.

Infective bursitis. This must be treated promptly in order to avoid any possible spread of the infection. It is necessary to establish drainage, if this is not already taking place naturally. Once the infection has been controlled, which may require the administration of appropriate antibiotics, treatment is similar to that for traumatic bursitis.

Rest is an important element in the treatment of bursitis, but this does not usually imply complete immobility, which is rarely practicable. Sufficient immobilisation can be secured by the use of protective padding which protects the tissues from further mechanical injury. Protective shields and footwear modifications should be prescribed to prevent recurrence. If conservative measures prove inadequate, surgical excision of the bursa, together with surgical correction of the underlying deformity, may be required.

Tenosynovitis

Tenosynovitis (inflammation of a tendon sheath) occurs infrequently in feet and almost invariably arises from mechanical strain. The extensor tendon sheaths in front of the ankle are sometimes affected. At the back of the ankle, the Achilles tendon has no true sheath but may suffer strain with inflammation (tendinitis) from overuse. Bursae around the Achilles tendon are subject to acute bursitis from the same cause. The symptoms of tenosynovitis are usually mild, with some swelling, stiffness, pain and crepitus on movement.

Treatment

Treatment is directed at immobilisation with padding and strapping, together with cold or heat therapy to resolve the inflammation. Tendinitis of the tendo Achilles may be caused by overactivity, such as over-enthusiastic athletic training, which should be suspended temporarily. If associated with an ankle equinus, however, the footwear should be suitably modified by a permanent increase in the height of the heel.

The tendon of the long extensor of the great toe is particularly prone to inflammation in cases where the hallux is hyperextended, as, for example, in pes cavus. The tendon then stands out from the dorsum of the foot and is liable to be irritated by the crease in the upper of the shoe. A small heloma may develop first, and enucleation may expose a sinus, leading to the tendon sheath. This cavity may be repeatedly plugged by dried exudate, forming an apparent heloma, but infection may occur through the sinus.

It may prove difficult to remove completely the source of irritation. The footwear is commonly implicated: the shoe may be too loose or a deep fold in the upper can arise due to surplus material in an oversized or otherwise ill-fitting shoe. A change to more suitable footwear or modifications to existing shoes may be indicated. Protection for the tendon is provided by appropriate padding. A permanent shield made from latex or silicone may be required.

Ganglion

A ganglion is a firm swelling protruding from a tendon sheath or joint capsule which has herniated, allowing synovial fluid to escape and form a rigidly encapsulated cyst. Ganglia are not inflammatory and the swelling may be hard or soft and fluctuant. They occur fairly commonly on the dorsum of the foot, around the lateral aspect of the ankle, over the calcaneocuboid joint and around the first metatarsophalangeal joint. At this latter site, pressure may cause the fluid contents to track anteriorly or posteriorly in relation to the joint. On examination, the swelling can be related to the underlying joint or tendon structures from which it derives. The skin can be moved over the ganglion easily, but the cyst is usually tied firmly to its structure of origin so that it cannot be mobilised over the underlying bones and joints. A light passed into the cyst from a pocket torch causes the whole cyst to glow (transillumination) as the synovial contents of the ganglion readily transmit light.

Ganglia are often asymptomatic and may be left alone. If symptoms are produced, usually because of pressure from the shoe, then surgical removal is indicated. It is not possible to aspirate ganglia, because they frequently prove to be internally divided into cavities by multiple connective tissue septae, and the aspiration needle cannot be directed to each minute locule of synovium. Occasionally, they prove to be attached extensively and surgical removal may not be straightfoward.

CONDITIONS ARISING FROM INFECTIONS

Bacterial infection

Minor infections of the foot are common. However,

early treatment and antibiotic therapy, when necessary, usually prevent the spread of infection from the initial location. Most bacterial infections of the foot are, therefore, relatively easily resolved and do not require antibiotic treatment but can be managed with simple local measures.

Predisposing factors are extremely important when considering bacterial infections. Such infections are generally more prevalent in older people and in association with debility and systematic illness, poor hygiene, inadequate nutrition and anaemia. In some instances, medicines such as corticosteroids, and immunosuppressive and cytotoxic drugs may contribute to reduced resistance. Coexisting illnesses may be of significance since they may be associated with an increase in the incidence and severity of bacterial infection. Amongst such disorders, diabetes mellitus is the most frequent from the viewpoint of the podiatrist. Ischaemic disorders, due to changes in the arterial wall leading to occlusive arterial disease (atherosclerosis), represent a further important risk group.

The skin of the human foot supports a relatively large microflora. This is due to the effect of occlusion in footwear and the associated moisture retention, particularly in the interdigital spaces and toe webbing. The specialised thick stratum corneum of the plantar skin acts as a barrier to the ingress of otherwise commensal organisms and pathogens. The relative absence of hair on the dorsal thin-skinned areas of the foot reduces the possibility of bacteria gaining access via the hair follicle. Footwear is a relevant factor in the aetiology of many of the common lesions of bacterial origin occurring in the foot. Shoes create an environment which is high in humidity and temperature and therefore conducive to the establishment of large populations of bacteria. Ill-fitting footwear tends to produce abrasions and other mechanically induced lesions, which represent a route of entry for bacteria. Occlusive footwear tends to produce increased numbers of organisms which would normally be present in smaller numbers. There are also factors, such as the prolonged use of corticosteroids, antibiotics and immunosuppressive medicines, which alter the immune response of the host to infection. These may also alter the normal relationship and therefore equilibrium of the skin flora, so that changes in populations of microorganisms may become significant. This is the case when there is an overgrowth or increase in the number of potential pathogens due to an alteration in environmental conditions which favours proliferation. Organisms which are a normal part of the skin flora (commensal) can, due to rapid colonisation, act as opportunistic pathogens.

Erythrasma

Erythrasma is the most common bacterial infection of the foot. It is a mild infection, affecting body folds as well as the toe webs. In those sites, usually intertriginous, in which colonisation by *Corynebacterium minutissimum* occurs, a well circumscribed dry lesion appears with discoloured brownish patches covered by a fine scaling. In toe webbing the picture is less clear and erythrasma appears simply as maceration and fissuring. Because of its rather nondescript appearance in the interdigital site, this most common bacterial infection may be misdiagnosed as simple intertrigo or as an interdigital dermatophyte infection. This infection may account for the large number of apparent fungal infections which prove to be negative on culture and in which no mycelia can be demonstrated.

Treatment consists of the application of topical keratolytics, e.g. salicylic acid, or the use of broad-spectrum antiseptics. If infection is persistent, then erythromycin given as a daily dose of 1 g for between 7 and 10 days is indicated, and is virtually always curative. The significance of erythrasma, which is a common bacterial infection of the foot, should not be underestimated since its differential diagnosis should be considered carefully in cases of apparent interdigital mycosis.

Aetiological factors in erythrasma include occlusion and increased humidity. It is likely that a break or damage to the epidermis is necessary for increased colonisation by the multiple members of the diphtheroid group of bacteria, collectively referred to as *C. minutissimum*. Only then will clinical manifestations of the disease become apparent. These organisms are also noteworthy because they are fluorescent. When viewed under Wood's ultraviolet light, they fluoresce coral red.

Intertrigo

This is not principally a bacterial infection since it is due to the effects of mechanical forces on contiguous skin surfaces, increased friction and environmental factors such as increased temperature and moisture. Lesions occur only on contiguous skin surfaces and this includes the toe webbings of the feet. The early signs are redness and maceration, but later there may be marked surrounding inflammation with a white centre and exudation. At this stage, numerous secondary bacteria may colonise the area and so aggravate the lesion and prolong its course. No single organism can be identified as the main colonising agent, but a number of different bacteria, fungi and yeasts may be involved as secondary contaminants.

Treatment is designed to separate and dry the contiguous skin surfaces by the application of absorbents simultaneously with a disposable interdigital wedge. Specific treatment may be indicated to eradicate secondary infection if this is severe.

Staphylococcal infections

Staphylococcus pyogenes can be considered the most frequent cause of pyogenic infection of the foot. Infections involving *Staph. pyogenes* frequently follow puncture wounds, abrasion, surgical incision and indeed any trauma to the foot. They also occur as secondary infections in cases of dermatophytosis. Often, this organism is responsible for infections in heloma durum, which, for one reason or another, become damaged, allowing the ingress of this colonising pathogen. Lesions are typified by localised inflammation, abscess formation or discharge. *Staphylococcus pyogenes* has an extremely wide distribution, and as organisms of this species are the most common cause of pyogenic infection, and the majority of them involve the skin and its appendages, they are of considerable importance to the podiatrist. The species is typified by the ability of the organism to form an enzyme which is similar to thrombin; this is called coagulase and it produces clotting of citrated plasma.

All those staphylococci which produce coagulase (coagulase-positive) belong to the species *Staph. pyogenes*. They may occur as commensals as well as in lesions but are regarded in that situation as potential pathogens. Coagulase-negative staphylococci are commonly found on the skin but are either non-pathogenic or only low grade pathogens.

Occasionally, infection with *Staph. pyogenes* may occur on the dorsum of the foot due to colonisation of hair follicles. The resulting folliculitis may be superseded by the development of a furuncle (a boil or carbuncle). These lesions occur only in areas where there are hair follicles, and are therefore confined to the dorsum of the foot. The clinical picture is typical, and the site tends to point to the diagnosis since there is an obvious association with one of the small areas of hair on the dorsum of the foot and toes. All the signs of inflammation are present, and a tender nodule appears which becomes a fluctuating swelling over a period of 3–4 days.

Treatment is by the administration of antibiotics of a penicillinase-resistant type, e.g. flucloxacillin, in a dose of 1 g per day for 7–10 days. When there is outright suppuration and the swelling becomes fluctuant,

carefully timed surgical incision may be indicated so that drainage of the lesion may be achieved.

The most common staphylococcal infection to present in the podiatrist's surgery is that of an infected heloma durum, the causes of which have already been considered. The treatment of this lesion serves to typify the approach which should be made to virtually any localised infected lesion of the foot. The principles therefore apply to infected lesions of types other than the infected heloma durum, which may be accompanied by an underlying abscess.

Commonly, an aseptic necrosis, which occurs due to the continuous pressure exerted by the nucleus of an heloma, leads to maceration of the overlying hyperkeratosis. This produces an opportunity for *Staph. pyogenes* to gain entry into the deeper layers of the skin and subsequently to produce an abscess underneath the lesion.

The principal steps in treatment are:

1. Cleanse the area surrounding the lesion and finally the lesion itself.
2. Establish drainage by removal of the overlying tissue or by incision.
3. Clean out the abscess cavity by irrigating with sterile saline solution.
4. If there is considerable inflammation or if it proves difficult to expel all the pus from the abscess, a hypertonic saline foot bath may be used. The foot is immersed in the solution which is maintained at 43°C for 10–15 minutes.
5. After the footbath, the lesion is again thoroughly irrigated with a sterile solution to ensure that the abscess cavity is clean.
6. Apply a sterile dressing (see also Ch. 9). The use of topical antibiotics is never indicated. The narrow spectrum of activity provided by antibiotic preparations limits their value. If a local medication is used, a broad-spectrum antiseptic such as chlorhexidine should be selected. Staphylococci have an ability to develop a resistance to antibiotics, which provides a further good reason for avoiding topical application of systemically effective medicines. Hypersensitivity reactions to topical antibiotics are also too frequent for their use to be indicated, except in unusual circumstances. This is not to say that antibiotics are never indicated in the case of staphylococcal infections. In the case of the old, debilitated, diabetic or immunosuppressed patient, or in individuals who have a history of recurrent infection for any reason, antibiotic therapy may be indicated, but this would usually be by parenteral administration.
7. Protective padding is required to distribute pres-

sure away from the lesion, if this has been an antagonising factor. Appropriate padding will depend upon the site of the infected lesion.

8. Follow-up should usually take place twice weekly until healing is complete.

These procedures are repeated until the infection has cleared. A final check made 2–3 weeks after the inflammation has subsided is prudent.

Collections of pus due to staphylococcal infection close to the nail plate and associated with the sulci or proximal to the eponychium are fairly common and need to be differentiated from paronychia due to *Candida albicans*. The treatment of these superficial infections follows the above pattern. The secondary infection associated with onychocryptosis is usually due to *Staph. pyogenes*, although numerous organisms will colonise a long-standing onychocryptosis.

Mechanical factors may be significant, particularly in relation to lesions on the dorsum of the toes, over the first metatarsophalangeal joint and on the lateral aspect of the fifth metatarsophalangeal joint. In all dorsal, medial and lateral sites, modifications of footwear may be useful. These range from simply cutting a hole in an old shoe to accommodate a deformed joint which has developed an infected lesion, to the provision of a balloon patch or some other more permanent adaptation to accommodate deformity (see Ch. 14).

Streptococcal infections

The group of commonly occurring streptococci, *Streptococcus pyogenes*, which may be carried by healthy individuals in the throat or nose, or on the skin surface, are potentially extremely pathogenic, although they may be found occasionally as harmless commensals. The aerobic strains are classified according to their haemolytic activity on a blood agar plate. All strains of *S. pyogenes* are β-haemolytic, i.e. they can lyse red cells and decolourise haemoglobin in culture. It is with this group that the podiatrist should be concerned. *Streptococcus pyogenes* does not remain localised in the same way as *Staph. pyogenes*, since the streptococcus is able to produce a number of enzymes which facilitate its migration into the tissues. Of the six or so enzymes produced, the most important in relation to the spread of infection from the skin into the connective tissues are streptokinase, hyaluronidase and streptodornase. In consequence, infections with *S. pyogenes* tend to spread rapidly into surrounding tissue. The action of several enzymes allows the organism to spread in this way from the primary lesion into the connective tissues and from

there into the lymphatic system. If unchecked at this point, spread may continue into the bloodstream. The conditions which occur as this process of extension takes place are describe below.

The primary lesion. Due to rapid spread away from the site of initial infection, the primary lesion may be unremarkable and consist of a brief inflammatory reaction which shortly gives way to the signs of spreading infection.

Cellulitis. This presents with localised redness, heat, pain and diffuse oedema of the skin. It represents a spreading of the infection into the connective tissue subjacent to the skin. The infection may be arrested and resolved at this point by the vigorous inflammatory response. Alternatively, spread may continue from the connective tissue into the smaller lymphatic vessels of the greater or lesser saphenous systems, producing lymphangitis.

Lymphangitis. This is typified by the appearance of a red line which conforms closely to the route of the saphenous vessels. Because most of the foot and all of the forefoot is drained by the greater saphenous system, lymphangitis will usually occur along the system of vessels which passes in front of the medial malleolus and then up the anteromedial aspects of the leg. Infections occurring in a small area, confined mainly to the lateral and posterior aspects of the heel, may produce lymphangitis of the lesser saphenous vessels, which run posteriorly to the lateral malleolus and up to the popliteal fossa, where the short vessels terminate.

In patients suffering from cellulitis which does not rapidly resolve, and more particularly in those suffering from lymphangitis, systemic symptoms become quite marked, with pyrexia and other signs of toxaemia. If the infection is not halted at this stage, spread of infection may occur into the lymph nodes, producing lymphadenitis.

Lymphadenitis. The lymph nodes become inflamed and tender and ultimately, if the infection persists, these may deteriorate into a series of abscesses. This is more likely to occur in the greater saphenous system, thereby implicating the inguinal lymph nodes, but it may occasionally involve the popliteal lymph nodes. Spread beyond the lymph nodes results in the appearance of *S. pyogenes* in the bloodstream (bacteraemia), and possible spread via the bloodstream (septicaemia).

In practice, it is extremely unusual for streptococcal infections to pass beyond the stage at which cellulitis is the clinical manifestation. Since β-haemolytic streptococci are sensitive to penicillin, antibiotic treatment should quickly eradicate the infection. Following treatment, care should to be taken to identify the means whereby infection became established and to prevent recurrence as far as possible.

Pseudomonas pyocyanea (Ps. aeruginosa)

This is a Gram-negative bacillus which is pathogenic and tends to be resistant to the commonly used antibiotics. For this reason, it may give rise to persistent infections and these may occur on the foot. It may invade accidental or surgical wounds and give rise to a characteristically discoloured blue-green pus, which is further characterised by its smell. Since this organism is a contaminant of abraded wounds, it must be differentiated from staphylococcal infections. While both produce localised inflammation and pus, the blue-green discolouration of the discharge and the musty-sweet smell produced by *Ps. pyocyanea* infections readily indicate its presence.

Treatment. Since *Ps. pyocyanea* is resistant to a wide variety of antibiotics, this infection may be persistent. Treatment by the local application of dilute acetic acid may be sufficient to eradicate superficial infections. Broad-spectrum antiseptics may be effective, provided adequate drainage and debridement are first carried out.

Pseudomonas pyocyanea commonly occurs as a secondary bacterial infection in nails affected by one of the dermatophytes, when it tends to discolour the nail plate dark blue to black.

Bacterial paronychia

While a number of different bacteria may be involved, including staphylococci, streptococci, *Escherichia coli* and *Ps. pyocyanea*, the presence of *Candida albicans* is most likely to produce chronic paronychia. Secondary bacterial infection is the usual cause of acute inflammatory exacerbations which occur during the course of chronic paronychia.

Treatment consists of dealing first with the secondary bacterial infection and then with the *Candida* infection. Clotrimazole 1% cream or solution, and miconazole nitrate cream 2% are effective against fungi, including the yeasts, and are useful following treatment with broad-spectrum antibacterial medicaments.

Verrucae

Verrucae, or warts, particularly affecting the hands and feet, represent one of the most common viral infections of the skin. The frequency of this lesion seems to be related to the provision and use of shared facilities in swimming baths, sports centres and gymnasia. Management of viral infection calls for an understanding of the causative organism, and any attempt at treatment should take into account the natural history of the infection. It is important to consider the normal outcome of this infection in view of its frequency and the consequent costs of providing treatment.

Warts are caused by the human papilloma virus (HPV), which induces benign spontaneously regressing epithelial tumours in the skin and mucosa (Jablonska & Orth 1983). The virus is widely distributed in nature and has been the subject of considerable study. It is an isometric virus with a constant 72 units in its capsid (outer coat). A number of HPV types are recognised and classified according to molecular differences of nucleotide sequencing. There appears to be a preferential association between given HPV types, lesion morphology and location. However, because there may be some plurality of lesion type associated with HPV infection, relating specific viral types to particular lesion morphologies may not be sound.

The deep endophytic plantar or palmar wart is associated with HPV 1. The common wart, affecting the dorsal or palmar surface of the hands and the face, and the mosaic wart, of the plantar surface, are associated with HPV 2. The small keratosis punctata, like lesions of the plantar and palmar surfaces, are associated with HPV 4. Histological features of each type of wart, and variations in immunity and regression are associated with HPV type.

HPV is found in large numbers distributed throughout the cells of the prickle cell layer in infected tissue, and there is no difficulty in demonstrating its presence by electron micrography, particularly in lesions of under 18 months' duration. The plantar wart occurs as a sharply circumscribed tumour with a hyperkeratotic covering which tends to obscure the typically papillomatous dermal component. The cells of the germinal layer appear normal. There is abnormal mitotic activity which leads to hyperplasia of the prickle cell layer (acanthosis). Other histological features include the presence of vacuoles in affected cells and remarkable changes in the morphology of the dermo-epidermal junction, with gross enlargement and elongation of the rete pegs. The hypertrophic rete pegs converge in a characteristic centripetal fashion, i.e. they tend to become aligned between the superficial peripheral margin and a point deep in the centre of the lesion (Fig. 7.7A).

In the earliest stages, the lesion may be represented by the minimal disturbance of the papillary structure,

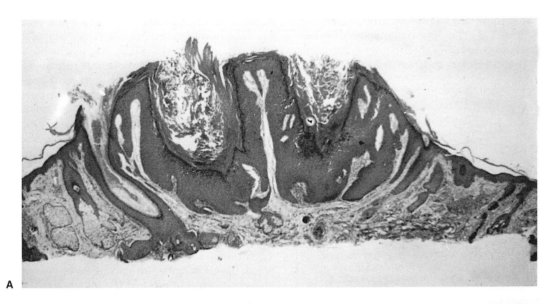

A

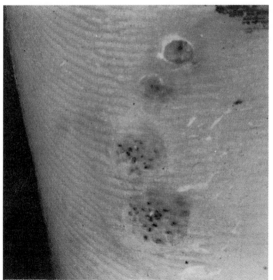

B

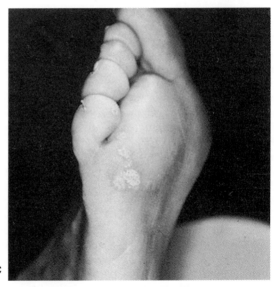

C

Figure 7.7   A: Transverse section of wart, demonstrating acanthosis and hyperkeratosis. B: Plantar warts—multiple. C: Plantar warts—mosaic.

appearing not unlike a small vesicle, but, characteristically, the primary dermal ridge involved is sharply interrupted. Later there is a cessation of the normal pattern of dermal ridging at the periphery, with a cloud-like or cauliflower pattern representing the papillomatous part of the lesion. Dilated capillaries may appear as red spots within the lesion, and darker brown or black spots and streaks are seen in regressing lesions due to the presence of extensive microvascular thrombosis affecting the small vessels within the wart.

These changes are not neoplastic but represent an example of focal reactive hyperplasia of the epidermis. Warts due to HPV 1, HPV 2, and HPV 4 do not undergo malignant conversion.

Morphologically, there is considerable variation in the clinical appearance of warts. Weight-bearing sites on the plantar aspect of the foot modify the appearance of the lesion by forcing its mass into the dermis and leaving only the hyperkeratotic overlay exposed. For this reason, verrucae may be mistaken for heloma durum or discrete areas of callus, from which they may be differentiated by close examination of the papillary structure after removal of the overlying callus. Other differential factors are given in Box 7.1.

Box 7.1 Points in differential diagnosis: verrucae vs heloma

---

1. The speed of onset: warts being much more rapid in their development than heloma durum, which are associated with chronicity.
2. Site: warts may occur at any site, whereas heloma occur only at sites of intermittent compression and friction.
3. Age: warts usually affect children and young adults, while heloma are more common in middle-aged and older people.
4. In the case of warts, when the lesion surface is cut, bleeding tends to occur quite freely from the cut ends of dilated capillaries. In the case of heloma, capillary bleeding is not usual when the overlying hyperkeratosis is removed.

It is emphasised that these factors (Box 7.1) are only indicators and that diagnosis should be made on the basis of examination of the papillary structure of the skin using a $10\times$ power magnifying glass if necessary. On non-weight-bearing sites, the warty appearance of the papilloma, which projects in a dome-like fashion above the surface, tends to be much more obvious and the differential diagnosis presents few problems.

Warts may occur as single or multiple tumours affecting any aspect of the foot. Not uncommonly, the lesion is shallow and covers a wide area. This so-called mosaic pattern is brought about by infection with HPV 2, whereas the deep endophytic type of plantar wart is caused by HPV 1. The mosaic wart tends to be shallow and pain-free, while the deep plantar wart can be extremely painful (Fig. 7.7B & C).

HPV is probably inoculated mechanically through micro-injury of the skin. This may easily take place during barefoot activities, especially when the skin has been wet for some time, as in swimming, or due to sweating after intense exercise followed by showering. Such factors could well be associated reasons for the gently fluctuating endemic status of plantar wart infections. These considerations will tend to suggest means for controlling local epidemics in schools and similar situations where it is feasible to isolate and treat the infected group, while regularly checking the others. However, it is almost impossible to apply this technique to a larger population and it is doubtful whether the practice of foot inspections at swimming

baths achieves anything, since the virus will have spread quickly before a lesion becomes clinically obvious.

Since there is an immunological response to this infection, which confers some degree of protection after first infection, the anxiety which surrounds the appearance of this common foot lesion is not justified. It has been shown that humoral antibodies can be detected in the serum of individuals who have wart infection and that high levels of wart virus-specific IgG are associated with regression of the lesion. The relationship between the appearance of humoral antibodies and the cell-bound immune reactions which must occur prior to regression are not clear. However, there is abundant supportive evidence to show that regression is the normal outcome of infection and tumour development due to wart virus. Some patients with warts have been shown to have a defect of non-specific cell-mediated immunity.

Regression takes place usually within 6–8 months of onset and persistence beyond this time must be considered an indication that treatment may be necessary. Pain or disability for any reason constitutes the main indication for active treatment. In the case of pain-free lesions of recent onset in children and young adults, explanation of the expected outcome is preferable to immediate and possibly unnecessary treatment. Confusion can sometimes arise because the regressing wart tends to become painful or tender and may be inflamed for about 2 weeks prior to a sudden abatement of the discomfort. This painful phase may be misinterpreted and treatment begun. In fact, shortly after this phase there will frequently be extensive microvascular thrombosis of the vessels running through the lesion, so that they appear as black or red lines and streaks radiating from the centre, and the surrounding hyperkeratosis shows a yellow discolouration (Fig. 7.8).

Treatment

When treatment is indicated there are two potential avenues of approach:

1. the use antiviral medicines
2. the destruction of all the cells involved in the lesion, guaranteeing that virally infected cells do not survive.

In practice, the first of these has not proved to be effective. Clinical trials with the antiviral drugs idoxuridine in dimethylsulphoxide (DMSO), rimantadine hydrochloride and xenazoic acid have been disap-

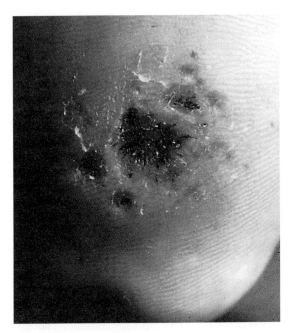

Figure 7.8 Regressing wart. Note the dilated vessels filled with coagulated blood. The thrombotic vessels appear to radiate from the centre.

pointing. The most promising of these, idoxuridine, has been investigated in clinical trials, but the results are no better than with existing treatment. There is a serious pharmacological drawback since idoxuridine works by incorporation into the DNA of replicating virus, and in the case of an established wart there is not likely to be any increase in the number of virus particles, and therefore no active replication takes place. Gluteraldehyde solutions have been used widely but have proved to be less effective in clinical trials than keratolytics.

This leaves destructive techniques to eradicate the viral-infected tissue and thus remove the cause of the lesion. All the techniques employed have in common one underlying principle: that the wart, together with a small margin of unaffected tissue, is destroyed and removed. Only the means of tissue destruction varies, and the various techniques are described in Chapter 12.

Tinea pedis

The most common fungal infections of skin are those which occur on the feet. Footwear creates the necessary conditions of moisture and warmth between the toes, and communal activity permits the spread of infection. Swimming baths and shared bathing facilities in schools and other communal situations are often the most frequent locations of small-scale epidemics. Tinea pedis in its chronic form is largely a disease of adults, while acute episodes of athlete's foot are more common in school-age children. There are three common forms, which show the following characteristics:

1. Maceration and desquamation in the lateral toe spaces (Fig. 7.9); this is the prevalent type and can be caused by any of three common organisms: *Trichophyton (T.) rubrum, T. interdigitale* and *Epidermophyton (E.) floccosum.*

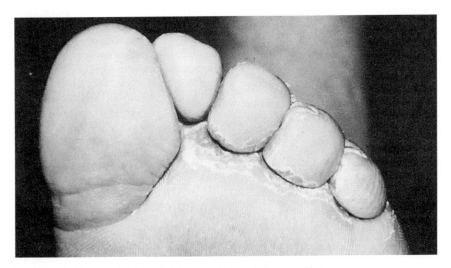

Figure 7.9 Tinea pedis: interdigital maceration and desquamation.

2. Episodes of unilateral acute vesiculation on the soles, which are usually caused by *T. interdigitale* or *E. floccosum*.
3. Dry redness and diffuse scaling over the soles, the so-called moccasin type, is usually caused by *T. rubrum*.

Fungal hyphae are also capable of invading the nails (see Ch. 8). Acute tinea pedis may be followed by a vesicular eruption on the hands from which no fungus can be isolated. The term *trichophytide* is used to describe this reaction.

The clinical diagnosis of a fungal infection can be confirmed by microscopic examination of skin scrapings and the type of fungus can be identified by culture of the scales. A single species is usually grown, but mixed infections occasionally occur.

Clinical trials of topical treatments have not demonstrated any one to be greatly superior to the others. Traditional remedies include Castellani's paint and Whitfield's ointment. Newer topical agents include tolnaftate, clotrimazole and miconazole, which are more acceptable to the patient, and the latter two are also active against yeasts. These should be used twice daily. Widespread severe infections and those involving the nails are treated with systemic griseofulvin, terbinafine or the imidazoles.

Toenail infections may take more than 18 months to clear, as the drug is incorporated only into newly formed nail. Griseofulvin is normally well tolerated and active against most dermatophyte infections. Oral ketoconazole may be considered where griseofulvin causes an adverse reaction or the infection proves resistant to its use. It is now thought that long-term ketoconazole for dermatophyte nail infection is unacceptable as a first line treatment because of the risk of hepatic toxicity. Ketoconazole is active against both yeasts and dermatophytes, but griseofulvin is only active against the latter. Terbinafine, a newer systemic agent, has also produced promising results and is claimed to have a more rapid effect than griseofulvin. Until the infection has been cleared, patients should not go barefoot in places where they would expose others to the fungi, e.g. changing rooms and swimming baths. They should not allow anyone else to use their towels, shoes and socks. A non-absorbent bath mat, which can be cleaned with disinfectant, should be used. Antifungal powders may be used regularly inside the shoes as a prophylactic measure.

DISORDERS OF SWEATING

Hyperhidrosis

Excessive production of sweat from the palms and soles does not usually imply any disease process but is a physiological phenomon. Emotional disturbances however, worsen the problem. Sweat may be produced continuously or intermittently, usually less in the winter than in summer.

Hyperhidrosis may affect either sex and often starts in childhood or adolescence. Young adult men are particularly prone to hyperhidrosis of the feet and there may be a family history of this condition. Clothing and shoes can become saturated and pools of sweat may form. The risk of developing pompholyx (q.v.) and contact eczema (q.v.) is increased by hyperhidrosis.

Treatment is often unsatisfactory, but reassurance should be given that improvement will normally occur in the mid-20s. There are a number of useful over-the-counter antiperspirants and absorbent powders available. Aluminium chloride hexahydrate in alcoholic solution may be effective, but often requires prolonged periods or overnight application; sometimes added polythene occlusion may be necessary. Iontophoresis with tap water or a solution of the anticholinergic drug glycopyrrhonium bromide may give a good response. The side-effects of medicines that reduce sweating, such as propantheline, make them too troublesome for routine use. Sympathectomy, the surgical division of the nerve supply to the sweat glands controlling secretion, is rarely indicated.

Bromhidrosis

Malodour of the feet is usually the consequence of keratin decomposition in the presence of hyperhidrosis. Particularly around the toes and on the weight-bearing areas, this may be visible as multiple superficial pits, giving rise to a 'worm-eaten' appearance caused by corynebacterial overgrowth and known as pitted keratolysis. Fungal colonisation of the skin will worsen the situation. Measures to reduce sweat production and to control secondary infection will effect some improvement. Talcum powder, spray deodorants and absorbent insoles are simple remedies which the patient is likely to have tried before seeking advice. Regular washing and the avoidance of occlusive footwear are important adjuncts to treatment. Boric acid footbaths or 3% formalin soaks may also be helpful.

Anhidrosis

When sweating does not occur, the term anhidrosis is used. Unlike hyperhidrosis, it is usually associated with organic disease. It may occur as an isolated symptom and there is an age-related decline in sweat gland activity, so that the skin of older people is drier than that of the young.

Anhidrosis can originate at any of the stages involved in sweat production. Table 7.1 summarises some of the more important causes. Treatment will be directed towards the basic cause if possible. Failing this, the regular use of emollients such as lanolin or soft white paraffin may reduce discomfort and the tendency for dry skin to become fissured, especially around the margins of the heels. The use of creams containing 10% urea has also proved to be effective in treating anhidrotic skin.

Erythema pernio (chilblains)

Chilblains represent an abnormal vascular reaction to cold. They may be produced on rewarming after exposure to cold, when there is more rapid dilatation of the constricted arterioles than of the draining venules. This leads to reactive hyperaemia and the exudation of fluid into the tissues. Chilblains occur at any age but are most common in children and young people, especially young women. They start in early winter, but outdoor workers may develop them as late as springtime.

Itching and erythema are followed by swelling of the subcutaneous tissues on the dorsum of the proximal phalanges of the toes, on the heels, the lower legs, the fingers, nose or ears. Chilblains may be single or multiple and usually subside in 2–3 weeks. Sometimes the reaction is more intense, with ulceration and irreversible necrosis. Acrocyanosis or erythrocyanosis may be associated features.

Prevention by wearing warm clothing, avoiding cold and damp, taking adequate exercise and a good diet is much more effective than local treatment used once the lesions have appeared. A local antipruritic such as menthol in aqueous cream may help. In the most severe cases, sympathectomy has been employed and there are reports of benefit from oral slow release preparations of nifedipine.

Table 7.1   Some causes of anhidrosis

Site	Causes
Brain	Hypothalamic disease
Spinal cord	Trauma, including surgery, syringomyelia
Peripheral nerve	Sympathectomy, drugs, leprosy, diabetes
Sweat glands	Absence, congenital ectodermal dysplasia, atrophy, scleroderma
Sweat ducts	Prickly heat, eczema, psoriasis

Trophic ulceration

Damage to the sensory nerves of the skin leads to anaesthesia and an increased liability to injury. Persistent painless ulceration may result on the pressure areas of the feet, under the metatarsal heads and on the heels. This can be precipitated by ill-fitting shoes or inexpert enucleation of heloma.

Some conditions predisposing to the formation of trophic ulcers are listed in Box 7.2. Similar, but usually painful, ulceration may be induced by vascular disease or irradiation.

The skin surrounding a trophic ulcer is hyperkeratotic and anhidrotic. Sinus formation and osteomyelitis of an underlying tarsal or metatarsal bone may follow the inadequate treatment of infections. Management depends on the relief of pressure, the correction, if possible, of the underlying disorder and the eradication of infection. Surgical intervention, e.g. the removal of a metatarsal head, may be required.

Box 7.2   Some causes of trophic ulceration

- Diabetic peripheral neuropathy
- Trauma to spinal cord or peripheral nerves
- Spinal vascular disease
- Syringomyelia
- Poliomyelitis
- Neurosyphilis (tabes dorsalis)
- Polyneuropathy
- Tuberculoid leprosy
- Congenital absence of pain sensation

OTHER SKIN CONDITIONS AFFECTING THE FEET

It is not the intention in this section to describe all the skin disorders which may affect the feet; reference should be made to textbooks of dermatology for more information. Those skin diseases which are common or of particular importance in managing foot disorders are summarised. Only the main clinical features will be given, as in most cases investigation and treatment will be described in detail in standard texts.

Psoriasis

Psoriasis is a common condition, affecting approximately 1 person in 50. Onset is rare under 3 years of age and is most common between 15 and 40, but can occur at any age. The cause of psoriasis is unknown but a predisposition to the disease can be inherited. Several factors are known to provoke attacks.

Psoriasis varies greatly in its extent and appearance. It can be recognised by its clearly marginated red plaques with large silvery scales that are easily detached. On the soles, scaling may be thicker and more waxy. Thick fissured areas may mimic a hyperkeratotic eczema, but the presence of lesions elsewhere assists in the diagnosis. The commonest sites are the elbows and knees. About 25% of patients show nail abnormalities, most commonly as tiny pits (see Ch. 8). Onycholysis commonly begins distally. Finally, the nail may become greatly thickened and turn a brownish yellow with much subungual hyperkeratosis. Psoriasis may be associated with an arthritis, usually of the distal interphalangeal joints of the fingers and toes. A distorted nail is usually present beyond the swollen painful joint. Patients with psoriasis can also develop coincidental rheumatoid arthritis or osteoarthrosis.

Palmoplantar pustulosis (pustular psoriasis)

The soles and palms are particularly liable to develop this variant of psoriasis, in which sterile yellow pustules turn to yellow-brown surface flakes as they age, before being shed (Fig. 7.10). If pustules erupt without other manifestations of psoriasis, the differentiation from infected eczema of the palms and soles may be difficult. Pustular psoriasis is often chronic and responds poorly to treatment.

Reiter's disease

This disorder is a triad of urethritis, arthritis and conjunctivitis, but it may also include mucous membrane lesions and, rarely, an eruption on the soles (*keratoderma blenorrhagica*), which may resemble pustular psoriasis. Most cases follow a non-specific venereal infection but occasionally dysentery precedes its onset.

The fully developed skin lesions show irregular, heaped-up yellowish masses of hyperkeratosis on the soles but pustulation is not always seen. The nails may also be involved, leading on occasion to their destruction. These changes subside over a period of months.

Eczema and dermatitis

The terms *eczema* and *dermatitis* are best regarded as being synonymous. Eczema is sometimes used to imply a constitutional process, and dermatitis a reaction to an external agent. Nevertheless, the distinction is by no means rigid and it is advisable to use the term eczema when speaking to patients as it does not carry the same industrial connotations to the lay person.

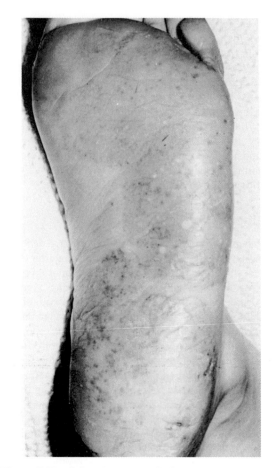

Figure 7.10 Palmoplantar pustulosis.

Acute eczema starts with erythema, vesiculation, oozing and crusting, whereas the skin in chronic eczema is dry, scaly and thickened.

Atopic eczema

The skin changes may or may not be accompanied by other manifestations of atopy, such as hay fever and asthma, and these disorders may also affect others in the family. This type of eczema often starts on the scalp or face, as early as 3–4 months of age, and later spreads to involve the limb flexures and napkin areas. Itching is severe and, with constant rubbing, a dry scaly erythema develops in the flexures, with an increase in skin markings known as lichenification. Lesions occur less frequently on the feet than on the hands but the ankle is commonly involved (Fig. 7.11). The skin elsewhere tends to be dry.

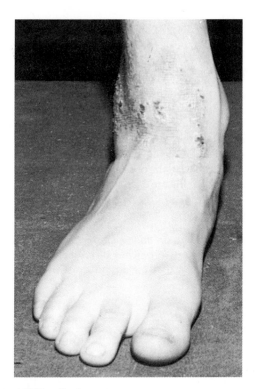

Figure 7.11   Atopic eczema.

Fortunately, atopic eczema tends to remit spontaneously and a proportion will clear each year from the age of 2 upwards. Sometimes atopic eczema does not develop until puberty or even later and then it can pursue a very chronic course.

Eczema of the palms and soles

Some patients experience recurrent episodes of irritable vesiculation of the palms, soles and the sides of the digits. These blisters may be larger than those usually seen in eczema and resemble sago grains. The term pompholyx is sometimes used to describe this pattern.

Another constitutional pattern of chronic eczema seen on the palms and soles is characterised by an initial microvesiculation and later by stubborn hyperkeratosis and fissuring (Fig. 7.12). In these cases, no precipitating cause can generally be found, but allergic contact eczema and fungal infection must be excluded.

Irritant dermatitis

A single massive exposure, or more commonly recurrent exposure of the skin to mild acids, alkalis or degreasing agents, produces an irritant dermatitis. The mistaken regular bathing of the feet in antiseptics may give rise to this condition. Housewives' dermatitis of the hands is another well-known example.

Allergic contact dermatitis

True sensitisation of the skin can be produced by a wide variety of substances. Once this allergy is established, further exposure to the chemical will lead to an

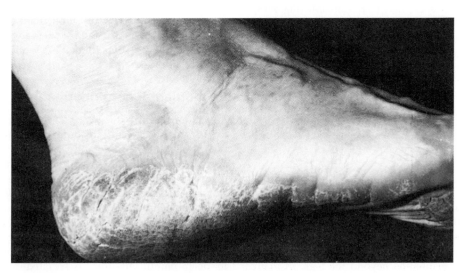

Figure 7.12   Chronic hyperkeratotic eczema.

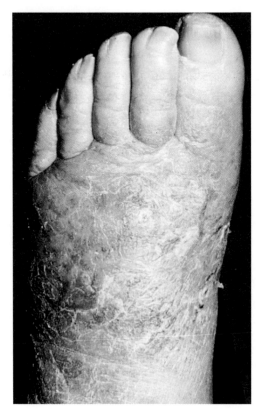

Figure 7.13 Allergic contact dermatitis.

eczematous reaction. On the feet, chemicals added to rubber, chrome used to tan leather, nickel in shoe buckles or dyes in socks may be responsible (Fig. 7.13). The pattern of involvement, e.g. the weight-bearing area of the sole in rubber sensitivity, will assist in the diagnosis. Allergy to various components of medicaments, including preservatives and antibiotics, may exacerbate a pre-existing eczema.

The offending substance can be identified by the application of patch tests to normal skin on the patient's back. Positive reactions usually occur within 48 hours.

Varicose eczema

Impaired venous drainage leads to a variety of skin changes. Increased pigmentation and purpura appear along the lines of the veins and around the ankles. Eczematisation may follow and sudden exacerbations can lead to dissemination beyond the legs. In many chronic cases, white scarring (*atrophic blanche*) and

ulceration ensue, the latter often beginning after a minor injury.

Lichen simplex

A localized area of dry thickened skin showing lichenification is referred to as lichen simplex or circumscribed neurodermatitis. Itching is always prominent and the thickening is due to repetitive, at times almost violent, scratching. As a result, the surface may show fresh excoriations or haemorrhagic crusting. The lower leg and ankle are especially common sites.

Discoid eczema

The terms *discoid* or *nummular eczema* are used to describe the coin-like patches of erythema, vesiculation and crusting that are found most often on the limbs of adults.

Infective dermatitis

This is most commonly seen in those adolescent boys who pay little attention to hygiene and have a problem with hyperhidrosis. It starts on the dorsum of the foot near the toes and spreads towards the ankle. Bacterial infection plays an important part in its perpetuation.

Juvenile plantar dermatosis

This recently described condition affects the weight-bearing areas of children's forefeet. The involved parts of the sole and undersurfaces of the toes show a glazed, scaly, sometimes fissured erythema. The heels and insteps are less often involved (Fig. 7.14). Its cause remains in some doubt, but the irritant effect of new synthetic materials in children's footwear may be important, though some think it is a localised manifestation of atopic eczema.

Palmoplantar keratoderma

Punctate or diffuse thickening of the palms and soles occurs in a variety of disorders. The term tylosis describes a diffuse dominantly inherited type. Keratoderma associated with structural and functional foot disorders has been described in an earlier section. One common acquired pattern is *keratoderma climactericum*. This is seen in middle-aged, often obese women. The thickening is most marked on the sides of the heel and extends over the sole to the metatarsal heads (Fig. 7.15). Splitting and cracking of the keratin result in deep painful fissures. Associated hyperhidrosis may produce an unpleasant smell.

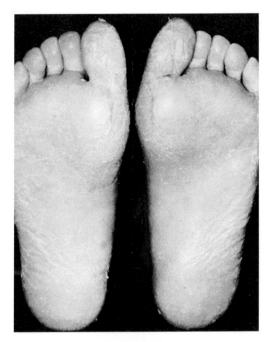

Figure 7.14   Juvenile plantar dermatosis.

Lichen planus

The cause of lichen planus is unknown. The common sites are the wrists, forearms, lower abdomen, back, legs and the mucous membranes. Both the dorsum of the foot and the soles may be affected. Individual lesions consist of itchy, flat, polygonal, violaceous papules that may be small and discrete, or fused to form larger plaques. The surface may show a network of fine white lines called *Wickham's striae*.

In about 10% of cases, the nails are affected. The majority of these show only reversible longitudinal ridging, but cuticular hypertrophy may result in a triangular central projection, known as a pterygium, growing along the nail (see Ch. 8). This causes considerable deformity, and occasionally permanent nail destruction ensues.

The eruption usually subsides spontaneously, though only after months or even years. Brown macules often remain but may fade eventually.

DISORDERS OF THE BLOOD VESSELS

Urticaria

Urticaria, or nettle-rash, consists of short-lived itchy weals which vary in diameter from a few millimetres to several centimetres. Individual lesions tend to fade

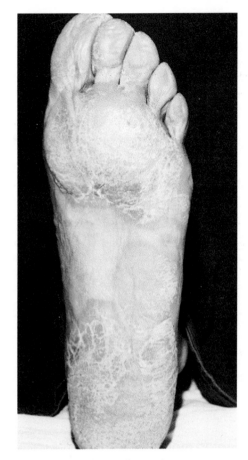

Figure 7.15   *Keratoderma climactericum.*

after 8–24 hours, but purpura is occasionally left on dependent parts of the body. In chronic cases, episodes recur at variable intervals.

Urticaria may be the result of an allergic reaction to a food substance or drug. Aspirin can exacerbate urticaria whatever its original cause; however, the precise cause in the majority of cases cannot be found.

The feet may be involved as part of a generalised eruption but are particularly affected by a rare pressure urticaria. Here, painful swelling of the soles occurs some hours after the repetitive pressure of walking or running. Manual labour may lead to the same appearance on the hands. The underlying mechanism of this and other physical urticarias is not known. It can be long-lasting and disabling.

Purpura

Purpura is the consequence of spontaneous bleeding

into the skin. Small lesions a few millimetres in diameter are described as *petechiae* and larger lesions as bruises or *ecchymoses*. These areas are identified by their purplish colour when fresh, and by failure to blanch on pressure.

A wide variety of disorders of the blood, blood vessels or the tissues supporting them may produce purpura. Elucidation of its cause depends on detailed medical investigation. Purpura is particularly liable to develop on the lower limbs because of the effects of gravity and varicose veins, factors which increase the pressure exerted on vessel walls.

Talon noire (black heel)

In this condition, groups of bluish-black specks appear on the heels, usually just above the thickened horny edge of the sole. It is believed to be due to the rupture of small capillaries by repetitive shearing stresses often exerted by particular footwear. It is most commonly seen in fit young persons and is entirely benign.

TUMOURS

The feet can be the site of birthmarks, e.g. linear naevi which appear as warty overgrowths of the epidermis, and can extend the whole length of a limb.

Pigmented moles

These are fairly common on the feet, and although they have a very small chance of becoming malignant, the risk is increased on the sole, the toes and beneath the nails. The possibility of a malignant melanoma must be considered if a pre-existing mole grows rapidly, changes colour, begins to bleed or shows evidence of a surrounding inflammatory reaction (Fig. 7.16). Any patient with a suspect mole should be referred, without delay, for excision and histological examination.

Haemangiomas

These are vascular malformations. The familiar port wine stain or capillary haemangioma appears at birth or in the first few weeks of life. An acquired haemangioma, called a pyogenic granuloma, may occur at the site of a trivial penetrating injury. The cherry-red friable vascular tumour grows rapidly and requires removal under a local anaesthetic by curettage and cautery. Recurrence is not uncommon but the lesion is benign.

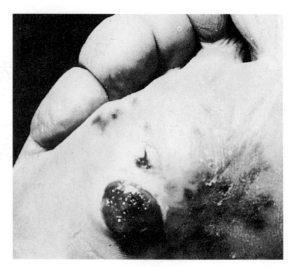

Figure 7.16   Melanoma.

Bullous disorders

Primarily blistering disorders are rare, and do not selectively involve the feet, although these may be involved as part of a generalised eruption. An exception to this is epidermolysis bullosa. The dominantly inherited variant may cause blistering only on the feet and this may first be noticed when the infant begins to crawl or walk. In mild forms, the onset may be delayed until adolescence. Trauma induces clear tense blisters which eventually heal without scarring. Recessively inherited forms of epidermolysis bullosa are much more severe with widespread involvement of the skin and mucous membranes. Considerable scarring ensues and lethal complications may eventually arise.

Granuloma annulare

Granuloma annulare consists of a group of small pink or skin-coloured nodules, usually forming an arc or complete ring, varying from 1 cm to several centimetres across. The lesions are asymptomatic and may be single or multiple. Although the hands are the most common site, the feet are affected in 20% of cases, usually in children. Granuloma annulare eventually fades but this may take some years.

DRUG ERUPTIONS

Adverse reactions to drugs are common and are frequently seen on the skin. The rashes vary considerably and may mimic common primary skin disorders. Very few drugs cause specific eruptions and a detailed history of medication is essential for diagnosis.

The feet are often involved as part of a widespread eruption. Occasionally, however, isolated lesions occur in the same places whenever a particular drug is taken. These *fixed drug eruptions* appear as a disc of erythema that fades on withdrawal of the drug, often leaving a patch of pigmentation.

FURTHER READING

Almeida J D, Goffe A P 1965 Antibody to wart virus in human sera, demonstrated by electron microscopy and precipitin tests. Lancet II: 1205

Baran R, Dawber R P R 1984 Diseases of the nails and their management. Blackwell, Oxford

Bunney M H 1982 Viral warts: their biology and treatment. Oxford University Press, Oxford

Gold S 1973 The enigma of viral warts. Practitioner, Nov

Jabonska S, Orth G 1983 Human papovaviruses. In: Champion R H (ed) Recent advances in dermatology. Churchill Livingstone, Edinburgh, p 1–36

Johansson E, Pyrohonen S, Rostila T 1977 Warts and virus antibodies in patients with systemic lupus erythematosus. British Medical Journal 1: 74–76

Le Rossignol J N 1980 An encyclopaedia of materia medica and therapeutics for chiropodists. Faber, London

Le Rossignol J N, Holliday C B 1963 A pharmacopoeia for chiropodists, 7th edn. Faber, London

Levene G M, Calrian C D 1974 A colour atlas of dermatology. Wolfe, London

McMillan S A, Haire M 1975 Smooth muscles antibody in patients with warts. Clinical and Experimental Immunology 21: 339–344

Matthews R S, Shirodaria P Y 1973 Study of regressing warts by immunofluorescence. Lancet, March

Morrison W L 1976 Cell-mediated immune responses in patients with warts. British Journal of Dermatology 93: 553

Ogilvie M M 1970 Serological studies with human papova (wart) virus. Journal of Hygiene 68: 479

Pyrhonen S, Perittinen K 1972 Wart virus antibodies and the prognosis of wart disease. Lancet Dec 23

Read P J 1972 An introduction to therapeutics for chiropodists, 2nd edn. Actinic Press, London

Reid T M S, Fraser N G, Kernolien I R 1976 Generalised warts and immune deficiency. British Journal of Dermatology 95: 559

Rook A, Wilkinson D S, Ebling F J G, Champion R H, Burton J L 1986 Textbook of dermatology, 4th edn, vols I, II, III. Blackwell, Oxford

Shirodaria P V, Matthews R S 1975 An immunofluorescence study of warts. Clinical and Experimental Immunology 21: 329–338

Sneddon I B, Church R E 1983 Practical dermatology, 4th edn. Arnold, London

Solomons, Bethel 1983 Lecture notes on dermatology, 5th edn. Blackwell, Oxford

8

The human nail and its disorders

M. Johnson

Keywords

Embryology
Eponychium
Granulation tissue
Growth and development
Hippocratic
Hyponychium
Involution
Lovibond's angle
Matrix
Onychauxis
Onychocryptosis
Onychocytes
Onychodermal band
Onychogryphosis
Onycholysis
Onychomycosis
Paronychia
Pterygium
Subungual exostosis
Subungual heloma
Sulci

The human nail is a hard plate of densely packed keratinised cells which protects the dorsal aspect of the digits and greatly enhances fine digital movements of the hands. Nails are descendants of claws used for digging and fighting, but now only serve as a protection for the digit and to assist in basic behaviour such as scratching and picking up small objects.

The nail is a flat, horny structure, roughly rectangular and transparent. It is the end product of the epithelial component of the nail unit, the *matrix*. The nail plate moves with the nail bed tissues to extend unattached as a free edge, growing past the distal tip of the finger or toe. The nail bed is normally seen through the plate as a pink area due to a rich vascular network. A paler crescent-shaped *lunula* is seen extending from the proximal nail fold of the hallux, thumb and some of the larger nails. At the lunula, the nail is thin and the epidermis is thicker, so that the underlying capillaries cannot be seen. It is less firmly attached to the bed at this point and light is reflected from the interface between the nail and the bed, making the lunula appear white.

In profile, the nail plate emerges from the proximal nail fold at an angle to the surface of the dorsal digital skin. This angle is commonly called *Lovibond's angle* (Fig. 8.1A) and should be less than 180°. Only in abnormal circumstances, e.g. clubbing, is this angle greater (Fig. 8.1B).

The nail grooves mark the limit of the nail, are separated into proximal, distal and lateral grooves (sulci), and are best seen when the nail is avulsed. The distal groove situated at the hyponychium is covered by the nail plate, and lying immediately proximal is a thin pale translucent line known as *Terry's onychodermal band* (Fig. 8.2).

The proximal nail fold (PNF) is an extension of the skin of the surface of the digit and lies superficial to the matrix, which is deeper in the tissues. It has a superficial and deep epithelial border, the latter not

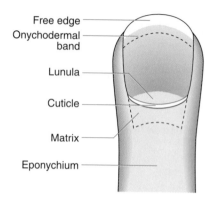

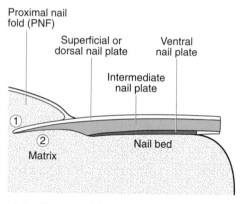

Figure 8.2 Structure of the human nail. 1, superficial layer of nail; 2, deep layer of nail.

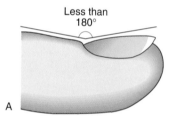

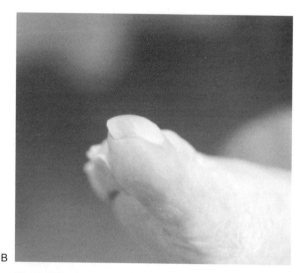

Figure 8.1 A: Lovibond's angle. B: Clubbing.

being visible from the exterior. The PNF extends its stratum corneum onto the nail plate as a cuticle, which remains adhered for a short distance before being shed. The function of the cuticle is unclear—it may prevent bacterial access to the thinner and more delicate tissues of the ventral PNF epidermis or it may help in forming a smooth nail surface.

The superficial skin of the PNF, extending from the distal interphalangeal joint to the nail plate, is devoid of hair follicles and is thinner than the dorsal skin of the digit. At the tip of the PNF adjacent to the cuticle, capillary loops can be seen and, if proliferative, can be associated with certain disease states, e.g. lupus erythematosus, dermatomyositis and phototoxic conditions.

The ventral PNF is thinner than the superficial PNF; it does not have epidermal ridges and may be the portal of entry for bacteria and/or irritating chemicals which produce *chronic paronychia*. It is continuous with the matrix epithelium but has a stratum granulosum which may be differentiated on staining.

EMBRYONIC DEVELOPMENT AND NAIL GROWTH

The earliest anatomical sign of nail development occurs on the surface of the digit of the embryo at week 9, appearing as a flattened rectangular area. The primary nail field is outlined by grooves which are the forerunners of the proximal and distal grooves and lateral sulci (Zaias & Alvarez 1968). The nail field mesenchyme differentiates into the nail unit structures and the fully keratinised nail is complete in week 20 of gestation. Toenail formation usually occurs 4 weeks later than that of the corresponding fingernail.

The theories proposed to explain the formation and growth of the human nail have polarised between a single source of matrix production from the lunula (Zaias & Alvarez 1968, Norton 1971, Achten 1982) and a trilamellar structure where, in addition to the lunula, the nail bed and proximal nail fold contribute as the nail plate grows out (Lewis 1954, Lewin 1965, Hashimoto et al 1966, Jarrett & Spearman 1966, Samman 1990, Johnson et al 1991).

Zaias (1990) stated that the nail plate is a uniform structure produced solely by the matrix, with onychocytes genetically directed diagonally and distally, and not shaped or redirected by the PNF. The proximal portions of the matrix form the superficial nail plate and the distal matrix forms the deepest portion of the plate. As the nail produced from the lunula is in advance of that from the proximal matrix, this supports the theory that nail plate shape is related to lunula shape. Zaias (1990) also demonstrated a direct relationship between nail plate thickness and the length of the matrix.

However, the exact structure of the nail plate is still disputed, as Achten (1982) claimed that nail embedded in paraffin and stained with the periodic acid shift method (PAS), toluidine blue and the sulphydryl groups reveals three layers with differential staining. The most proximal cells of the matrix form the superficial layer of the nail, while the distal cells form the deeper nail layer, which is thicker (Fig. 8.2). As the nail grows distally and comes to rest on the nail bed distal to the lunula, a thin layer of keratin from the bed attaches to the undersurface of the nail. Achten argued that this keratin does not form an integral part of the nail, but migrates with it and remains firmly attached to it even when the nail is surgically avulsed. Measurements of progressive thickness of the nail from the proximal lunula to the point of detachment at the onychodermal band have shown that about 19% of nail mass is formed by the nail bed as the nail grows out along it (Johnson et al 1991).

The nail bed has a surface with numerous parallel longitudinal ridges which fit closely into a similar pattern on the underside of the nail plate, thus ensuring a very strong cohesion between the two surfaces.

The three nail layers are often described as the dorsal, intermediate and ventral nail plates and each is physicochemically different. Seen in transverse and longitudinal sections, the cells of the nail plate are arranged regularly and interlock like roof tiles, with the main axis horizontal. In the superficial layer, cells are flatter and closer together, and in the nail bed they are more polyhedral and less regularly arranged.

It is thought that the layers stain differently due to variations in the composition of the main polypeptide chains and the number of lateral bonds in the keratin molecule (Achten 1982). The more numerous the lateral bonds, the fewer free radicals are available to combine with different stains. In softer keratin there is less bonding and therefore more staining (Fig. 8.3). Studies on the chemical composition of nails show moderately

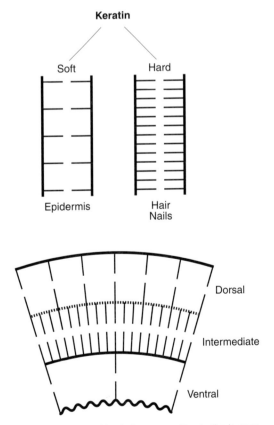

Figure 8.3 Polypeptide chain composition in the human nail.

high concentrations of sulphur, selenium, calcium and potassium.

BLOOD SUPPLY AND INNERVATION

In the foot, the nail is supplied by two branches of the dorsal metatarsal artery and two branches of the plantar metatarsal artery, lying at the laterodorsal and lateroplantar areas of each toe. They form an anastomosis at the terminal phalanx, the plantar arteries supplying the pad of the toe and the nail bed.

Innervation of the proximodorsal area of the nail and bed is provided by two small branches from the dorsal nerves (superficial peroneal, deep peroneal and sural), while the medial and lateral plantar nerves provide a medial and lateral branch to each toe to supply the plantar skin, and extend to supply the anterodistal area of the nail bed and superficial skin.

Growth of the nail is continuous throughout life, the rate being greatest in the first two decades when the nail plate is thin (Hamilton et al 1955). The rate of growth decreases with age, and ultimately in the elderly the nail plate loses colour and may thicken and develop longitudinal ridges. The normal development of the nail depends on the matrix and nail bed having an adequate nerve and blood supply, and interference with either will affect growth. Some systemic disorders may cause a reduction or an increase in the growth rate. Other factors which, directly or indirectly, have a detrimental effect on the development and growth of the nail are trauma, infection, nutritional deficiencies and some skin diseases. Congenital and inherited factors are not common.

Nail growth is continuous throughout life, with peak rates of elongation in the 10–14 year old group and a steady decline in growth rate after the second decade (Hamilton et al 1955); therefore, periodic cutting is necessary and incorrect performance of this task leads to onychocryptosis (ingrowing toe nail), one of the most painful conditions affecting nails. The free edge of a nail should never be cut so short as to expose the nail bed, but should be cut straight across or slightly convex with all rough and sharp edges smoothed. The overall aim should be to ensure that the nail complies with the shape of the toe.

INVOLUTION (pincer, omega nail)

This term describes a nail which increases in transverse curvature along the longitudinal axis of the nail, reaching its maximum at the distal part (Fig. 8.4). Three types of this condition exist (Fig. 8.5) and they produce a variety of symptoms.

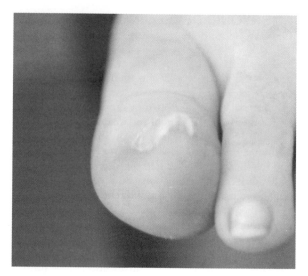

Figure 8.4 Involution.

Tile-shaped nails often occur in association with yellow nail syndrome, affecting both finger- and toenails. The nail increases in transverse curvature, while the lateral edges of the nail remain parallel (Baran et al 1991). The condition rarely produces symptoms.

Plicatured nails occur where the surface of the plate remains flat while one or both edges of the nail form vertical parallel sides hidden by the sulcus tissue. Toenails and fingernails are affected and the condition causes considerable pain in the foot if the nail is thickened and subjected to shoe pressure, with the development of onychophosis.

Pincer (omega, trumpet) nail dystrophy shows longitudinal curvature, which ranges from a minimal asymptomatic incurving to involution so marked that the lateral edges of the nail practically meet, forming a cylinder or roll; hence the names for this deformity. Lateral compression of the nail may result in strangulation of the soft nail bed tissues and the formation of subungual ulceration as the circulation to the nail bed and matrix is reduced. In all stages of the condition, the sulcus may become inflamed and may ulcerate, causing considerable pain.

Aetiology

Although the precise cause of involution is unknown, in toenails it is often associated with constriction from tight footwear or hosiery. In fingernails, an association with osteoarthritic changes in the distal interphalangeal joint has been shown (Zaias 1990) and heredity may play a part, particularly where all nails are affect-

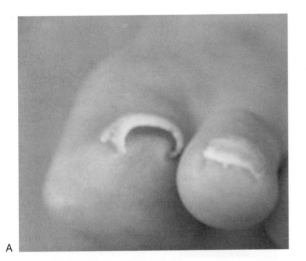

A

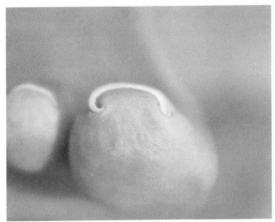

B

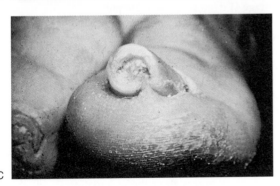

C

Figure 8.5   Types of involution. A: Tile-shaped.
B: Plicatured. C: Pincer.

ed (hidrotic ectodermal dysplasia, yellow nail syndrome). Some severe cases of involution have an underlying exostosis of the terminal phalanx which must be excised.

Treatment

In minor degrees, involution produces little or no discomfort and the main consideration is to ensure that the nail is cut so that it conforms to the length and shape of the toe. The incurved edges, if thickened, should be reduced, and advice given about correctly fitting footwear and hosiery.

More severe cases may be treated conservatively with careful clearing of the sulcus and the fitting of a nail brace. This is made from a short piece of 0.5 mm gauge stainless steel wire which applies a slight upward and outward tension to the nail edges to correct them gradually. The nail must be of adequate length to allow correct fitting of the side arms of the brace, and good contact of the nail plate with the nail bed is essential to allow effective tension for correction.

The brace is formed using a length of wire approximately 1.5 cm greater than the width of the nail. At the middle of the length of the wire, a 'U' loop is formed in the horizontal plane so that the open end of the loop faces towards the free edge of the nail. With round-nosed pliers, a small hook is made at each end of the wire, lying in the frontal plane and being large enough to accept the thickness of the nail edges. The ends of the wire must be rounded and filed smooth before finally fitting. Each arm of the brace from the hook to the central loop is shaped to conform to the curvature of the nail (Fig. 8.6).

The brace is applied by engaging each hook over the appropriate edge of the nail, and tension is obtained by closing the long side of the loop as far as possible, without applying so much tension that the nail splits. A light packing of cotton wool and suitable antiseptic, e.g. Betadine solution, may be inserted into each sulcus if necessary. The brace should be kept in position for at least 1 month and then reassessed for correction achieved by caliper measurements; tension can be adjusted throughout the period of the treatment.

Other derivatives of the nail brace are now available in plastic and are adhered to the nail directly, exerting tension upwards and outwards because of their preformed shape or via rubber bands fitted to small plastic hooks. These are reported to be very successful where good adherence is achieved.

Severe and painful involution is likely to require a unilateral or bilateral partial nail avulsion with destruction of the matrix. Where lateral compression causes painful nail bed constriction and ulceration, a total nail avulsion with matrix destruction is the only means of providing relief.

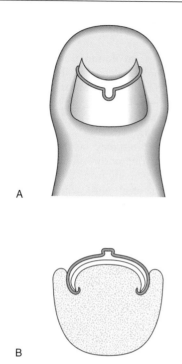

Figure 8.6   Involution. A: Nail brace in position, dorsal view.

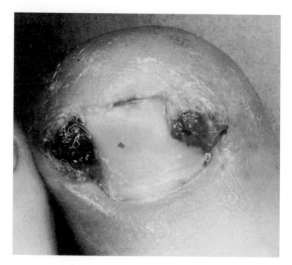

Figure 8.7   Onychocryptosis with hypergranulation.

If an underlying subungual exostosis is detected, this needs to be surgically excised (see Ch. 19).

ONYCHOCRYPTOSIS (ingrowing toenail)

Onychocryptosis is a condition in which a spike, shoulder or serrated edge of the nail has pierced the epidermis of the sulcus and penetrated the dermal tissues. It occurs most frequently in the hallux of male adolescents and may be unilateral or bilateral. Initially, it causes little inconvenience, but as the nail grows out along the sulcus the offending portion penetrates further into the tissues and promotes an acute inflammation in the surrounding soft tissues which often becomes infected (*paronychia*).

The skin becomes red, shiny and tense and the toe appears swollen. There is throbbing pain, acute tenderness to the slightest pressure and a degree of localised hyperhidrosis. The continued penetration of the nail spike prevents normal healing by granulation of the wound in the sulcus, and a prolific increase of granulation tissue is common (*hypergranulation*). This excess tissue, together with the swollen nail folds, overlaps the nail plate, sometimes to a considerable

extent, partially obscuring it (Fig. 8.7). Since infection is almost always present, pus may exude from the point of penetration in the sulcus and may be seen as a pocket lying beneath the sulcus epidermis or beneath the nail plate.

Zaias (1990) describes three stages of the condition with individual treatment regimes for each stage.

Stage I is the first sign of ingrowing, with minimal injury to the sulcus tissue but with symptoms of pain, slight swelling, oedema, varying degrees of redness and hyperhidrosis. Elevation of the nail with non-absorbent cotton wool corrects the condition in 7–14 days.

Stage II demonstrates acute pain, erythema, hyperhidrosis, granulation tissue from the ulcerated sulcus tissue, a seropurulent exudate and a fetid odour. The latter may be the result of Gram-positive or colonic bacterial growth on the surface of the granulation tissue. Topical high potency steroids or intralesional corticosteroid injection of 2 mg/ml triamcinolone acetonide are reported to clear the granulating tissue, and the condition clears with further cotton wool packing as in stage I.

Stage III. The symptoms present at stage III are those described for stage II, with the addition of an epidermal overgrowth of the granulation tissue, thus making elevation of the nail out of the sulcus impossible. Surgical intervention with excision or cauterisation of the granulation is recommended (Fig. 8.8).

Aetiology

The most common predisposing factors are faulty nail cutting, hyperhidrosis and pressure from ill-fitting

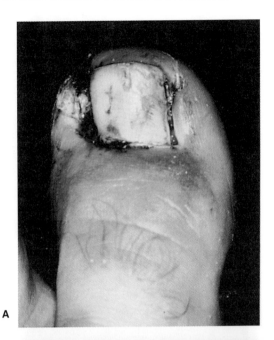

A

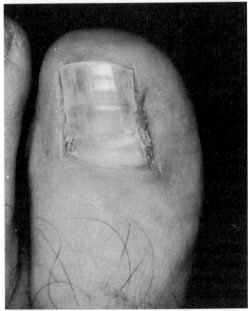

B

Figure 8.8 A: Onychocryptosis with hypergranulation. B: Same case as A, 8 weeks after partial nail avulsion. The nail plate is permanently flattened and narrowed after excision of the involuted nail edges.

footwear, although any disease state which causes an abnormal nail plate, e.g. onychomycosis, or onychorrhexis, may promote piercing of the sulcus tissue by the nail.

If a nail is cut too short, the corners cut obliquely, or if it is subjected to tearing, normal pressure on the underlying tissue is removed and without that resistance, the tissue begins to protrude. As the nail grows forward, it becomes embedded in the protruding tissue. Tearing of the nails has a similar effect to cutting obliquely across the corners of the nail plate. Both are likely to result in a spike of nail left deep in the sulcus, especially if the nail is involuted. Any spike left at the edge of the nail increases the risk of sulcus penetration as the nail grows forward. Maceration of the sulcus tissue is commonly due to hyperhidrosis in adolescent males but may also arise from the overuse of hot footbaths in the young or elderly. Moist tissue is less resistant to pressure from the nail such as that caused by lateral pressure from narrow footwear or abnormal weight-bearing forces, e.g. pronation or hallux limitus, and as compression forces the lateral nail fold to roll over the edge of the nail plate, the sulcus deepens and the nail may penetrate the softened tissues.

Hamilton et al (1955) showed that the nails of adolescent males increased in lateral width disproportionately to the increase in length of the nail plate. This together with hyperhydrated tissues, abnormal foot function and/or pressure from footwear may lead to onychocryptosis. However, the relationship between toenail length and width in adolescents has not been further investigated.

Treatment

If the onychocryptosis is uncomplicated by infection, the penetrating splinter may be located by careful probing and then removed with a small scalpel or fine nippers. Extreme care must be taken to avoid further injury to the sulcus and to ensure that a spike of nail is not left deep in the sulcus. The edge of the nail can be smoothed with a Black's file, although this should be avoided if the nail plate is extremely thin or shows signs of onychorrhexis. The area is then irrigated with sterile solution and dried thoroughly. It should then be packed firmly with sterile cotton wool or gauze, making sure that it is inserted a little way under the nail plate to maintain its elevation. An antiseptic astringent preparation, such as Betadine, is applied to the packing and the toe is covered with a non-adherent sterile dressing and tubular gauze.

It is sometimes necessary to make use of an interdigital wedge to relieve pressure on the distal phalanx from the adjacent toe. In approximately 3–5 days, the nail should again be inspected and re-packed, and then again at appropriate intervals until the nail has regained its normal length and shape. If there is associated hyperhidrosis, this requires an appropriate regime while the onychocryptosis is being treated.

When onychocryptosis is complicated by infection and suppuration is present, it is important to remove the splinter of nail, facilitating drainage and allowing healing to take place. Hot footbaths of magnesium sulphate solution or hypertonic saline solution may be used to reduce the inflammation and localise the sepsis before removal of the splinter is attempted.

Location and removal of the penetrating nail may cause considerable pain and, if there are no contra-indications, a local anaesthetic should be given. The injection should be made at the base of the toe, well away from the infected area. After the splinter is removed, the edge of the nail should be left smooth, and the area irrigated thoroughly with a sterile solution and dried carefully. A light packing of sterile gauze or cotton wool with a suitable broad-spectrum antiseptic agent can be applied and the toe covered with a sterile non-adherent dressing and tubular gauze.

The patient should be advised to rest the foot and, if necessary, to cut away the upper of the slipper or shoe to remove all pressure from the toe. The patient should return the following day for the renewal of dressings, and this must be continued until the sepsis is cleared.

If hypergranulation tissue is present, it may be excised when the splinter of nail is removed, taking care to control the profuse bleeding which often results following excision. Small amounts of granulation tissue may be reduced by repeated applications of silver nitrate, taking care to avoid its introduction into the sulcus.

Following this treatment the prognosis is good, but the patient must be given clear guidance on the predisposing factors so that they can avoid recurrence. If the condition does not respond, it is likely that there is still a small nail splinter embedded in the sulcus, and further careful investigation must be undertaken to locate the remaining piece of nail. Where it is obvious that the onychocryptosis results from a minor involution of the nail, the application of a nail brace will flatten out the nail plate and reduce the involution. If conservative treatment of severe involution does not provide long-term relief, nail surgery will invariably be necessary. This involves partial or complete avulsion of the nail and the destruction of part or the whole of the nail matrix (see Ch. 19).

SUBUNGUAL EXOSTOSIS

Subungual exostosis (Fig. 8.9) is a small outgrowth of bone under the nail plate near its free edge or immediately distal to it. Most frequently, it occurs on the hal-

A
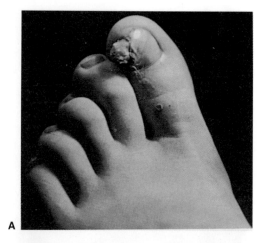

B
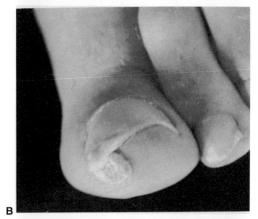

C
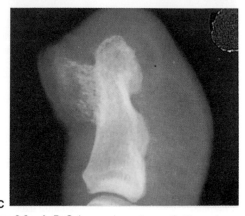

Figure 8.9 A, B: Subungual exostoses. C: X-ray shows elevation of nail plate by exostosis.

lux in young people, is slow-growing and is a source of considerable pain in the later stages. Trauma is a major causative factor (Baran et al 1991), although this is disputed by some authors (Cohen et al 1973). Repeated trauma, though slight, from shoes which are too short, too shallow or excessively high-heeled, is a common finding in podiatry.

As the outgrowth increases, the nail becomes elevated and displaced from the nail bed and the tumour may emerge from the free edge or destroy the nail plate. If the nail is eroded, the nail bed tissue ulcerates and may become infected. The protuberance offers a hard resistance to pressure and there is usually a clear line of demarcation around the area. As the exostosis increases, a fissure may develop at the edge of this line of demarcation with a serous or purulent exudate.

The epidermis covering the tumour becomes stretched and thinned and takes on a bright red colour which blanches on pressure. When the exostosis protrudes distal to the free edge, the bright red gives way to a more yellow colouration, which must be differentiated from subungual heloma and psoriasis. Accurate diagnosis of this condition requires X-ray examination, which shows trabeculated osseous growth, expansion of the distal portion and a radiolucent fibrocartilage cover.

Pathology

Following an injury to the periosteum of the distal phalanx, a periostitis occurs. Initially, there is an outgrowth of cartilage which later ossifies.

Treatment

Temporary relief may be given by means of protective padding and advice on footwear, but surgical excision is always the most satisfactory treatment (see Ch. 19).

ONYCHAUXIS (hypertrophied nail)

This is an abnormal but uniform thickening of the nail, increasing from the nail base to the free edge, which is commonly seen in podiatric practice. It may be accompanied by slight brown colour changes in the nail plate and enlargement of the sulci due to the thickened lateral edges of the nail. Often, only the nail of the hallux is affected but the disorder may appear in other nails. The excessive growth makes nail cutting difficult and this is often neglected, with the result that subsequent shoe pressure may cause pain and discomfort. Unremitting pressure from footwear may lead to the development of subungual aseptic necrosis, especially in the elderly. A differential diagnosis must be made from pachyonychia congenita, in which all the nails are affected and nail bed hypertrophy is a major feature.

Aetiology

Onychauxis occurs following damage to the nail matrix, for which there may have been one or more of several causes:

1. single major trauma from a heavy blow or severe stubbing, or repeated minor trauma from shallow shoes or pressure from footwear on long and neglected nails
2. fungal infection of the nails and chronic skin diseases such as eczema, psoriasis and pityriasis rubra pilaris
3. poor peripheral circulation, especially in the elderly
4. some systemic disturbance, e.g. Dariers disease; this may be suspected when several or all of the nails are affected.

Pathology

Trauma to the nail matrix results in the excess production of onychocytes and the nail becomes progressively thicker as it grows along the nail bed. Why this increased production is permanent is as yet unresolved as very little research into the condition has been undertaken. Rayner (1973) reported that the proximal nail fold was shortened and everted and therefore unable to exert pressure on newly formed cells, but also that there was a greater vascularity of the nail fold and nail matrix areas, together with an enlarged artery a short distance proximal to the angle of the nail matrix. Furthermore, it was shown that the nail matrix produced an epidermal type keratin which increased the thickness of the nail plate and resulted in a thicker but softer intermediate nail layer.

Baran et al (1991) described hyperplasia of subungual tissues, seen in histological sections, as homogeneous oval-shaped amorphous masses surrounded by normal squamous cells and separated from each other by empty spaces (+ve PAS stain).

Treatment

Irrespective of the cause, the nail should be reduced in size to as near normal as possible at each visit, in order to relieve pain caused by pressure on the nail bed tissues. Footwear should be examined for correct fitting, but as the damage to the matrix is irreversible, regular treatment is necessary. In some cases where the cause

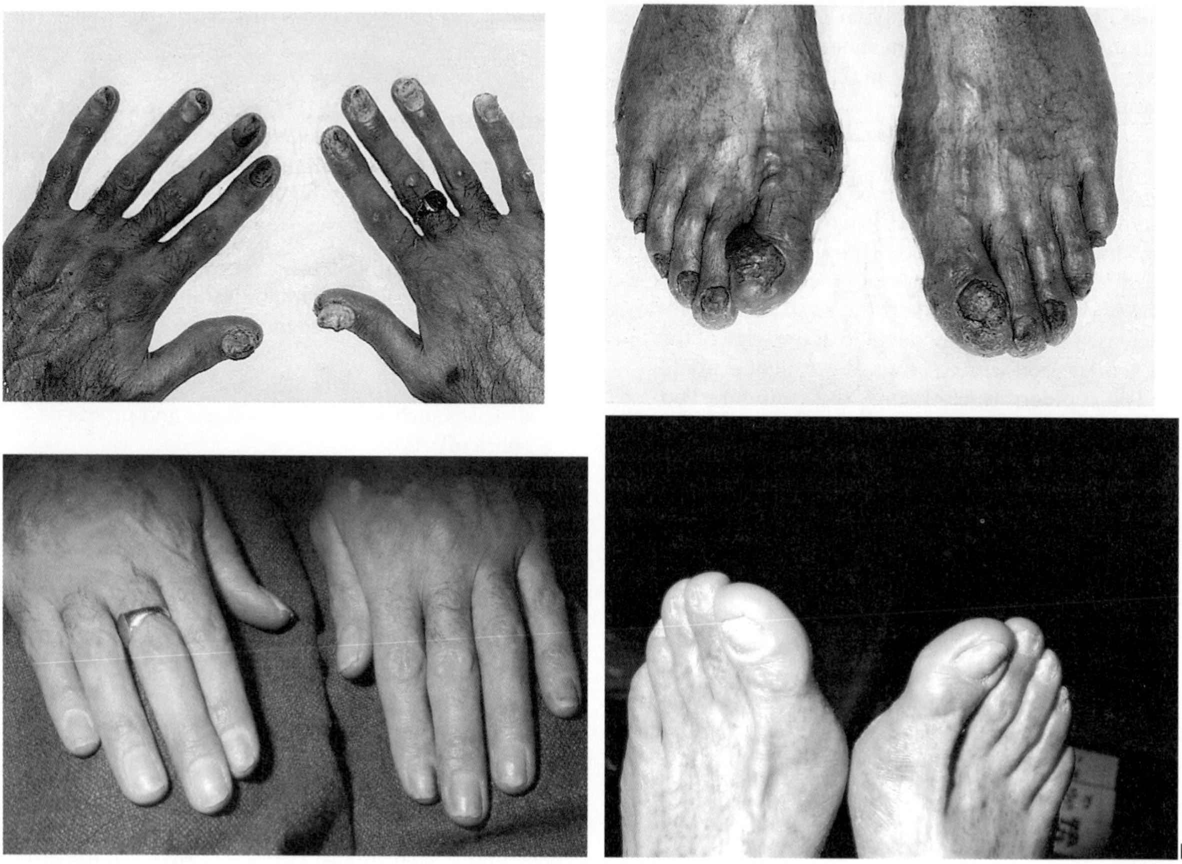

Figure 8.10 Onychauxis with eczema. A: Hands before (top) and after (bottom) treatment of eczema. B: Feet before (top) and after (bottom) treatment of eczema.

is linked to a skin disease such as eczema, stabilisation of the skin condition results in a remarkable improvement in the nails of both the hands and the feet (Fig. 8.10).

If the patient is young and the condition is confined to one toenail only, and if there is no contraindication, avulsion of the nail and destruction of the matrix provide the most satisfactory treatment.

ONYCHOGRYPHOSIS (ram's horn, Ostler's toe)

Onychogryphosis is readily distinguishable from onychauxis since, as well as hypertrophy, there is gross deformity of the nail which develops into a curved or 'ram's horn' shape (Fig. 8.11). The nail is usually a dark brown or yellowish colour, with both longitudinal and transverse ridges on its surface. Commonly, only the great toe is affected, since from its size and

prominence it is the one most prone to injury, but the condition may also arise in other toes.

Aetiology

Any one of the aetiological factors involved in the development of onychauxis may be the cause, but by far the commonest cause is a single major trauma arising from a heavy blow or a severe stubbing of the toe. It is sometimes the result of neglect and the consequent increasing impaction from footwear against the lengthening nail. This may cause the nail's free edge to penetrate the soft tissues of the affected toe and perhaps also of the adjacent toe, resulting in an area of ulceration.

Pathology

It is believed that the spiral-like appearance of ony-

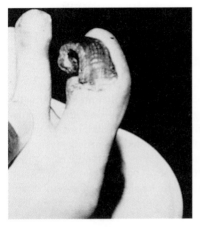
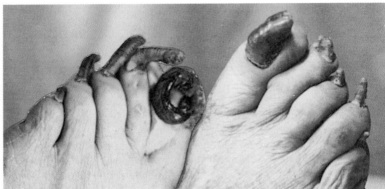

Figure 8.11 Onychogryphosis.

chogryphosis is due to an uneven production of cells from the nail matrix, the damaged side of the matrix producing cells at a slower rate (Zaias 1990). However, if the faster-growing side determines the direction of the deformity, it would be unlikely that the same side would be damaged in each nail. The most commonly seen deviation in onychogryphosis is towards the median of each foot (Fig. 8.11) and the most probable explanation for this is shoe pressure.

Treatment

Palliative treatment consists of reduction of the hypertrophy, taking care to prevent haemorrhage from any nail bed tissue which has been caught up in the malformed nail. Throughout this treatment, it is important to hold the toe firmly to avoid excessive pull on the underlying soft tissue. Footwear should be examined to ensure adequate fitting. This treatment, if repeated at regular intervals, is usually sufficient to give the patient freedom from discomfort. In a young person, especially when only one toe is affected and when palliative measures have been tried, avulsion with matrix destruction is the most satisfactory method of providing long-term relief.

ONYCHOPHOSIS

Onychophosis is a condition in which callus and/or the formation of an heloma occurs in the nail sulcus, which may result in the sulci becoming swollen and inflamed. In a mild case the effect is little more than irritating, but it can develop to a degree where even slight pressure to the nail plate or the sulcus wall gives rise to acute, sharp pain. There may be associated hypertrophy of the shoulders of the nail plate.

Aetiology

1. Lateral pressure from constricting footwear or from an adjacent toe which has some structural abnormality, e.g. hallux abductovalgus
2. Unskilled nail cutting, particularly if the lateral edges of the nail have been left rough or jagged, which may irritate the epithelium of the sulcus and give rise to callus or heloma formation
3. Unnecessarily harsh probing of the sulcus may lead to excessive thickening of the stratum corneum.

Treatment

It is sometimes necessary to soften onychophosis to facilitate its removal. This may be achieved by the application of a soak of hydrogen peroxide (3 vol) left in situ for several minutes; the callus can then be carefully cleared with a small scalpel and checked for the presence of helomata, which must be enucleated.

If removal is not possible after such a soak, it may be necessary to pack the sulcus with a keratolytic, such as 10–15% salicylic acid in collodium, and left in situ for no more than 7 days. Reduction of the callus and full enucleation can than be carried out, leaving a smooth edge to the nail plate. If the lateral edge of the nail is thickened, this should be reduced with a Black's file or a pencil burr. Dependent on skin texture, an antiseptic astringent or an emollient should then be applied and a cotton wool packing inserted between the nail edge and the sulcus.

If it is necessary to reduce pressure from an adjacent toe, an interdigital wedge, made from semi-compressed felt or a long-lasting silicone material, may be inserted. Footwear should always be examined to ensure adequate fitting, and advice on the care of the nails should be given.

SUBUNGUAL HELOMA (corn)

As the term implies, a subungual heloma is the development of a nucleated keratinised lesion under the nail plate. It may occur on any part of the nail bed. As the lesion increases it detaches the nail from the nail bed and is seen clinically as a small area of onycholysis, although it assumes a yellowish grey colour. The colour does not change under pressure and this distinguishes a subungual heloma from a subungual exostosis. A further aid to diagnosis is that a subungual heloma will yield slightly to pressure, while the subungual exostosis presents hard resistance. Once the condition is fully established, pain in the area is acute and may prevent wearing of shoes with an enclosed toe box. Even slight pressure from bedclothes will elicit extreme, sharp pain.

Aetiology

1. Trauma which may be slight but prolonged, from shoes which are too short or too shallow, or sometimes from high-heeled shoes which produce abnormal pressure on the nail plate
2. Forefoot deformity, such as hallux limitus/rigidus with hyperextension of the hallux, or overlying toes in association with hallux abductovalgus; each incurs increased pressure from the shoe onto the nail plate, resulting in keratinisation of that particular part of the nail bed.

Treatment

If the heloma is near the free edge, an area of the nail plate can be removed to enable it to be enucleated. A suitable antiseptic emollient can then be applied together with protective padding, if necessary, and the dressing held in place with tubular gauze.

Where the heloma is located towards the proximal half of the nail, it is necessary to carefully reduce the nail thickness overlying the lesion with a nail drill. Care must be taken not to drill into nail bed tissue. The remaining thin shell of nail can then be removed with a scalpel and the area enucleated and dressed as before.

Treatment may require to be repeated, especially if the heloma forms proximally, and it is essential to eliminate the cause or provide permanent protection to prevent recurrence, pain and the possible formation of an aseptic necrosis. Modification of footwear may accommodate the deformity but there are cases where surgery is indicated.

PARONYCHIA

Paronychia and onychia frequently occur together. The former is characterised by inflammation of the tissues surrounding the nail plate, and the latter by inflammation of the matrix and the nail bed. Both may be acute or chronic conditions and are always potentially serious as they arise most commonly from either a bacterial infection or a systemic disease. Acute paronychia begins with local redness, swelling and throbbing pain at the side of the nail; gentle lateral compression of the digit produces a droplet of pus at the lateral or posterior fold. Chronic paronychia develops insidiously and may not be noticed by the patient. Redness and mild swelling of the proximal nail fold are the earliest signs, which progress slowly to resemble a semicircular cushion around the base of the nail (Fig. 8.12). The cuticle is detached and eventually the nail shows transverse ridging and becomes friable, which may cause shedding of the entire nail plate, beginning at the proximal margin.

Aetiology

Any traumatic incident to the toe which might facilitate the entry of bacteria or a foreign body into the tissues can predispose to paronychia. There are many causes, which include severe stubbing of the toe, slight injury to the periungual tissue, unskilled treatment with a scalpel and untreated ingrowing toe nail. The condition may be a manifestation of some systemic disease, such as diabetes mellitus, collagen vascular disease, sarcoidosis or vasculitis.

There is always the possibility that the infection will

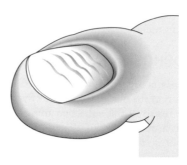

Figure 8.12 Paronychia with swelling of the PNF and transverse ridging of the nail plate.

become widespread, and therefore it is advisable to suggest that the patient consult a physician. Spreading infection is particularly likely when more than one nail is affected. Chronic paronychia most often occurs in the fingernail, particularly among persons whose occupation entails regular immersion of their hands. e.g. bar staff, fishmongers and confectioners, thus rendering them more likely to infection, even after slight trauma. Young women are more susceptible to the condition.

Pathology

Once bacteria or some foreign body have gained access into the tissues, the natural defensive reaction of the body induces a local inflammatory response in the area, which becomes red, swollen and extremely painful. The oedema separates the nail fold from the proximal nail plate, allowing further ready access to bacteria, which are commonly of the staphylococcal or streptococcal type. Infection leads to the formation of pus, which may be expressed from the nail fold. The yeast *Candida albicans* can also infect the tissue.

Treatment

Paronychia should always be regarded as potentially serious and it must be ascertained whether the condition is acute or chronic.

Acute paronychia is mainly the result of local trauma and treatment is directed primarily towards the prevention of infection, if this is not already present, and towards the reduction of inflammation and congestion. Cold compresses of Burow's solution every 4 hours for 24 hours should be applied to relieve congestion. This is followed by an application of an antiseptic agent and a suitable protective dressing. The treatment should be repeated at frequent intervals until the symptoms subside. It is important that the patient be advised to rest the foot as much as possible and avoid the causative action, if practical to do so. Usually, if infection is not present, the condition will resolve satisfactorily.

If infection is present, the first principle is to promote drainage of any pus by means of a hot antiseptic footbath, repeated at home at 4-hourly intervals, or by surgically removing the nail plate. Arrangements should be made for the patient to obtain appropriate systemic antibiotic therapy from the doctor, while podiatric dressings continue at frequent intervals. Drainage, once established, must be maintained until all pus has been cleared. The insertion of a piece of sterile ribbon gauze, to prevent premature closure of the wound, will assist this process. Once complete

drainage has been achieved the lesion can be thoroughly cleansed with a sterile saline solution and dried. To promote healing, an antiseptic of wide antibacterial spectrum should be applied covered by a sterile dressing. Such treatment is usually adequate, but the condition may progress to become chronic, when further medical advice should be sought.

ONYCHIA

Onychia is an inflammation of the matrix and nail bed and frequently originates from paronychia. The clinical features of both conditions are similar and they should always be regarded as serious. Local infection will cause suppuration, which produces a discolouration of the overlying nail plate (yellow, brown, black or green, depending on the infecting organism). A throbbing pain, which increases in severity, is the common symptom, relief only being obtained by drainage of the pus.

Aetiology

1. Any traumatic incident which introduces bacteria or a foreign body into the tissues; the condition will probably be confined to one toe
2. Any one of a number of systemic diseases; it is likely that several of the toes will be affected.

Pathology

Onychia can, and often does, result from paronychia (q.v.) and the pathology is similar. Bacterial invasion results in a purulent infection which collects beneath the nail plate, causing pressure and onycholysis (seen as separation of the nail from the nail bed).

Treatment

Immediate relief of acute pain will be obtained by removal of as much as necessary, or even all, of the nail plate to provide drainage of the underlying pus. Once this is achieved, the further treatment is the same as for paronychia.

ONYCHOLYSIS

Onycholysis is defined as separation of the nail from its bed at its distal end and/or its lateral margins (Baran et al 1990). It may be idiopathic or secondary to systemic and cutaneous diseases, or it may be the result of local causes. Air entering from the distal free edge gives a greyish-white appearance to the nail plate and forms variably shaped areas of detachment. If a sharp sculptured edge is present, it is likely to be self-induced by harsh manicuring. It is more common in fingernails than toenails and affects women more frequently than men.

Aetiology

1. Idiopathic—Baran et al (1991) suggest that idiopathic onycholysis of women and sculptured onycholysis are probably the same condition
2. Systemic disease, such as poor peripheral circulation, thyrotoxicosis and iron deficiency anaemia
3. Cutaneous diseases, which include psoriasis, eczema, hyperhidrosis
4. Drug-induced, due to the administration of bleomycin, retinoids, chlorpromazine, tetracyclines or thiazides
5. Local causes, such as trauma, where only one nail will be affected, or local infections, e.g. fungal, bacterial and viral. External irritants also result in onycholysis, the most common being prolonged immersion in hot water with added detergents, solvents such as petrol and cosmetic nail polishes.

Pathology

Separation of the nail is usually symptomless, but as the condition progresses, the space becomes filled with hard keratinous material from the exposed nail bed. The increased subungual pressure caused by this excess tissue may give rise to inflammation and very rarely becomes liable to infection.

Treatment

If a systemic cause is suspected, the patient should be advised to consult a physician. The single most important step in the treatment of onycholysis is to remove all of the detached nail at each visit. This prevents trauma from hosiery and bedclothes, allows possible mycotic material to be taken from the most proximal lytic area for culture, allows the nail bed to dry out where *Candida albicans* is the infecting organism and permits application of a suitable antifungal preparation at the active edge of the disease. Within 3–4 months the nail should resume a normal, fully attached appearance (Zaias 1990).

ONYCHOMADESIS (onychoptosis, aplastic anonychia)

This condition involves spontaneous separation of the nail, beginning at the matrix area and quickly reaching the free edge. The separation is often accompanied by some transient arrest of nail growth, characterised by a Beau's line.

Aetiology

1. Trauma, resulting in a subungual haematoma, or from repeated minor trauma, e.g. sportsman's toe
2. Serious generalised diseases, e.g. bullous dermatoses, lichen planus or drug reactions
3. Local inflammation, e.g. paronychia or irradiation
4. Defective peripheral circulation or prolonged exposure to cold
5. It may be an inherited disorder (dominant) and shedding will occur periodically.

Treatment

If a newly formed subungual haematoma is present, treatment should be aimed at relieving pressure, which may necessitate puncturing the nail.

For those cases where trauma can be excluded, the podiatrist can merely protect the nail with simple tubular gauze dressings or an acrylic resin plate, which prevents snagging on bedclothes and hosiery until the nail regrows fully.

ONYCHATROPHIA (anonychia)

The term onychatrophia is used to describe a nail which has reached mature size and then undergoes partial or total regression. The term anonychia is reserved to describe a nail which has failed to develop. However, the two conditions are difficult to differentiate.

Damage to the nail matrix resulting in onychatrophia is caused by lichen planus, cicatricial pemphigoid, severe paronychia, epidermolysis bullosa dystrophica or severe psoriasis. Anonychia occurs with rare congenital disorders, e.g. nail–patella syndrome.

ONYCHORRHEXIS (reed nail)

This condition presents as a series of narrow, longitudinal, parallel superficial ridges. The nail is very brittle and splitting at the free edge is common. Ridging naturally becomes more prominent with age but can be initiated by lichen planus, rheumatoid arthritis and peripheral circulatory disorders.

BEAU'S LINES

First described by Beau in 1846, these transverse

ridges or grooves reflect a temporary retardation of the normal growth of the nail. They first appear towards the proximal nail fold and move towards the free edge as the nail grows. The distance of the groove from the PNF indicates quite accurately the length of time since the illness or trauma (nail growth being about 1 mm per week).

Aetiology

Any condition or disease which may temporarily affect nail production from the matrix can be responsible. A single groove is usually the result of a severe febrile illness, although they have also been noted postnatally and in many other non-specific events. When the transverse ridges are due to paronychia or repeated minor trauma, they often have a rhythmic, rippling appearance.

Treatment

No specific treatment, other than reassurance, is necessary, as the nail condition will resolve once the aetiological factor has been removed.

HIPPOCRATIC NAILS (clubbing)

Hippocratic nail is the term used to describe an exaggerated longitudinal curvature of the nail, sometimes extending over the apex of the toe, which gives the digit a 'clubbed' appearance. The disorder is usually associated with some long-standing pulmonary or cardiac disorder and has been linked with thyroid disease, cirrhosis and ulcerative colitis (Fig. 8.13).

KOILONYCHIA (spoon-shaped nail)

This condition is more frequently met in fingernails than toenails. The normal convex curvature is lost and, instead, it becomes slightly concave or spoon-shaped. In infancy, koilonychia is a temporary physiological condition, but there is a proven correlation between koilonychia and iron deficiency anaemia. Thin nails of any origin, occupational softening and congenital forms are all aetiological factors (Fig. 8.14).

ONYCHOMYCOSIS (tinea unguium)

Onychomycosis is a fungal infection of the nail bed and nail plate. Fungi are microscopic vegetable organisms possessing no chlorophyll, which can only exist by utilising other organic matter for food. Certain groups of fungi, which are generally classified as dermatophytes, possess the ability to metabolise keratin and thereby grow and proliferate in the presence of protein. The human nail and its nail bed provide an exceedingly suitable environment in which the dermatophytes can flourish, and once these fungi have established themselves in that situation, the condition is known as onychomycosis. Since dermatophytes can utilise keratin as a source of food, it follows that any one or all of the nails will be liable to attack.

An infected nail plate becomes thickened and quite brittle and takes on a yellowish-brown colour, eventually developing a 'worm-eaten' or porous appearance.

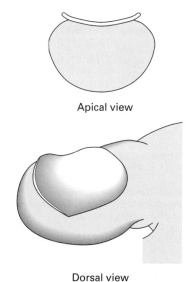

Apical view

Dorsal view

Figure 8.14 Koilonychia (spoon-shaped nail).

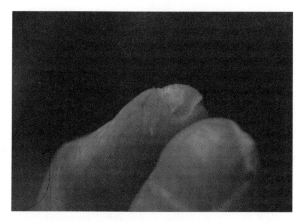

Figure 8.13 Hippocratic nail.

Aetiology

It is not always possible to pinpoint the actual source of the infection but one of the predisposing factors is failure to maintain a good standard of foot hygiene. Hyperhidrosis, communal showers, failure to dry the feet thoroughly following sporting activities and spread of an existing skin infection are all factors to be considered.

Pathology

Of the dermatophytes associated with onychomycosis the most frequently identified in practice are *Trichophyton rubrum* and *T. interdigitale*. Infection usually commences at the distal edge of the nail and gradually spreads over the entire nail plate and nail bed. Eventually, the nail plate becomes onycholytic as subungual debris increases. White marks, indicating fissuring, may appear on the nail plate.

Treatment

To halt, and perhaps ultimately to eradicate, a fungal infection of the nail plate requires continuing careful treatment over many months. A full explanation of the treatment regime should be given to the patient, as success will depend largely on patient compliance. Treatment involves the use of topical fungicides, and to facilitate their full potential the nail should be thinned as far as is practicable before the preparation is applied. Alternatively, the nail plate can be cut away so that the medicament can be applied directly to the active edge of the infection. The patient should repeat the treatment daily for 1 month or until new nail growth shows no signs of fungal infection. Thereafter, treatment should continue for up to 3 months to prevent reinfection.

Systemic fungal treatment with griseofulvin has been disappointing to date, with side-effects which cause the patient to discontinue treatment after a short time. However, recent evidence suggests that terbinafine (Lamasil) will clear onychomycosis within 12 weeks with no reported side-effects (Dykes et al 1990).

Advice must emphasise the spread of the infection via towels, hosiery and shoes, together with vigilant attention to drying and general personal hygiene.

LEUCONYCHIA

This is characterised by white markings on the nail in lines (*striata*), dots (*punctata*) or extending over the entire nail plate (*totalis*). They usually indicate minor trauma, e.g. as a result of short shoes or sporting activities, but rarely result from an illness.

YELLOW NAIL SYNDROME

In this disorder, the rate of nail growth reduces greatly and sometimes almost ceases. All the nails become a yellowish-green colour; they also thicken and display an increased longitudinal curvature with some evidence of onycholysis. The condition is almost always associated with some underlying respiratory or lymphoedema abnormality. Spontaneous recovery occurs in 30% of cases and the use of intravenous vitamin E is said to give beneficial results (Zaias 1990).

PTERYGIUM

Pterygium is adhesion of the eponychium to the nail bed following destruction of the matrix due to diminished circulation or some systemic disease. The entire nail plate is eventually shed.

REFERENCES

Achten G 1982 Histopathology of the nail. In: Pierre M (ed) The nail. G.E.M. Monograph 5. Churchill Livingstone, Edinburgh

Baran R, Barth J H, Dawber R P R 1991 Nail disorders. Common presenting signs, differential diagnosis and treatment. Martin Dunitz, London

Cohen H J, Franck S B, Minkin W, Gibbs R C 1973 Subungual exostosis. Archives of Dermatology: 431–432

Dykes P J, Thomas R, Finlay A Y 1990 Determination of terbinafine in nail samples during systemic treatment for onychomycosis. British Journal of Dermatology 123: 481–486

Hamilton J B, Terada H, Meistler G E 1955 Studies of growth throughout the lifespan in Japanese: growth and size of nails and relationships to age, sex, heredity and other factors. Journal of Gerontology 10: 401–415

Hashimito K, Gross B G, Nelson R, Lever W F 1966 The ultrastructure of the skin of human embryos, III. The formation of the nail in 16–18 week old embryos. Journal of Investigative Dermatology 40: 143–145

Jarrett A, Spearman R I C 1966 The histochemistry of the human nail. Archives of Dermatology 94: 652–657

Johnson M, Comaish J S, Shuster S 1991 Nail is produced by the nail bed: a controversy resolved. British Journal of Dermatology 125: 27–29

Lewin K 1965 The normal finger nail. British Journal of Dermatology 77: 421–430

Lewis B L 1954 Microscopic studies of fetal and mature nail and surrounding soft tissue. Archives of Dermatology 70: 732–747

Norton L A 1971 Incorporation of thymidine-methyl-H^3 and glycine-2-H^3 in the nail matrix and bed of humans. Journal of Investigative Dermatology 56: 61–68

Rayner V R 1973 An investigation into nail hypertrophy. Chiropodist, September: 288–302

Samman P D, Fenton D A 1986 The nails in disease, 4th edn. William Heinemann, London

Zaias N 1967 The movement of the nail bed. Journal of Investigative Dermatology 45(4): 402–403

Zaias N (ed) 1990 In: The nail in health and disease, 2nd edn. Appleton and Lange, Norwalk, Connecticut

Zaias N, Alvarez J 1968 The formation of the primate nail. An autoradiographic study in the squirrel monkey. Journal of Investigative Dermatology 51(2): 120–136

FURTHER READING

Baden H P 1987 Diseases of the hair and nails. Year Book Medical Publishers, Chicago, Illinois

Baran R, Dawber R P R 1984 Diseases of the nails and their management. Blackwell, Oxford

Baran R, Dawber R P R, Levene G M 1991 A colour atlas of the hair, scalp and nails. Wolfe, London

Burton J L 1991 Textbook of dermatology, 5th edn. Blackwell, London

9

Management of high risk patients

B. Wall

Keywords

Categories
Cleansing/desloughing agents
Diabetes mellitus
General management
High risk patients
Prevention
Wound assessment
Wound dressings
   Alginates
   Conventional dressings
   Foams
   Hydrocolloid
   Low adherence dressings
   Semi-permeable hydrogels
Wound history
Wound management

All patients are at risk of acquiring complications following podiatric treatment, the possibilities being minimised by the podiatrist adopting stringent aseptic techniques before, during and after treatment. Various pathological conditions can reduce the individual's healing potential or produce an increased susceptibility to infection and/or necrosis and ulceration. The patient group frequently cited as being at high risk are diabetics, but there are other systemic and local pathologies that place patients in the high risk category (Box 9.1).

Diabetes mellitus affects approximately 750 000 individuals in the UK (1–2% of the population). It is estimated that 6% of people over 65 years of age are diabetic. The podiatrist is part of the multidisciplinary diabetic team caring for the patient. Diabetes is a multisystem disease; without close liaison between all those involved in the patient's care, treatment will be submaximal. The diabetic care team ideally comprises the podiatrist, diabetologist, specialist nurse, vascular and orthopaedic surgeons, radiologist, orthotist, microbiologist, general practitioner and the patient

---

Box 9.1 Sources of high risk categories

1. *Vascular disorders:*
   Arterial, venous and lymphatic
   Macrovascular and microvascular, i.e. ischaemia
2. *Neurological disorders:*
   Peripheral and central nervous systems, i.e.
   sensory loss, deformity, alterations in gait
3. *Compromised immunity to infection:*
   Primary pathology, e.g. AIDS, diabetes mellitus
   Secondary to drug therapy, e.g. steroid therapy
4. *Arithritides*
   e.g. rheumatoid arthritis
5. *Oedema:*
   e.g. in association with venous incompetence,
   chronic cardiac failure. Oedema prevents the
   normal exchange of nutrients and metabolites
   between blood vessels and skin, because the
   excess fluid compresses capillaries and increases
   the distance between the capillary and the
   superficial tissues
6. *Metabolic disturbances:*
   e.g. diabetes mellitus
7. *Malnutrition:*
   This may occur more frequently than is supposed,
   particularly in the elderly of limited means or when
   religious or cultural conventions govern diet
8. *Psychological disturbances:*
   These can make it difficult for patients to care for
   themselves, e.g. depression. Patients with mental
   disability may require additional help in recognising
   and preventing foot problems

Box 9.2 Secondary disorders associated with diabetes mellitus that may affect the feet and lower limbs

1. *Vascular:*
   Accelerated atherosclerosis
   Microvascular changes
2. *Altered blood constituents:*
   Red blood cells become 'stiffer' and cannot flow
   easily through the capillaries; oxygen is not given
   up so readily by the haemoglobin
   Abnormal white cells which are not so effective in
   phagocytosing and destroying pathogenic
   microorganisms
3. *Neuropathic:*
   Abnormal conduction in motor, sensory and
   autonomic nerves, resulting in deformity and
   alteration in appreciation of damaging stimuli.
   Autonomic neuropathy will lead to anhidrotic skin
   and alteration in blood flow to the foot as a result of
   sympathetic nerve damage
4. *Increased susceptibility to infection:*
   As a result of the factors mentioned above
5. *Impaired eyesight:*
   Diabetic retinopathy and cataracts may limit the
   patient in looking for signs of damage to the feet
6. *Kidney disease:*
   This may result in oedema and increased
   susceptibility to infection
7. *Abnormal non-enzymatic glycosylation of various proteins:*
   This can include collagen, leading to abnormal
   wound healing and soft tissues

---

and her carers. 'Shared care' of diabetic patients, between the hospital and the general practitioner, should still allow multidisciplinary cooperation between professionals.

The complications associated with diabetes that can affect the feet are summarised in Box 9.2. Recently, it has been shown that diabetic complications can be reduced substantially by strict control of blood glucose concentrations (Diabetes Control and Complications Trial Research Group 1993).

In the future, podiatrists and colleagues from other medical disciplines will be under increasing pressure to preserve tissue viability in diabetics; for example, the St Vincent Declaration aims to reduce all diabetic lower limb amputations (resulting from gangrene) by 50% over 5 years (Diabetes Care and Research in Europe 1990).

AIMS IN MANAGING HIGH RISK PATIENTS

The main aims when managing high risk patients, be they diabetic or not, are:

1. to prevent complications (e.g. infection or injury)
2. to effectively manage established wounds, infection or necrosis.

Prevention of complications

History-taking and assessment

Obtaining a detailed medical history is paramount; this is accompanied by a vascular, neurological and biomechanical assessment. History-taking includes recording medical and surgical details. Any drug therapy (including non-prescription medication) taken by the patient is noted and checked with a current edition of the British National Formulary. It is important to make enquiries regarding drug therapy, as the underlying condition for which the drug is being administered may impair wound healing, e.g. vitamin B injections for pernicious anaemia. Alternatively, the drug itself may impair wound healing potential, or compromise the patient's immune system, e.g. corticosteroids.

Investigation of vascular and neurological systems does not need to be complicated; methods of performing simple routine tests are detailed in Chapter 2. Non-invasive methods of vascular assessment, such as estimation of ankle brachial systolic pressure indices, are relatively simple to perform. The use of forceplates can be helpful in locating areas of high pressure loading, particularly in the neuropathic foot.

Simple urinalysis and/or estimation of blood sugar levels, using a correctly calibrated glucometer, are indicated when there is a family history of diabetes, or when the patient presents with signs and symptoms of diabetes, for example with recurrent episodes of infection.

Patient education regarding the relationship of their primary systemic pathology to foot health is vital; many excellent educational packs are available, but they must be accompanied by explanations appropriate to the individual patient. Whenever possible, carers should attend and be involved in education sessions.

General points regarding treatment

The practitioner must pay close attention to aseptic techniques. The use of autoclaves for instrument sterilisation is now legally mandatory. Meticulous pre-operative preparation of the patient's skin is necessary to effect a rapid reduction in the number of pathogenic transient flora, and to remove gross contamination. The most important pre-operative cleansing routine is a thorough application of an alcohol-based preparation; any antiseptic added to the alcohol provides limited improvement to the solution's activity.

Padding must be accurately shaped, avoiding creases and irregularities. Strapping should be non-constrictive. If caustic medicaments are used, they must be applied with great care and their actions monitored closely. Detailed advice regarding suitable footwear and hosiery is essential and is considered in other chapters. Minor surgical procedures are performed as a last resort, and only after consultation with the patient's general practitioner.

Management of established wounds, infection or necrosis

An ulcer is an example of a wound that, for various reasons, will not heal. Most research pertinent to wound healing is not restricted to ulcers; the general term 'wound' is used in preference to 'ulcer' in the following discussion.

The following wound management strategies are considered:

- examination of the wound
- the use of antiseptics and topical medicaments
- the use of dressings.

Examination of the wound

A detailed history and examination of the wound should take place at the initial consultation (Box 9.3). At each subsequent visit the wound and the patient's general condition are assessed, with any changes being recorded with meticulous care. The points that will be observed by the podiatrist are summarised in Box 9.4 and Figure 9.1. Photographs provide a detailed permanent record, although this recording method is not always practical during routine clinical practice. However, special pieces of transparent film are available for marking the area of a wound accurately, without the risk of contamination and cross-infection. At each visit, a subjective, as well as an objective, assessment of the wound and the whole patient should be made (plantar wounds are shown in Figs 9.2 and 9.3).

Swabs are taken from exuding wounds and sent for microbiological examination. It is vital that microbiological specimens are collected in the correct manner, and all paper work completed accurately. Advice from a microbiologist will be invaluable in both these matters. All wound surfaces are populated by microorganisms, but not all of these *contaminated* wounds are clinically *infected*. Microorganisms obtained from swabs taken from the deepest part of the wound are more likely to be of clinical significance than those obtained by superficial swabbing. The recent increase in multiple antibiotic-resistant strains of microorganisms, for example, methicillin-resistant *Staphylococcus*

Box 9.3 History of the wound

1. The *duration* of the wound
2. Any changes in the *size or appearance* of the wound?
3. Any change in the *number* of lesions/wounds?
4. Any *previous incidents* of similar lesions?
5. Any *pain or altered sensation* associated with the lesion?
6. The presence of other *signs and/or symptoms* that may be related to the wound, e.g. ischaemic changes
7. Does the patient know the *cause* of the wound?

Box 9.4 Points to be observed when examining a wound

1. The precise *anatomical site* of the wound
2. The *size* of the wound. This should be measured accurately using a commercial device
3. The *general appearance* of the wound and the surrounding tissue, e.g. presence of callus or maceration. Special note should be made of signs of local or spreading infection (cellulitis, lymphangitis, lymphadenitis)
4. The *sides* of the wound. When the walls are undermining the viable tissue, the true extent of the wound must be assessed by the careful use of a sterile probe
5. The *base* of the wound, for the presence of slough, granulation tissue or deeper structures such as bone or tendon. Radiographs are necessary if deeper structures are thought to be involved. The wound *depth* should be assessed. Chronic lesions are associated with fibrous bands tying the base to underlying structures; by gentle manipulation of the wound, the degree of fibrosis may be estimated
6. Any *discharge* should be noted and a specimen sent for microscopy and culture. The colour, consistency and odour of discharge should be recorded. The quantity may be approximated by observing dressings and finding out how often they require renewing

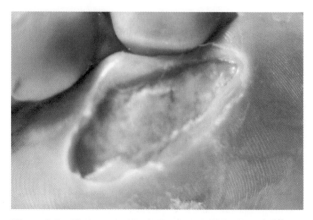

Figure 9.2 Plantar wound proximal to the toe webbing. The wound has walls that undermine surrounding tissue, making its true size difficult to ascertain. Slough covers its base. The surrounding tissues are macerated.

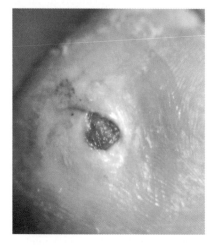

Figure 9.3 Plantar wound under the first metatarsal head. The wound is shallow and its walls are not undermining surrounding tissue. The base is covered with granulation tissue.

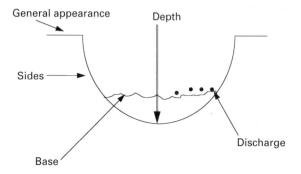

Figure 9.1 Points to observe when examining a wound.

aureus (MRSA), dictates that systemic antibiotics must not be prescribed indiscriminately. However, for heavily infected wounds (particularly diabetic neuropathic ulcers), antibiotic coverage will include drugs active against Gram-positive staphylococci and streptococci, Gram-negative species and anaerobes (for example, *Bacteroides fragilis*). Where infection has become chronic, or when deeper structures are thought to be involved, radiographs are required to exclude soft tissue infection or osteomyelitis.

Management of wounds

There has been much debate about the use of surgical masks, sterile gloves, hats and plastic aprons whilst treating wounds. Historically, face masks were worn to prevent contamination of wounds by droplets disseminated from the practitioner's nasopharynx. Surveys demonstrate that the incidence of hospital-acquired infection is not affected by the use of face masks (Orr 1981). It is concluded that masks contribute little to protecting wounds and may increase transmission of *Staph. aureus*, by encouraging shedding of colonised skin squames through the rubbing action of the mask on the face (Infection Control Nurses Association 1984). The most effective method of preventing contamination is to reduce conversation whilst attending to the wound and to effect a well organised treatment. Sterile surgical gloves may be worn, but clean latex gloves are acceptable. The practitioner's hands are the main vehicles of cross-infection (Sims 1980). By adopting a standardised hand-washing technique, using soap and water, the number of pathogenic transient organisms is reduced. Hand rinses containing 70% ethanol are very effective in removing transient organisms (Rotter 1984). Paper hats can prevent skin squames from the scalp contaminating wounds.

Single-use plastic aprons may be worn to prevent contamination of permeable cotton clinic coats. Studies demonstrate a 50% reduction in the number of organisms recovered from clean plastic aprons when compared to the number isolated from a clean cotton garment; the moisture content of cotton supports the growth of bacterial colonies (Infection Control Nurses Association 1984)

The use of pre-packed, sterile instruments, medicaments and dressings is strongly recommended. When treating open lesions, aseptic techniques should be employed correctly and with care. It has been shown that such techniques can be become ritualised, and potentially dangerous, unless employed logically and with some thought (Merchant 1988). Disposal of soiled dressings must follow local infection control guidelines.

The use of instruments on any wound, and the amount of tissue debrided, will depend on the aetiology and clinical state of the lesion at the time of treatment. Diabetic ischaemic ulcerations must be treated conservatively; conversely diabetic neuropathic ulcers require maximum debridement to encourage healing. It is important when treating neuropathic ulcers with undermining walls to ensure full exploration of the site and to identify the full extent of the wound.

Cleansing and desloughing agents

Wounds require cleansing and there are many products available for this purpose. Slough (a collection of necrotic material, leucocytes and microorganisms) can become a medium for further bacterial growth; in many cases it is important to try and remove it. In ischaemic wounds, slough tends to be firmly attached to the base of the wound, whereas slough in neuro-

pathic wounds may be less adherent and easier to remove. It is important to recognise the intimate physical relationship that exists between slough and granulation tissue; the problems of disturbing the latter whilst removing the former must be considered before deciding upon a treatment method.

Cleansing agents commonly used include sterile isotonic saline (0.89%), chlorhexidine gluconate, cetrimide (quaternary ammonium compound) and povidone iodine. Most of these medicaments are available in sterile, single-use sachets, the use of which is strongly advocated. Solutions are applied to the wound site using sterile gauze or cotton wool; solutions may be applied to difficult sites via a sterile syringe barrel, without the needle attached.

Sterile aqueous solutions of chlorhexidine gluconate are suitable for cleaning wounds. Chlorhexidine is effective against a wide range of Gram-positive bacteria, but it is less effective against Gram-negative species and fungi, and ineffective against bacterial spores or viruses. Cetrimide possesses a moderately wide range of activity against microorganisms. It demonstrates less activity against Gram-negative bacilli than against Gram-positive species. Cetrimide's detergent action makes it suitable for cleaning exceptionally contaminated wounds. Cetrimide may be combined with chlorhexidine gluconate in varying concentrations (Steripod chlorhexidine/cetrimide solution, Tisept: Seton Healthcare). The regular use of cetrimide on wounds is not recommended, as it has been shown to have deleterious effects on healthy tissues, even at low concentrations (Thomas 1990).

Iodophors are complexes of iodine and solubilisers (for example, povidone iodine) and are found in many products. Povidone iodine has a wide range of activity against microorganisms, including a sporicidal action.

Older, traditional cleansing agents, such as proflavine, are not recommended as their role has been superseded by newer medicaments. Hydrogen peroxide (up to 10 volumes or 3%) has limited antiseptic properties; any beneficial effects are due to mechanical bubbling resulting from the liberation of oxygen gas.

Experiments have demonstrated that all the medicaments discussed above, with the exception of isotonic saline, can produce transient closure of capillaries (Brennan et al 1986). Chlorhexidine's effect was minimal. However, in clinical practice, the reduction of capillary blood flow is of very short duration, although the use of sterile isotonic saline is suggested for cleaning the majority of wounds.

Desloughing/cleansing agents include the hypochlorite group of chemicals and enzymes that allow autolytic breakdown of slough by-products generated from the patient's own leucocytes. Other methods use dextronomer beads and occlusive dressings.

The hypochlorites were introduced into clinical practice by Semmelweis (1818–1865). The hypochlorites interact with protein and it is this reaction that imparts their antibacterial role. It should be noted that the British National Formulary (September 1994) stipulates that neither chlorinated lime and boric acid solution BP (Eusol) nor chlorinated soda solution, surgical BPC (Dakin's solution) is suitable for use as cleansing agents, due to their irritant effects.

Preparations containing enzymes are used for desloughing wounds (Forsling 1988). Enzymes such as streptokinase and streptodornase degrade fibrin and remove DNA from cell nuclei. Most enzyme preparations are presented as dry powders, which are refrigerated until application, when they are reconstituted with sterile isotonic saline (e.g. Varidase: Lederle). The solution can be held in contact with the wound using gauze and a film dressing, or it can be injected under tough necrotic slough using a syringe.

Organic acids held in propylene glycol (Aserbine: Forley) cause swelling of necrotic tissue, without affecting healthy tissue; this encourages preferential removal of slough from the wound base.

Agents such as Debrisan (Kabi Pharmaceuticals) are composed of sterile beads of dextranomer (between 0.1 and 0.3 mm in diameter). The beads exert a hydrophilic action, acting as absorbents; they also help to remove debris and bacteria from the wound surface by capillary action. Paste formulations have helped in applying the product to the foot. It should be noted that if the beads are spilt on the floor the environment becomes dangerously slippery. Cadexamer iodine (Iodosorb: Perstorp Pharmaceuticals) is similar to Debrisan in appearance, although it is chemically different. The product contains 0.9% w/w of iodine. The beads swell under the influence of exudate and release the iodine.

Dressings

There is an abundance of new wound dressings, and as technology moves forward, more are to be anticipated. It should be stressed that in many chronic wounds, the failure of a wound care product to work is the result of underlying pathologies, stressing the need to assess the patient's general health before deciding on a management strategy. No dressing will heal a wound whilst the local microenvironment is unsuitable (e.g. oedema and local infection). It is unrealistic to expect all chronic wounds to heal. Turner (1979) encapsulates this concept by emphasising the

need to consider, before predicting the likely prognosis for wound healing:

factors which will produce a micro-environment associated with the wound that will allow healing to proceed at a maximum rate commensurate with the age and physiological condition of the patient.

The literature accompanying a product must be consulted, to ensure the suitability of the dressing for individual patients and their wounds. Unfortunately, the price and availability may restrict the use of some products.

The properties of the 'ideal wound dressing' are considered before describing the various groups of products.

The criteria for the 'ideal wound dressing' are:

1. the ability to remove exudate
2. the ability to maintain humidity at the wound/dressing interface
3. permeability of the dressing to gases
4. the ability to maintain a suitable pH
5. the ability to maintain a suitable temperature at the wound surface
6. the ability to maintain low adherence at the wound/dressing interface
7. the ability to be free from contaminants
8. the ability to be impermeable to microorganisms
9. other factors, including ease of application, patient acceptability and comfort, and cost.

The ability to remove exudate. The removal of excess exudate from the surface of the wound is important for three main reasons:

1. exudate can act as a hospitable medium for pathogenic growth
2. exudate can macerate the wound. Enzymes present in exudate can produce autolysis of surrounding tissues
3. exudate can soak dressings and 'strike-through' occurs; this allows entry of pathogens, from the outside of the dressing onto the wound surface, by capillary action.

It should be noted that exudate also possesses desirable actions. Various substances found in exudate, for example growth factors, are necessary for successful wound healing.

The ability to maintain humidity at the wound/dressing interface. Until Winter's seminal work, wounds were kept dry. The rationale for this regime was to discourage bacterial invasion. In 1962, Winter showed that epithelial movement across a wound was compromised by thick scab formation. Epithelial cells seek a moist surface for movement, and thus in dry wounds the suitable environment is deep under the scab; in this case re-epithelialisation is a slow, energy-consuming process (Winter 1962). It should be noted that dressings that allow strike-through can dehydrate wound surfaces.

Permeability of the dressing to gases. The importance of atmospheric oxygen varies with different stages of wound healing. Early dressings such as Opsite (Smith & Nephew) were gas permeable. Under this type of dressing, the number of neutrophils in the exudate increased, and regeneration of epithelial cells increased 10-fold—both these events are beneficial to wound healing.

The effects of hypoxia (reduced oxygen levels) can aid the healing process. Neo-angiogenesis (the production of new capillaries, a major component of granulation tissue) is increased in hypoxic environments. Reduced oxygen concentration stimulates macrophages to produce molecules able to stimulate new vessel growth (Silver 1994). Hypoxia is reported to decrease pain, possibly by interfering with the production of prostaglandins and other chemicals.

The ability to be impermeable to microorganisms. The dressing should be impermeable to the entry of pathogenic microorganisms onto the wound surface; this situation is most likely to occur during *strike-through*.

The ability to maintain a suitable temperature at the wound surface. After routine cleansing, it takes 40 minutes for the surface of a wound to regain its original temperature, and 3 hours for normal cell mitotic function to return (Myers 1982). It is therefore advisable to leave wounds exposed for the minimum time possible during redressings (also reducing the risk of cross-infection). It is also wise to avoid using cold solutions for irrigation and cleaning lesions.

Oxygen dissociation from haemoglobin is impaired when the temperature is reduced by 10°C. Thus dressings that allow *strike-through* not only allow contamination, and encourage dehydration of wounds, but can cause temperature loss by convection.

The ability to maintain low adherence at the wound/dressing interface. Dressings that adhere to wound surfaces damage delicate granulation tissue and epithelium when removed. These dressings can become incorporated into granulation tissue and produce foreign body reactions. In addition, patients may experience distress and pain during the change of dressings, if the material has become adherent.

Some low-adherence dressings can be responsible for autolytic damage to tissues around the wound site. This is because exudate is unable to travel through the pore structure of the dressing's plastic film interface.

The ability to be free from contaminants. The dressing must be constructed from material that can be sterilised and kept in that condition until it is used. Dressings should not contain substances able to cause toxic reactions, or adversely interact with the wound surface. Particulates or fibres shed from a dressing can become incorporated into granulation tissue and produce foreign body reactions.

The ability to maintain a suitable pH. Oxygen dissociates from haemoglobin most efficiently in an acidic environment (Bohr effect). A low pH (acidic) is important in stimulating neo-angiogenesis.

Other factors, including patient acceptability, ease of application and comfort, and cost. Some early dressings (particularly the occlusive hydrocolloids) were unacceptable to patients because of malodour and exudate formed by the interaction of the dressing components and the wound.

Some dressings are difficult to apply to the contours of the foot as they are designed for use on larger, flatter body surfaces. The judicious use of strapping and conforming bandages helps to overcome these problems. The cost and availability of some dressings may prohibit their use; however, the cost-effectiveness of a product should always be fully researched.

Types of dressing for use in podiatric practice

The introduction and accessibility of new dressings is changing at such a prodigious rate that detailed description of individual dressings is inappropriate. This section will describe the features of groups of products currently available. It is stressed that, before using any wound care product, practitioners make themselves fully aware of the product's indications and contraindications, by consulting either the manufacturer or a current edition of the British National Formulary.

Conventional dressings

Examples: Gauze swabs BP.

The majority of podiatrists use gauze swabs, mainly because of availability and low cost. The disadvantages associated with gauze dressings include: 'strike through', the shedding of fibres, adherence and incorporation into the wound surface (these problems are discussed above).

The use of paraffin gauze (the older name for which is tulle gras) reduces some of the adverse effects of using gauze; however, granulation tissue can grow through its structure and incorporate the paraffin gauze into the wound.

Low adherence dressings

Examples: Bioclusive (Johnson & Johnson), Tegaderm (3M Healthcare), Melolin (Smith & Nephew).

The first low adherence dressing was Opsite (Smith & Nephew), developed originally as an adhesive incise drape for general surgery. This type of film dressing is gas- and water vapour-permeable, but is impermeable to water. It has no fibres that can be shed into wounds; it is transparent and allows monitoring of the wound site. However, semi-permeable films are non-absorbent. Some other low adherence dressings are prepared from knitted viscose and may incorporate an antiseptic, but are not absorbent (Inadine: Johnson & Johnson), requiring a secondary dressing to absorb exudate. Others incorporate an absorptive backing, e.g. Melolin (Smith & Nephew), Telfa (Kendall) and Release (Jonhson & Johnson). Newer dressings incorporate silicones to facilitate removal (Silicone NA: Johnson & Johnson).

Semi-permeable hydrogels

Examples: Geliperm (Geistlich), Intrasite Gel (Smith & Nephew).

Structurally, these products are hydrophilic polymers that contain a high percentage of water. There are two basic presentations of semi-permeable hydrogels: the first type is in a sheet form (not dissimilar to a thin slice of table jelly); the second are known as amorphous hydrogels and resemble wallpaper paste in texture. Both forms are absorptive; the first group retain their gross structure but swell, while the second group absorb exudate until their substance becomes dispersed in water.

The sheet form of hydrogels consist of approximately 96% water (percentage varies with individual products), and are transparent, flexible and easily moulded, with mechanical properties that protect delicate granulation tissue. They are gas-permeable but impermeable to water. This form of hydrogel will dehydrate and must be either replaced or rehydrated with sterile isotonic saline to prevent fragmentation of the product. The percentage of water in the original dressing dictates its absorptive power.

The amorphous hydrogels can be used to remove slough by rehydrating dry, necrotic tissue. This group is effective in absorbing exudate, and it is proposed that they reduce local oedema. Hydrogels are kept in situ by applying gauze, or another secondary dressing, over them and then applying conforming bandage.

Hydrocolloids

Examples: Granuflex (Convatec), Comfeel (Coloplast), Tegasorb (3M Healthcare).

These are referred to as 'interactive' dressings. They are composed of hydrogels combined with substances such as elastomeric compounds, adhesives, polysaccharides and proteins. The constituents adhere to, and interact with, the wound surface; these are held on a water-repellent, flexible foam backing which should not require a secondary dressing. In early versions of hydrocolloid dressings, interaction between the dressing and wound surface produced a yellow, semi-liquid and malodorous substance. Contemporary products are more sophisticated. The semi-liquid produced at the dressing/wound interface is protective and absorptive, provides a moist and insulated environment, and forms an impermeable layer. This layer results in an acidic and hypoxic environment conducive to neo-angiogenesis. The occlusive environment contraindicates the use of hydrocolloids when a wound is clinically infected particularly when anaerobe species are isolated. The use of hydrocolloids may also be contraindicated for treating diabetic ulcers.

Hydrocolloids are available in other presentations (e.g. pastes), which are used in wounds supporting a heavy slough. Most manufacturers produce 'wound management systems'; these involve using desloughing agents and specific types of dressing at different stages of wound healing.

Alginate dressings

Examples: Kaltostat (BritCair), Sorbsan (Steriseal).

These products are manufactured from alginates derived from seaweed. They represent a very old treatment: sailors used seaweed for dressing wounds and effecting haemostasis centuries ago.

When in contact with blood or exudate, alginate fibres convert, via calcium/sodium ion exchange, into a hydrophilic gel. The gel is absorbent and provides a protective, moist interface to the wound. Generally, alginates are relatively easy to remove, provided the area is irrigated with sterile isotonic saline; however, some situations will require the use of forceps to complete removal of the dressing. Theoretically, the fibres associated with the dressing present no hazard as they are biodegradable. There have been some reports of patients experiencing a mild burning sensation when alginates are applied; this could be due to the intensely hydrophilic properties of the product causing a rapid dehydration. The effect can be minimised by moistening the dressing with sterile isotonic saline before application.

Foams

Examples: Lyofoam (Seton Healthcare), Allevyn (Smith & Nephew).

Marine sponges were probably the earliest form of foams used as wound dressings: in 1884, Joseph Gamgee introduced an artificial absorbent sponge.

Foams are indicated for treating wounds with moderate amounts of exudate. The manufacturing process produces a dressing with a smooth, low-adherent hydrophilic inner layer and an outer layer of untreated hydrophobic foam. The construction of the outer layer helps reduce strike-through, although a secondary dressing may be required. Foam dressings are very permeable to gases and allow adequate hydration of the wound surface. They also provide extremely effective thermal insulation.

Other dressings—the way forward?

Almost every substance imaginable has been used as a wound dressing at some point in history. Some of these older remedies are currently being reassessed using modern scientific methods. Honey, for example, has an acid pH (approximately pH 3.7) and this may encourage wound neo-angiogenesis as well as being bactericidal. Sugar may act in a similar way to dextranomer beads (discussed above).

Other approaches involve seeding the patient's own epithelial cells onto a suitable culture medium and using the resultant culture on their wounds (Shakespeare 1991). Platelet-derived growth factors and cytokines (e.g. transforming growth factors α and β) have been used to treat diabetic ulcers (Holloway et al 1993).

Other aspects of management

The use of antiseptics on wounds is disputed. Most antiseptics have a deleterious effect on the wound microenvironment: they can interfere with wound healing, produce resistance in some microorganisms and produce skin sensitivities if used for long periods of time. The use/non-use of antiseptics is, however, a matter of personal choice and circumstances. The use of topical antibiotics is totally contraindicated; antibiotics should be delivered systemically, but only after the causative microorganism has been identified, and its sensitivity to a specific antibiotic ascertained.

The use of padding and orthoses to protect wounds may be indicated; each patient will require a specific prescription, and therefore only general comments can be made.

Soft cushioning padding materials will be indicated rather than firm redistributive materials; the use of the latter can compromise capillary blood flow to the edges of the wound. Accurate positioning of pads is vital, and is not always an easy task, particularly when large dressings have been applied. As little adhesive as practically possible should be placed on the skin; conforming bandages (e.g. Kling: Johnson & Johnson) or plastic film sprays can be used to protect vulnerable areas of skin from adhesives.

When specific areas of high pressure loading are identified, casted insoles constructed from composites of low, medium and high density thermoplastics are helpful. These customised insoles are valuable in preventing initial damage occurring. Footwear and hosiery must be carefully selected, and, if necessary, modifications such as stretching or balloon patching can be executed.

Slippers, often a popular choice with patients, are not recommended unless they are well-fitting, as they produce shearing stresses that cause movement of dressings, predispose to falls and reduce activity of the calf muscle pump. Bootees made from low density thermoplastics may be suitable for an immobile patient. Bespoke or semi-bespoke footwear is the answer to many chronic foot problems, or can be used as a preventative measure. The orthotist is an important link in the provision of special footwear when caring for patients in a hospital setting.

Total contact casting may be indicated when treating neuropathic ulcers. The technique has several variations that allow removal of the cast for inspection of the wound site. The technique must be taught correctly before practitioners attempt to use total contact casts on patients.

The patient is advised to rest and elevate the affected limb, but the danger of immobility producing a deep vein thrombosis cannot be overlooked. Other problems of immobility are the development of pressure sores and, if the limb is insufficiently elevated, oedema may ensue.

Patients must be discouraged from smoking. Smoking adversely affects wound healing in several ways: it causes vasoconstriction, reduces macrophage and epithelial cell function and reduces IgG levels (Siana et al 1992). However, it should be recognised that the patient's quality of life and compliance with treatment may be adversely affected unless a compromise between ideal and realistic advice is made.

Consideration of the role of multidisciplinary care of the patient is crucial during treatment of wounds. This is also important once improvement of the wound occurs, so that the patient is monitored by professionals, such as district nurses and the general practitioner, who can liaise with each other and the podiatrist in providing patient care.

CONCLUSIONS

High risk patients and their wounds provide a challenge to the podiatrist; the adage of 'prevention being preferable to cure' holds true for this group of patients. The challenge is minimised by adopting a multidisciplinary approach to patient care, using expertise gained by other health care professionals and by colleagues. It is important that other professions understand the role of podiatry in the care of the high risk patient, and it is incumbent upon the podiatrist to ensure that this information is forthcoming.

Patient education is important, but only if patients and their carers understand the rationale behind the information that is provided—the responsibility for this lies with the podiatrist.

When wounds develop they must be treated on an individual basis, and only after a full medical history and physical examination of the patient and the lesion have been carried out. When selecting wound care products, the practitioner will be aided by an understanding of the normal wound healing process and by frequent consultation of the medical and nursing press for new developments.

REFERENCES

Brennan S, Foster M E, Leaper D J 1986 Antiseptic toxicity in wounds healing by secondary intention. Journal of Hospital Medicine 8: 263–267

Diabetes Care and Research in Europe 1990 The Saint Vincent declaration. Workshop report. Diabetic Medicine 7: 360

Diabetes Control and Complications Trial Research Group 1993 The effect of intensive treatment of diabetes on the development of long-term complications in insulin dependent diabetes mellitus. New England Journal of Medicine 329: 977–986

Forsling E 1988 Comparison of saline and streptokinase-streptodornase in the treatment of leg ulcers. European Journal of Clinical Pharmacology 33: 637–638

Holloway G A, Steed D L, De Marco et al 1993 A randomised, controlled, multicenter, dose response trial of activated platelet supernatent, topical CT-102 in chronic, nonhealing diabetic wounds. Wounds: A Compendium of Clinical Research and Practice 5(4): 198–206

Infection Control Nurses Association Working Party 1984 Report on ward protective clothing. Infection Control Nurses Association

Merchant J 1988 Aseptic technique reconsidered. Care – Science and Practice 6(3): 74–77

Myers J A 1982 Modern plastic surgical dressings. Health and Social Services Journal March: 336–337

Orr N 1981 Is a mask necessary in the operating theatre? Annals of the Royal College of Surgeons 63: 390

Rotter M 1984 Hygienic hand disinfection. Infection Control 5: 18

Shakespeare P 1991 Cultured human skin epithelium for wound repair. Journal of Tissue Viability 1: 19–20

Siana J E, Frankid S, Gottrup F 1992 The effect of smoking on tissue function. Journal of Wound Care 1(2): 37–41

Silver I A 1994 The physiology of wound healing. Journal of Wound Care 3(2): 106–109

Sims W 1980 The problem of cross infection in a dental surgery with particular reference to serum hepatitis. Journal of Dentistry 8: 20–26

Thomas S 1990 Wound management and dressings. Pharmaceutical Press, Royal Pharmaceutical Society, p 79

Turner T D 1979 Products and their development in wound management. Symposium on wound healing, Espoo, Finland

Winter G D 1962 Formation of the scab and the rate of epithelialisation of superficial wounds in the skin of the young domestic pig. Nature 193: 293–294

FURTHER READING

Ayliffe G A J, Lowbury E J L, Geddes A M, Williams J D 1992 Control of hospital infection, 3rd edn. Chapman and Hall, London

Duckworth G J, Lothian J L E, Williams J 1988 Methicillin resistant *Staphylococcus aureus:* report of an outbreak in a London teaching hospital. Journal of Hospital Infection II: 1–5

Foster A, Greenhill M, Edmonds M 1994 Comparing two dressings in the treatment of diabetic foot ulcers. Journal of Wound Care 3(5): 224–228

Levin M E, O'Neal L W, Bowker J H 1993 The diabetic foot, 5th edn. Mosby, St Louis

Pickup J C, Williams G 1994 Chronic complications of diabetes. Blackwell Scientific, Oxford

Taylor L J 1978 An evaluation of handwashing techniques. Nursing Times 74(54): 108

Underwood J C E 1992 General and systemic pathology. Churchill Livingstone, Edinburgh

Watkins P J, Drury P L, Taylor K W 1990 Diabetes and its management, 4th edn. Blackwell Scientific, Oxford

10

The ageing foot

G. J. French
S. J. Braid
A. M. Barlow

Keywords

Domiciliary care
Foot deformity in the elderly
General physical/mental influences
Institutional care
Mobility
Neoplasia
Night pains
Non-malignant lesions
Podiatry provision for the elderly
Steroids
Systemic medication
Ulceration
Vascular impairment

The last two decades have seen a great increase in the volume of literature published about the elderly. This has included surveys to determine the medical and social needs of this section of the population, and has also described the effects of ageing on body systems. The process of ageing is no longer considered to be anything other than a normal phenomenon. However, ageing is often accompanied by more severe degenerative changes which may manifest as specific diseases.

One omission from the literature has been an attempt to define the term *ageing* itself. It appears to be generally accepted that the term *elderly* is associated with age in terms of years, and that the retirement age, i.e. 60–65 years, is the age at which one makes the transition from middle age to elderly. Hamdy (1984) states:

Any population can be divided into three main groups: a financially productive working population, which supports a young dependent population, and an elderly population which has retired from active wage-earning employment.

The elderly population is continuing to increase, although it is expected that the balance of different age groups will change.

Those aged 65–74 are projected to make up 53% of the population aged 65 and over in the year 2001, and there will be a dramatic increase among those aged 85 or over, who are projected to make up 11% of the elderly in 2001 compared with just over 8% in 1984 (OPCS 1986).

It is also interesting to note that 64% of disabled people in Britain are over the age of 75.

Podiatry has a key role to play in this scenario. The most expensive patient is the one who occupies a hospital bed. The independent mobile person, who can attend local health care facilities, requires only minimal public expenditure. Adequate appraisal today of the determinants of this dependency spectrum will lower the costly manpower requirements of tomorrow.

Resistance to health-threatening factors diminishes progressively through life and the function of the podiatrist in the geriatric field can become progressively demanding. Broadly, the task is to maintain mobility, and to delay the semi-mobile from becoming the expensively nursed immobile. Ederly age must not be considered as being synonymous with disease and disability. Many elderly people differ from the young only by being somewhat slower and having a reduced fatigue threshold.

Age can also influence a person's willingness to accept treatment. Anxiety about the procedures which are (often wrongly) imagined to be painful can delay the timely removal of onychogryphosis and cutaneous lesions, which again can be precursors of ulcerative and infective states. Reassurance by the podiatrist is needed, together with the willingness to spend extra time, especially when some of the more bizarre looking hypertrophies require attention. Patient confidence may need to be captured by spreading treatments over a series of attendances in much the same manner as is sometimes necessary with children.

SKIN AND NAIL CHANGES

Both Gilchrist (1979) and Gibbs (1975) stated that the most common signs of ageing skin are dryness, scaling and atrophy, and that the most common change in pedal skin as a result of ageing is hyperkeratosis.

Structural and functional alterations caused by intrinsic ageing, and independent of environmental insults, are now recognised in the skin of elderly individuals. Structurally, the aged epidermis becomes thinner, the keratinocytes become less adherent to one another, and there is flattening of the dermo-epidermal interface. The number of melanocytes and Langerhans cells is decreased. The dermis becomes atrophic and it is relatively acellular and avascular. Dermal collagen, elastin and glycosaminoglycans are

altered. The subcutaneous tissue is diminished in some areas, especially the face, shins, hands and feet, while in others, particularly the abdomen in men and the thighs in women, it is increased.

Due to the loss of elasticity, the atrophic skin and the subcutaneous tissues take longer to regain their normal configuration when pinched between thumb and forefinger. The number of eccrine glands is reduced and both the eccrine and apocrine glands undergo attenuation. Sebaceous glands tend to increase in size, but paradoxically their secretory output is lessened. The nail plate is generally thinned, the surface ridged and lustreless, and the lunula is decreased in size. Functional alterations noted in the skin of elderly persons include a decreased growth rate of the epidermis, hair and nails, delayed wound healing, reduced dermal clearance of fluids and foreign materials, and compromised vascular responsiveness. Eccrine and apocrine secretions are diminished. The cutaneous immune and inflammatory responses are impaired (Fenske & Lober 1986).

Skin atrophy can take the form of insidious thinning, which requires nothing more than woollen hosiery, fleece-lined shoes or slippers, or, occasionally, polyurethane foam pads to cushion and protect potential decubital lesions.

Where vascular insufficiency is an added feature, the slow erosion of terminal phalanges through digital apices, or the prominence of the styloid process of either of the malleoli through the overlying skin can be encountered. These states normally tend to be painful at night.

A further type of skin atrophy is associated with steroid therapy, usually systemic but occasionally topical. Thick plantar skin does not usually succumb to steroid abuse, but drugs prescribed for a non-infective itch–scratch–itch cycle, such as neurodermatitis, may be misapplied to abrasions and other trivial lesions on the dorsal or lateral areas of the foot. Persistent mistreatment of such a nature causes skin atrophy in association with telangiectasis, ecchymosis and cyanosis or pigmentation. Recovery of skin texture is poor and telangiectasis continues, but the cyanosis may fade if bland antiseptic barrier cream is used under a non-occlusive, ventilated dressing.

Fungal infection of the skin in the elderly does not usually present as an urgent problem but may be encountered as a chronic recurring condition in those who have previously been infected in early life. In contrast, fungal infections of the nails appear to be more common. English (1976) found that over 40% of elderly patients attending a chiropody (sic) clinic with thickened nails were microscopically positive for ony-

Table 10.1   Frequency of first nail conditions by sex (535 patients). From *Clinical Rehabilitation* 4: 217–222 (1990)

	Onychauxis	Onychogryphosis	Onychomycosis	Involution
Female	80 (20.8%)	40 (10.4%)	57 (14.8%)	61 (15.9%)
Male	1.7 (11.3%)	20 (13.2%)	35 (23.2%)	27 (17.9%)
Total	97 (18.1%)	60 (11.2%)	92 (17.2%)	88 (16.4%)
Significance	6.01 $P < 0.05$	0.63 NS	4.78 $P < 0.05$	0.20 NS

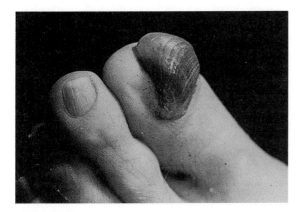

Figure 10.1   Onychogryphosis typical of those which reveal subungual ulceration.

chomycosis. Cartwright & Henderson (1986) observed thickened nails in over 40% of cases. This was consistent with the findings of Barlow (1987) (Table 10.1).

Both onychauxis and onychogryphosis are common in the elderly and may become more severe when neglected (Fig. 10.1). Shires (1988) examined 26 elderly patients and discovered 31 ulcerated nails, 23 of which were pain-free, so that patients were unaware of their existence. These ulcers occur as a result of pressure and may be described as sterile subungual pressure necrosis. When the nail is cut at the free edge, or reduced in thickness by the drill, a serous or watery discharge occurs. Occasionally this may be spontaneous, when it gives rise to alarm on the part of the patient or carers. The fluid pressure does cause discomfort in some cases, but release of the fluid gives immediate relief. Provided that the nail is reduced in thickness and the appropriate measures are taken to avoid infection, these cases resolve satisfactorily, but those patients who have vascular or sensory impairment need to be monitored very carefully.

The onset of psoriasis is rare in the elderly, although exacerbation of the disease occurs with emotional stress, and occasionally a mild localised psoriatic patch will become rapidly generalised as a result of the stresses encountered by such events as the loss of a marriage partner or the need to move into a different home. Extreme forms of the disease may present as an acute exfoliative dermatitis. Generally, eczema is said to be rare in the elderly. However, the localised form of neurodermatitis described as nummular or discoid eczema is not unknown and may also be associated with anxiety states. This condition is frequently accompanied by intense itching.

Itching without any obvious lesions is a symptom often complained of by the elderly. This condition, known as senile pruritus, is thought to be affected by air conditioning and central heating, with the hot or cold dry air demoisturising the already atrophic skin. Pseudokeratoses or stuccokeratosis, in which plugs or plaques of keratinised skin develop, are benign conditions easily removed or relieved by the application of mild emollients and moisturisers.

Verrucae are rare in the elderly and, unless they cause undue discomfort, are probably best left untreated. They should always be monitored carefully as occasionally they mask malignancy.

FOOT DEFORMITY IN THE ELDERLY

There is a high incidence of foot deformity among the elderly, females being almost twice as likely to have foot deformity than males. The commonest deformities found among the elderly are hallux abductovalgus (Table 10.2) and lesser toe deformities, (Figs 10.2 and 10.3), both of which have been found to be significantly more prevalent in females than in males (Braid 1987). These findings are consistent with the random survey of the elderly carried out by Cartwright & Henderson (1986).

Table 10.2 Prevalence of deformities. From *Clinical Rehabilitation* 4: 217–222 (1990)

	Hallux abductovalgus	Hallux rigidus	Hammer second toes	Clawed/retracted toes	More than one deformity
Female	238(61.8%)	52(13.5%)	91(23.6%)	139(36.1%)	198(51.4%)
Male	47(31.1%)	32(21.1%)	13(8.6%)	42(27.8%)	47(27.8%)
Total	285(53.2%)	84(15.7%)	104(19.4%)	181(33.8%)	245(45.7%)
Significance	$\chi^2 = 40.22$ $P < 0.001$	$\chi^2 = 4.23$ $P < 0.05$	$\chi^2 = 14.81$ $P < 0.001$	$\chi^2 = 2.67$ NS	$\chi^2 = 17.2$ $P < 0.001$

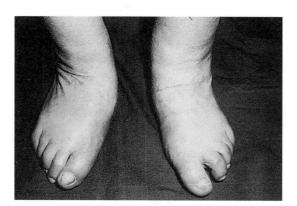

Figure 10.2 Generalised osteoarthritic changes and deformity in the feet of an elderly female patient.

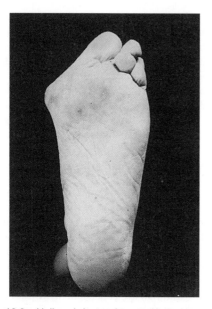

Figure 10.3 Hallux abductovalgus and lesser toe deformities typical of those found in the elderly.

Foot deformity in the elderly is often fixed by osteoarthritic joint change, and further complicated by an inability to accommodate the feet in suitable footwear. Fixed deformities of the toes can lead to soreness and heloma formation interdigitally, and moist fissures may develop either because the toes are fixed or because the elderly person is physically unable to dry between the toes after bathing. Pressure points and heloma formation commonly occur over the interphalangeal joints of the toes and may develop over the medial exostosis in hallux abductovalgus. An associated bursa develops infrequently, and bursitis and sinus formation over the medial exostosis are uncommon findings among this age group.

Plantar callosities and helomata develop as a result of incompetence of the first metatarsophalangeal (MTP) joint in hallux abductovalgus, and where subluxation of the toes occurs localised lesions may develop over the corresponding metatarsal head. Braid (1987) also compared the incidence of foot deformity between the sexes and found that whilst hallux abductovalgus was significantly more common in females, hallux rigidus was found to be significantly more common in males (Table 10.2). The condition may result in development of callosities and helomata over the interphalangeal joint of the hallux on the plantar surface of the foot, or over the fifth metatarsophalangeal joint (Fig. 10.4). This is consistent with the findings of Barlow (1987), who found that significantly more males than females had helomata formation over the fifth MTP joint. Where deformity is so severe as to render it impossible for patients to accommodate their feet in standard footwear, advice on extra-depth footwear or referral for orthopaedic/surgical footwear may be required.

Mobility

Mobility is of prime importance in the elderly. Senile ataxia, falls and fatigue can lead to a marked diminution of a person's self-confidence in their ability to walk. Careful attention to the feet is essential in this

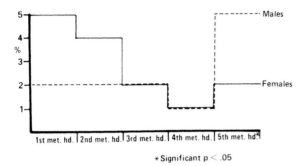

Figure 10.4 Frequency of plantar helomata. From *Clinical Rehabilitation* 4: 217–222 (1990).

type of patient, in order to ensure that the foot is not used as an excuse to avoid beneficial exercise. Footwear must be lightweight, supportive and well-fitting, and should hold the heel back into the heel cup. The number of elderly people whose mobility is impaired *solely* as a result of foot problems appears to be relatively small. Braid (1987) found that, of 536 elderly aged 75+ interviewed/examined, only 31 (5.8%) said that they felt that foot problems hindered their mobility. However, foot problems may arise as a result of hindered mobility due to generalised systemic disease, e.g. vascular disease, rheumatoid arthritis, etc., and the podiatrist has a vital role to play in maintaining the feet in as healthy a condition as possible in these circumstances, so that mobility is not further impeded.

Accurate assessment of ranges of joint motion is often difficult to carry out in the elderly patient. They may be unable to relax the foot sufficiently to allow an accurate assessment to be made and many resist passive motion of the foot. Osteoarthritic changes may result in slight to severe limitation of joint motion. Orthoses may be beneficial to the elderly patient. On the whole, these tend to be protective cushioning type devices, constructed from materials which are not likely to cause tissue irritation or to lead to possible necrosis. Lightweight walking frames and a trolley to carry small articles such as a tea tray will also provide the physical as well as psychological support for the housebound elderly person. Walking sticks with a non-skid ferrule and elbow and axillary crutches also have a place for some patients.

GENERAL PHYSICAL AND MENTAL INFLUENCES

Obvious *physical disabilities*, such as arthritis, amputation, stroke, respiratory disease or colostomy, will all impose burdens on mobility as well as upon general personality. Gross obesity, which may be related to bad dietary habits, lack of exercise, endocrine disturbances, or genetic factors affecting general metabolism, will adversely affect all weight-bearing structures, not least the feet. Conversely, grossly emaciated and cachectic patients will be poor risks, with impaired healing processes and vulnerability to infection and hypothermia.

Although each of the above states must remain the responsibility of the physician, the podiatrist should not automatically assume that the GP is aware of the condition. Some elderly people are proud of the fact that they have not troubled a doctor for years. Health and religious eccentrics, as well as immigrants with language problems, can be difficult to persuade that further medical help will benefit the local foot lesion.

Elderly people living alone understandably can be liable to neglect good *nutrition*—even where 'Meals on Wheels' are provided. A combination of apathy and poverty can lead to low grade vitamin deficiency; this state should be considered when delayed healing in the absence of other pathological processes is found.

Public awareness of *hypothermia* is greater today than in the recent past and it should be borne in mind when visiting the poorer sections of the community. Social services should be alerted, as well as the GP, when subjective appreciation of low skin temperature is impaired together with a low oral temperature, pulse and respiratory rate.

Mental health can affect the podiatric management of the aged. Chronically depressed and withdrawn patients are usually easy to treat since they tend to be submissive and to accept clinical attention almost with a sense of fatalism. However, such patients will not comply well with instructions concerning hygiene or routine medication; lay or professional aid will probably be needed for patients with ulcerative or infective lesions requiring simple dressing changes or saline baths.

Although they are few in number, the elderly hyperactive and manic patients can be a very serious risk both to themselves and to the operator. No treatment should be commenced until the podiatrist is satisfied that the previously requested sedative has been given by the patient's doctor—and that it is really effective.

Drug and alcohol abuse are not the exclusive prerogatives of the young, and the chronically addicted should be regarded with the same caution as the hyperactive and the athetotic, although many can be calmed and soothed by a carefully chosen approach. Applied psychology and the art of communication, especially where deafness or a language barrier is a feature, are skills which are usually acquired by practice and experience, and may be supported where necessary by a chaperone or an interpreter. The construction of questions in taking the history may need to be tailored to the mental capacity of the patient. Some will be able to cope with open-ended enquiries, while others will need the more closely filtered questions which require only a yes/no response. The podiatrist should liaise with relatives or carers of the elderly in order that effective treatment may be provided.

SYSTEMIC MEDICATION

It is necessary for the podiatrist to ascertain the nature of any regular medication which the patient is taking. Questions put to patients should always be phrased in an easily understandable form and this is perhaps even more important when taking a case history from the elderly patient. Weekly injections, e.g. vitamin B_{12} (Cytamen), may not be thought of necessarily as medication because it is neither drunk as medicine nor swallowed as tablets. The elderly respond better to individual questions, e.g. 'Do you take any tablets for anything?', 'Do you take any medicine for anything?', rather than to a blanket question covering all three of the above: 'Are you taking any medicines at all?' The response may reveal:

1. A general systemic disease, e.g. diabetes, collagen disorder, anaemia, heart disease, infection, pulmonary disorder
2. Drugs which have the potential to modify or mask signs and symptoms which could be present in the feet. Anti-inflammatory drugs (steroidal and nonsteroidal) can suppress an inflammatory response which may precede ulceration/infection. Diuretics may mask oedema, either totally or in degree of severity.

Prolonged antibiotic therapy reduces the numbers of commensal bacteria present on the skin surface. This, therefore, can create the right conditions for fungal infections to flourish, although they are seldom seen in the skin of the elderly.

Steroids

This group of drugs can be particularly important in podiatry. Although prolonged medication is undesirable, there are some life-threatening conditions, such as leukaemia, which leave little alternative. They are also used long-term where pain is an intractable feature and where the sedative effects of powerful analgesics are unacceptable, as in rheumatoid arthritis. Cushing-type mooning of the face, often with telangiectasis, should be a warning sign of the need for care. Skin thinning and atrophy commonly present on the lower leg and foot, and demand scrupulous bland antiseptic therapy. Antibacterial drugs should be a first line of attack, but liaison with the physician may paradoxically require an increased dosage of the steroid together with antibiotic reinforcement. Patients in this category are usually issued with a blue card to warn other practitioners, such as dentists and podiatrists, that this is an 'at risk' patient. A few, those treated at home for example, may not receive this warning card.

Although as a general maxim steroids, because they potentiate infection, should not be used in infected states, sometimes there are agonising decisions to be taken which involve a balance of risks. The podiatrist in this situation should be fully aware of infection risks and meticulous in ensuring that he or she does not contribute to them. No one can be expected to memorise the details of every drug, and it is reasonable to check in *MIMS* for details of toxicity, side-effects and contraindications for drugs commonly encountered in general practice. The podiatrist can sometimes assist the general practitioner by reporting any unexpected clinical findings if these are of significance, so that the drug may be changed, or perhaps the current 'yellow card' system of reporting to the Committee on Safety of Medicines may be used.

VASCULAR IMPAIRMENT

Geriatric vascular insufficiencies range through a broad spectrum, with mild chilling and acrocyanosis at one end and gangrene at the other. They include:

- *Drainage defects*
  (i) Venous incompetence
    — varicosity
    — phlebitis
    — thrombosis
  (ii) Lymphatic blockage
  (Combinations of the above, all exhibiting oedema, can be associated with back pressure arising from congestive heart failure.)
- *Supply defects*
  (i) Vasospastic
    — Raynaud's phenomenon
  (ii) Arterial occlusion
    — atheroma
    — arteriosclerosis
    — thrombosis.

Drainage

Very few of the lymphatic and venous states encountered in podiatry pose threats to the survival of the foot. Many, however, do degenerate into eczematoid conditions which create difficulties with adhesive dressings. Gross *oedema* arising from venous back pressure or the presence of lymphatic failure can result in serous leakage through the skin, sometimes preceded by bulla formation. Although the leaks occur more commonly on the lower leg, they can, especially in those who wear only loose low-cut slippers, appear over the dorsal metatarsus.

Infection is not a common feature of these leaks because, although the fine breach in the skin continuity is a potential portal of entry, the high serous pressure maintains continuous drainage.

Supply defects

Mild arteriolar insufficiencies in the aged, such as complaints of coldness and chilblains, are treated exactly as in younger age groups. The principle is to promote internal heat production and to minimise external heat loss. Although other disabilities may prohibit vigorous exercise, this should not preclude the encouragement of extra movement. Tactful enquiries may need to be made about the adequacy of diet in the elderly housebound who live alone and cannot be bothered to look after themselves. These are the people who drift into the hypothermic risk category. Insulation involves not only the foot but the person as a whole and their living quarters. Liaison with the GP and the district nurse is necessary in these cases. Plastazote insoles are thermally beneficial and man-made materials can be better insulators than traditional wool and leather footwear.

More serious vascular insufficiency is evidenced in the foot by skin which is smooth, shiny, inelastic and hairless and by nail dystrophy. The long-term establishment of a collateral circulation may reduce the importance of pulse impalpability. Blanching of the skin by limb elevation, followed by observation of the speed and pattern of dependent rubor, can indicate the presence of ischaemia (Fig. 10.5). Engorged veins are evidence that blood is reaching the foot. Routine testing of digital capillary reflux time is a useful method of monitoring the adequacy of the circulation. Light digital pressure on the pulp or apex of each toe will cause blanching. In the elderly the reflux of blood upon release of pressure is approximately 3–4 seconds, although individual variations may be noted.

Before carrying out digital capillary reflux tests it is

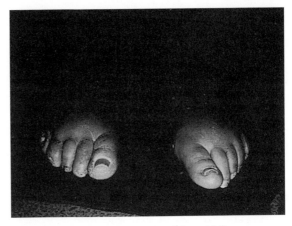

Figure 10.5   Red, shiny, swollen digits exhibiting severe ischaemia.

useful to ensure that the feet have acclimatised to ambient room temperature, since a false impression of the circulatory state will be obtained if the test is undertaken on a patient entering the clinic from outside, particularly in winter. The use of the ankle/brachial index test is a valuable means of obtaining a more accurate estimate of peripheral blood flow and should be used whenever the podiatrist feels that there is cause for concern.

Supporting the above signs will be a history of classical *intermittent claudication* affecting the calf muscles, the less well recognised cramp of plantar intrinsic muscles (rather akin to plantar digital neuritis, except that it does not possess a lancinating, electric shock character) and the significant complaint of night pain, insomnia and the need for nocturnal foot cooling.

Night pains

Night pains arise when the metabolic demands of the tissues of the foot exceed the competence of the available blood supply. Sufferers frequently discover for themselves that the metabolic demand rises when the foot becomes warm in bed. Metabolites accumulate from the higher level of cellular activity and, because of the vascular incompetence, they cannot be drained away fast enough. Since the metabolites are themselves cytoirritant or even cytotoxic, they promote a greater (unsatisfied) demand for blood and thus a vicious circle is established. Advanced cases of this type are helped by sleeping with the feet uncovered and exposed to the draught of an electric fan. Cold compresses and ice packs can damp down metabolic demands to a tolerable level but the prognosis is not good.

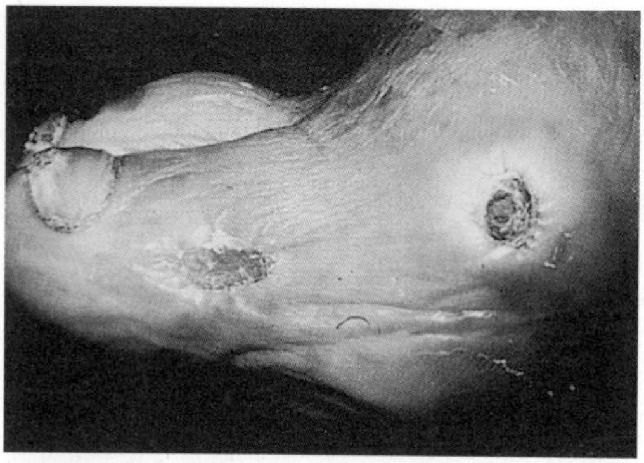

Figure 10.6 Ischaemic ulceration in the elderly patient.

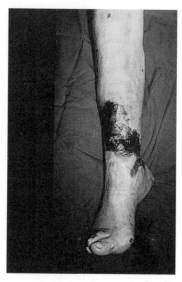

Figure 10.7 Onset of gangrene in the same patient as in Figure 10.6 following injudicious handling of the limb at risk.

General vasodilators are of doubtful value in peripheral ischaemia and for some patients they could pose a hypotensive threat. Empirically, a regular 'nightcap' of an alcoholic beverage promotes peripheral vasodilation, thereby relieving night pains and inducing sleep, but the cost is prohibitive to many. Apart from its well-documented property as an anti-inflammatory, phenylbutazone is occasionally prescribed for its less well reported side-effect of enhancing blood flow. Normally, one would advocate that cigarette smoking should be discontinued because of its known role in the pathogenicity of small vessel disease. Whether this would be humane counselling for a 90-year-old, confined to bed with very few pleasures in life, is a matter for the individual to decide.

Prolonged ischaemia is a pregangrenous state. It is characterised by toxaemia, which provokes weakness, incontinence, mental confusion and the destruction of morale. No podiatrist should witness these changes without summoning medical aid urgently (Figs 10.6 and 10.7; also Plates 4 and 5). The sequel is gangrene, which will be either dry and painful or moist and infected.

ULCERATION

Ulceration in the elderly is a condition which can have limb- or life-threatening consequences. Counsel of perfection is to treat the cause, but this is not always possible. Progressive obliterative vascular disease is irreversible, but careful assessment of the causation will assist in creating optimum management conditions and diminish the risk of avoidable tissue damage. The comprehension of the patient is important in securing patient compliance and cooperation. This will obviously vary across the whole spectrum of age and conditions. The alert and active insomniac receiv-

ing heavy nocturnal sedation who develops a lateral malleolar ulcer is likely to be more cooperative and helpful than the senile alcoholic with advanced peripheral neuropathy. The latter, together with senile demented patients, represent something of a challenge.

Aetiology

Listed below are conditions conducive to ulceration:

1. Ischaemia
   — atheroma
   — arteriosclerosis
   — Raynaud's phenomenon
   — diabetes
2. Neuropathy
   — diabetes
   — leprosy
   — syphilis
   — subacute combined degeneration of the cord
   — psychotropic drug abuse (including alcohol)
   — iatrogenic
3. Metabolic disorders
   — sequestration of gouty tophi
   — malnutrition
4. Intrinsic trauma
   — rheumatoid nodular and bursal erosions
   — bony sequestration
   — arthritic hyperostoses

— postural overload (secondary to obesity, surgery, etc.)
5. Extrinsic trauma
    — footwear
    — appliances (including splints)
    — dressings
    — bedsores
    — physical, chemical injury
6. Neoplasia—very uncommon but should be considered when all other factors have been excluded.

In all these conditions, infection may be a superimposed problem.

The evaluation of the quality of lower limb innervation in the elderly demands a recognition that degenerative processes will modify clinical responses which are demonstrable in the young. Some proprioceptive loss is normal. Diminution of the appreciation of vibration which would be significant in a 30-year-old may be compatible with normal ageing. The significance of motor fatigue has to be judged in relation to the patient as a whole person. Is it the harbinger of multiple sclerosis or attributable to a small cerebrovascular accident needing referral?

Ataxia and loss of confidence after a fall may be attributable to a foot lesion, but consideration should be given to defects arising in other systems. Apart from such obvious neurological possibilities as subacute combined degeneration of the cord, abnormalities affecting the eyes, ears or nutrition (avitaminosis) can all coexist with a foot problem which is regarded by the patient as the major cause of complaint. The physician will have a valuable ally if sensible early referrals arise from a judicious assessment of areas above the malleoli. It is unlikely that the podiatrist will be the first to be consulted for stocking and glove anaesthesia, but she may be the first to recognise early sensory loss which will degenerate into the potentially ulcerative neuropathy of diabetes (Fig. 10.8; also Plate 6). Leprosy, which was once very rare in the UK, is now seen more frequently among recent Afro-Asian immigrants.

NEOPLASIA

Malignant lesions

Malignancy affecting the foot is rare, and of those lesions which do occur the commonest are *melanoma* and *basal cell tumours*. Less common is *squamous cell carcinoma*.

Although melanoma may be a conversion from a formerly benign to a malignant state, it should be

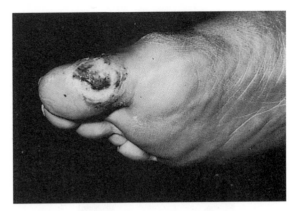

Figure 10.8   Neuropathic ulceration of diabetes.

remembered that it can arise spontaneously. All moles on the foot should be regarded with suspicion, and prompt surgical referral is required whenever there is a change in the character of a hitherto benign lesion. Such changes would include serous leakage, splitting, extension of the edge, bleeding, pitting or thickening. In the elderly, one sees an occasional melanoma which can simulate subungual haematoma. The tumour will present as a small filament, with no history of trauma, and will increase slowly in length and width. An intraepidermal haematoma can also mimic a melanoma, which is best examined by diascopy—the demonstration of melanotic grains seen through a microscope slide which is used to blanch the lesion and surrounding skin. Long-term steroid therapy can induce cutaneous skin fragility which sometimes causes laking of blood and a pseudohaematoma. These sharply circumscribed, often slightly elevated lakes, are seen on the lower leg and dorsum of the foot. The lakes are slightly fluctuant when newly formed, but can become consolidated by fibrosis or they can ulcerate spontaneously.

Basal cell epithelioma may arise in a setting of traumatic hyperkeratosis, which acts as a mask (Fig. 10.9; also Plate 7). It needs to be distinguished from mechanical extravasation arising as a sequel to faulty weight transmission through the skin. This seminecrotic extravasation is slightly 'mushy' in texture when the overlying hyperkeratosis has been removed and it may look like dull velvet with variable moisture. The basal cell lesion differs postoperatively by being startlingly red, very smooth and highly lightreflective. Lesions located within plantar callus can be complicated by the presence of white, shiny, fibrous material. Careful tissue reduction will reveal a sharply delineated edge which is sometimes rolled.

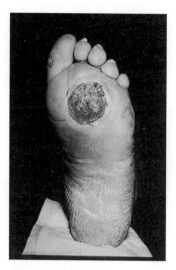

Figure 10.9 Basal cell epithelioma after reduction of plantar callosity.

Squamous cell carcinoma rarely develops in areas of normal-appearing unexposed skin. However, it may develop from burns, ulcers and osteomyelitic sinuses. Initially, it may be seen as a small erythematous nodule. The surface may be smooth or rough and may or may not be ulcerated/bleeding. Metastases occur more readily from areas that have been previously damaged; the frequency can be up to 50%.

Bowen's disease is a lesion of squamous cell carcinoma. It appears as plaques of reddish papules or nodules. A very low percentage of these areas metastasise.

Kaposi's sarcoma most commonly affects men in their 60s, although it is now becoming more common in younger men affected by HIV. It is a disease of multicentric origin which primarily affects the skin and often begins with non-pitting oedema of one ankle, which later becomes bilateral. This is then followed by irregular reddish-blue, purple or reddish-brown macules. These macules may grow into nodules and even become verrucous. A coalescence of lesions gives rise to irregular patches and plaques that most commonly affect the feet or thighs.

Neoplasia arising in any area may be moderated by immunosuppressive medication, which heightens the risk of infection. Operative procedures should be cautiously designed to produce minimal tissue damage compatible with the therapeutic aim. In such circumstances, the hazard of creating a potential portal of entry for pathogenic organisms must be weighed against the risk of neglecting a lesion which may deteriorate to a threatening level. Faced with such a dilem-

ma, a prudent podiatrist would seek the opinion of the prescribing physician.

Non-malignant lesions

A non-malignant tumour which does afflict the aged, especially in association with posterior nail folds, is *angiokeratoma*. This is a normal skin-coloured papilloma with a keratinised cap. The nail borders are equally the site of non-keratinised papillomata and skin tags. None of these lesions is dangerous, but some patients are concerned because they catch in hosiery as well as being cosmetically unacceptable. All can be treated by freezing with liquid nitrogen after a K-Y jelly thermocouple. When frozen solid, they are snipped off at the skin line with nail nippers and dressed with a non-adherent cover such as Micropad. If this is applied with moderate firmness before basal thawing has occurred, bleeding will not be a problem. They normally heal uneventfully in a few days.

PODIATRY PROVISION FOR ELDERLY PATIENTS

All health authorities provide podiatry for their elderly patients. There is a difference between authorities as to when a person becomes elderly: some may receive treatment at the age of 60, and some at 65. Many elderly patients prefer to attend for private treatment.

The treatment may take place in a health centre near to the patient's home, in the patient's home—whether it be a nursing home or their own house—or, in some areas, in hospital out-patient clinics, especially if the patient has a condition such as diabetes or rheumatoid arthritis. These latter clinics will be connected to relevant departments and treat patients of all ages.

In recent years, the hospital podiatrist has become an essential part of the team, working especially alongside rheumatologists and diabetologists in the management of the high risk patient, and in the facilitation of the multidisciplinary approach to patient care. It is important that community podiatrists and private practitioners maintain liaison with general practitioners, community nurses and social services in order that the patient derives the best possible care in the community. Equally, effective liaison must exist between hospital-based and community practitioners.

Domiciliary care

The treatment of patients in their own homes affords an ideal means of assessing the patient as a whole and their ability to cope with their condition and environment. For many elderly people, treatment at a clinic has a double value: not only does it provide care for the foot problem, it is also a psychological stimulus which boosts motivation. The effect is that the treatment is regarded as a trip or a day out. Extra care with personal grooming and dress can disguise a patient's true life style. The cheerful little elderly lady who brightly agrees to the suggestion in the clinic to have saline baths twice daily may, when visited because of intervening acute illness, be found to be housed in a single top-floor room with no adequate facilities for the regime prescribed.

Even without intentional snooping, it is difficult not to perceive likely sources of threats to general and foot health. If the basic requirements of food, warmth, dryness, shelter and sleep cannot be met, then the podiatrist should be familiar with the location of the agencies concerned with social welfare. Health and social workers are spread patchily over the country, and rural and urban communities will differ quite markedly in their allocation of resources. Local knowledge will guide and influence one in requesting aid from GPs, district nurses, health visitors, social services, home help departments and Meals on Wheels organisers. Contact with voluntary agencies such as Age Concern, WRVS or the Red Cross may well be useful. Basically, the GP should be the lynch-pin in the overall care of the patient and some will prefer the podiatrist to route calls for aid through them. Others will welcome the independent initiative of the podiatrist who solicits the aid of other public services—but a copy note to the GP is a courtesy as well as a helpful protective memorandum in the event of any later misunderstanding. Even in the best ordered communities, personality clashes with eccentric elderly people can lead to interprofessional criticism.

Unlike any other podiatry practice, domiciliary work demands a number of working compromises which involve a safe and comfortable operating position for the operator and the patient, and cleanliness of the patient, the immediate environment and the operator's hands. No compromise should ever increase the risk to the patient. Two questions are helpful:

1. What are the consequences of undertaking treatment in this environment ?
2. What are the consequences of *not* giving treatment?

As far as the consequences are predictable, they will be within an assessable time-scale. For example, suppose treatment is requested for an 80-year-old lady complaining of painful overgrown nails. On arrival, she is found to have moderate and uncomplicated bilateral onychauxis and one foot which is pale, painful and pulseless. The operating conditions are poor. It might just be possible to give treatment. It would be better, though, to recognise that the lady is suffering an acute obliterative arterial crisis and to telephone her GP as a matter of urgency. Such treatment as is possible should be provided and the patient should be reassured pending the arrival of the doctor. Obviously, the visiting podiatrist must make strenuous efforts to ensure such cases are followed up by the appropriate agencies.

It is especially in the domiciliary situation that the use of foot care assistants (FCAs) has given rise to great controversy. The majority of domiciliary calls may be of a more routine nature but the elderly are subject to multiple foot pathologies which require surveillance by a state registered chiropodist. Morris et al (1978) revealed that the majority of geriatric and psychiatric hospital patients had three or more podiatric conditions; 2% of patients were deemed to require no foot care and only a further 2% to be suitable for routine care by ward staff. Pelc (1979) surveyed 465 patients in clinics, surgeries and their own homes, of whom 423 were over the age of 65. Of the total, 82% were reported as having one or more general conditions which made it difficult or dangerous for them to attend to their own feet. These general conditions included poor peripheral circulation (46%) and diabetes (8%). However, in this study, clinic patients accounted for 199 of the total, and 58% of these who were free from such conditions were said to be suitable for care by FCAs. A further study revealing multiple pathologies in the elderly was conducted by Ebrahim et al (1981), and the undetected presence of subungual ulceration has been demonstrated by Shires (1988).

Calls for first aid figure slightly more frequently in domiciliary work with the aged. This is not just first aid for feet. The dropped frying pan and splash burns, and contused and fractured toes will be met, but heads, hands and knees—all areas commonly damaged in falls by the ataxic and partially sighted will also be presented. Simple dressings should be given as an act of humanity, especially where exposure to infection is a hazard. Clinical judgement will dictate whether further help should be summoned.

The advent of pre-packed sterile dressings and small dispensers for medicaments has made the adoption of sterile procedures more easy to accomplish in the domiciliary situation. Instrument packs are somewhat heavy on the domiciliary round and the introduction of portable sterilisers is a step forward.

The choice of items to be carried should be left to the individual practitioner, but it is possible in some cases that appropriate drugs and dressings may be supplied on prescription by the GP and left in the patient's home as a 'working pool' for visiting health care professionals.

Institutional care

Visiting elderly people in a non-domestic environment is much less taxing than domiciliary work. Some will be in well-appointed nursing homes and others in poorly equipped psychogeriatric units, both public and private. The great majority will be nursed and housed in conditions falling between these two extremes. Whatever the establishment, it is necessary to become familiar with the hierarchy of the institution. The matron, ward sister or warden—whoever is responsible for the nursing needs of the patient—should always know of the podiatrist's presence and the reason for calling. This opening courtesy is the passport to later cooperation if there should be a need to delegate dressing changes, footbaths or the routine application of external medication.

It will ensure that an angle-poise lamp, towels, receivers, nursing help with turning a patient in bed and sundry other services will be made available when possible. The podiatrist will also learn when is not an appropriate time to call. Ward rounds, cleaning, bed baths and similar activities which would be mutually exclusive and time-wasting are avoided. Some homes will be able to accept advice about nursing decubital lesions on autoclavable polyurethane sheets, gutter splints or heel cups. Although such items are the mutual province of nursing and podiatry, not all nursing establishments, especially the smaller private ones, are always conversant with new products.

Pressure sores occur not only on the feet, but also on the sacrum and elbows. If good podiatry secures the resolution of a heel or a malleolar lesion, one may be asked to apply those skills to other areas. It is a matter of assessing other calls upon available time which will determine the nature of what help can be given. At the very least, one can give general therapeutic advice about the merits of ripple beds, the advantages and disadvantages of water-repellent silicone creams for macerated lesions, or enzyme debriding agents where adherent necrotic slough is impairing resolution.

Apart from maintaining one's own record of the patient's progress, it is helpful to add a note of the foot condition and its treatment to the general ward notes and to avoid the use of podiatric jargon. This is particularly necessary if adhesive dressings should be left undisturbed during blanket baths, etc., or if routine simple dressing changes and medication are required. Access to the patient's general notes can save valuable time in taking a case history, and even if a clear diagnosis is not immediately apparent, a look at the medication regime can be informative.

The rest, repair and convalescence of the post-surgical patient can be much disturbed by uncomfortable nails. Nail pain to lay and nursing attendants can seem to be out of all proportion to the apparent signs. To an hitherto ambulant elderly person, the enforced bedridden state can focus attention almost to an obsessive degree upon overgrown nails with impacted sulci. Although plate length and dystrophy, together, perhaps, with hyperkeratotic sulci and subungual helomata, can be a source of much discomfort, a fair proportion of cases of onychauxis exhibit a sterile subungual pressure necrosis.

When surgery has affected weight distribution (such as in hip arthroplasty, amputation, spinal fusion, etc.), there is much to be said for early assessment of foot function before the patient returns home. Podiatrists and physiotherapists have an overlapping interest in this field. Whilst walking exercises and postural re-education are best supervised by physiotherapists, it should be remembered that their efforts will be undermined if foot support and padding needs are not fully recognised and met. The elderly amputee, particularly, can benefit by having good stabilising filler insoles for the surviving foot. In the early days when the stump is becoming reconciled to its new home in the pylon socket, the podiatrist can alleviate discomfort by adding padding to the prosthesis if necessary.

MANAGEMENT

The management of foot pathologies in the elderly is based upon the general principles of clinical management of any age group. Attention should always be given to the patient's medical and social status, since these factors may influence the selection of particular treatment regimes. Liaison with medical practitioners, district nurses and social services departments is often important when, for example, dressings need to be changed frequently, infection monitored and when patients are recommended to rest. Elderly patients with limited mobility and poor eyesight may have the greatest difficulty in replacing even a sterile pre-packed dressing in appropriate conditions. They may need antibiotics when control of infection is difficult to obtain by other means, and they may need additional help in the home or for basic shopping needs if they live alone and have been advised to rest.

It should also be borne in mind that, although most elderly patients will be cooperative and sensible in their attitude, some may be in the early stages of dementia and thus unable to recollect simple instructions concerning their foot problems. The more overt symptoms of senility are more easily recognised but bring their own problems of management. Apart from the sociomedical aspects of care, the management of foot problems in the elderly may be said to require:

- maintenance of sterility
- maintenance of tissue viability and/or promotion of tissue regeneration
- protection from pressure and compensation for tissue atrophy.

Maintenance of sterility

Standard measures of pre-operative and postoperative swabbing with a non-irritant antibacterial agent are sufficient in most cases, with 'no-touch' techniques used in the application of sterile dressings to ulcerated areas. Persistent infection which does not respond to treatment must be regarded with suspicion and every care taken to avoid cross-infection.

Antiseptic medicaments should be selected with care, bearing in mind that the skin is often denatured and atrophic. The continued use of medicaments to promote wound healing has recently been called into question. It has been suggested that many antiseptics are actually toxic to healing tissues (Leaper 1986, Anthony 1987). Traditional dressing materials, such as gauze and other dry dressings, may also be contra-indicated since current thinking favours the mainte-nance of a moist environment which nonetheless allows uptake and absorption of exudate and cell debris

(Turner 1979, Harding 1987). An extensive list of wound management products, including modern envi-ronmental dressings, was published by Morgan (1988) and a further review of their relative merits by Turner (1991) and Fotherby et al (1991) (see also Ch. 9).

The greater difficulty in achieving wound healing on the feet is probably caused by impaction of the dress-ing upon weight-bearing and by pressure from the footwear. In selecting appropriate forms of padding to relieve pressure, careful judgement must be applied in weighing up the merits of the accurate positioning of adhesive pads against the greater versatility of the replaceable variety (see also Chs 12 and 14).

It must always be borne in mind that the treatment of the elderly involves consideration of sociological, biological and physiological factors, which may influence not only the podiatric management but the overall health and well-being of the patient. Modern geriatric specialists regard their role as being more rehabilitative than custodial. Podiatry mirrors that philosophy. The maintenance and restoration of tissue function will contribute to remobilisation and the delay of immobility. Towards the end of life, comfort and protection are required; feet require the same con-siderations. The most appropriate care is ensured by the motivation of the patient, as well as by the motiva-tion of the podiatrist engaged in this clinically reward-ing field. The ultimate aim is to add years to the life and life to the years.

REFERENCES

Anthony D 1987 Pointers to good care. Nursing Times 83(34): 27–29
Barlow A M 1987 Skin and nail deformity in the elderly foot aged 75 years and over. MSc thesis, University of Manchester
Bond J, Bond S 1988 Sociology and health care, 2nd edn. Churchill Livingstone, Edinburgh
Braid S J 1987 The prevalence of foot deformity in the elderly aged 75 years and over. MSc thesis, University of Manchester
Cartwright A, Henderson G 1986 More trouble with feet. HMSO, London
Ebrahim S B J, Sainsbury R, Watson S 1981 Foot problems of the elderly: a hospital survey. British Medical Journal 283: 949–950
English M P 1976 Nails and fungi – an interdisciplinary collaboration. Chiropodist 31(9): 234–239
Fenske N A, Lober C W 1986 Structural and functional changes of normal ageing skin. Journal of American Dermatology 15(4): 571–583
Fotherby et al 1991 Effect of various dressings on wound healing. Journal of Tissue Viability 1(3): 68–70
Gibbs R C 1975 Skin and nail changes in the elderly foot. Journal of the American Podiatry Association 65: 471–474

Gilchrist A K 1979 Common foot problems in the elderly. Geriatrics, November: 67–70
Hamdy R C 1984 Geriatric medicine. Baillière Tindall, London
Harding K 1987 Wound healing. Chiropodist 43(10): 195–197
Leaper D 1986 Antiseptics and their effect on healing tissue. Nursing Times, May 28: 45–47
Morgan D 1988 Formulary of wound management products. Care Science and Practice 6: 4
Morris J B, Brash L F, Hird M D 1978 Chiropodial survey of geriatric and psychiatric hospital in-patients, Angus district. Health Bulletin, September. Scottish Home and Health Department
OPCS 1986 Mid-1986 Population estimates, Office of Population Censuses and Surveys, London
Pelc E 1979 Footcare assistants: how much would they help? Public Health, London 93: 306–310
Shires J 1988 Subungual ulceration . . . is there a need for health education? Chiropodist 43: 29–32
Smiler I 1979 Geriatric foot care: an ageing challenge. Pennsylvania Podiatry Association
Turner T D 1979 A look at wound dressings. Health and Social Service Journal, 4 May: 529–531
Turner T 1991 Surgical dressings in the drug tariff. Wound Management 1: 1

11

Sports injuries

P. M. Boyd
R. J. Bogdan

Keywords

Acute anterior compartment syndrome
Advice to athletes
Ankle sprains
Ballet
Basketball
Biomechanics
Equinus state
Football
Fractured sesamoid
Golf
Hamstring tendinitis
Heel spur syndrome
Leg length discrepancy
Osteochondritis dissecans
Overuse injuries
Pain in the forefoot
Podiatric approach
'Q' angle
Retrocalcaneal exostosis
Rugby
Runner's knee syndrome
Runner/patient history
Running cycle
Shin splints
Sports injuries
Sports shoes
Tendinitis
Tendo Achilles injury
Therapeutic modalities
Tibial/fibular stress fractures
Treatment/management
Young sportsperson

'There is a crack in everything God made,' said Ralph Waldo Emerson. Nowhere does this concept manifest itself to a greater extent than in the athlete. The 'athlete' today is the average man and woman engaging in activities that were formerly called 'minor sports'. Running, cycling, racquet ball, aerobic dancing and tennis are all examples of sports that many people pursue with determination to improve their physical and mental health.

It is this documented improvement in physical well-being that has been mainly responsible for the increased participation in sports. These athletes rarely pretend to be of world class or to have professional aspirations. They just enjoy athletics for the fun and competitiveness of sports, and especially for the physical fitness it bestows upon them. Athletes in these sports require medical care that allows them to continue training while alleviating any specific injury or problem at the same time. 'Sports medicine', as it is now called, is concerned with structural integrity, muscle balance and posture, rarely orthopaedic surgery.

The majority of athletic injuries are due to overuse syndromes arising from innumerable repetitions of some physical activity. The best treatment plan requires a knowledge of the particular sport, and of the anatomical areas and the mechanics involved. In addition to these areas of treatment determination, the practitioner must know the athlete. The training regimen and environment of the athlete are critical in determining a treatment plan, and the quantity and quality of the training are critical to evaluation of an injury. The athlete's environment includes such factors as shoe gear, running surfaces, diet and sleep, and they are all vital to correct diagnosis and treatment of the athlete's problem. For example, it is important to know which types of terrain produce which symptoms, if the patient is a runner, or which shoes provide adequate support if the patient is a basketball player. Evaluation of an athletic problem must also include proper evaluation of any relevant medical factors.

The following is an example of a special history questionnaire for athletes written by Kevin Kirby, DPM.

Runner/patient history

Training history

1. How long have you been running (in years)?
2. How many miles/day do you average?
3. How many miles/week do you run?
4. What's your longest run during the week?
5. What pace (in minutes/mile) do you average in your workouts?
6. Do you do intervals, long slow distance and/or long fast distance in your workouts?
7. What type of terrain do you usually run on (grass, dirt, concrete, asphalt, sand, hilly, flat, etc.)?
8. Do you run on any canted surfaces (on one side of the road, on beaches) or always around the track in the same direction?
9. What time of day do you normally run (a.m., p.m. or midday)?

Racing history

10. How often do you race?
11. What distances do you normally race at?

Running shoe history

12. What model(s) of running shoes do you train and/or race in?
13. How long have you had your present pair(s) of shoes?
14. Do you wear any orthotics, special arch supports, etc., in your shoes?
15. Do any of your pairs of shoes make the problem better or worse?
16. Do you 'build up' your running shoes to keep the soles from wearing out too quickly?
17. Where does the most outsole wear occur on your running shoes?
18. How do your shoes fit (too long, short, narrow, wide)?
19. Do you wear socks when you run? How many pairs?

Pre/post run-activities

20. Do you stretch before and/or after your run, and for how long?
21. What type of stretching do you do (describe it precisely)?
22. Do you warm-up/warm-down for your runs and for how long?
23. Do you do any muscle strengthening exercises (describe them)?
24. Do you participate in any other sports or any other physical activities?

Injury-related history

25. Did you modify your training/racing schedule prior to your injury?
26. Did you run a particularly hard race or have a hard workout immediately prior to your injury?
27. Did you switch to another pair of running shoes prior to your injury?
28. Did you modify your shoe gear prior to your injury?

29. Was there any direct trauma associated with your injury?
30. Did you have another injury or any discomfort in your feet or legs prior to your injury that you tried to train through?
31. Have you cut back on your mileage or pace since your injury? Any results?

Past treatment

This is essential information. With acute injuries, it is necessary to know what the patient may have done for it already. Many patients do not know the concept of RICE (Rest, Ice, Compression and Elevation—see also Ch. 15) and their self-treatment may have altered the condition. It is very important that their return to activity should be gradual.

With chronic injuries, the question arises as to why a condition has not healed properly, even if the patient has rested for a long period. Often it is because the patient has never properly re-strengthened the muscles. Atrophy occurs quickly, and if the muscle is not re-strengthened, it will be susceptible to injury. Scar tissue adhesions will also make swelling and stiffness prominent. Biomechanical problems, e.g. leg length discrepancies which are not treated, may also contribute to chronic, recurrent injuries. Tight muscles are also a factor.

Functional instability often requires bracing, without which recurrent injury occurs.

Current limitations

This is what the patient can or cannot do. In treatment, the patient must not attempt anything that causes pain. Temporarily, an alternative sport may be required to keep up fitness levels.

Patient constraints

The treatment plan must be realistic so that the patient can complete the treatment in the time available, (Appendix 4).

A sensible diet is necessary. Many patients will not rest.

To summarise: following a diagnosis, a treatment plan is started, possibly with a follow-up programme, and a prognosis is formulated. Then, after the patient's return, there are four possibilities for the patient's condition:

1. no improvement or worse
2. somewhat improved
3. greatly improved
4. completely better.

If the patient is completely better, a gradual return to activity is essential (Fig. 11.1).

THE RUNNING CYCLE

When playing sports, people utilise either the whole of the walking and running cycles or parts of them. Indeed, they may adapt them, as in the cases of hopping in the triple jump or maintaining foot-flat in downhill skiing. In the majority of sports, some form of running is required, so it needs to be analysed to understand what is required of the body.

The cycle of events in running varies from that in

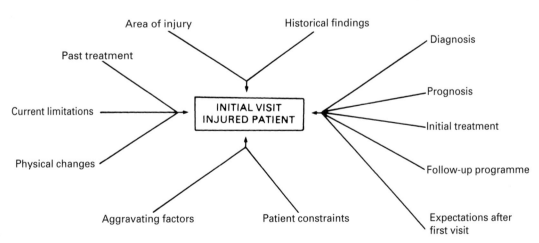

Figure 11.1 The full picture.

walking in several ways. Walking is characterised by heel contact, foot-flat and toe-off, with a base of gait of approximately 5 cm between the malleoli. There is a period of double support as weight is transferred from the trailing foot to the forward foot. One foot is always on the ground whilst the other is in the swing phase. As the pace of walking increases, the contact pattern persists but the contact phase becomes shorter, until finally, when running, the double support phase disappears completely and is replaced by a float phase when neither foot is on the ground.

In running, at heel contact the supporting foot must move beneath the centre of mass of the body for stability. This reduces the base of gait, which compels the limb to take a varus attitude requiring greater amounts of pronation at the subtalar joint to allow the foot to become plantargrade. The total range of motion of the subtalar joint, from initial contact to total pronation, can be as much as 18°. All the joints of the lower limb must move through a greater range of motion as speed increases. In running, the knee flexes through 35–40° at contact, compared with only 15° when walking. Because subtalar joint pronation is greater, it lasts longer in the running cycle and recovery into supination occurs much later—70% of the support phase. The foot is in adaptive mode for longer in the gait cycle and resupination has to occur much faster if it is to achieve its rigid structure for propulsion.

This support of the body during running, first by one foot and then by the other, means an increase in ground reaction forces. Up to two or three times the body weight passes through the loaded limb during the contact phase.

Some runners are categorised as 'heel strikers', or 'forefoot strikers', depending on which part of the foot first contacts the ground. Heel strikers have two impact peaks which occur in the weight-bearing phase. The first is at heel contact, when the heel first makes contact with the ground, and the second is at the propulsive stage, when most of the force is at the forefoot.

At heel contact, the heel striker has a straight knee, with the impact being reduced by subtalar joint pronation followed rapidly by knee flexion. Forefoot runners make the initial contact with the forefoot, either remaining on the forefoot or falling back to the heel. Impact forces have been shown to decrease with forefoot runners, as the Achilles tendon and calf muscles act as a shock absorbing system. The hips and knees are also flexed at contact, utilising the quadriceps for shock absorption. This reduces the transference of shock waves from the foot to the skull. However, this muscular effort requires an increase in oxygen uptake by as much as 50% and increases the tension taken by the Achilles tendon.

FOOTBALL

Other sports require different movements in addition to running. Footballers are notorious for their injured knees and ankles. Much of the game requires manoeuvering and manipulating of the ball with the foot, using ankle and subtalar joint motions, and tackling to gain the ball. Kicking the ball requires the foot to reach higher than the waist of the player if height and distance of the ball are to be achieved. Rapid changes of direction and acceleration indicate flexibility as a major component of successful play. Strength and endurance are important but not at the expense of flexibility; thus, where weight training is part of the training programme to increase strength and endurance, its effects on flexibility need to be monitored carefully.

BASKETBALL

Basketball is a sport which requires rapid acceleration and deceleration. The players must be able to reach, twist and change direction quickly. Leaping and landing hard onto a badly placed foot puts demands on tendons and ligaments at the ankles and plantar structures. Flexibility and quick reactions to avoid and evade fellow players are key factors in training methods.

RUGBY

Rugby has a history of being a macho sport where little attention has been paid to training methods, let alone 'warming up' and 'warming down'. Bad training methods have been self-perpetuating as retiring players take on the role of coaches and managers. Where training and preparation for sport are poor, more injuries are likely to occur.

The sport requires upper body strength and lower body power. However, speed is also required, with sprint running during which there is catching and passing of the ball requiring balance and coordination. Training is aimed at improving stamina and speed.

Recent studies show that injuries to the head and neck are not as prevalent as in the past, probably due to changes in the rules for tackling in the game.

GOLF

Golf is a sport where flexibility of the shoulders and

hips is of prime importance. To drive off, the golfer must strike the ball with the head of the club, which should pass through as perfect an arc as possible. It is also necessary that the feet of the golfer should move to the extreme limits of pronation and supination. The golfer walks many miles in pursuit of the ball, but this is mainly over soft undulating ground which is most suitable for human feet. Injuries tend to be pulled muscles, due to inadequate warm-up, and stress fractures and foot strain as a result of the large number of miles walked, particularly in competitions.

BALLET

The demands on ballet dancers in terms of choreography have increased considerably in recent years, so much so that the ballet dancer can now be considered an 'elite aesthetic athlete'. Dancers are very much prone to overuse injury, mainly because the preferred physique is one which includes a long back, long legs and hypermobility at the joints and a slim, lithe body. Ballet training results in muscle imbalance; plantar flexors that are stronger than extensors; external rotators of the leg that are stronger than the internal rotators; and vastus lateralis that is stronger than medialis. Overloading of the knees is common and, if exercises are not performed properly, serious twisting of the knees causing excessive torque can lead to patellar tracking problems.

One of the most important positions in ballet is the 'turn-out' of the feet. This movement should occur at the hips with lateral or external rotation. The plié exercise consists of deep knee flexion while maintaining 'toe-out'. The hips should be at 180° laterally rotated to each other. This is an extremely demanding exercise and places great strain on the knees. When the knee flexes to 130°, several times the body weight is applied to the knee joint. Should lateral rotation at the hip be limited, 'turn-out' is obtained by twisting the knees and pronating the feet. Considerable torque occurs at the knee and the feet undergo deforming pronatory forces. This is particularly harmful in young growing bodies.

Dance teachers are becoming more aware of the dangers of poor training and posture, and have changed the order of training and structure of classes in order to warm up and prepare the body before taxing exercises are attempted.

THE YOUNG SPORTSPERSON

Children are now beginning to present with overuse injuries at younger ages, due in part to the increased interest in sport by children and the intensity of training regimes. Misplaced enthusiasm and pressure from parents, coaches, teachers, etc., lead to excessive competition and training, which in the long run can lead to injury. This is seen, particularly, with football, where 'the earlier the better' philosophy and 'exercise is good for you' belief can put the young person at risk.

Four main causative factors for injury have been identified:

1. load—this is the amount of training and playing time
2. technique
3. posture, including biomechanical abnormalities
4. equipment.

In 1992, medical examinations for trialists trying to gain scholarships at the Football Association's School of Excellence found that 35% of them had overuse injuries. It was found that most of the injuries were of the low spine, which can have grave long-term effects and can terminate a career in sport.

The training and playing techniques of adults cannot be applied to young players. Between the ages of 11 and 15 years there is a significant amount of growing, often rapid and in spurts. Bone is immature and is not fully ossified until 18–21 years and can be stressed when muscles are relatively overdeveloped through excessive activity (Appendix 2).

Injuries often occur where ligaments and muscles attach to bone. Bone grows faster than soft tissue and often there are muscle imbalances and restrictions in motion for periods of time while soft tissues adapt to the new bony development. Epiphyses are particularly soft and weak during puberty, and again, at the end of the growing period they become vulnerable as they lose their elasticity.

The young person has to cope with adjusting to his new body shape, which continues to change and develop over a period of years. Coordination of the body's new dimensions and weight has to be relearned.

Biomechanical faults can also be responsible for overuse injuries. Excessive compensatory pronation for whatever structural problem can lead to stress on soft tissues as normal alignment is disrupted and shock-absorbing mechanisms are reduced. Young people respond well to biomechanical intervention with antipronatory devices. These restore good alignment and function of the limb and feet, and encourage healthy development of the body. Other factors which affect the growing body are puberty, diet and training schedules.

Common overuse injuries include traction apophysitis (Sever's disease), damage to articular cartilage of the knee joint and patella, osteochondritis dissecans, chondromalacia patellae, avulsion injuries, stress fractures, spondylosis and spondylolisthesis.

Signs and symptoms of overuse injury

The following signs and symptoms are characteristic of overuse injury. The injury develops slowly, seldom interrupting the playing or training schedule. Usually, the main complaint is of an ache after sport which takes some hours or days to disappear. There may be some stiffness or pain at the start of the activity but this eases as the sport continues. Usually there is not a history of direct injury or trauma, but there may be some tenderness to the touch and some swelling. The injury responds well to rest.

The Football Association recognises the seriousness of overuse in the young sportsperson and has published a booklet, as well as giving lectures, highlighting the problem to parents and coaches and those involved in training young people.

An awareness of the dangers is of prime importance in identifying overuse injury at an early stage. Steps to reduce the level of activity and to control functional abnormality will minimise potential problems and allow a full and enjoyable sporting life.

PAIN IN THE FOREFOOT

Pain in the ball of the foot can be very disabling for any athlete. Many sportspersons place a large proportion of the stress on the ball of the foot, and pain is usually due to unsupported loading of the area. The following list summarises the usual differential diagnostic considerations of a mechanical origin:

- sesamoiditis
- capsulitis
- bursitis
- neuroma
- stress fracture.

It is helpful to compartmentalise the forefoot into medial, central and lateral sections to aid differentiation. The medial section is the first ray, the central encompasses the second, third and fourth metatarsals, and the lateral is denoted by the fifth ray.

The most common complaints of the medial compartment are capsulitis of the first metatarsophalangeal joint, sesamoiditis, fracture of the sesamoid and osteochondritis dissecans of the first metatarsal head. Mechanical disability of the first metatarsophalangeal joint, as occurs in hallux abductovalgus, plantarflexed first ray and the use of improper shoe gear,

results in significant stress overload on this area. Proper treatment to eliminate inflammation and instability is necessary to return the athlete to his or her sport. Usually a supportive pad and strappings will ensure rest of the area while allowing for minimal function. Changes of terrain and shoes will also contribute to the success of this treatment.

A history of burning, numbness or radiating pain in this area would be unusual and might suggest some neurological involvement. Very rarely, neuromas have been found close to the fibular sesamoid in ballet dancers, footballers and hurdlers.

The central compartment provides more clinical entities and diagnostic challenges because of its participation in the stability of the foot during propulsion. In some foot types, the metatarsals move excessively in both the sagittal and transverse planes. This movement contributes to compression of the intermetatarsal nerves and bursae. With tight shoes or thin soles, and with unshod feet, extreme forces may create pain and swelling sufficient to cause the athlete to limp.

Most commonly, the third intermetatarsal nerve develops such symptoms. The joining of the branches of the medial and lateral plantar nerves gives rise to a larger nerve about the fourth toe which can easily be traumatised. This is the classical Morton's neuroma. Its symptoms can be very debilitating to the sprinter, tennis player, ballet dancer or runner. Cushioning of the forefoot by means of metatarsal supports and orthotics is necessary. Anti-inflammatory agents, such as ice, ultrasound, cortisone injection or vitamin B_{12}, may be necessary as intermediate stages during the 4–8 weeks of treatment. If all else fails, surgical excision may be necessary. However, even after surgery, treatment for the lack of stability is of the utmost importance to prevent further complications.

Metatarsal stress fracture is an equally debilitating condition. This occurs most commonly in the central portion of the forefoot. The fracturing of the bone is due to the stress of continual pounding and vibration through the tissues during a repetitive sport. Cracks result in the crystalline meshwork, which the bone consistently attempts to remodel, but remodelling is never properly achieved, and a fracture is precipitated. The symptoms of a stress fracture differ from those of other forefoot conditions in that they are more intense, come about more quickly, and demonstrate significant swelling.

X-rays are essential in the evaluation of the stress fracture but it may take up to 2 weeks for the fracture line to show. It may also be necessary to go one stage further and to arrange for a bone scan.

The best treatment for the stress fracture is avoidance of any activity that causes pain. Many patients can be treated with a change in activity, rest, stiff supportive shoe gear and plenty of ice treatment. However, at times, plaster casting and crutches may be the only therapy to resolve the immobilisation of the sportsperson. Returning to activity should be delayed until further X-rays and a simple jump test prove negative.

Osteochondritis dissecans

This condition is most commonly found at the second metatarsophalangeal joint but can affect any metatarsophalangeal joint. It produces a softening of the subchondral bone at the distal end of the metatarsal. The softened bone undergoes moulding during normal function and becomes flattened as the bone finally hardens again. The flattened metatarsal head no longer conforms to the adjacent bony surface of the proximal phalanx, particularly in full extension of the joint in propulsion. Impingement of the joint occurs with the thickening, reducing the range of motion and producing pain on extension. Sports usually require a full range of motion at this joint and this deformity seriously impairs foot function. The condition can mimic the clinical features of a stress fracture of the neck of the second metatarsal, and an X-ray is required to differentiate the conditions. Treatment usually requires surgery either to replace the joint or to remove the proximal phalanx of the toe.

Evaluation of the dynamics of the forefoot overload and how it may be reduced is essential for complete control of the clinical problem. The key to success is prevention of the overload.

Fractured sesamoid

Pain in the first metatarsophalangeal joint can be experienced where the athlete is required to remain on the balls of the feet for given periods of time. Ballet dancing, aerobics and callisthenics, hurdling and running are examples of activities with this requirement.

The main complaint of a fractured sesamoid is an aching pain that comes on with exercise and with dorsiflexion of the hallux. The symptoms are due to the irritation to the sesamoidal joint cartilage and plantar cartilage of the first metatarsal head. Symptoms are like those of osteoarthritis or gout of this joint. X-rays (medial oblique and axials) are required for the differential diagnosis. Appropriate lateral X-rays should also be obtained. They will show either of the sesamoids to be in pieces.

The forefoot valgus foot types and plantarflexed first ray deformities predispose to sesamoid fracture. Treatment is with some type of immobilisation. Rest with accommodative padding should be the first line of treatment.

Persistent symptoms may require referral to an orthopaedic surgeon for a below-knee walking cast. Surgical removal of the sesamoids can lead to hallux abductovalgus or trigger toe deformities. The sesamoids act as mechanical fulcrums and are responsible for giving the intrinsic muscles of the foot stability as they function round the first metatarsophalangeal joint.

HEEL SPUR SYNDROME

This is the most common disorder found in the heel and ankle area. It makes up about 12% of injuries in the foot and is found mostly in race walkers, runners and basketball players. It is a debilitating problem for any individual, the causes of which may be mechanical or systemic.

Pain is located in the region of the plantar surface of the medial tubercle of the calcaneus. The pain is often described as deep and aching, or burning. It is due to an overuse traction of the thick medial band of the plantar fascia, which originates at the medial tubercle of the calcaneus. It may also be associated with the bursa found in this area.

On X-ray, in many cases, a spur of bone will be seen arising from the origin of the fascia. This is not diagnostic and is merely a sign of pronation of the subtalar joint. Table 11.1 shows the differential diagnosis, which is important as there are several possible medical reasons for the symptoms of mechanical spur syndrome.

Nerve entrapment syndrome can produce pain in the heel area, entrapment being of the tibial nerve or either of the medial or lateral plantar nerves, producing neuritis.

Enthesopathy is a term which describes inflammation and cystic degeneration that occur at the junctions between a muscle tendon or ligament and the perios-

Table 11.1 Differential diagnosis for mechanical heel spur syndrome

- Arthritis
- Neuritis
- Enthesopathy
- Insufficient fatty pad
- Osteoid osteoma
- Poor shoe gear
- Calcaneal stress fracture

teum to which the tendon or ligament attaches. Excessive strain and traction on that insertion give rise to degeneration and pain. This can occur at any junction, and is commonly found in the knee and ankle.

Insufficient fat pad on the plantar surface of the heel can produce pain. The fat pad should be approximately 1 cm in thickness on weight-bearing and is built to absorb up to 12% of the shock that the heel receives. Reduced subcutaneous fat allows the heel to become bruised and inflamed, giving rise to pain and discomfort. Icing and anti-inflammatory therapy should resolve this problem, combined with a heel cup orthosis, which concentrates the remaining fat pad beneath the heel and provides extra shock absorption.

Injury from a direct blow or a traumatic bursitis or fracture are all possible causes of pain in the heel region. Rheumatoid arthritis and other systemic diseases should be ruled out before finalising diagnosis. Referral to the patient's GP for laboratory tests may be necessary.

Mechanical heel spur syndrome is produced by excessive pronation at the subtalar joint and subsequent supination of the midtarsal joint round its longitudinal axis. Because of its attachments, the plantar fascia is elongated with pronation and shortened with supination. In a foot that abnormally pronates through the gait cycle, no resupination can occur at toe-off and the plantar fascia remains stretched and undergoes strain (Box 11.1).

Football, rugby, baseball and cricket players require good support for the medial column and shock absorption in the heel. Most have a very flexible shoe which may require stiffening in the shank to support this area of the foot to prevent the mechanical heel spur syndrome.

Basketball is a traumatic sport with a lot of jumping and landing flat on the foot. Sudden deceleration also adds to the pull on the plantar fascia. Side-to-side sports such as tennis cause traction on the plantar fascia; as the player reaches and lunges, the foot is required to flatten along the medial column.

A hypermobile forefoot valgus foot type most commonly predisposes to the heel spur syndrome, particularly in women who have a high degree of genu valgum.

Long-term therapy

Prevention of recurrence is important and steps can be taken to ensure this. Evaluate the surface the sport is being played on. It may be hard and unforgiving. Footwear may be inadequate and non-shock-absorbing, and may not give enough stability to the foot. An orthosis is necessary if a mechanical anomaly is present in the foot to stabilise the medial column. This stabilisation of foot function may need augmentation with shock-absorbing materials such as heel pads and other devices for the shoes (see also Table 11.2).

THE EQUINUS STATE

Equinus is defined as limitation of ankle dorsiflexion to less than 10°. Normal gait requires 10° of dorsiflexion, and without it the function of the foot and structures within the lower limb are radically altered.

Equinus can be caused by several entities. These include congenital shortness of the gastrocnemius muscle, obliquity of the ankle joint or a congenital osseous block. Dorsal lipping may occur at the neck of the talus, preventing free movement within the ankle mortice in sports that require jumping, such as football, basketball and ballet. Other possibilities are: injuries to the posterior muscle group or myositis resulting in fibrosis and contracture of the muscle belly; athletic hypertonicity due to overuse in a new training programme, allowing metabolites to build up and cause contracture of the muscle; growth spurts in

Table 11.2 Heel spur syndrome: treatment

Initial visit
Three positional Achilles stretch
Ice massage × 10 minutes × three daily
Self-tape midtarsal strapping
Antipronation shoes if patient runs
Heel accommodation if plantar pain
Contrast foot baths if swelling present× two daily

Second visit
Orthotic evaluation and casting
2 weeks anti-inflammatory medication
2 weeks ultrasound if chronic, or EGS if acute
Cut activity to pain-free level only

Third visit
Dispense orthosis
Continue therapy
If bursal, consider cortisone therapy
X-rays

If not improving significantly or re-flare occurs as activity is increased:

Fourth visit
Cortisone injections
Check orthotic control
Bone scan
BK cast × 4 weeks

If not helped:

Fifth visit
Surgical discussion

children where long bones outgrow the muscles; adaptive shortening of the muscle in women who wear high-heeled shoes; and gastrocnemius muscle tightness and relative shortness in association with generalised ligamentous laxity.

Clinical features of ankle equinus

Equinus compensation can manifest in many ways. Because the required 10° of dorsiflexion is absent at the ankle joint, this motion is obtained by adaptations from other parts of the lower limb, particularly the midtarsal joints. Gait adaptations include abducted feet with the hips functioning in an externally rotated position; short stride; early heel lift; knee flexion throughout the gait cycle; an abductory twist of the

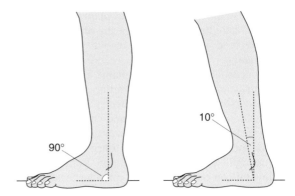

Figure 11.2   Ankle motion.

foot and forefoot subluxation, giving a break in the medial column. Footwear shows minimal lateral wear with excessive wear at the ball of the shoe.

The patient complains of leg cramps, digital deformities and hindfoot pain. There may be knee subluxation, which also gives rise to pain.

The ankle joint must be tested for range of motion with the knee in the flexed and extended positions, to determine whether the equinus is of a bony or soft tissue nature (Fig. 11.2).

Treatment for osseous deformity is with heel lifts. Soft tissue deformity can be helped with heel lifts and stretching exercises. With athletic hypertonicity, various forms of heat will stimulate the circulation and flush away metabolites.

TENDO ACHILLES INJURIES

Achilles tendinitis is an extremely common injury among sportsmen and sportswomen. A study of over 300 athletes at a medical research unit showed that 14% of all the injuries were of the Achilles tendon. It is found most frequently in joggers and sports where running plays a major part, such as tennis. Competitive sportsmen and women are particularly prone to this injury. Its cause appears to be due to overuse, with biomechanical faults being found in 66% of sufferers.

The area of the Achilles tendon that causes most complaints is the zone 8–10 cm proximal to the top of the posterior aspect of the calcaneus. There is an increase in calcaneal tendon disorders in individuals over the age of 35 years. The circulation in this area decreases by about 40% at this time.

The tendon comprises two muscles that are the main decelerators of the leg, in all activities. It is also a supinator of the subtalar joint and plantarflexor of the ankle. In activities such as ballet, the muscle group is also involved in sustaining various positions and movements.

Pain is usually the main complaint, at the insertion, along the tendon or at the myotendinous junction, and is due to a strain of these structures.

Aetiological factors are many and varied. Variations in the surfaces on which the sport or activity is carried out, or inclination of running surfaces, can alter the torque applied to the Achilles tendon. Running uphill or downhill, or on canted roads, can alter the direction of the torque; low or negative heels can cause excessive torque on the tendon. Flexibility of the shoe at the metatarsal break is very important and inflexibility can cause increased strain. Hamstring and iliopsoas muscle tightness should be evaluated to ensure that they are not contributing to the condition.

The tendo Achilles (TA) has a poor circulation and requires special warm-up and stretching. In side-to-side sports such as tennis, lunging forward is an important factor in rupturing the TA where there has been inadequate warm-up. Tennis shoe soles are made of soft material, and on weight-bearing can give the same effect as a negative heel, and a greater range of motion for the TA.

In 'contact' sports like basketball and rugby, a direct blow can cause a tendinitis. Basketball also requires spurt running and rapid deceleration, and the triceps surae group is put under strain. A full study of the sport and playing surface is necessary to establish the aetiological factor.

Biomechanical aetiology

Functional overuse of the tendon obviously plays a major role in the aetiology of Achilles tendinitis, but mechanical overuse also needs to be investigated. In one particular study, 90% of cases were shown to have structural abnormality of the lower extremity, the most common faults being forefoot varus and limited subtalar and ankle joint motions.

Tightness of the triceps surae predisposes them to tearing. During running the heel usually strikes the ground first, followed by the forefoot. The momentum of the body drives the leg over and forward of the weight-bearing foot in preparation for propulsion. The ankle becomes maximally passively dorsiflexed by the combined action of the body weight travelling forward and the ground reaction forces resisting the movement of the foot. The more force exerted by the runner moving forward, either by running faster or with a longer stride, the greater the force pushing the ankle into dorsiflexion. This causes stress on the posterior soft tissues, including the TA. A forefoot varus deformity adds further stress to the triceps surae. This group of muscles helps to change the foot from a stable base at the end of midstance to a rigid lever in propulsion. The pull of the tendon on the inverting calcaneus causes rapid supination of the subtalar joint, and ground reaction forces on the lateral side of the foot cause pronation of the forefoot, locking the bones into a rigid structure. Rigidity is necessary to maximise efficiency in the transfer of energy and to minimise risk of injury to the joints and soft tissues during propulsion.

Where there is a structural deformity of the forefoot, as with a forefoot varus deformity, compensatory subtalar joint pronation occurs as the forefoot loads in midstance and into propulsion. The supinatory inversion of the calcaneus at heel lift cannot occur because the calcaneus is everting. As the triceps surae fail to initiate heel lift, the pull of the Achilles tendon enhances the evertory movement at the subtalar joint by everting the calcaneus further. This twisting action produces a torque within the tendon, stretching the medial side and compressing the lateral side, which causes stress. The normal locking of the forefoot to the hindfoot does not occur and rigidity of the foot is not achieved.

Tendinitis

Any of the above aetiologies may be responsible for an inflammation of the tendo Achilles.

Clinical features

Acute stage. Presentation is usually unilateral. The affected tendon is two or three times the normal size and there is crepitus, soft swelling and a torpidity on movement. Examine for any nodules above the insertion, the presence of which indicates rupture of some of the fibres. An X-ray with soft tissue density will show that the tendon is affected. The area will be hot and painful.

Treatment

Acute stage. Apply ice to the affected part three to four times per day for 10 minutes' duration. Apply strapping to the foot and ankle to prevent movement and put a heel lift in the shoe to rest the part. Once the swelling is down, start mild stretching with ultrasound therapy two to three times per week for

3 weeks. Rest from the athletic activity will be necessary for 4–6 weeks, and then it can be restarted gradually.

Chronic stage. This is generally the stage at which patients present with the condition having attempted to treat the condition themselves or having been referred from a physiotherapist or GP. The condition has probably responded well to physiotherapy treatment but recurs on a return to activity (Table 11.3).

Examination may not show acute signs, such as redness or swelling, but there may be some residual thickening along its length. The patient usually complains of pain after activity but not during sport. There is some stiffness of the tendon on rising in the morning, which usually eases on walking. The pain may progress to being present during sport and may eventually be present all the time when walking. It may never reach or even pass through the acute stage, presenting only as a chronic condition. It is necessary to carry out a full biomechanical evaluation to determine the treatment necessary to correct the foot function, the aim of which is to control abnormal pronation and to encourage some supination during the propulsive stage of gait, thus reducing the torque in the tendon.

RETROCALCANEAL EXOSTOSIS (Haglund's bump)

This is a hypertrophy of the posterior–lateral shelf of the calcaneus, with or without a bursa. It is due to mechanical irritation during the gait cycle. The triceps surae muscles act as decelerators of the body as it moves forward over the foot. During the propulsive phase of the cycle, the heel is in constant contact with the counter of the shoe and it is this stress that gives rise to the exostosis. Other factors that influence the formation of the exostosis are: the inclination angle of the calcaneus—this can vary from heel to heel and cause the exostosis to cover a large area of the posterior aspect of the calcaneus; the pitch or degree of adduction of the calcaneus, which may cause the exostosis to be situated more laterally; and the amount of hindfoot varus, which will also influence the area and extent of the exostosis.

These bumps are difficult to deal with. Control with orthoses or lifting the heel with a lift in the shoe should be tried. Low counters or soft counters are also helpful. Excision may be necessary.

Such bumps are common in skiers and skaters and they may require orthotic control of the midstance or propulsive phase of gait. They are also produced in sports that require the plantarflexed attitude of the ankle and rapid changes of direction; these include ballet, football, rugby and American football. They are often associated with inversion sprains (Fig. 11.3).

ANKLE SPRAINS

Ankle sprains, especially sprains of the lateral liga-

Table 11.3   Achilles tendinitis: treatment

Initial visit
Check flexibility hamstrings: gastrocnemius, soleus stretches, heel lifts
Check shoes: heel to ball ratio, not worn excessively; check especially heel counter; stable or new shoes
Check for swelling, tenderness: EGS and ice
Ice massage at home
Check training habits, eliminate hill running and speed work
Gait observation, excessive torque, instability: varus wedge

Second visit
Re-check swelling, tenderness: ultrasound three times per week for 2 weeks
Re-check flexibility: hot water bath, hot/cold stretch routine
Orthotic casting
Alternative activity, no propulsion, bicycling, swimming
Continue stretches, ice massage
Check new shoes
Anti-inflammatory for 2 weeks
X-rays if suspect bony block (stretching only gently) or insertional tendinitis

Third visit
Dispense orthotic: check for control
Continue ultrasound and ice massage if helpful
Consider tendinosis, tenosynovitis, partial rupture, retrocalcaneal bursitis, gout, plantaris rupture, posterior ankle capsulitis, os trigonum, fracture of posterior lateral process talus

Subsequent visits
Consider immobilising using a cast
Last resort: surgery

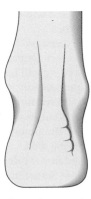

Figure 11.3   Retrocalcaneal exostosis (Haglund's bump).

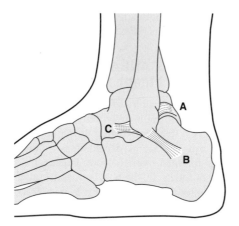

Figure 11.4 The lateral ligaments. A: Posterior talofibular. B: Calcaneofibular. C: Anterior talofibular.

ments, are very common injuries (Fig. 11.4). They are also the most missed and maltreated of the acute injuries in the casualty department. Ankle sprains require a lot of care and rehabilitation if the individual is not to be left with an unstable, weak ankle. Medial ankle sprains, are much rarer than lateral sprains, as the medial ligaments are thicker and stronger.

The lateral ankle ligaments are the calcaneofibular, the posterior talofibular and the anterior talofibular; in 20% of the population the anterior talofibular ligament is missing, which leads to instability and constant sprain of the lateral structures.

The position of the foot at the time of sprain will determine which ligament will be damaged. In the supinated position, the calcaneofibular ligament lies parallel with the ankle and subtalar joint axes, and therefore has no counter action to the motion of supination. In this situation, the anterior talofibular ligament is the one that is strained. In the dorsiflexed position, the calcaneofibular ligament is the greatest restrainer of inversion and will be the structure that is damaged in this situation.

Identification of the damaged ligament is important if treatment is to be correct. Palpation will localise the pain, but pain and swelling will limit manipulation of the joint. X-ray is undoubtedly the best method of evaluation if rupture and fracture are to be ruled out.

Most lateral sprains occur in side-to-side sports like tennis and football, as the peroneals quickly fatigue and no longer control the ankle. A hindfoot varus of 5–10° or a plantarflexed first ray deformity will predispose to lateral sprains. Sometimes just stepping on something uneven, pivoting, trauma or running will result in a sprain.

Residual pain about 1 month after the sprain may be due to an inflammation of the internal interosseous ligaments. Palpation of the area over the sinus tarsi elicits pain, and inversion of the subtalar joint is also painful. The internal ligaments may have been ruptured during the sprain and may have healed poorly, resulting in malalignment and some capsular inflammation and fibrosis. It is a difficult injury to treat and may require referral for manipulation under local or general anaesthetic.

Treatment of any sprain depends very much on the severity. When total rupture or fracture has occurred, referral to an orthopaedic surgeon is necessary.

Sprains short of rupture can be treated by the podiatrist (Table 11.4).

For the first 36–48 hours, icing to reduce swelling should be carried out as often as possible. Strapping to prevent movement in the frontal plane should be applied and the limb elevated as high as can be tolerated. Once the acute stage has passed, weight-bearing can be resumed with supporting strapping, which should be such as to allow the patient, however slow-

Table 11.4 Ankle sprains: treatment

Initial visit
Determine severity, mechanistic: X-rays if fracture suspected
fifth metatarsal base, beak of calcaneus, fibular neck
EGS with ice if acute or swelling
Contrast footbaths; ultrasound if chronic swelling
Compression stocking with horseshoe pads on malleoli
Weight-bearing as tolerated with crutches

Second visit
Continue contrast footbaths, compression wrap
Increase range of motion (draw alphabet in warm water)
Begin stretching exercises, especially Achilles tendon
Observe gait for compensation (stop any compensation)
If swelling is down, test for ankle instability and ankle strength

Third visit
Begin ankle strengthening (progressive programme)
Increase range of motion
Continue contrast footbaths
Start toe raises, comparing affected and unaffected sides

Fourth visit
Progressive ankle strengthening, especially peroneals
Continue contrast footbaths, stretching range of motion
Teach strapping
Encourage high top shoes, ankle brace, ankle strapping
Consider orthotics if foot type is a factor
Begin BAPS or straight line running: progress to cutting drills (side-to-side running)

Subsequent visits
Test ankle strength
If chronic re-sprain, consider stabilisation

ly, to use a normal walking action. The importance of this should be stressed to patients so that they maintain as normal a gait as is possible. This is to be preferred to limping, even though the patient may move more quickly that way.

Strengthening of the muscles should begin, particularly the lateral muscles. Apply heat to the area to stimulate circulation, using heat, ice or ultrasound. Rehabilitate with exercises such as drawing with the toes, and use a wobble board or isometrics (15 repetitions three times per day with weights). Stabilise the foot with orthotic therapy using flat posts. For lateral instability, use a higher heel cup and lateral flare up to 1–2 cm.

SHIN SPLINTS

This is a vague term describing many possible anomalies that arise as a stress reaction in the lower leg. Bone, muscle, tendon or insertion may be the source of pain.

To determine which structure is involved, it will probably be necessary for the podiatrist to watch that person perform the sport, or at least to see how that sport is normally performed. This may give an indication as to which structures become fatigued. Shin splints can be categorised according to the compartments of the lower limb (Fig. 11.5).

Anterior compartment

Pain is normally felt along the inner distal two-thirds of the tibial shaft. There is inflammation, stiffness and an ache which is present at the beginning of the activity. Pain may be present with no activity, as swelling may be causing increased pressure on nerve endings. On examination, the patient may limp or walk with a stiff-legged gait.

The most commonly involved anterior muscles are the extensor hallucis longus and the anterior tibial muscles. These are decelerators of the foot at heel strike and can be overused in situations such as downhill running, running on hard surfaces, or over-striding. They decelerate foot slap. These muscles also decelerate pronatory motion. They can become overworked or fatigued with exaggerated limb varus or foot types such as forefoot varus or supinatus, or forefoot equinus.

Lateral compartment

The peroneus longus and brevis muscles are those overworked with lateral compartment shin splints. They become fatigued in side-to-side sports, classical-

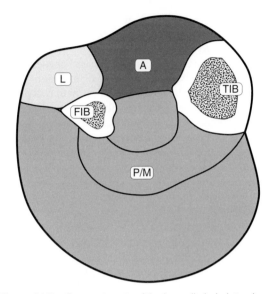

Figure 11.5 Compartments of the lower limb. L: lateral; A: anterior; P/M: postero/medial; FIB: fibula; TIB: tibia.

ly tennis, but also aerobic dance with much hopping from one foot to the other. A hypermobile first ray can also cause fatigue of the peroneus longus. Pain is experienced around the lateral malleolus and the distal one-third of the fibula.

Posterior and medial compartment

The posterior tibial is the muscle most commonly affected of all the posterior/medial muscles. Its main actions are to decelerate pronation around the oblique axis of the midtarsal joint, and also to decelerate the internal rotation and forward momentum of the tibia. It also tries to accelerate resupination of the subtalar joint. The stress on this muscle in a sport depends on the amount of utilisation of the midfoot.

A runner can stress this muscle because running prolongs the amount of pronation in the gait cycle. More pronation requires more supinatory effort by the posterior tibial muscle.

Pain is frequently felt at the lower one-third of the tibia with posterior/medial shin splints. This is almost certainly an enthesopathy, and pain is due to periostitis at the muscle attachment. There is a fibrocartilage breakdown and a cyclic reaction is set up.

If the shin splint syndrome is due to a mechanical disorder producing abnormal pronation, fatigue of the muscle leads to less shock absorption. Shock waves passing up the leg destroy bone cells and prevent the remodelling of the damaged bone. Stress fracture may occur. Therapy is aimed at preventing the excess pronation, thus lessening the shock and allowing muscle and bone to recover.

A subtalar varum or tibial varum predisposes to this syndrome. The available amount of eversion at the subtalar joint may be entirely used up with compensation for the subtalar varum or tibial varum, and there will thus be none left for shock absorption in normal gait. The posterior tibial muscle is the one that gets fatigued as it tries to maintain the function of shock absorption of the subtalar joint.

Treatment (see Table 11.5)

Sporting activity should be stopped until the patient has spent 2 days being able to walk without pain. Patients can then restart the activity until a feeling of tightness arises. The muscle should then be iced and stretched. Limit the activity to a walk/run cycle. Allow patients to run only 10% of their normal distance and then to gradually build up the amount of activity. Restrict the activity to an even terrain and ensure that the footwear is adequate with sufficient shock-absorbing ability. Orthotic therapy to reposition the subtalar joint will be necessary.

ACUTE ANTERIOR COMPARTMENT SYNDROME

From Figure 11.5, it can be seen that the nerves, blood vessels and muscles are enclosed in a compartment surrounded by virtually non-stretchable structures.

Any ordinary activity, such as walking or running, will result in increased capillary filtration to nourish the muscles, and they will expand by 20–25% of their normal resting volume. Anteriorly, the crural fascia can expand to allow for this increase in bulk.

However, an activity such as running down a steep incline for too long can cause fatigue to the anterior muscle group as it tries to prevent foot slap. The muscles become less efficient, foot slap increases and shock waves reverberate up the leg. An inflammatory tendinitis or myositis sets up, increasing the extracellular fluid within the compartment.

Another explanation by F A Matsen suggests that veins are collapsible tubes and that a patient's veins cannot have internal pressures less than those in the tissues around them. Thus local venous pressure rises with local tissue pressure. This causes a local anterior venous gradient, resulting in reduced capillary flow; as a result tissue perfusion occurs.

Acute anterior compartment syndrome can result.

Table 11.5 Shin splints: treatment

Initial visit
Ankle strapping, strengthening exercises for ankle invertors
Ice massage to painful areas of shins
Neoprene shin sleeve
Varus heel wedges
Change of shoes to antipronation if a runner
X-ray if chronic swelling
Activity modification to avoid pain

Second visit
2 weeks of physical therapy with ultrasound
X-ray evaluation if stress fracture suspected
Continue all home treatments
Consider functional orthoses if excessive subtalar joint pronation noted
Strict guidelines on activity based on presence of pain
Consider strong anti-inflammatory medication

Third visit
Functional foot orthoses dispensed
Continue physical therapy to remove any residual swelling and as much tenderness as possible
Re-test muscle strength and consider manual resistance exercises, isotonic to increase strength if that is the problem
Consider bone scan if question of stress fracture still present

Fourth visit
If not improving, question closely about type of pain if this is still continuing and consider compartment syndrome
Bone scan indicated to see radioactive uptake pattern
Check to ensure functional foot orthoses are properly controlling motion with the current shoes

Fifth visit
If pain continues, consider test for compartment syndrome and, if positive, consider surgical intervention with fascial stripping
If bone scan negative, consider prolonged rest
Continue to treat any signs of swelling and tenderness with therapy
Question about any alternative exercises patient can participate in to maintain physical fitness

This is an emergency situation which can lead to drastic complications. Increased pressure against the vascular bundles causes ischaemic pain and discomfort. Continuation of the activity increases the damage occurring within that compartment. Following the pain, there will be numbness and tingling on the dorsum of the foot which spreads proximally. The foot feels cold, and numbness on the dorsum makes the shoe feel loose. Motor control is lost and the foot is dragged.

On removal of the shoe, the foot and toes appear white and cool. The shin will be throbbing. These are symptoms of a 'shut-down' syndrome.

Emergency treatment in a hospital is required to save the foot. Slitting of the crural fascia is the only remaining action. Permanent damage may have been caused, paralysing the anterior tibial or extensor hallucis longus muscles.

Chronic or recurrent anterior compartment syndrome is less severe and has no drastic results. It can be prevented with the use of orthotic therapy to avoid foot slap and by warning the athlete about the potential dangers of downhill running and excessive fatigue. Orthoses may be necessary to control the foot at heel strike right through to propulsion in cases of limb varus or hindfoot varus. Shock-absorbing materials are useful, and even limiting the amount of activity may be necessary to avoid symptoms. Ultimately, surgical fasciotomy may be the only treatment when all else fails.

TIBIAL/FIBULAR STRESS FRACTURES

The main aetiological factor in these conditions is poor shock absorption, whether of the limb with a mechanical disorder, where the foot is excessively pronated or supinated and rigid, or where muscle fatigue can no longer work the shock-absorbing mechanisms of joints, such as in downhill running. Inadequate footwear may cause stress, in that it may be worn down, non-shock-absorbing, or inadequate for the particular activity. The athlete may be unfit for prolonged activity or it may be the start of a new training programme.

Clinical features

There will be pain in the area of fracture which can be of sudden or gradual onset. Pain may be sharp or a deep ache. Swelling will be present if the bone fracture is near the skin surface. An X-ray or bone scan will be diagnostic.

Symptoms can be confused with shin splints or deep myositis.

Treatment (Table 11.6)

Rest is necessary for 6–8 weeks, and occasionally 12 weeks, to allow the fracture to heal. Rest in a plaster cast may be the answer in keen athletes. Determine the aetiology of the stress and take steps to prevent recurrence. Suggest swimming or cycling to maintain fitness.

THE KNEE

The knee is a complex joint and it is not within the scope of this chapter to describe its function in detail. However, it is vulnerable to overuse syndrome where the normal function of the foot has been disrupted by structural abnormalities, be they intrinsic or extrinsic,

Table 11.6 Tibial stress fractures: treatment

Initial visit
X-ray evaluation if pain has been present for 2–3 weeks
Bone scan evaluation if X-rays are inconclusive or pain present less than 2 weeks
2–3 months' rest to allow fracture to heal
Local physical therapy techniques to help remove swelling and muscle soreness during rest
Make another appointment when the patient has been free of pain for 2 weeks to re-evaluate the situation and analyse possible biomechanical problems causing inadequate shock absorption

Second visit
Check for poor mechanics with inadequate shock absorption
Recommend shoes with better shock absorption
Consider sorbothane or spenco padding for the shoes
Outline gradual return to activity programme at this time
Have patient stay off downhill runs and not wear unsatisfactory shoes
If pain returns with activity, arrange a follow-up appointment

Third visit
Re-take the X-ray to see if the fracture is not healing: 'dreaded black line'
Consider if source of pain is elsewhere, e.g. from compartment syndrome or shin splints
Treat the localised tenderness and swelling, and when pain-free start on a walk/run programme
If pain persists with a return to activity, arrange a follow-up visit

Fourth visit
Consider testing for compartment syndrome
Consider pain referred to leg from the low back
If X-ray evaluation inconclusive, consider a bone scan if not taken previously; also consider prolonged period of rest

and so the functional interrelationship between the foot and the knee requires some description.

The foot, through the subtalar and ankle joint complex, has a direct effect on the tibia and thus the knee joint. Weight-bearing motions of pronation and supination of the subtalar joint are passed on to the tibia at the ankle joint, making it rotate internally and externally, respectively. Internal rotation of the tibia initiates flexion of the knee, and external rotation completes knee extension during walking. Knee flexion occurs just after heel contact to absorb shock, aiding the subtalar joint in its shock-absorbing capacity. The knee flexes again during swing as the foot clears the ground. Knee extension occurs after the foot-flat phase when the weight-bearing limit takes the full load of the body. The tibia and the femur rotate externally, locking the knee in full extension until toe-off stage.

Rotations of the tibia on the femur can occur because of the lateral condyle. They are also asymmetrical in terms of their articular surfaces. This partly facilitates the knee to function in two planes, sagittal and transverse, rather than one, as in the case of a simple hinge. The effect of this incongruity of the articular surfaces seems most marked when the knee flexes through its first 15° of flexion. It is at this point that the tibia appears to rotate on the femur. With each degree of flexion, there is 1° of internal rotation of the tibia, up to about 10–15°.

When the foot supinates and the knee extends, the knee locks and is stable, but when the subtalar joint pronates, the tibia rotates internally and the knee flexes and other structures such as muscles and ligaments have to stabilise it. In the sagittal plane, the quadriceps contract eccentrically and the tensor fascia latae and pes anserinus muscles decelerate the rotational movement of internal tibial rotation, aided by the anterior and posterior cruciate ligaments.

Overuse knee injuries

Overuse knee injuries can occur when the normal synchronous movements of the foot and lower limb are disrupted. Disruptive elements can include footwear, rough terrain, playing/training techniques, equipment or biomechanical causes.

Biomechanical causes

These occur most commonly when the foot has to compensate for structural deformities in the leg or foot. This compensation usually takes the form of abnormal subtalar joint pronation, increasing the speed, or altering the amount, of pronation, or altering the time at which it normally occurs in the cycle of events (Fig. 11.6). These motions of the subtalar joint affect the functioning of the limb as a whole and can give rise to pain in or around the knee. When subtalar joint pronation compensates for a hindfoot deformity such as hindfoot varus, the amount of pronation is greatly increased. The normal recovery time of the subtalar joint to the neutral position at the end of midstance is extended and may not even be achieved. The subtalar joint remains pronated and maintains the tibia in its internally rotated position, and as the heel lifts and the limb prepares for propulsion, the normal locking of the knee in extension cannot occur.

In preparation for propulsion, the pelvis is externally rotating, and the femur in phase with it is rotating similarly. The tibia should also be rotating externally but is inhibited from doing so by the pronated foot. A torque is set up within the knee, with the proximal end of the joint rotating externally and the distal end either rotating internally or being prevented from

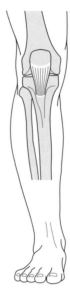

Figure 11.6 Torque of the knee produced by overpronation of the foot.

rotating externally. The effects of this torque are most marked and damaging when compensating pronation in the foot occurs late in the gait cycle, i.e. after midstance.

Subtalar compensation for forefoot varus, ankle equinus and ligamentous laxity may also produce pronation late in the gait cycle. Late stage pronation causes the strongest opposing forces to external rotation of the femur at a time when the ground reaction forces peak for a second time in the gait cycle. It thereby increases the forces through the flexed unlocked knee which is depending on soft tissue structures to give it stability.

Any of the structures in and around the knee can be strained or become injured due to the malalignment and increased torque (Fig. 11.7), particularly with the added demands of sport. The injuries that can occur are named according to the structures involved or the syndrome produced. However, it is sometimes difficult to be precise about the structures which are involved, as the following description of overuse injury suggests.

Definition of overuse knee injury

Overuse knee injury is a chronic, non-traumatic injury giving pain around the knee, and is often associated with sport. Generally, there is not a history of any specific trauma and examination does not show insta-

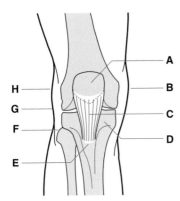

Figure 11.7 Overuse knee injuries: patellofemoral syndrome (A); semimembranosus/semitendonosus tendinitis (B); patellar tendinitis (C); tibial plateau stress fracture (D); Osgood–Schlatters' disease (E); biceps femoris tendinitis (F); popliteal tendinitis (G); iliotibial band friction syndrome (H).

bility of the joint due to ligamentous damage; neither is there locking of the joint or major swelling which could be caused by loose bodies within the joint or meniscal damage. There may be a mild puffiness around the knee joint. Investigations with X-ray or arthroscopy usually do not show abnormalities.

Symptoms

Pain is present in the knee, which is made worse with activity. The location of the pain varies with the individual syndrome and may be inconsistent from day to day. Sometimes there is a localised tenderness or even pain on resisted movement.

The nature of the pain is often described as a sense of weakness, aching or stiffness which may occasionally be sharp or severe. It responds to rest but will quickly restart with a return to sporting activity. The patient is often able to carry out other sporting activities without pain. The patient is often able to recall a trigger episode or one which varies from the normal routine, such as an increase in mileage or speed; a return to activity following a period away from sport; a change in footwear; downhill running or hiking; a change in training surface, such as going from grass to clay courts.

Signs

Often, examination will reveal some form of malalignment of the lower limbs or feet: femoral anteversion, genu valgum or varum, tibial varum, subtalar varus, forefoot varus or valgus. Sometimes there will be atro-

phy of the quadriceps, but on the whole the knee is considered normal with no signs of ligamentous or meniscal insufficiency and an absence of swelling. From a physiotherapist's point of view, it is a frustrating condition to treat and it may be referred to a podiatrist.

Treatment

It is important to identify the cause of the abnormal pronation and to re-establish a more normal pattern of foot function so that the lower limb and knee can lock and become stable in propulsion. Some form of functional orthosis will be necessary to compensate for the structural abnormality.

The patellofemoral joint

This joint is commonly affected by mechanical overuse injuries. The patella is the sesamoid of the knee (Fig. 11.8), which works in a pulley-like groove on the femur and is a fulcrum for the action of the quadriceps muscles. It can adapt to forces that act upon it and is an external braking mechanism, producing a dynamic balance between hamstrings and quadriceps. It has a full 1.5 cm of cartilage on the posterior surface to deal with the forces it endures.

The 'Q' angle

The 'Q' angle is still cited as being one of the main causes of patellar subluxation, although other factors, such as vastus medialis weakness, patella alta and abnormal pronation, are recognised as causative factors. This is an angle between a line drawn from the anterior superior iliac spine to the dorsal surface of the ipsilateral patella and a line bisecting the patellar liga-

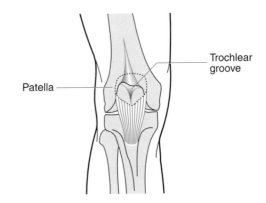

Figure 11.8 Patella and trochlear groove.

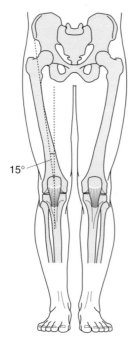

Figure 11.9 The 'Q' angle.

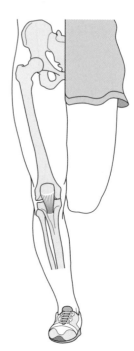

Figure 11.10 Limb varus while running.

ment (Fig. 11.9). It indicates the relationship between the pull of the quadriceps muscles and the position within its normal limits at about 15°. Any more than this and the change in direction of the pull of the quadriceps will cause the patella to be dislocated from the femoral groove. Uneven vectral forces prevent the vastus medialis from balancing the pull from the lateral muscles. A lateral shearing stress is set up on the posterior surface of the patella. Any sport that requires running will intensify these detrimental forces.

Runner's knee syndrome

This is a mild lateral subluxation of the patella and is *not* chondromalacia, for which it is commonly mistaken. It can be caused by an excessive Q angle or excessive pronation of the foot. Lateral stress causing subluxation over a period of years establishes a new position for the patella, creating an uneven pressure on the lateral surface. The shape of the patella changes as it adapts to these stresses and new position. Abnormal pronation causes internal rotation of the tibia; this produces pain.

The syndrome is frequently experienced by runners; the running motion and limb varus produced by running exacerbates the patellar dislocation (Fig. 11.10). Women, in particular, suffer with this problem because

of their anatomical disadvantage, i.e. wider hips and higher Q angle.

Orthotic therapy can realign the foot and prevent the changes that occur at the knee.

Compensatory internal rotation of the femur: a theoretical model (Tiberio 1987)

This theory sets out to explain the mechanical causes of subluxation of the patella and the injuries that ensue. It is generally recognised that abnormal pronation of the subtalar joint delays the external rotation of the tibia during the propulsive phase of the gait cycle. This sets up a dilemma for the knee joint, which should extend but is unable to do so without the external rotation of the tibia that is required for extension. The theory presented here is that the femur should internally rotate on the tibia, providing the necessary alignment for extension. Since the foot is fixed on the ground, the body can move to accommodate the knee joint.

However, this alters the patella femoral tracking. During extension of the knee, the patella is gliding on the femur and the quadriceps are contracting. When the femur internally rotates, the compression between the lateral femoral condyle and the lateral articular surface of the patella is increased. This results in relative lateral tracking of the patella when the knee is near full extension. This may produce symptoms, depending on the extent of the pronation, the degree of internal femoral rotation, the amount of activity, etc.

Chondromalacia patellae

This condition is commonly associated with vastus medialis tendinitis. It is described as a blistering, cystic change of the patellar cartilage and it usually affects the medial facet of the patella.

It is caused by the combination of several factors which ultimately push the patella out of its groove on the femur. These factors include weakness of the vastus medialis muscle; a high Q angle, which causes vastus imbalance and overaction of the lateral vastus; malalignment produced by pathomechanics of the foot, leading to abnormal excessive pronation and internal rotation of the tibia. Finally, aberrations of the anatomy can lead to malfunction, such as irregular-shaped facets on the patella or an abnormally high vastus medialis insertion.

On examination, the patient will complain of a generalised, deep knee pain. The knee may be swollen with a chronic effusion of synovial fluid, and there will be a positive patellofemoral grinding test when the condition is severe. The patella will appear out of alignment and there may well be a high Q angle. The vastus medialis will be weak. X-rays will occasionally show spurring and the patient will be unable to do squats.

Before diagnosing chondromalacia patellae, several other anomalies should first be eliminated. These include chronic synovitis, causing swelling, chronic meniscal injuries, plica syndrome and sprain of the retinaculum. Treatment involves ice and ultrasound, massage of the painful areas and realignment of the maltracking of the patella. This may be achieved with orthotic therapy, otherwise referral to an orthopaedic surgeon may be necessary for surgical management (Table 11.7).

Ankle equinus and knee pain

A short posterior muscle compartment or a bony block at the ankle producing ankle equinus can be responsible for knee pain. Ten degrees of ankle dorsiflexion is necessary for normal gait. When this is reduced, one of the body's compensations is to lift the heel early during the walking cycle. The heel lifts slightly at midstance and the knee functions in an excessively flexed position.

Table 11.7 Chondromalacia patellae: treatment

Initial visit
Ice pack to knee
Activity modification to decrease any painful activities
EGS and ice if swelling is present on the knee
Quadriceps stretching programme, five times daily
Neoprene knee brace with lateral patellar buttressing

Second visit
Consider functional foot orthoses if excessive pronation is present
Decrease activities further
Review all first visit recommendations and increase any not fully carried out
X-ray evaluation including sunrise view and lateral knee to look for spurring and degeneration of posterior aspect of the patella

If knee pain still persists:

Third visit
Consider gastrocnemius and soleus stretching programme and heel lifts
Check function of foot orthoses and increase subtalar joint control if necessary
Continue to concentrate on knee swelling if still present

If not improving significantly:

Fourth visit
Consider an orthopaedic consultation with a view to possible surgery

The more the knee is flexed, the greater are the forces at the articulating facets of the patella. In joggers and long-distance runners this mechanism produces aching and discomfort during and after running. This is a satisfactory condition to treat as it responds well to heel lifts fitted in the running shoes combined with posterior muscle group stretching. Occasionally, flexed knee position is due to tight hamstrings or iliopsoas muscles.

Plica

This commonly occurs in individuals, causing no symptoms whatsoever, although it can also, in some cases, cause a great deal of pain and discomfort. In the embryo, the kneecap is surrounded by a large bursa which differentiates into the pre-patellar, the suprapatellar and the infrapatellar bursae (Fig. 11.11). These can resorb completely in the adult and fall into folds laterally, superiorly and medially. With trauma, overuse or running, the structure can become inflamed, thickened and fibrosed, and can become almost ligamentous in nature. This can fold under the patella and displace it laterally. The vastus medialis is not powerful enough to pull the patella into its ideal situation

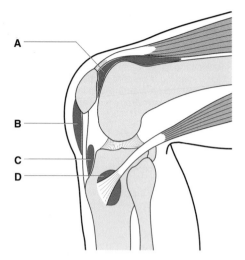

Figure 11.11 The bursae at the knee. A: Suprapatellar. B: Pre-patellar. C: Infrapatellar. D: Pes anserinus (lateral view).

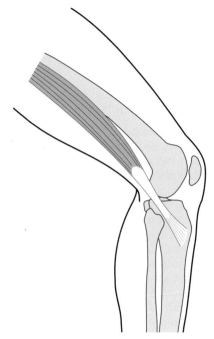

Figure 11.12 Insertion of the iliotibial band (lateral view).

and it subluxates. It can cause pain and clicking in the knee and can mimic other knee disorders.

Iliotibial band friction syndrome (ITBFS)

This is a painful, debilitating condition affecting a significant number of runners, especially the endurance runner. It is caused by friction of the iliotibial band as it passes back and forth over the lateral femoral epicondyle during flexion and extension of the knee (Fig. 11.12). The condition tends to occur mainly from overuse.

The iliotibial band is a thickening of the fascia lata that extends from the iliac crest to insert into the lateral tibial condyle. The band receives insertions from the tensor fascia lata and gluteus maximus muscles. Excessive amounts of friction occurring during flexion and extension movements of the knee may produce mechanical irritation, leading to inflammatory reactions within the iliotibial band, the underlying anatomical bursa, if present, and/or the periosteum of the lateral femoral condyle.

Clinical presentation is of pain on the lateral aspect of the knee close to the lateral femoral epicondyle and it may extend along the iliotibial band. On occasion, soft tissue swelling is present at this site. The pain is usually aggravated by repetitive knee movements in running, but not in walking. Running downhill and over-striding also induce pain as the iliotibial band is compressed by the lateral femoral condyle. Side-to-side sports such as tennis and basketball do not aggra-

vate the condition. The area is tender. The diagnosis can be confirmed by the use of the compression test. With the knee flexed at 90°, pressure is applied over the lateral femoral epicondyle or just proximal to it. The knee is then extended slowly. At approximately 30° of flexion, a severe pain should be elicited, which patients will describe as the same pain as they get when running.

Thorough examination of the knee should be performed to rule out other pathology which could include cysts, meniscal tears and chondromalacia. Treatment emphasises a decrease in the amount of distance the patient is running. To stop completely is best, but most runners will not do this. Running on flat soft surfaces, reducing speed and running to tolerance without pain should reduce symptoms. Ice massage, ultrasound and stretching will help (Table 11.8).

If the patient cannot run without pain, other training programmes should be instituted, such as swimming and weight training. The muscles to be strengthened are the quadriceps, hamstrings and abductors. Re-introduction to running should be slow and gradual.

HAMSTRING TENDINITIS

Strain of a hamstring is a common injury as it is one of the flexor muscle groups and hence a group prone to

Table 11.8 Iliotibial band syndrome: treatment

Initial visit
Iliotibial band stretching programme
Quadriceps strengthening programme with adductor
strengthening programme
Ice massage to injured area
Rule out meniscal disease and others in differential diagnosis
Check for excessive rotation or varus stress situation in
biomechanics

If not improving significantly or re-flare with activity:

Second visit
Apply physical therapy, usually ultrasound, followed by ice
massage
Consider testing excessive rotation factor with ankle taping
If excessive varus stress is considered, exclude such
possible causes as short limb, worn out shoes, etc.

If re-flare with return to activity:

Third visit
Consider possible lateral meniscus problems and
orthopaedic referral
Consider the use of knee arthrogram to check for possible
tear in lateral meniscus

Table 11.9 Hamstring tendinitis: treatment

Initial visit
Hamstring stretching programme, five times daily
Ice packs to injured area three times daily but especially after
activity
Activity modification to reduce painful activity (especially hill
and speed work)
If extremely tender, EGS and ice treatments three times a
week until symptoms resolve
If rupture is suspected or chronic problems, initiate hamstring
strengthening exercise

If re-flare with return to activity:

Second visit
Quadriceps and hamstring dynamometer testing for strength
ratios
Do not allow return to activity until flexibility and strength are
normal
Consider functional foot orthoses if rotation is a significant
problem
Check for history of sciatica and low back problems, possibly
causing hyperinnervation of hamstring muscles and chronic
tightness
Heel lifts to take some pressure off tendo Achilles and
hamstrings
Evaluate for leg length discrepancy with hamstring tendinitis
on side of long leg

If re-flare with return to activity:

Third visit
Consider prolonged rest

shortening. It should be carefully stretched before any sport but particularly sprinting or running.

It is possible for a muscle or a tendon of this group to be damaged at any part along its length, whether at the muscle belly or its tendon attachment at the ischial tuberosity.

A strain is normally caused by the sudden over-extension of a tight hamstring, whether at the hip or knee, with over-striding or sprinting. A hamstring that has previously been injured is never as strong again and predisposes to further damage.

On examination, the hamstring will appear to be tight; there will be swelling and bruising only if some fibres have been ruptured. Pain will be present at the site of the sprain, e.g. at the ischial tuberosity, but most commonly mid-thigh. Pain will increase if the muscle is contracted against resistance. The individual may have to walk with a fixed-knee position.

Chronic hamstring pulls should alert the podiatrist to the possibility of the cause being of mechanical origin. The malalignment produced by excessive subtalar pronation can also affect hamstring alignment. Where internal rotation of the tibia occurs, well into the propulsive stage of the running cycle, a twist between origin and insertion of the hamstring will also occur. This is exaggerated with sport and often the sport is blamed as the cause.

In chronic cases, mechanical evaluation is essential to ensure sound foot function and realignment of the muscle groups. In acute cases, the key factor is to

stretch the hamstring muscles to ensure no further injuries. Ice should be used directly after the injury to keep down swelling and inflammation. After the acute stage, ultrasound and heat followed by massage will stimulate healing (Table 11.9).

Finally, it may be necessary to change the style of running to avoid sprinting or over-striding and down-hill running. Daily exercises and stretching should be part of the warm-up routine to prevent injury recurring.

GROIN STRAIN

Groin strain is a painful and debilitating injury and seems to be common among rugby players, sprinters and joggers. The term *groin strain* encompasses a number of conditions which can produce pain in the groin area, i.e. the curved area forming the junction between the anterior abdominal wall and the front of the thigh lateral to the peroneal area, although the pain may be ascribed to an area which extends a little beyond these boundaries. Any structures in this area—adductor muscles, inguinal ligaments, abdominal muscles, etc.—may be injured and be the reason for the pain

---

> **Box 11.2** Case history: groin strain
>
> A male, aged 32, who was a very keen sportsman in good general health, presented with groin strain of 2 years' duration. His sporting activity included cycling to and from work each day, a distance of 5 miles (8 km) each way; a lunch-time run three times a week for half an hour; an 8-hour hill walk at the weekend or a 50-mile (80 km) cycle ride; and, finally, swimming in the evening each week. His activity was purely recreational but occupied a major part of his life.
>
> His groin strain started slowly; after a lunch-time run he felt an ache at the top of the adductor muscles on his left leg. The pain subsided after 2 or 3 hours but returned towards the end of his next run. Gradually the pain became worse and there was stiffness in the muscle in the morning when walking after rising from bed.
>
> He attended the local sports injury clinic and was shown stretching exercises and received a course of ultrasound treatment. To begin with, this was helpful, but the pain always returned with running. Running was stopped and he consulted his GP, who referred him to see a consultant orthopaedic surgeon whose diagnosis was groin strain. The surgeon prescribed physiotherapy treatment, which did not have any effect, and then steroid injections were given. At this stage, pain was apparent during hill walking and eventually even during walking, so he resorted to cycling only.
>
> Further physiotherapy treatment was given and a second opinion was sought from another orthopaedic surgeon, who also diagnosed chronic strain of the muscles. At this stage, even cycling was producing pain and the only form of activity left to the patient was swimming in the evenings. He became extremely depressed by his inability to participate in sport and as a last resort was referred to a podiatrist who found on examination that there was a limb length discrepancy of 2 cm on the left side. He was also found to have bilateral forefoot varus, which was more pronounced on the left side. Functional orthoses were prescribed which had a heel raise of 1/4 inch on the left foot. These were worn for progressively longer periods over 3 weeks until fully in use when the symptoms began to subside. Steadily, over the next 3 months, the pain reduced during walking and the stiffness in the muscle in the morning ceased to be present. Cycling and hill walking were resumed without the return of the symptoms and the patient's mood of depression lifted.
>
> When the patient was reviewed after 6 months, all the former sports could be attempted without the return of pain, with the exception of jogging. This latter brought about some tightness of the muscle with resultant stiffness, suggesting that it may take some time before this last activity can be resumed.

(see Box 11.2). Often it is not possible to identify accurately the structure involved. Groin strain generally presents a pattern which starts as a mild ache following activity, which is relieved by rest but returns with the next period of activity. Gradually the pain becomes worse, beginning earlier in the activity and taking longer to subside, until it does not disappear at all. At this stage the pain may be present even with normal walking or getting in and out of cars, and may even be aggravated by coughing or sneezing.

This injury, unless it is due to a sudden or violent trauma, is most usually biomechanical in origin and bears the hallmark of an overuse injury—slow onset which subsides with rest and physiotherapy but returns with activity. The biomechanical cause is often limb length difference, where the foot on the anatomically shorter leg pronates longer than the foot of the longer limb. This excessively pronated foot causes more internal rotation of the limb, which in turn tilts the pelvis forward on that side. The overall effect is to produce a limb where the muscle groups, including the adductor group of muscles and iliopsoas, now function with a twist, as the pelvis lists downwards. The adductor group of muscles are important in giving stability to the pelvis, particularly in fast and long-distance running. When having to contract with the pelvis listing to one side, they now have to twist from origin to insertion and they have to work harder. Rest or stretching will not allow the condition to heal unless there is action to control the basic structural abnormality.

The aim in treatment is to restore good functional biomechanics by limiting pronation of the foot to within normal limits. This will resolve the twist in the leg and reduce some of the effects of limb length difference by correcting the functional element. Orthoses will achieve this effect and will also straighten the pelvis to a certain extent. Next, if not contraindicated by other unwanted effects, a small heel raise can be added to the orthoses to compensate for the discrepancy of the limb length on the shorter side.

LEG LENGTH DISCREPANCY

During running, forces of up to three times body weight are transmitted through the feet and the lower limb. When a sport involves leaping and jumping, these forces can reach seven or eight times body weight.

A limb length difference starts to be significant at around 3 mm. With a leg length difference of 6 mm, the mere shifting from one side of the body to the other, plus the added stress of a sport, can cause the equivalent of 2 cm difference. Given this difference, a sport such as cycling, skiing, rugby or basketball will produce a significant difference in function on one side of the body compared to the other, resulting in fatigue.

Leg length difference can be anatomical or physiological:

1. Anatomical leg length difference describes a true anatomical difference that exists between two legs. It is measurable without variation. The difference is found in both neutral calcaneal stance position and relaxed calcaneal stance position. The height of the femoral heads on X-ray is diagnostic.

2. Physiological leg length difference results when some other body structure or aberration affects the leg length measurement. This may include scoliosis, muscle imbalance or abnormal biomechanics of the foot, and may originate above the pelvis or below the malleoli.

Functional leg length difference may occur in unilateral sports where overdevelopment of one-half of the body produces a significant discrepancy. Symptoms produced by leg length differences include snapping of the iliotibial band, bursitis on the lateral aspect of the knee and low back complaints. There may also be unilateral knee pain and asymmetrical function of the feet. Below the knee, medial shin splints, Achilles tendon pain and ankle pain are also problems.

These symptoms are usually unilateral and should suggest some asymmetry of the body. It is necessary to carry out a full biomechanical examination to determine where the asymmetry lies.

A biomechanical examination should include measurements of the limbs (Fig. 11.13) in order to quantify the difference. The measurement is taken from the anterior superior iliac spine to the medial or lateral malleolus. The femoral component should be measured at the joint line of the femur and tibia. Measuring can be difficult if bony landmarks are hard to find. The examination should include the comparison of ranges of motion of the joints, their flexibility and quality of motion, both weight-bearing and non-weight-bearing. Measurements of limb and limb segments, neutral and relaxed stance measurements, will eliminate the foot as a cause of discrepancy. Examine forefoot to hindfoot position. Look at the ankle axes and the subtalar joint axes. Determine whether there has been soft tissue injury or surgical intervention which might cause asymmetry.

One of the simplest forms of examination is to examine the patient standing (Figs. 11.14 and 11.15) and walking in a swimsuit, so that body proportions and attitudes can be observed. Look at the head, the neck and the back. Shoulders may tilt on the shorter side. In adults, the head will not tilt; it will straighten so that the eyes are parallel to the horizon, but look to see if the neck is curved. If a double scoliosis is

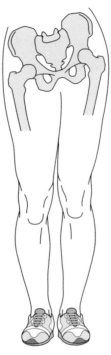

Figure 11.13 Limb length difference syndrome leading to groin strain.

present, the shoulders will level out. These are compensations which occur in the body and can give rise to pain. Elbow and hand positions may appear lower on the longer sides, and indentations and folds on the back will also appear on this side. On the posterior aspect, muscle compartments may be bulkier or even in spasm. Draw a line down the spines of the vertebrae and, using a goniometer, measure the degree of deviation. Look at the scapulae and sacral dimples.

Twists and rotations may be in the transverse plane; women are more prone to scoliosis than men. Arm swing can show up an asymmetry of the pelvis—the opposing arm will swing more with the shorter leg.

Compensations for leg length difference can take place in the feet. On the short side, the foot will supinate and maintain weight-bearing on the outside of the foot in an attempt to lengthen the limb. It may also function in an equinus position to prevent too much dorsiflexion and shortening occurring. The opposite will happen on the long limb. There will be excess wear on the inside of the shoe as the foot pronates and shortens that limb; 4–6 mm of shortening can occur with pronation at the subtalar joint.

Finally, go and watch the patient in action; watching

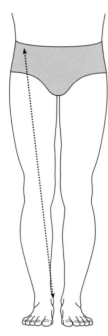

Figure 11.14 Measuring limb length.

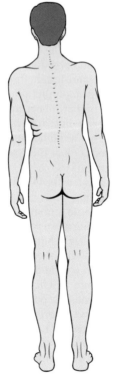

Figure 11.15 Examination of the patient standing.

patients and the sport they are involved in may be a vital clue to diagnosis.

A runner complaining of unilateral knee pain should immediately suggest a leg length discrepancy (see Box 11.3). There are, of course, other aetiological factors for unilateral knee pain and these should be eliminated. Examples of these are strain of the medial collateral ligaments of the knee; strain of the pes anserinus muscles insertion, i.e. gracilis, semitendinosus, sartorius; bruising from a traumatic injury, patellar subluxation and strained vastus medialis muscle; the plica syndrome.

Box 11.3   Case history: leg length discrepancy

A 36-year-old male runs 30–50 km a week at a rate of 6 minutes/km. He complains of pain on the medial aspect of his left knee, which started after an especially long run. The pain is present during the day, when activity is low, and becomes quite sharp when he changes direction. He warms up well, stretches well and warms down after his run. He finds the pain gets worse when he runs on harder surfaces. He has tried changing his running shoes; various shock-absorbing materials in the shoes, icing and ultrasound have all been to no avail.

He has noticed that the right leg of his trousers is a bit longer on that leg, and recently he has noticed some stiffness and discomfort in the right back and shoulder and in the lower back. On examination of his shoes, there is asymmetrical wear. They are worn out laterally on the right shoe and medially on the left shoe.

Once these have been eliminated, the reason for the leg length difference must be determined. The knee pain in this situation is a result of the pronated position of the foot on the longer leg. Pronation causes internal rotation of the tibia, increased flexion of the knee and more stress on the posterior aspect of the patella. The shorter leg is also prone to stress fracture because of the lack of shock absorption in the supinated foot and the position of the acetabulum directly over the femoral head.

Treatment of leg length discrepancies

1. Anatomical leg length discrepancy, once it has been determined, is reduced by a simple shoe lift or heel lift. It may be necessary to have some manipulative therapy to aid the readaption of body structures to the new position.

2. Physiological leg length difference may require an orthosis as well as a heel lift if poor foot mechanics are the aetiological factor.

Special exercises may be necessary to strengthen or stretch certain muscle groups that are unbalanced. The individual should be reassessed regularly to ensure the deforming force does not cause the condition to recur. Care should be taken to avoid over-correction of leg length discrepancy, and it may be necessary to refer the patient to a manipulative therapist or physio-therapist for their expertise.

SPORTS SHOES

There is a wide variety of sports shoes available cur-rently, with 200 styles devoted to running and many others for specialist use. The pace of change in styles and technology is rapid, so it is wise to seek advice from specialist footwear shops and particularly those who deal with particular sporting activities. Sales staff may not be experienced enough or may not under-stand the needs of particular activities, and may thus suggest footwear because it is popular and not because it is the correct shoe for the sport. Podiatrists specialising in the treatment of sports injury would be well advised to liaise with specialist sports shoe retail-ers to learn about particular types of footwear.

Over the last 30 years the manufacturing emphasis in running shoes has changed from durability and the length of time for the outer sole to wear, to the need for shock absorption and cushioning from the mid-sole, to finally that of foot function. This latest move has changed the emphasis to the uppers and how the shoe fits. Because of the commercial pressures that manufacturers face to market their particular brands, most of them incorporate many 'high-tech' features into their products to encourage sales. Such features include shock-absorbing mechanisms, stabilisers, and antipronator and antisupinator mechanisms, etc. It is in the identification of features such as these that a good sales assistant will help the individual select the shoe for the sporting activity.

Shoe manufacture

Special shoes are manufactured for running, tennis, cycling, skateboarding, javelin throwing, pole vault-ing and high jumping. Although the detailed specification for these shoes differs widely, the funda-mental structure of the shoes is very much the same (Fig. 11.16).

Lasts

As with most other footwear, sports shoes are made

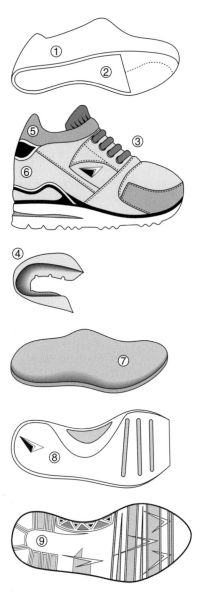

Figure 11.16 Parts of the sports shoe. 1, last; 2, combination last construction; 3 upper—synthetic material and mesh for ventilation; 4, motion control device; 5, Achilles flex notch; 6, heel counter; 7, inner sole—removable; 8, midsole; 9, outsole.

on lasts which may be either wooden or plastic foot-shaped models. The process which follows may be *slip lasting*, where the upper of the shoe is stitched around the last with the closure being along the length of the sole. This can be seen if the inner sole is removed; the stitches will be revealed running along the length of the foot from the heel to the toe. The shoes made from this process are flexible and lightweight; they do not give much control of the foot and are usually chosen for racing.

Another process is *board lasting*, where the upper is stitched to a board that has the shape of the inner sole. This method of construction can also be seen with the removal of the inner sole. It produces a much firmer type of shoe, which may require some time for the shoe to be 'worn in', and as a result gives the foot much more stability and is a good base for orthotics.

A third form is *combination lasting*, where the front part of the shoe is slip lasted and, from just behind the metatarsal heads to the heel, it is board lasted. This combination gives good stability, but because of the more flexible forepart is not so heavy and difficult to wear at first (Fig. 11.17)

Shape of the last. There are three basic last shapes, the first of which is the *straight* or *semi-straight last*. This has only the slightest inflare along its medial border and is considered the most supportive, and should be chosen for the overpronating low-arched and pronating feet.

The second and most common shape is the *semi-curved last*, which has a greater degree of inflare along the medial border. It offers some medial support but not quite as much as the straight last, and is used for the greater majority of the population.

The third last type is the *curved last*, which is used for racing shoes and lightweight trainers as it has the greatest amount of inflare along the medial border and provides the least amount of support. It is chosen for the higher arched feet which tend to be more rigid and for mid- to forefoot strikers. The shoe is flexible and lightweight (Fig. 11.18).

Other factors

The heel counter. This part of the shoe probably gives the shoe most of its stability; if the counter is soft and flexible then stability at the heel is lost, however well the rest of the shoe is built. It is usually made from a board type of material or a plastic and should not compress with manual pressure.

The tongue. This is designed to protect the foot from the laces but is tending to be excluded from shoe design at present as a separate entity, and is being incorporated into the upper or the inner sleeve of the shoe. Its function remains the same.

Insole. This is usually a moulded or contoured thin piece of material, often made from EVA (ethyl vinyl acetate), with a towelling or fleecy top cover which conforms to the sole of the foot. It provides comfort and gives some stability, and stops the foot from moving within the shoe. It is often removable and can easily be

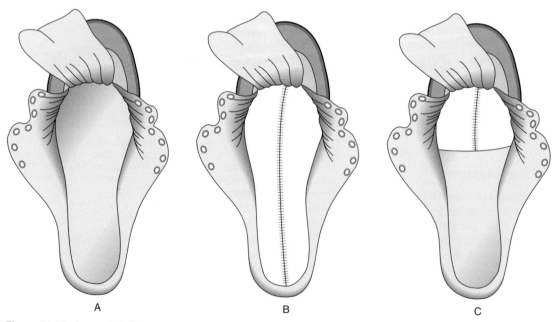

Figure 11.17 Lasts. A: Fully board lasted. B: Slip lasted. C: Combination lasted.

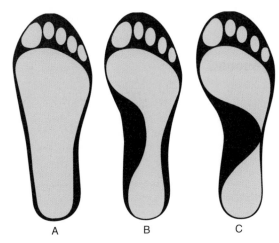

Figure 11.18   Lasts. A: Semi-straight last. B: Semi-curved last. C: Curved last.

replaced with shock-absorbing materials and orthotics.

Outsole. This is sometimes referred to as the top sole, since, in the method of construction, it is one of the final components to be added when the shoe is on the last and upside down. It provides the grip and durability, with differences in tread and pattern which can be chosen to respond to different needs. Treads with wider spaces are less easily clogged when running off-road. The materials are usually carbon rubber, which is a heavy and durable material for weighty people or rugged activity, or blow rubber, which is lighter and less durable but has more cushioning and is suitable for racing and lightweight people and activities.

Midsole. This is often considered the foundation of a running shoe which gives cushioning and stability. It can be made from EVA (which provides more cushioning) or polyurethane (which has greater durability) or combinations of both, and may have various devices added. These can include gel, air sacs, tubes and other such mechanisms, all of which can add to the cost of the shoe. The durability of the midsole depends much on the weight of the individual, the mileage covered and biomechanical problems.

Upper. This is mostly made from synthetic material and mesh to produce ventilation and a lightweight shoe. Recent materials include lycra and neoprene, which are comfortable, durable and supportive. Recent advances using these materials have seen the introduction of a sleeve or semi-sleeve, which encloses the foot within the shoe rather like a glove and allows the standard shoe to fit many more foot shapes.

Laces have been replaced with many other types of fastenings and closures, including velcro, straps, belts,

screws and wheels. One shoe even includes a canister of carbon dioxide which inflates on the inner sole to improve the fit of the shoe around the foot.

Scientific evaluation

Shoe manufacturers invest much time and money in testing shoes and materials for their shock-absorbing properties and ability to reduce trauma. There is an awareness of the causes of trauma and attempts are made to incorporate materials which will reduce it; similarly, they have gained an awareness of the effects of foot function, mechanics and overpronation as a cause of injury, and attempt to incorporate mechanisms to improve foot function and control excessive pronation. Much dependence is placed on current computer technology and efforts are being made to produce more reliable data concerning the function of the foot in the shoe.

Features of a good sports shoe

1. Select a shoe with a toe box which has adequate height over the toes and 2 cm of length from the ends of the toes.

2. There is not a standard width or length fitting to cover all makes of shoe; therefore, the selection of the shoe remains a matter for the judgement of the person who is going to wear it. The correct width is necessary to avoid squeezing the forefoot, and it should not be too loose as this will cause fatigue problems of the forefoot. It should be possible to 'pinch' 2 cm of the upper material over the ball of the foot to ensure a good fit.

3. Balance and equilibrium in the shoe are necessary to avoid excessive stresses and forces which could interfere with the normal motion of the foot and limb during running. If the shoe tilts towards the medial border, most of the motion will be in that direction, causing overuse syndrome. Always check that the heel counter is perpendicular to the supporting surface of the shoe.

4. Good flexibility at the ball of the shoe is important to avoid fatigue of the muscles of the lower leg and to avoid tendon strains. If the shoe does not flex at the correct position, arch fatigue or footstrain may result. A shoe should bend easily at the ball of the shoe using the power of one finger alone.

5. The position of the heel counter and its rigidity are important factors for controlling the direction of forces on the foot during the heel contact phase of the running cycle.

6. Weight and softness of the shoe are closely relat-

ed as most lightweight shoes are usually made from soft midsole materials. Such shoes are adequate for a lightweight person who has good foot structure and who hits the ground hard, but they tend to fatigue and warp after 300–400 km of use. With less midsole protection, the insoles must be made from soft resilient materials, especially at the forefoot.

7. Shoes have a shelf-life after which their component materials, such as EVA in the midsole, become hard and the glues harden and become brittle. It is not necessarily wise to purchase two pairs of shoes unless they are used concurrently.

THERAPEUTIC MODALITIES

The use of heat and cold as therapy for sports injuries can prevent potentially debilitating and chronic conditions from arising. Once their action on blood vessels, skin and other structures is understood, their application can speed rehabilitation, lessen scarring and fibrosis, and prevent sprains and strains. Heat and cold can be applied in various forms and they are easy to apply either at home or at the surgery. The details of theory and practice of these and other physical therapies are discussed in Chapter 15.

Cold

Cold can be used on acute injuries, such as sprains and strains, to reduce inflammation, suppress fluid build-up and swelling in the tissues and prevent scarring and adhesions. It can also be used as a mild analgesic in painful conditions.

Acute injuries, sprains and strains require immediate application of cold to prevent swelling. Cold in the form of an ice pack, for example, should be applied for the first 36–48 hours after injury.

Cold, if applied for 3–6 minutes, can also be used to give vasodilatation (Hunting response or effect). This can be applied and combined with massage to produce stimulation of the circulation locally.

Heat

Heat should not be applied until 48 hours after an injury, and should not be used on areas which are oedematous. It can be used combined with cold in the form of contrast baths to produce the Hunting effect, which stimulates venous pumping and the removal of excess tissue fluid. Contrast baths should be followed by compressional strapping and elevation of the part

to above the level of the heart. This procedure should be followed several times during the day.

Ultrasound

Ultrasound has a mild analgesic effect. It disrupts fibrous tissue which has formed after injury and so breaks up adhesions. It can be used to disrupt and break down a haematoma that has congealed. Its analgesic and heat-producing effect can also be used to relax muscle spasm. Details are discussed in Chapter 15.

Contraindications

Ultrasound should not be used in the eye area, with heart or vascular disease, where there is embolism or haemorrhages, on anaesthetised skin, on the epiphyseal area in children or on bony prominences such as the spine. For best effects it should be used once or twice a day, three to four times per week. It must be used at least six to eight times before it is discarded as being ineffective. A dosage of 1 W/cm^2 for 10 minutes is required to produce an effect. The time period should be gradually increased. Some individuals are more sensitive than others to its effects.

Medical diathermy

This is an electromagnetic wave force generated between two pads applied one on either side of the injured part; it produces a deep heat. It can be used to treat deep bruising or tendinitis.

It especially stimulates the lymphatics and the collateral circulation, and is a good method of treatment for traumatic inflammatory processes: myalgia, neuralgia, muscle spasms, adhesions and chronic infections.

Contraindications

Diathermy should not be used on haemorrhages, acute inflammatory processes, malignant tumours or burns.

Treatment

Application should be for 20–30 minutes, three times daily for 3–4 days. The patient will feel a deep warm 'glow' at the site of application. Fibrotic lesions may need longer treatment.

ADVICE TO ATHLETES
Stretching exercises

Before an individual attempts any form of sport, he or

she must first warm up with a series of stretches and exercises. Many injuries, such as tears, sprains and strains, can be avoided by taking time to stretch muscle groups, to set the circulation going and to prepare the body for action.

In modern life, the human body is curled into a sitting position for many hours of the day: at work behind a desk, in the car and watching TV. The muscles on the flexor surfaces shorten and require lengthening, while those on the extensor surfaces require strengthening.

The reason for stretching exercises is to stimulate blood flow through the muscles, which function best when stretched to 110% of their resting length, and also to get the synovial fluid in the joints flowing. Exercises also increase flexibility if carried out over several months, improving function and the ability to carry out the sport.

Exercises can be devised for a general warm-up and for specific sports. A sound knowledge of anatomy and of the origins and insertions of muscle groups will be required if the exercises devised are to be effective in stretching particular muscles. There are many exercise books on the market, which are easy to follow and can be used as the basis for a warm-up programme.

When following an exercise plan, start distally and work proximally. Probably the most important muscle group to stretch is the triceps surae, followed by the hamstrings. Adductors and abductors need stretching in long-distance runners, and adductors in cyclists, skaters and hurdlers. These muscles are stabilisers of the hip.

When stretching a muscle, it is important not to bounce the muscle. This stimulates the stretch receptors in the muscle to fire off and the muscle will contract rather than stretch. Go into the stretch slowly and hold for 10–15 seconds. Repeat this 15 times.

Warming up the muscle beforehand makes the stretch easier. A warm bath or spa bath for 10 minutes is a good preparation before starting on a new activity or sport. Heat can be applied locally by heat pad on areas that have been injured in the past or on a tendo Achilles injury where some fibrosis has formed. Ice for 3–6 minutes also stimulates the circulation to a specific area.

Yoga and ballet are excellent activities for maintaining strength and suppleness, and it may be beneficial for a runner to take up one of these as an extra activity to maintain flexibility.

A common complaint from runners who have recently taken up the sport is pain in the calf muscles. Metabolites build up in these muscles and the muscles go into contraction, causing a false equinus. Heat and stretching exercises can overcome this problem.

Strengthening exercises

Strengthening exercises for the muscular system play an essential role in podiatric therapy. All types of exercise must be used in the correct proportion in athletics. The focal points should vary according to the individual athlete's constitution and condition, and the types of sport.

Types of strengthening methods

1. Isometric
2. Isotonic
3. Isokinetic.

Isometric exercise should form the first part of active therapeutic treatment after athletic injuries, such as sprains, tears, dislocations or fractures which are conservatively treated.

Isometric means 'same length'. Isometric contraction is an active contraction which produces no motion of the part. There is no work accomplished, but power is exerted against a fixed resistance.

The advantages of isometric exercise are as follows:

- no cost for equipment
- no equipment space required
- it does not put a muscle or joint through a range of motion. It will allow particular strength only at a specific angle. This is good for rehabilitative runner's knee or athletes in a cast
- it helps stabilise a joint.

The disadvantages of isometric exercise are:

- it is not so good for older patients: it raises the blood pressure so may put strain on the cardiovascular system
- it does not develop or strengthen muscle power throughout the range of motion.

Isotonic conditioning is a type of exercise in which the muscle goes through a range of motion with a fixed weight. This is a dynamic exercise. There are two sub-categories of isotonic exercise:

- *concentric* strengthening—where a weight is lifted with the force of muscle contraction
- *eccentric* strengthening—where the contraction force of the muscle is against an overpowering weight resistance.

Concentric exercise is the best means of producing strength with safety. During rehabilitation, the correct formula of repetitions to sets and repetitions to weight must be determined. The determination of endurance versus hypertrophy of the muscle is essential. The athlete's injury and sport will dictate this.

Eccentric exercise is the best means of producing strength but it is very dangerous. It can be termed dynamic negative work; however, during this form of exercise, muscular tension two or three times greater than normal can be created. This is very important for the sports podiatrist, as much of the extrinsic musculature to the foot and ankle applies decelerating forces on poorly stabilised fulcrums.

Isokinetic or 'same speed' strengthening is exercise where the speed is set so that a specific range of motion is executed per unit time. The speed of some of the machines can be set from 0° to 300° (Cybex or Orthotron). The machine also pushes back against the operator as hard as he or she is pushing against it. It matches the user's strength through the muscle/joint range of motion.

The settings of the machine can be adjust according to the type of strength the user wishes to develop. If hypertrophying of muscle is desired, slow speeds (0–100°) are utilised. To increase speed and power, speeds above 120° are set.

Many of the isokinetic machines have instructions to demonstrate a range of motion and strengths within that range of motion. Universal and Nautilus machines are less sophisticated but attempt to accomplish a similar goal or resistive exercise throughout the range of motion.

The following is a suitable regime for starting a rehabilitative strengthening programme:

1. electromuscular stimulation (EMS) to maintain tone in the injured musculature (see Ch. 14)
2. isometric exercise programme involving all muscles about the joint
3. isotonic exercises of the above muscles
4. ultimately, isokinetic training while the athlete returns to athletic activity; this may require 3–4 months of follow-up.

FURTHER READING

Bale R L, Denton J A 1985 Functional foot orthoses for athletic injuries. Journal of the American Podiatric Medical Association 75 pp. 359–363

Botte R R 1981 An interpretation of the pronation syndrome and foot types of patients with low back pain. Journal of the American Podiatric Medical Association 71

Cavanagh P R 1980 The running shoe book. Anderson World, California

Francis V 1994 Runners' shoe guide April.

Frankel V H 1980 Biomechanics of the skeletal system. Lea and Febiger, Philadelphia

Hammer W I 1992 Chiropractic sports medicine 6(3): 97–101

Heil B 1992 Lower limb biomechanics related to running injuries. Physiotherapy 78(6): 400–405

Helfet A J, Gruebel Lee D M 1980 Disorders of the foot. Lippincott, Philadelphia

Hlavac H F 1977a The joints of the ankle. Williams and Wilkins, Baltimore

Hlavac H F 1977b The foot book. World Publications, California

Hodson A 1994 Too much too soon. Sportscare Journal 1(6): 19–23

Inman V T, Ralston H J, Frank T 1981 Human waltzing. Williams and Wilkins, Baltimore

Jahss M A 1982 Disorders of the foot. Saunders, Philadelphia

James L, Bates B T, Ostering L R 1978 Injuries to runners. American Journal of Sports Medicine 6: 40–50

Kirby K A, Valmassey R L 1983 The runner-patient history. Journal of American Podiatry Association 73(1)

Krist M 1991 Achilles tendon injuries in athletes, An Chir Gynaecol 80(2): 188–201

Lea R B, Smith L 1972 Non-surgical treatment of tendo Achilles rupture. Journal of Bone and Joint Surgery 41B

Lutter L D 1982 Running athletes in office practice. Foot and Ankle 3(153): 48–51

Mann R A 1982 Biomechanics of running: the foot and leg in running sports. Symposium of American Academy of Orthopaedic Surgeons. Mosby, St Louis.

Orava S, Leppihihti J, Karpakka J 1991 Operative treatment of typical overuse injuries in sport. Ann Chir Gynaecol 80(2): 208–211

Perry J, Antonelli D, Ford W 1975 Analysis of knee joint forces during flexed knee stance. Journal of Bone and Joint Surgery 57A(7): 961–967

Power R A Greencross P 1991 Lower leg compartment syndrome. British Journal of Sports Medicine 25(4): 218–220

Rist R A 1994 Children and exercise. Sportcare Journal 1(6): 4–7

Root J L, Orien W P, Weed J H 1977 Clinical biomechanics, vol 11. Normal and abnormal functions of the foot. Clinic Biomechanics Corp, Los Angeles

Seaton S 1994 Runners' shoe guide (April)

Sgarlato T E 1978 Compendium of podiatric biomechanics. California College of Podiatric Medicine, San Francisco

Subotnick S I 1975 Podiatric sports medicine. Futura Publishing, New York

Tiberio D 1987 The effect of subtalar joint pronation on patella–femoral mechanics: a theoretical model. Journal of Orthopaedic and Sports Physical Therapy: 160–165

Williams J G 1986 Achilles tendon lesions in sports medicine 3(2)

Williams P L, Warwick R (eds) 1989 Gray's Anatomy, 37th edn. Churchill Livingstone, Edinburgh

12

Clinical therapeutics

M. O'Donnell
D. L. Lorimer
D. E. Neale

Keywords

Anhidrosis
Chemical cautery
Digital padding
Dressings
Electrosurgery
Footwear advice
Fungal infections
Heloma durum
Home treatments
Hyperhidrosis
Hyperkeratoses
Inflammatory conditions
Medicaments
Operating
Padding and strapping
Plantar fasciitis
Review periods
Plantar metatarsal padding
Single treatment techniques
Sinus formation
Therapeutic caustic agents
Ulceration
Verruca pedis

THERAPEUTIC MANAGEMENT OF SUPERFICIAL LESIONS

The superficial lesions of the feet are often a source of much pain, disability and partial loss of, or altered, foot function. These lesions are frequently the initiating factor in the patient seeking podiatric advice. Many are unique to the feet and deserve particular consideration as clinical entities in their own right. Their efficient and effective treatment must always be a first priority in management, whether or not the underlying deformity or dysfunction of which they may be symptoms is amenable to correction. The patient's first concern is to obtain relief from pain and anxiety. The podiatrist's ability to treat such conditions successfully may well determine the patient's willingness to cooperate in further therapeutic measures, such as changes of footwear, which may be necessary to deal with the underlying problem. Psychosocial factors must be considered with empathy and tact. An holistic view is an essential element in management.

The range of therapeutic measures available includes careful operating, discriminatory medication, applications of heat and cold, therapeutic laser therapy, protective dressings, padding and strapping. The use of such measures in a number of common conditions is discussed to exemplify effective management, it being presumed that any underlying pathology or other causative factor such as footwear will also be appropriately managed.

Padding and strapping, in most cases an integral part of clinical therapies, may also be used as the sole therapeutic method. The principles upon which it is based provide the rationale for orthoses in the continuing management process. Although the basic padding and strapping methods are discussed, the biomechanical abnormality should be taken into consideration and any padding modified where possible to encompass the underlying cause.

Operating

Nothing is more important for the quick relief of pain related to skin and nail pathologies than skilful operating, and this aspect of podiatric management should never be underestimated or undervalued. Pain during operating should in most instances be negligible, and almost immediate relief should be provided unless the tissues are inflamed. Essential elements in painless operating are, therefore, maximum immobilisation of the area being reduced by correctly applied skin tension, the accurate selection of instrumentation and the optimum level of reduction. When painless reduction is impossible because of the nature of the condition, as in heloma neurovasculare and verruca pedis, operation should be reduced to the minimum, with recourse to caustics and exfoliants to facilitate the desired result or to allow further reduction on the return visit.

Protective padding and strapping will also assist in relieving pain when accurately applied. Alternative measures under these circumstances may be the use of transcutaneous electrical nerve stimulation (TENS) to reduce pain whilst operating, or pre-operative analgesia may be achieved, either by topical application or by injection, to allow complete enucleation.

Medicaments

With the exception of local anaesthetics, medicaments used in podiatry are used as topical applications. They may have a specific function, as in the case of chemical caustics (many of the medicaments which the podiatry profession refers to under the heading of caustics are in fact inaccurately categorised), antifungal agents and antiseptics, but they generally have a palliative effect. Topical therapy can be said to provide relief of symptoms and protection while the skin heals itself. Many of the agents used lack scientific explanation of their mode of action and are used because they are known to have been effective in the past. The fact that suitable agents may be selected and used empirically should not detract from their credibility but should encourage the practitioner to establish links which may add to the understanding of their mode of action. The form in which an agent is used, its method of application, the state of the substrate, the site of the lesion, and the patient's state of health are all factors to be considered in selection. The paramount concern should be to treat the lesion quickly and to use the minimum quantity of medicament to achieve the desired effect.

Long-term use of medicaments should be avoided, as some agents may cause allergic contact dermatitis. Where long-term application is unavoidable, as in the case of emollients or keratolytics in hyperkeratosis, the practitioner should be aware of this possibility and should minimise the risk by careful monitoring and suggesting alternatives at regular intervals. In the treatment of specific conditions, such as fungal infections and verrucae, the patient should be advised to follow the recommended treatment regime and not to supplement, reduce or vary the treatment in terms of medicaments or time.

Dressings

Dressings give protection to an area from friction, pressure and infection. Dressings are normally sterile and are mainly used on areas where the epidermis has been breached. Sterile dry dressings are available in a variety of sizes and are individually packed to facilitate the 'no-touch' technique. These dressings may be used with the addition of an appropriate medicament. The availability of a wide selection of environmental and interactive dressings for use on open lesions is worthy of consideration since many disadvantages are ascribed to traditional dressings. Hydrocolloid dressings are now quoted as being of therapeutic value in a variety of conditions. Tubular gauze dressings are an effective method for retaining sterile dressings on the digits.

Padding and strapping

Many foot problems are biomechanical in origin, and mechanical therapy therefore has a vital role in their management, whether or not surgery is also required. Therapy includes both short-term treatment with adhesive padding and strapping and long-term management by orthoses with footwear advice, modification to footwear or specialised shoes. In the immediate short-term, adhesive padding, correctly chosen, properly designed and accurately applied with appropriate strapping, almost invariably gives immediate relief from pain. This padding can, in many instances, be adapted into replaceable clinical padding until the longer-term orthoses have been manufactured. The continued use of clinical padding is inefficient in terms of time, durability and hygiene. The combination of both methods affords the most effective, comprehensive and economical means of controlling biomechanical foot disorders. The management process should be carried out speedily, efficiently and effectively with the full understanding and cooperation of the patient. Patient compliance is an absolute essential to effect the best possible result in any treatment strategy.

Adhesive padding protects by one or more of several methods: correction, deflection, cushioning or removing tensile or shearing stresses from the epidermis and subcutaneous tissues. Corrective padding is normally used when there is sufficient joint function available to realign the joint to a relatively normal position. It will therefore improve anatomical alignment and reduce or eliminate abnormal stresses. Appropriate strapping is applied with the padding to assist in the corrective role. Padding which protects by deflection or cushioning is also adhered by strapping, but in this instance there is little or no alteration to the position of the underlying deformity. The role of strapping is then only to secure padding closely to the foot in its correct position. Padding or strapping used to remove either shearing or tensile stresses from the epidermis is normally of a thin stretch-type material.

Clinical padding may be applied directly to the foot in either an adhesive or a replaceable form; it may be fitted into the footwear as an insert, or built into a corrective or protective orthosis. The wide range of materials available to the podiatrist provides a choice of thickness and densities from the very firm to the very soft, the choice depending on the therapeutic objective. Firm materials are required for correction and deflection. Soft materials are required to provide shock absorption or cushioning for tissues which are subjected to abnormal stresses, or where there is atrophy of the subcutaneous tissues due to age, or to debilitation by disease, and the area is subject to trauma and ulceration. A combination of high and low density materials is often required for optimum effectiveness and good tolerance by the patient. Silicone and thermoplastic materials can also be used at the chairside as a longer-term alternative to clinical padding and strapping (see also Ch. 14).

Review periods

Review at each stage in the management process is an essential factor in clinical practice. The overall management of podiatric conditions is dependent on the practitioner's ability to assess progress and to change or modify treatment strategies as required. Review periods are variable dependent upon a number of factors which need to be considered in any strategic management plan. This hinges on the practitioner's ability to communicate effectively, assimilate and evaluate information. The review process is facilitated by full and accurate case notes, which may be supplemented, in some instances, by photographs or accurate charting (see also Ch. 8). Consideration must also be given to the legal issues relating to the recording of treatment strategies and the regular updating of medical disorders and drug therapy.

Change of treatment strategies may be required if additional information or a change in medical or social circumstances is subsequently given by the patient. If there is no improvement in the condition, then the podiatrist is required to reconsider the original treatment strategy decided upon or the diagnosis reached. Lack of success following an initial review may lead to adaptations of the management strategy, or referral to another professional in the medical field may be required.

CONTROL AND TREATMENT OF THE HYPERKERATOSES
Pathological callus

This, the most common sign of malfunction, should be carefully removed with a suitable scalpel in order that the areas are clear of thickened stratum corneum. It is often considered by some practitioners that callus which produces no discomfort and is functionally of a protective nature should not be removed. This may be referred to as 'physiological' callus. Care should be taken if this decision is reached to ensure that the patient does not have a loss of sensation due to an underlying medical condition. A common cause of sensory loss to the feet is diabetes, and if callus is not removed, it may lead to breakdown of tissue if there is compression of underlying blood vessels, leading to a local ischaemia.

Emphasis must be placed on an accurate and detailed medical history and examination, with regular updating. Visual or mechanical methods of gait analysis should also be undertaken (see Ch. 2) to enable the practitioner to arrive at an accurate diagnosis.

Postoperatively an antiseptic is required. The choice is dependent on the state of the patient's skin. The base in which the antiseptic is dispensed will have implications for its action. Some antiseptics are inactivated in the presence of blood, serum or pus, while others will inhibit most bacterial organisms but will be bactericidal to one specific type. The time during which an antiseptic will act on bacteria is important. Depending on the activity required, the choice may be an antiseptic which acts immediately and has a long duration of action, or a medicament whose action builds up slowly to optimum effectiveness in its activity and has a long-lasting action. Consideration should be given to the action required of the antiseptic, the nature of the substrate, the optimum time desired of the antiseptic action, the concentration of the antiseptic and the nature of any infecting organism, before deciding on the appropriate medicament.

There is a wide variety of postoperative antiseptics from which the practitioner may choose, such as chlorhexidine gluconate 0.5% in 70% isopropyl alcohol, povidone-iodine in various preparations, and tincture of benzoin compound. The last of these is said to prevent loss of moisture from the tissues, but painting with flexible collodion is better for that purpose.

On dry skin, the preferred method is to use emollients to soften the skin and retain moisture. To be effective, most agents need to be applied by the patient at least twice a day, preferably after a footbath. Many proprietary medicaments are available for this purpose; they are, inter alia, E45 cream, lanolin (which may have the addition of 3% salicylic acid) or calmurid. Where the hyperkeratosis is widespread and associated with extreme anhidrosis, the use of an emollient with occlusion overnight may be required.

On moist skin, astringent agents should be used to improve the state of the skin. This is essential to prevent secondary problems, such as fissuring, blistering, bacterial or fungal infection, from arising. Mild astringents in solution, such as 3% salicylic acid, potassium

permanganate or limited applications of 3% formalin, may be applied. Alternatively, footbaths containing the latter two may be used if the hyperhidrosis is affecting the whole foot and is not limited to specific areas. Localised moistness of the tissues underlying the callus may require more astringent applications of silver nitrate solution at strengths of 25% or 50%. The eschar formed produces a protective film over the area and it has been suggested that silver nitrate may inhibit the process of keratinisation by coagulation of the protein content of the reproductive cells or the intracellular fluid which feeds them. Another theory is that silver nitrate constricts the orifices of the sweat glands and prevents the infiltration of sweat and increased fluid pressure within the tissues. Since sweat is a stimulant to the growth of the epidermis, then, theoretically, by reducing sweat output, a reduction of epidermal growth should ensue.

The only evidence to support the view that silver nitrate is beneficial is empirical. The effectiveness of silver nitrate is dependent on its application at frequent intervals to an area which has been thoroughly reduced of stratum corneum. Owing to its rapid short-lived action, there is little advantage to being in contact with the tissues for long periods of time between treatments. The eschar should be removed at frequent intervals if continuity of action is required.

Following reduction of the lesion and the application of the medicament of choice, appropriate padding and strapping should be applied.

Helomata durum of the digits

These commonly occur on the dorsal aspect and apices of the lesser toes, in the nail sulci associated with pressure from the nail plate, or at the lateral edge of the nail, particularly the fifth. Since footwear pressure is the initiating factor in the majority of cases, advice in this respect is mandatory. It is essential to eradicate the nucleus with a scalpel at the earliest stage possible. Enucleation should remove all the keratinised epidermal cells so that the underlying tissue can be restored to a better condition. Enucleation can usually be accomplished without difficulty at the first visit, provided there is not extreme pain and tenderness due to inflammation. Difficulty in removal due to hard impacted keratin may be facilitated by the application of 5% potassium hydroxide solution for a few minutes prior to reduction. This has the effect of softening the keratinised tissue by a keratolytic action.

The enucleation may be followed by the application of chemical cautery to minimise the possibility of recurrence. With little underlying fibro-fatty tissue, the choice of caustic agents is limited, with the more penetrating caustics being contraindicated. If complete reduction has not been achieved, the application of 15–30% salicylic acid ointment in a lanolin or white soft paraffin base may be used. This keratolytic, used at the above percentages, will produce a slow and painless structural alteration of keratinised tissue, softening and macerating it. The action of this medicament is slow and cumulative, rather than immediate, and for this reason it should be left in situ for a period of 5–7 days, and the coagulum left by the acid should be completely removed before further treatment is initiated. This treatment may be necessary two or three times at weekly intervals to ensure complete enucleation. Prolonged treatment with salicylic acid may cause skin dermatitis. Application should be with a masking plaster as this is necessary to prevent spread to surrounding healthy tissue. When the application of salicylic acid in ointment form is not practical, the base may be changed to collodion or spirit and can be applied directly to the area, by means of an applicator stick without masking the surrounding tissues. This method may also be used in the nail sulcus in low percentages. The addition of padding to deflect pressure away from the area, in conjunction with footwear advice or modification, is necessary. When complete reduction has been achieved, 25% or 50% silver nitrate solution may be applied. This protein precipitant will 'shrink' the walls of the cavity, and repeated applications in conjunction with expert scalpel action will return the tissues to normal, provided compressional stress to the area has been eliminated. Thereafter, patients should be encouraged to restore elasticity to the area by the regular use of emollients applied with a gentle kneading action to release any subdermal adhesions. This is done by applying firm pressure while moving superficial tissues to and fro over the underlying bone.

The presence of peripheral neuropathy, vascular insufficiency or impaired immune response, or the effects of long-term steroid therapy on healing, will make the application of caustics or any medicament with the ability to cause breakdown of tissue undesirable, but a mild exfoliant such as 10% salicylic acid in collodion can be used to facilitate enucleation.

Electrosurgery (described later) can also produce good results with intractable lesions in carefully selected patients.

Helomata durum on the plantar metatarsal area

These are usually chronic in nature when they are of several years' duration and they may be associated with common structural deformities, such as pes cavus (under the first and fifth metatarsal heads), with hallux limitus/rigidus (under the second or fifth metatarsal heads and the interphalangeal joint of the hallux), and with hallux abductovalgus (under the second and third metatarsal heads). The chronic nature of these lesions results from fibrosis of the underlying dermal tissues because of traumatic inflammation over a long period caused by overloading due to abnormal gait patterns. Such lesions may prove difficult to eradicate successfully because the tissues at the weight-bearing area have lost their elasticity. They will respond to a certain extent to attempts to increase pliability, but the main emphasis in management must be on deflective and protective padding and orthotic therapy.

After careful reduction, the use of 20% pyrogallic acid with 20% wheatgerm oil in white soft paraffin is said to be effective in inhibiting the formation of fibrous tissue. A similar effect is reputed to be achieved with ultrasound therapy, due to the micro-massage effect. There is no objective evidence to support this view, but it is possible that the increased frequency of treatment which is necessary for the application of pyrogallic acid ensures that the nucleus is brought under control, giving the appearance of a cure. The use of wheatgerm and pyrogallic acid should be limited in the same way as for the application of pyrogallic acid alone. If used, it can be alternated with plain buffering ointments. However, where there have been large 'fibrous' lesions, the plantar tissues never seem to fully regain their elasticity. When the lesions are of a relatively short duration and the superficial tissues have not been subjected to long-term trauma, the outlook is much brighter. Silver nitrate and salicylic acid may be used as a caustic treatment in a similar method to that discussed in the previous section on digital lesions.

Interdigital helomata

These are evidence of abnormal compression usually occurring between opposing interphalangeal joints due to abnormal digital alignment or to the base of a proximal phalanx pressing on an adjacent metatarsal head with subsequent pressure on the overlying tissues. These lesions may be exacerbated in some cases by hypermobility and lengthening of the feet through excessive abnormal pronation and consequent constriction of the toes from footwear. Although a lesion may be limited to the 4/5 interdigital space, it should be borne in mind that the causative factor may well be a biomechanical problem in the rearfoot, such as a rearfoot varus, and that complete resolution depends on the elimination of the biomechanical problem, which is not always possible. They may also be associated with hyperhidrosis, which determines their consistency as hard (helomata durum) or soft (helomata molle), and which, if present, needs to be controlled. Their enucleation requires skilful operating, especially when they are situated in the fourth web space.

Helomata molle respond well to the application of 20% silver nitrate solution following enucleation. As previously discussed, this has the apparent effect of reducing sweat production. It also toughens up the epidermal tissue of the helomata molle lesion and makes reduction easier on the return visit. Silicone orthodigital splints or interdigital wedges are the most effective form of padding when the lesion is due to pressure from opposing interphalangeal joints. When the lesion is in the web space, realignment of the metatarsal to the base of the opposing phalanx is required. This can be achieved with a short shaft or a dumb-bell pad, but consideration must also be given to rearfoot/forefoot biomechanical problems.

Vascular and neurovascular helomata

Lesions of this type are found over interphalangeal joints and plantar to the metatarsal heads. They are characterised by the protrusion of vascular and neural structures into the overlying hyperkeratosis and the objective of treatment is to destroy these elements by cauterisation. The presence of nerve filaments and capillaries close to the surface makes these lesions highly sensitive and liable to bleed. Operating on these lesions is extremely painful and this prevents complete reduction. Superficial callus should be reduced without causing haemorrhage, but should this occur, treatment with caustics must be delayed until the wound has healed. Any essential operation may be assisted by the pre-operative application for 5 minutes of 5% potassium hydroxide solution to soften the overlying callus. These lesions often have multiple small nuclei which cause further problems in reduction. Pain from the neural elements during operating is reputed to be controlled by the use of TENS, as discussed earlier. Rarely, a local anaesthetic by nerve block or infiltration may be indicated if extensive excision or electrosurgery to the lesion is contemplated, but progressive cauterisation is the less traumatic treatment of choice. Whichever method is chosen, these lesions are, by the nature of their pathology, extremely difficult to eradicate.

In vascular lesions, applications of 50% silver nitrate solution, following reduction without haemorrhage,

are effective over several weekly visits. This method may cause intense pain when used for neurovascular corns and is not recommended. An alternative is to apply 20% pyrogallic acid ointment, which is reputed to have analgesic properties, but since these lesions are frequently associated with devitalised tissues this must be used with extreme care. Only a small amount of the ointment should be smeared over the area and applied via a masking plaster. After 7 days, the eschar should be removed and treatment repeated, but this should not be carried out on more than three consecutive visits. Pyrogallol is cumulative and continuous in its action and can penetrate deeply, causing severe breakdown of tissue. This breakdown can in fact be a cause of neurovascular lesions, and leaves scarring. Its use should be avoided under several circumstances, including patients with circulatory impairment, peripheral neuropathy, diabetes, rheumatoid arthritis, elderly and debilitated patients, and areas with little subdermal tissue. Salicylic acid, as previously discussed, is also of use in lower percentages when tissue breakdown is unlikely, and where there is impairment of the blood supply.

Electrocautery may also be used in the treatment of such lesions. Local impairment of circulation may make its use more problematical and, while early results seem encouraging, longer-term evaluation needs to be made. Vascular and neurovascular corns are often associated with a loss of subdermal tissue, and it is possible that any long-term improvement may need to be coupled with silicone implants, which remain controversial.

Helomata miliare

These lesions are commonly associated with anhidrosis and may appear on any area of the plantar surface of the feet. They are not associated with pressure, and common sites are the medial longitudinal arch and the heel. They often present difficulties in management due to high recurrence rates, regardless of a high level of expertise in enucleation. Some authorities suggest that, if pain is not a feature, treatment should consist of control by the application of emollients or of the urea-containing compounds, such as 10% urea cream, which affect the keratin linkages and increase the moisture content of the epidermal cells. However, success is more likely if the corn is reduced prior to treatment with a medicament. The area can be softened pre-operatively with 5% potassium hydroxide or postoperatively with salicylic acid preparations. The percentage and base of the salicylic preparation will be dependent on the nature and site of the lesion, and on the vascular and neurological status. A short review date is necessary with this form of treatment. Alternatively, patients are advised on the use of emollients in the long term.

Palmoplantar hyperkeratosis

This condition and its associated punctate form present problems in management. It is described by Thomson & Cotton (1983) as follows:

Palmoplantar hyperkeratosis is a minor feature of several more generalised genetic disorders as in Darier's disease, recessive ichthyosis and congenital ectodermal dysplasia. There is also a group of genetic diseases in which palmoplantar hyperkeratosis is the major presenting feature.

These conditions produce keratotic thickenings which can cause severe discomfort and interfere with the gait cycle. Much research into the genetic influence on autosomal dominant ichthyosis vulgaris has not yet revealed causative factors. When it appears in large plaques surrounded by an inflammation, its operative removal is often limited by the discomfort, which may be minimised by the application of 5% potassium hydroxide solution. This also helps when reducing the punctate form by scalpel, but it is seldom possible to remove all the hypertrophic material. In many instances, complete removal causes the patient discomfort, if not pain, for several days following treatment.

The management of this condition consists of simple reduction of the hyperkeratotic areas, and the daily use by the patient of emollients or salicylic-based preparations, either by rubbing in daily or by occlusion overnight. The use of a cushioning insole often gives added relief from pain.

SHORT-TERM PADDING THERAPY
Digital padding for the lesser toes

The application of ointments to digital lesions necessitates appropriate padding to contain the medicament. In most instances this should be used either to redistribute the pressure from the lesion or to correct toe function.

The common deformities of the lesser toes are hammer, mallet, clawed, retracted and digiti quinti varus. These deformities may be purely local, as a result of footwear restrictions over a period of years, or secondary, due to a rearfoot or forefoot structural pathology.

Regardless of the cause, conditions such as clawed or retracted toes arise because of excessive extension or flexion. In addition there may be degrees of axial

rotation and medial or lateral deviation. Digital padding should be designed to exert maximum correction on such malalignments, since they are only rarely fixed and some degree of correction is almost always possible. The correction achieved in the majority of cases is functional and not structural. Permanent correction can only take place when the foot is held in the correct position by ligamentous and muscular action without any external help. However, in the young supple foot, opportunities for full correction are increased. These conditions do not usually affect one digit in isolation, and although one digit only may be affected with a hard corn, functional correction is obtained in most cases by regarding the middle three toes as one functional unit and, where necessary, correcting and protecting all three simultaneously through one device.

The common and major element in claw and retracted toes is an imbalance between the extensor and flexor muscles, and it is logical to control these elements by combined dorsoplantar splints (Fig. 12.1A & B). This will exert a reciprocal corrective pressure on the deformities. In a full dorsoplantar splint for the middle three toes, the dorsal pad exactly covers the proximal phalanges and controls any excessive flexion. The plantar pad underlies the intermediate and distal phalanges and controls any excessive flexion. Body weight immobilises the plantar pad against the sole of the shoe, and the dorsal pad is held firmly by pressure from the upper. The whole splint is thus securely in contact with the toes, correcting unwanted deviation in the interphalangeal joints, while the metatarsophalangeal joints are left to function normally. If there is limitation, particularly of dorsiflexion, at the metatarsophalangeal joints, then plantar padding is required in addition to the digital padding. This takes the form of a metatarsal bar (Fig. 12.2) or a plantar metatarsal pad behind metatarsals two, three and four (Fig. 12.3) to realign the metatarsophalangeal joints and deflect pressure away from the metatarsal heads, if they are receiving excessive pressure. In addition, where there is some contracture of soft tissue, exercises or manual stretching should be initiated to encourage an increase in the range of motion.

The clinical padding used to manufacture these temporary pads is firm felt and adhesive strapping. Although a standard format can be seen in Figure 12.1A, the basic shape can be adapted to deflect pressure from lesions on the dorsal aspect or the apices of the digits (Fig. 12.1B). The plantar pad can be extended as a prop under the fifth toe, or under the proximal phalanx of the hallux to correct hyperextension of the

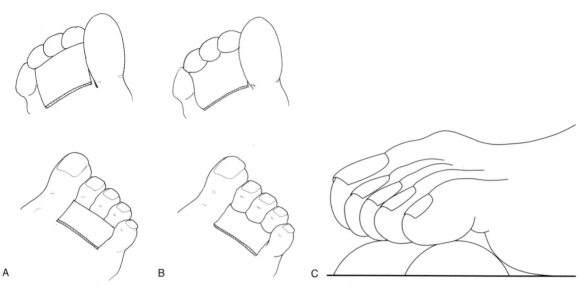

A   B   C

Figure 12.1   A: Combined dorsoplantar splint. B: Adapted combined dorsoplantar splint to obtain deflection from dorsal to apical lesions. C: Bolster pad for digits 2–4 when correction cannot be achieved. The bolster deflects pressure away from the apices.

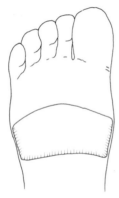

Figure 12.2   Metatarsal bar.

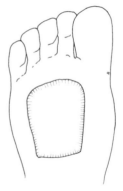

Figure 12.3   2–4 plantar metatarsal pad which may be placed over the metatarsal heads or immediately proximal to them.

distal phalanx. In addition, the splint can be made replaceable, although slippage may reduce the functional correction. The shape and thickness of each pad are determined by the needs of the individual patient, as is the relative degree of correction or protection required.

Felt padding is a relatively short-term measure for these splints and it is more efficient and effective to manufacture them in silicone. This material moulds itself into retaining grooves interdigitally and this controls any axial rotation and medial or lateral deviation of the digits. The digits must be held in the corrected

position until the silicone hardens. This is a minor disadvantage which requires considerable manual dexterity, but the advantages of holding the digits in their corrected position more accurately, being more durable and washable, outweigh the disadvantage (see Ch. 14). Because of the need for precision in the sizing and fitting of orthodigital splints, several important points need to be observed when this technique is used:

1. The full thickness of the dorsal pad must not extend any further proximally than the base of the

proximal phalanges, nor any further distally than the proximal interphalangeal joints (except if it is extended to include an oval cavity pad to protect a lesion).

2. The proximal edge of the plantar pad should conform to the plantar fatty pad of the foot, particularly where the fatty pad has been pulled distally due to the toe deformities. The full thickness of the pad should fit behind the pulp of the toes.

3. The pads must be thick enough to engage the pressure of the sole of the shoe on the plantar prop and the pressure of the shoe upper on the dorsal shield in order to maintain correction of the digits.

4. The medial and lateral edges of the pads should not overlap onto the first and fifth toes when all the toes are in a normally constricted position inside the footwear.

5. Good positional control for the plantar prop is maintained by allowing a concavity in each side of the pad to accommodate the pulp of the first and fifth toes.

6. Footwear should be of adequate length to accommodate the increased length of the foot with the toes in the corrected position, particularly if combined with a plantar pad to realign the metatarsophalangeal joints. In order to prevent crowding of the toes, the toe box of the shoe must be of the correct dimensions. Other points of well-fitting footwear are mandatory.

In fixed deformities of the lesser toes in the older patient, the splints are primarily for protection, by deflecting pressure away from dorsal and apical lesions, and will have no functional correction; they may, however, prevent further deformity. These pads are of similar dimensions but are shaped to mould to the position of the digits (Fig. 12.1C) and to act as a 'bolster' on the plantar surface of the digits, removing the pressure from the apices. In children, this form of padding should be firm and slightly oversized to ensure maximum correction. Photographic records are an excellent method of referencing correction under these circumstances, as are digital alginate casts taken at 3-monthly intervals.

Single-digit padding is sufficient when there is a fixed hammer or mallet deformity affecting only one digit. The fifth toe is particularly susceptible to pressure on the dorsal aspect from footwear when the digit is subluxated or in an adducted and varus position. Single padding will primarily have a protective role for dorsal, apical or interdigital lesions. These can take the form of oval cavity pads, crescent pads, 'U' pads (which may be in replaceable form) or props to the plantar surface of the toes, which may be shaped in the form of a crescent at the distal portion to protect lesions (Fig. 12.4). Silicone therapy should be initiated

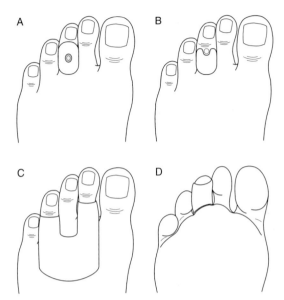

Figure 12.4 Single-digit padding. A: Oral cavity pad. B: Crescent pad. C: 'U' pad. D: Single prop. This padding is generally used to protect a lesion by deflection.

as soon as possible for the reasons stated above. It is moulded directly to the foot and this obviates any need for casting. An alternative to silicones for patients who have difficulty tolerating this form of orthosis is to cast the digit or digits in alginate and to manufacture a latex device incorporating the appropriate padding.

Plantar metatarsal padding

The range of movement in the metatarsophalangeal joints is crucial in determining the therapeutic objective and, consequently, the function, shape and material of the padding required. In the presence of chronic fixation, subluxation or dislocation of these joints, plantar metatarsal padding (PMP) is designed to palliate the consequential overloading of particular metatarsal heads, by redistributing the excessive load or by protecting them with a cushioning material. Cushioning is particularly important in the elderly when there is atrophy of the fibro-fatty pad underlying the metatarsal heads. In cases of mobile toe deformities in which the metatarsal heads are plantarflexed by the retracted phalanges, metatarsal padding assists in correcting the alignment of the affected metatarsophalangeal joint, particularly if combined with the use of digital dorsoplantar splints.

Footwear must be examined prior to the application of any padding and strapping to assess its suitability. It is essential that the footwear worn by the patient will accommodate the increased bulk of any padding and the increased length of the foot which results when corrective padding is applied. Initially, plantar metatarsal padding is most frequently used in its adhesive or replaceable form, but it is readily convertible for long-term use into the more durable form of metatarsal braces, or as one component of an accommodative insole or functional orthosis as appropriate.

The basic PMP (Fig.12.3) is shaped to cover the heads and approximately two-thirds of the shafts of the middle three metatarsals, in order that, on weight-bearing, they are relatively dorsiflexed, provided they are sufficiently mobile. The shape conforms closely to the underlying metatarsals, avoiding impinging on the first and fifth metatarsal heads, and taking into account variation in the metatarsal formula. The full thickness of the pad lies directly under the metatarsal heads and it is bevelled off from there in all directions, being carefully graduated on its proximal and distal edges to ensure that it is securely adhered, without any irregularities to cause discomfort under load. In addition to improving the alignment of the middle three metatarsals, it provides slight deflection away from the first and fifth metatarsal heads and it relieves symptoms of metatarsalgia. The improvement in the position of the clawed or retracted toes needs to be maintained with digital dorsoplantar splints.

In conjunction with plantar padding, metatarsal strapping is used to control excessive splaying of the forefoot. The strapping encircles the metatarsus immediately behind the first and fifth metatarsal heads, non-stretch material normally being preferable. A 'half-met' strapping may often be sufficient. This leaves the dorsum free, the ends terminating on the dorsum of the first and fifth shafts after traversing the plantar surface. Felt padding should be occluded with strapping; this is achieved by the application of two or three 5 cm wide straps, half-overlapping each other, and their lateral edges covered with 'side straps' with good anchorage to the skin (Fig. 12.5).

Adaptations from the basic PMP include single-wing pads (SW/PMP; Fig. 12.6A), double-wing pads (DW/PMP; Fig. 12.6B) and U-section cut-outs (U/PMP; Fig. 12.6C).

Winged pads are designed to protect either, or both, of the first and fifth metatarsal heads from overloading. This pad will deflect pressure from the first and fifth metatarsal heads onto the second, third and fourth metatarsal heads and down the shafts. When adhered to the foot, the wing is reverse bevelled, the

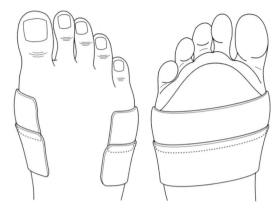

Figure 12.5 Strapping for plantar metatarsal padding.

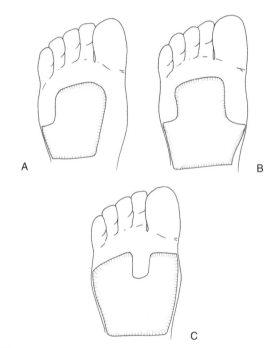

Figure 12.6 Plantar metatarsal strapping. A: Single-wing PMP to the fifth metatarsal head. B: Double-wing PMP to the first and fifth metatarsal heads. C: U-shaped PMP.

thickness of the wing fitting immediately around and behind the metatarsal head or heads concerned. For a SW/PMP to the first metatarsal head, the lateral edge of the pad is located over the area between the fourth and fifth metatarsal shafts. The medial edge of a SW/PMP to the fifth metatarsal head is located over the area between the first and second metatarsal shafts. With a medial wing, the overall width of the pad must conform closely to the medial curve of the footwear, so that no overlap of full-thickness material on the upper of the shoe is permitted, as this would unnecessarily tighten the vamp. The extra width required for anchorage is well bevelled and moulded around the metatarsal shaft. Full thickness will normally be provided under the middle metatarsal heads. This pad can be adapted to further increase metatarsophalangeal function by the addition of a metatarsal bar, or, if the first and fifth metatarsals are plantarflexed, by the addition of adapted shaft pads to those metatarsals, the distal aspect of the shafts stopping immediately proximal to the metatarsal heads.

The U-section pad is similar to the basic PMP but is extended across all five metatarsals, with the U-shaped section reverse bevelled and cut out over any one of the middle metatarsal heads. The function of this pad is to deflect pressure from a particular metatarsal head to the other metatarsal heads and down the shafts. A modified shaft pad may also be added behind the U-section to dorsiflex the metatarsal if motion is available. This pad follows the line of the toe webbing, but enough space is left distally to accommodate the strapping and it extends approximately two-thirds of the way down the shafts.

Metatarsal bars (Fig. 12.2) are functionally corrective pads and are designed to realign the metatarsophalangeal joints, increase toe function and deflect some pressure from the metatarsal heads down the metatarsal shafts. They are ineffective in high-heeled shoes. When adhered to the foot, the distal margin of the pad is reverse bevelled, the full thickness of the pad fitting immediately behind the metatarsal heads. The pad is contoured to the metatarsal formula and extends two-thirds of the way down the metatarsal shafts. It is adhered with non-stretch occlusive strapping, the toes being held in the neutral position when the distal strapping is applied.

Shaft pads (Fig. 12.7) may be used to any metatarsal (although the most common is to the first) and can be described as either long or short shaft pads. Long shaft pads (Fig. 12.7A) are used almost exclusively to the first metatarsal and extend to the interphalangeal joint at which point they are normally crescent-shaped and reverse bevelled. The purpose of a long shaft pad is to increase the weight-bearing through the metatarsal head, limit motion at the metatarsophalangeal joint and deflect pressure away from the interphalangeal joint. They are commonly used in hallux limitus/rigidus. Short shaft pads (Fig. 12.7B) stop distal to the metatarsal heads, the convex contour mimicking the metatarsal head, with the full thickness of the pad lying directly over the metatarsal head. They are

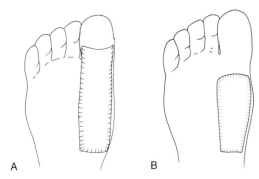

Figure 12.7 Shaft pads. A: Long shaft pad to the first metatarsal and proximal phalanx. B: Short shaft pad to the first metatarsal.

designed to increase the load to a particular metatarsal and realign the metatarsophalangeal joint. Perhaps the most common use is with a first metatarsal that is incompetent, for whatever reason. They are used in conjunction with interdigital wedges to treat interdigital corns in the web space.

VERRUCA PEDIS

Verrucae were thought to regress naturally after some months, thereby reducing the case for active treatment if they were not causing pain. Every practitioner knows, however, that they can remain unresolved for several years. Verrucae may be single, multiple or mosaic. Active treatment is indicated when pain is acute; when spread of the virus to other areas of the foot is observed; when the risk of cross-infection is high, as for other members of the same family; and when non-treatment would entail unacceptable limitations on activities such as swimming, games and athletics. Plastic waterproof socks are available for such activities to guard against cross-infection but are of little value in keeping dressings dry.

If treatment is to be commenced, it should be carried out quickly and effectively. The longer the time taken to reach a satisfactory conclusion, the greater the risk of producing a verruca resistant to treatment and causing pain to the patient. Most of the skin warts are caused by human papilloma viruses HPV 1, HPV 2, HPV 3 and HPV 4. Plantar warts associated with HPV 3 are thought to be particularly resistant to treatment. If the host immune response system is diminished, it allows the virus to replicate; however most people with verrucae have no major immune defect. In many cases, therefore, it is not an ineffective approach on the part of the practitioner that causes the verrucae to fail to resolve. Although only one foot may be affected, both feet should be kept under observation during treatment as a check against cross-infection.

Measures for the treatment of verrucae are centred on cell destruction techniques. Efforts to employ antiviral agents have not been successful. Existing methods include chemical cautery, cryotherapy, electrosurgery and laser therapy. In some instances, interactive dressings, astringents and homeopathic remedies are used when possible tissue breakdown is not desirable, as in the case of the 'at risk' patient. A growing number of practitioners are using actual cautery or curettage, with promising results.

Chemical cautery

This retains an important place in the treatment of verrucae and, properly employed, produces rapid results with minimal discomfort to the patient. Emphasis must be placed on the fact that chemical therapy can and does on occasions cause extreme pain and tissue breakdown. The stronger acids, such as monochloroacetic acid and pyrogallic acid, are particularly liable to cause tissue breakdown and pain. Although these acids can be accurately confined to the lesion on initial contact, whether in ointment or solution, when absorption into the tissues occurs there is no control over spread or depth (Fig. 12.8). Extreme care should be employed in their application.

The substances available for use include various preparations of salicylic acid, pyrogallic acid, monochloroacetic acid, trichloroacetic acid, nitric acid and potassium hydroxide, their caustic actions being strictly confined on application to the verruca tissue. The choice of agent depends on a number of factors, as all of the above have different actions and penetration potentials.

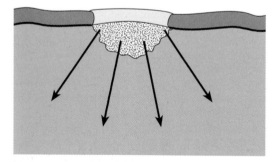

Figure 12.8 Absorption of acid into the tissues (arrows show directions of spread). Although medicament is confined at the surface, spread cannot be accurately controlled through the tissues.

Site. A lesion on a non-weight-bearing area is usually superficial, so liquid caustics are useful, e.g. salicylic preparations in collodion, trichloroacetic acid solution or a saturated solution of monochloroacetic acid used sparingly. A verruca on a weight-bearing area is relatively deeper, and thus both liquid and ointment preparations are suitable. However, care must be exercised in the use of caustics where there is little underlying adipose tissue, in order to avoid causing a severe breakdown or producing an inflammatory reaction in an underlying joint. In such a situation, less penetrating caustics or strong astringents are indicated. In certain cases where the verruca is on a site unsuitable for padding, treatments involving ointments cannot be carried out.

Number and size. These influence the form and strength of the medicament to be used. Large verrucae respond well to ointment preparations. However, when numerous growths are present, masking is difficult and pyrogallic acid may produce tissue toxicity if used in large quantities. A large growth surrounded by smaller satellites may be treated with 60–75% salicylic acid or 20–40% pyrogallic acid ointments, and the satellites with either salicylic, trichloroacetic, nitric or monochloroacetic acid solutions, or with toughened silver nitrate alone or in conjunction with trichloroacetic acid. In general, over a series of treatments, caustic ointments or solutions are indicated for one or more large growths, while multiple small verrucae are more easily treated with solutions. Cryotherapy or electrotherapy offer alternative single treatments for any type of verruca.

Skin texture. If moist, solutions of caustics are preferable, since there is no necessity to confine them within padding which would be contraindicated in the presence of hyperhidrosis. Fair-skinned people seem to be less tolerant to the action of acids and often react adversely to pyrogallic acid and silver nitrate. Tissues which are thin, dry and atrophied due to age or a systemic disorder do not tolerate acids and are liable to breakdown.

Circulation. When the arterial supply is reduced, as with a diabetic or atherosclerotic patient, ulceration of the area must be avoided since healing is delayed in these circumstances and bacterial infection could supervene. For the same reasons, similar care must be taken to avoid ulceration in the case of impaired venous circulation, which results in the tissues being oedematous. In such instances, caustics should be avoided and astringents or mild keratolytic agents employed.

Neuropathy. An inability to experience pain is a contraindication to any medicament likely to cause an inflammatory action or tissue breakdown. Astringents or mild keratolytic agents should again be employed.

Availability of patient. When powerful acids are used, it is essential to ensure that the patient is able to return within 7–10 days. Otherwise, an alternative form of treatment, such as cryotherapy or mild keratolytic agents, would be advisable. Home treatment is another possibility, provided the patient will adhere to the treatment regime.

Age. Very young children are often nervous, as well as seeming to have low pain thresholds. Skin texture also tends to be hyperhidrotic and they are normally very active with swimming or various other sporting activities.

Previous treatments. Where possible, the practitioner should establish which medicament has been used previously in order to reduce the risk of continuing a non-effective treatment or a treatment where there has been an adverse reaction.

All of the above and many other factors must be taken into account when deciding on the preferred method of treatment. Ointments or pastes will spread to normal surface tissue unless contained by careful masking of the adjacent healthy tissue. The surrounding skin is first masked by thick waterproof adhesive through which a hole, slightly smaller than the surface area of the verruca, has been cut. (A light application of silver nitrate to the periphery of the lesion by means of 95% silver nitrate stick gives added protection to the tissues.) The ointment is then applied through the hole to the verruca and sealed in with waterproof strapping to ensure its close contact. Alternatively, if more medicament is required after the initial masking tape is in position, a felt pad with an aperture of the same size is place over the verruca and the aperture filled with the ointment. If the first method is adopted then padding with a cavity to deflect pressure away from the area of the verruca and to relieve pain is applied, particularly if the lesion is on a weight-bearing area. The padding is totally covered with zinc oxide plaster, left in position for up to 7 days and kept dry to prevent spread of the acid (Fig. 12.9).

An appropriate instruction sheet must be given to patients receiving verruca treatment. This should include hygiene issues, method of treatment, specific instructions relating to the antidote to the medicament applied, keeping the area dry, and so on.

At the second and subsequent visits, the necrosed tissue is removed under strict antiseptic conditions. It is unlikely that one application will have resolved the verruca tissue, and subsequent applications of the caustic should be made and repeated as necessary

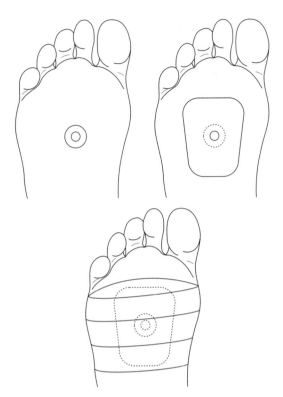

Figure 12.9   Masking of the tissues. Padding and occlusive strapping are used in the application of ointments in the treatment of verrucae.

until complete resolution has been achieved. The state of the skin should be taken into account when continued treatments are required, since maceration, either with the spread of salicylic preparations or with continual application of plaster to the skin, may require a different approach for a period of time.

The objective of treatment with acids is to produce an aseptic necrosis and resultant sloughing of the verruca tissue. With carefully controlled dosages and spacing of treatments, this is normally a painless, if prolonged, process. If tissue breakdown does occur, further applications of an acid should be stopped until healing has occurred. The resultant ulcer, although sterile, should be treated appropriately with a suitable antiseptic to prevent infection, or with one of the environmental dressings. Care should be taken when pyrogallic acid has been applied since, as the action is cumulative, residual action of the agent may continue. For this reason, pyrogallic acid should not be used on more than three consecutive visits.

It may be difficult to cope with the inevitable patient frustration when treatment is protracted. An initial explanation to the patient regarding the nature of the verruca, the treatment strategies available, and the difficulties in projecting a time for cure should ensure patient compliance.

Fewer practitioners than ever before are consistently using chemical therapy in the treatment of verrucae, because of the observable disadvantages to both practitioner and patient. Many routine practices with chemical therapy are now being re-examined and evaluated in the light of much research into the effectiveness of the various treatment modalities now available with the progress in biomedical science. Financial constraints, workloads and patient expectations have also had an impact in furthering research in this area.

Disadvantages of treatment with chemical therapy

- Treatment is time-consuming for both the practitioner and the patient, with continual short review dates of 7 days when using acids in ointment form. This is expensive for all concerned and is not cost effective.
- Padding applied continually over a period of time leaves the tissues macerated.
- Hygiene is problematical since the area must be kept dry.
- Penetration of the acid cannot be controlled and there is therefore the possibility of tissue breakdown which may leave scarring.
- No one chemical treatment can guarantee rapid results.
- All forms of treatment will cause a degree of discomfort or pain and inconvenience.
- Hyperhidrosis is a contraindication to the use of ointments, since padding containing the acid will not be secure on a moist skin and will lead to spread of the acid to normal tissue.

Therapeutic agents

Salicylic acid. This is one of the main agents used in the treatment of verrucae since it is available in many forms (ointments, pastes, solutions and collodion) and percentages (from 20% to 75%). It may be combined with 5% chloral hydrate for its analgesic effect. This acid became available over a century ago and is used widely by podiatrists and dermatologists in the treatment of verrucae. It is readily available in many proprietary forms from chemists for home use. The action of salicylic acid is primarily keratolytic. It causes a slow structural alteration to keratinised tissue, and in higher percentages produces an increasingly potent and rapid keratolytic effect on the stratum corneum. This causes maceration and epidermolysis. On non-keratinised tissue it has a destructive action, which as yet is not fully explained, and causes breakdown of tissue. This can be observed when reducing a verruca. The epidermal tissues appear intact to the practitioner, and when they are removed tissue breakdown is observed in the deeper tissues.

In solution or collodion bases, only a limited amount of the salicylic acid comes into contact with the verruca at any one time; it is easily confined to the area of the verruca and will produce a mild localised action. It is most commonly used on small lesions where there is little subcutaneous tissue, or on sites where padding is difficult, e.g. in the nail sulcus. These preparations are normally applied by the patient on a daily basis, and provided the application is restricted to the area of the verruca, it has a slow painless action. The resultant coagulum should be removed by the podiatrist every 14–21 days. This obviates the need for very short time-consuming return visits, the patient can bathe daily prior to application and there is no need for padding, although the area should be covered by a small plaster to prevent cross-infection. The ointment or paste forms are used in higher percentages and must be confined by masking the area and the use of padding. They produce a more localised drastic action when used on single verrucae on a site where there is adequate fibro-fatty padding. The action of salicylic acid can be enhanced by combining it with monochloroacetic acid. This can produce a violent reaction and should only be used with care on carefully selected patients. The monochloroacetic acid is usually used in saturated solution form and should be applied first. Continued use of salicylic acid may lead to a local dermatitis.

Monochloroacetic acid. This is available in solution or crystal form. It acts by hydrolysing proteins, converting the protein to soluble amino acids and peptides. It has a rapid penetrating action and may cause considerable pain. It is not unknown for patients to suffer from lymphangitis following too rigorous a treatment with this acid. It should only be used where there is adequate subcutaneous tissue; its use should be avoided over joints (periostitis or synovitis may result) and is contraindicated in the very young or elderly patient. It should never be used on a diabetic patient or those with peripheral vascular disease, or where healing is impaired due to the high risk of tissue breakdown. Prior to application, the superficial keratinised layers should be removed with no haemorrhage. The saturated solution should be carefully applied by means of an applicator stick directly and accurately to the verruca. Care must be taken to confine the application exactly to the verruca tissue, not allowing it to run over on to the surrounding skin. If deemed necessary, the surrounding skin can be protected by petroleum jelly as a masking material until the solution has been absorbed. If applied with care, this treatment is useful in the treatment of large single verrucae where padding is contraindicated, such as in hyperhidrotic states. If circumstances permit, padding may be applied to minimise pressure on the area. An alternative to the application of a saturated solution is to rub a crystal into the area for 30–60 seconds. This is a difficult procedure since the crystals are very friable. Crystals can be combined with the use of salicylic acid ointment but the practitioner should be aware of the depth which a combination of the two may achieve. The result may be a very deep penetrating ulcer with excessive destruction of tissue. The antidote to the action of monochloroacetic acid is 5% potassium hydroxide or sodium bicarbonate (1 in 80 solution), provided it is applied before the acid has been completely absorbed into the tissues. If the patient complains of pain some hours after application of the acid then a saline footbath should be recommended and a return to the practitioner to review the situation. Pain in such a short time is indicative of a violent inflammatory reaction associated with tissue breakdown.

Pyrogallic acid. This preparation is now becoming less readily available in the UK because of limitations on its manufacture imposed by the Medicines Act 1968. Its most common concentrations are 20%, 40% and 50%. Pyrogallic acid is a reducing agent which has a relatively slow cumulative action but has the ability to penetrate deeply. It should be used with care and, similarly to monochloroacetic acid, should not be used over large areas, near joints where there is a lack of subcutaneous tissue, on patients suffering from diabetes or peripheral vascular disease, or on the elderly or debilitated patient. Breakdown of tissue with the overuse of this medicament is likely to leave scarring. It should be limited to three consecutive applications. It should be applied with careful masking of the surrounding tissues.

Nitric acid. This is prepared from Chile saltpetre (sodium nitrate) or synthetically from nitrogen gas. The strong solution contains 70% nitric acid, and fumes when exposed to the air. On application it turns the tissues a yellow-brown colour. It is classed as an oxidising agent but it also precipitates the albumin of the tissues, thereby limiting its penetration; it then transforms the precipitated protein to other insoluble substances, which form an even greater barrier to the penetration of the acid. It therefore has a very localised surface action but a highly powerful one and must be applied strictly to the verruca tissue. It will not give rise to much pain if applied in small amounts. It can be used with care on shallow growths. Careful patient selection allows this medicament to be applied at home on a daily basis. Application is by means of an applicator stick directly to the surface of the verruca. It leaves a hard eschar. It is unsuitable for large deep growths as the action is very superficial.

Trichloroacetic acid. This is a protein precipitant which forms a barrier to its own penetration and is superficial in its action. Its action is slow and controlled. It can be used as a saturated solution where there is little adipose tissue between the verruca and underlying joints. It is ideal on shallow growths and mosaic verrucae and can be used by the patient at home. The application is as for nitric acid.

Potassium hydroxide. This is prepared in pellet form and it contains 85% potassium hydroxide. It is an extremely strong alkali which penetrates very deeply and is indicated in the treatment of large single verrucae when rapid action is required but the patient is unable to return at regular intervals, and provided there is adequate adipose tissue underlying the site of the verruca. The action of the caustic is stopped before the patient leaves the surgery. It is a method which does not require padding or strapping and therefore can be used in the presence of hyperhidrosis. As with any penetrating caustic, it should not be used on the previously quoted 'at risk' patients. Since it absorbs water to dissolve itself, the following method of application is appropriate.

All overlying callus should be reduced and the foot soaked in water for 5 minutes prior to application. The skin surrounding the verruca should be protected with Vaseline, petroleum jelly, or similar, to prevent spread of the potassium hydroxide to healthy tissue. The pellet is held with plastic forceps or with a specially designed applicator (for potassium hydroxide in 'stick' form) and is rubbed into the verruca for 2 minutes. The tissues will rapidly develop a white macerated appearance. If the application causes extreme pain, it should immediately be stopped. Following the 2-minute application, the foot should again be immersed in tepid water for a few minutes and on removal the resultant 'jelly-like' tissue should be carefully removed with a scalpel. The area should then be examined with a magnifying glass to establish if total clearance has been achieved. If there is any remaining verruca tissue, a small reapplication of potassium hydroxide should suffice. The area is then treated with 5% acetic acid to neutralise any remaining potassium hydroxide. This is not an infallible 'one-off' treatment since it is very difficult to distinguish any remaining verruca tissue with the naked eye. Following treatment, the area should be covered with an antiseptic dressing to prevent infection. The patient should be reviewed within 1 month, or sooner if any adverse reaction is noted by the patient.

Single-treatment techniques

These modalities are becoming more frequent in their use in the management of verrucae. They produce faster results in all but the most intransigent lesions, and the function of return appointments is to evaluate the success of the treatment and to dress any ulceration. Although classed as single-treatment techniques, there is not an absolute guarantee that this will be achieved.

The following methods fall into this category:

- cryotherapy, utilising liquid nitrogen or nitrous oxide
- electrosurgery, using coagulation, desiccation or fulguration (by 'hot-wire' cautery or with electrosurgical units)
- curettage
- laser emission.

Cryotherapy

Cryotherapy is a method of treatment which utilises profoundly low temperatures to destroy the tissues. Patients should be carefully selected prior to this procedure and those who have poor healing abilities for any reason, low pain thresholds and abnormal sensitivity reactions to cold should be excluded. It can be applied to a verruca of any size and on almost any site, since the depth of destruction can be controlled. The debate on the advantages, disadvantages and efficacy of this form of treatment continues, the major disadvantages being seen as the painful nature of the treatment, unforeseen adverse reactions with severe inflammatory states in some patients, and the initial monetary outlay for the equipment. These are offset by the relative safety of the procedure, since the operator can observe the growth of the ice-ball, knowing that the zone of demarcation will approximate to it. The area of cryonecrosis is of an inert quality. A sharp zone of demarcation is formed with a normally minimal inflammatory response. When the blister has resolved, there should be no scarring, and there is less danger of infection if the blister remains intact until healing has occurred. It is easy to use on difficult sites where oint-

ments are not indicated. It has a high success rate, is not time-consuming and does not entail frequent return visits. Padding is only necessary to relieve pressure after treatment if the verruca is on a weight-bearing area.

There are two main methods available to produce localised freezing of tissue (a third method is the use of carbon dioxide snow but this has been overtaken by more efficient methods and is now only of historical interest):

- *Nitrous oxide*, with a release of temperature of −88.5°C, which is employed in sophisticated apparatus using the Joule–Thompson principle. The various probe sizes available allow great accuracy in application and safety in use, but they also lose a significant temperature advantage. (Studies of over 100 applications show an average probe temperature of −52.4°C). Continued refinements to the apparatus are said to have largely overcome this problem although it is useful to be aware of a potentially significant rise in temperature.
- *Liquid nitrogen*, which has an operating temperature of −196°C. The apparatus available for its use is similar to the type of equipment available for nitrous oxide, and recent advances in manufacturing have made this technique more easily used. Due to the low release temperature, it would be expected that it is a more efficient modality than nitrous oxide, but empirical observation over a period of several years has not noted any appreciable difference in results between the two methods.

For cryosurgery to be successful the rate of freezing must be rapid, and all of the cells to be destroyed must reach a temperature of less than −20°C. This should achieve the intracellular formation of large ice crystals, which are necessary to rupture the cell membrane and cause the death of the cells. If the freezing rate is slower, the ice crystals may form in the intercellular spaces and the cell may survive. In recent experiments it has been shown that a repeat freeze technique induces immediate cell death.

Prior to the application of cold, all overlying callus must be reduced to facilitate the conduction of cold into the tissues. The following procedure may then be adopted:

1. A detailed explanation of the treatment should be given to the patient, including appropriate instructions to be followed after treatment (see Ch. 6). This should include the use of analgesics for any postoperative pain associated with the inflammatory reaction which will occur, and advice on self-treatment to burst

the blister if it becomes excessively filled with fluid and causes pain.

2. The apparatus should be checked for the correct pressure prior to commencement of treatment in order to achieve a fast freeze. The manufacturer's instructions should be adhered to in this respect.

3. A probe size equivalent to that of the verruca should be selected and a conducting medium such as KY jelly applied to the probe tip. The probe is applied with a slight pressure at right angles to the verruca. If the pressure is too great, the tissue surrounding the verruca will be blanched and it will be difficult to determine the 'halo' when it appears.

4. Begin the freeze, and release the slight pressure when the KY jelly turns white. This should not be mistaken for the 'halo', which is seen as a yellowish white ring to the outside of the frozen KY jelly. This halo identifies the extent of the tissue being frozen and is also referred to as the ice-ball. At this point the probe tip will be adhered to the tissues and cannot be removed until the probe tip has defrosted. Normal time of freeze is between 30 seconds and 2 minutes, depending on the size of the lesion and the modality chosen. Liquid nitrogen requires less freezing time than nitrous oxide. Timing of the freeze should begin once the halo is seen. A cryonecrosis depth of greater than 2–3 mm is not usually possible because the ice formed within the tissues acts as an insulator to further penetration of cold. Skin is thermally more resistant than mucosa.

5. Allow the tissues to thaw at normal room temperature. When normal colour returns, a repeat freeze should be carried out. A repeat freeze is more destructive of tissue than a single freeze. A third freeze is not normally required unless the lesion is very large or the freezing rate has been slow. Thaw cycles are normally of 1–2 minutes. Freeze times are longer on the plantar aspect of the foot where the epidermis is thicker. On the dorsum of toes, 30 seconds is often adequate. In this area, because of the thinner epidermis, the cold passes more quickly through the tissues and this can be observed by the growth of the ice-ball. If this extends beyond the margin of the verruca by more than 2 mm, freezing should be discontinued.

6. Silver nitrate may be applied over the verruca if desired, to harden the superficial tissues and prevent rupture of the blister. If necessary, apply a protective dressing to the area.

7. The patient may be seen again in 1 week to assess the effectiveness of the treatment. At this stage a blister should have formed around the entire lesion. The lesion may be cut out at this stage and the remaining ulcer treated with an appropriate antiseptic until healing is complete. Alternatively, the patient may be left for up to 6 weeks, when the blister will have resolved, and the dead verruca tissue removed with a scalpel. There are two schools of thought on which method is preferable. The advantage of the latter is that there is less danger of infection if the blister remains intact.

There are few dangers associated with cryosurgery other than accidental spillage of liquid nitrogen or accidental contact with freezing probes. The use of nitrous oxide equipment produces large volumes of the gas which must be vented outside the building. The risk of some genetic irregularities has been noted in anaesthetists of child-bearing age, due to prolonged exposure to nitrous oxide gas.

Electrosurgery

The term electrosurgery essentially describes three different types of procedure which utilise electricity in the performance of surgery—*electrocautery*, *electrolysis* and *high frequency electrosurgery*. However, electrosurgery is generally regarded as being synonymous with high frequency electrosurgery. With the advent of new equipment the latter type of electrosurgery is becoming the norm and it operates using a high frequency alternating current of above 0.1 MHz.

The most frequent application of electrosurgery is in the treatment of cutaneous lesions. Electrosurgery, particularly electrodesiccation, provides a simple and rapid method for the treatment of a wide variety of benign cutaneous lesions, such as verrucae and helomata. When using electrosurgery as a treatment modality, it is necessary to use local anaesthesia.

High frequency currents produce a rapid to and fro motion of molecules; friction from tissue resistance to this motion results in the production of heat. The amount and depth of heating are determined by the voltage and amperage of the current, the duration of application, resistivity of the tissue (bone has a greater resistivity than muscle) and the method of application. In electrosurgery, the current is emitted through a small electrode, producing a high intensity of the current, and is dispersed through a large electrode or plate, preventing unwanted damage to the tissue.

Safety. As with all electrical equipment, regular checks should be carried out and basic safety precautions, such as the removal of oxygen cylinders from the immediate vicinity, should be taken. Great care should be taken to ensure that the large dispersal plate makes good contact with the patient's skin. In podiatric procedures, a good area to apply the plate is to the posterior aspect of the calf. This large electrode offers a return pathway of least resistance for the current should the equipment malfunction or the patient touch a conductive surface during an electrosurgical procedure.

The use of electrosurgery is contraindicated where patients, or others, have cardiac pacemakers, particularly of the demand type. Extensive scar tissue or replacement joints between the two electrodes may intensify the current and cause tissue damage. Silastic implant joints may become distorted.

It has been shown that bacteria and viruses can survive on the emitting electrode, and therefore it is advisable to sterilise this probe after use.

High frequency electrosurgery. There are four forms of administration of electrosurgery: *fulguration*, *desiccation*, *coagulation* and *electrosection*. More recent equipment has been developed which combines desiccation and coagulation.

1. Fulguration. In this technique, the therapeutic probe is passed over the lesion to be treated at a distance of about 2 mm, so that the current arcs between the probe and the patient. This mode requires a higher voltage setting and produces wide sparks which result in superficial necroses which have the appearance of an eschar produced by silver nitrate. The necrosed area can be removed using a scalpel, thus making it possible to check the result and reapply the treatment. The lesion should be left as a necrosed surface, which need not be covered with a dressing, for 2–3 weeks and the result checked. This method of application is particularly suitable for superficial mosaic verrucae.

2. Desiccation. The probe is in contact with the lesion and the sparks produced are much less evident. It produces a deeper necrosis which is still confined to the epidermis and still has the appearance of an eschar produced by silver nitrate. This area can be removed with a scalpel and the procedure reapplied. It should be reviewed as above and is mainly used for the removal of mosaic and superficial verrucae.

3. Electrosection. Electrosection or the cutting of the tissues is achieved by the use of a very fine emitting electrode resembling a fine chisel or maybe a loop of wire. This electrode acts in the same way as a scalpel and allows accurate dissection of a lesion.

4. Combined electrodesiccation and coagulation. This type of unit has been developed for use in podiatry for the treatment of verrucae, fibrous plantar helomata or vascular and neurovascular lesions. The same electrode may be used in both modes, and output is varied by changing the setting on the unit. Electrodesiccation is particularly useful for the treatment of superficial cutaneous lesions, as it has the effect of removing moisture from tissue cells caus-

ing separation at the dermo-epidermal junction. Following removal of the lesion, the output may be altered to produce coagulation and the probe used to control any bleeding.

Before treating a lesion such as a heloma or verruca with a combined unit, it must be reduced in the normal way with a scalpel and a local anaesthetic administered. The unit is then set to desiccation mode and, keeping the tissues moist with sterile saline solution (to maximise the effect), the probe is held against the epidermis. Flow of the current produces a blanching of the tissues which should be repeated until the whole lesion shows this change. A separation at the dermo-epidermal junction causes a blister, the roof of which can be removed, leaving a clean sterile wound. The unit can then be set to coagulation mode and the electrode used to coagulate the base of the blister. A dry dressing may then be applied, together with any deflective padding which is indicated. Healing is usually quite rapid but a hard eschar may result, which should be removed with a scalpel.

Electrosurgery is a quick and relatively simple way of treating some of the most intractable podiatric lesions. For these reasons, it is becoming more widely used in the profession of podiatry.

Local anaesthesia and electrosurgery. The use of local anaesthetics to facilitate electrosurgery requires additional consideration, as the electrical current used to cauterise can stimulate nerve impulses to surmount the local anaesthetic blockade. It is recommended that the level of block be made more profound by the use of agents such as bupivacaine.

For verrucae or heloma durum on the digits, a digital nerve block is required, but local infiltration should suffice for any on the dorsum of the foot or on the non-weight-bearing plantar areas. The weight-bearing area where most verrucae occur is difficult to anaesthetise using local infiltration techniques, and it is usually better to employ a tibial nerve block to anaesthetise most of the plantar surface. If the verruca is on the lateral aspect of the heel, it may be necessary to block conduction in the sural nerve. The same criteria would also apply to plantar heloma durum.

Curettage

This technique tends to be regarded in an unfavourable light, but without adequate reason. There is some risk of scarring, but handled skilfully, curettage can give satisfactory results in the treatment of stubborn verrucae. The technique requires the administration of a local anaesthetic and, depending on the site, it may be convenient to apply a pressure cuff to control bleeding. The infiltration of local anaesthetics with a vaso-constrictive additive may also be used, to limit bleeding, if the site is suitable.

The edges of the verruca are located with a scalpel and, with a suitably sized Volkmann spoon, the wart can be scooped out of its location. Because this causes gross disruption of the papillae, it is necessary to apply a styptic, the most effective agent being 95% silver nitrate. It is wise to use a longer-lasting anaesthetic either at the outset or as a supplement. A sterile dressing and protective padding should be applied and the patient seen again in 3–7 days, and again after 1 month.

An alternative to the use of a Volkmann spoon is blunt dissection with a Macdonald's dissector. It is usually necessary to start the superficial separation with a scalpel, but blunt dissection is more accurate than cutting techniques and produces little postoperative bleeding. This method tends to be preferable when using electrosurgery, although some practitioners use sharp dissection coupled with forceps to elevate the tissue.

Laser emission

Laser (light amplification by stimulated emission of radiation) offers an alternative to electrosurgery. Laser emissions can be tailored to specific uses and have been employed with some success in dermatology and, more recently, in podiatry. Various types of laser are in use, the most commonly used, certainly in the dermatological field, being the carbon dioxide laser; more recently research has been carried out on the pulsed dye laser with good clinical results. The surgical laser is very versatile and allows more accurate localisation of tissue destruction than any previous technique. Surgery is conducted under local anaesthesia and the safety requirement for the use of class 4 surgical lasers must be observed: these include the use of protective goggles and a controlled environment with warning systems to indicate when the laser light is in use. The emission is directed onto the lesion and the tissue destruction is controlled by visual monitoring. The advantage of laser therapy is that the beam can be accurately controlled, with little or no resultant damage to the normal tissue surrounding the verruca. The area being treated remains blood-free due to immediate haemostasis, and therefore healing is rapid and postoperative pain and infection are diminished. In contrast, the disadvantages are a variation of penetration resulting from electrical wattage and focal distance, and the possibility of tissue damage because of excessive exposure leading to perma-

nent scarring. Other factors which prevent many practitioners from using this method are the initial cost of the laser and the adaptations required to the surgery to meet the health and safety requirements.

Therapeutic laser. This therapeutic modality is a low intensity laser therapy, and although its use in podiatry is relatively new, practitioners are recording satisfactory results with its use on various conditions, including verrucae. Other conditions suitable for its use are ulceration, inflammatory states, relief of pain in musculoskeletal disorders, both acute and chronic, and the reduction of oedema. Much of the therapeutic effect of low intensity laser therapy is by empirical observation or single case studies at present, but an increasing number of worthwhile scientific and medical research papers are becoming available (previously, a large number of research papers lacked validity), and in the foreseeable future it is set to become widely used in podiatry. There are a wide range of commercial systems currently available and a careful study should be made of the literature, the specifications supplied by the manufacturer and claims made regarding the efficacy of laser treatment (some of which are grossly exaggerated) before deciding on the laser of choice. The manufacturer's guidance should be followed for treatment times for verrucae. In practice the verruca tissue should be covered with an appropriate barrier film and the treatment probe placed directly onto the film at right angles to the skin surface directly over the verruca. The types of probe available include multiwave 'cluster' systems, which can contain up to 200 diodes, and single-diode treatment probes. Cluster probes are used to cover a large area in the case of multiple or mosaic verrucae, and the single probe is used for large single verrucae or in addition to the cluster probe for specific areas. This is not usually the first choice of treatment, but it is used for recalcitrant verrucae or where more vigorous methods are contraindicated, as in patients who are considered to be 'at risk'. However, caution should be exercised if treating patients with a decreased sensitivity to temperature or pain, even though this treatment modality is athermic and the danger of producing a burn in patients with a lack of sensitivity to heat is negligible.

Similarly, although no evidence exists to state that any damage is likely, treatment should be avoided over epiphyseal plates in children. With any relatively new treatment modality, the long-term effects are unknown. It is contraindicated in the presence of active malignant neoplasia, in patients who are photosensitive as in systemic lupus erythematosus, over areas of sensitised skin and in infected open wounds. A laser safety advisor should be consulted prior to the installation of the equipment, as local rules are variable.

Home treatments

Under certain circumstances, where patients are unable to attend on a regular basis and are unsuitable for, or do not wish to undergo, any of the above single treatments, verrucae may require to be treated with chemicals which can be safely used by the patient at home with only a limited amount of monitoring by the practitioner. The patient must be sufficiently cooperative to follow precisely instructions about the treatment. The problems with self-treatment are: patients must be motivated to carry out the treatment on a daily or twice daily basis; they may have difficulty restricting the medicament precisely to the verruca tissue; most treatments require the area to be covered with a plaster and this leads to maceration; spillage may occur and cause damage to clothing, etc. (for which the practitioner is not responsible). Some of these problems can be overcome with proprietary medicaments which come in containers with nozzles or applicators and in a quick-drying collodion gel base.

The most popular home treatments are salicylic acid preparations, gluteraldehyde and homeopathic preparations such as thuja occidentalis (available in ointment, solution or oral therapy). Podophyllum resin is present in some preparations incorporated with salicylic acid, but this can, on occasion, cause severe irritation and pain.

The actions and uses of salicylic have been discussed previously.

Gluteraldehyde (available as Glutarol solution— 10% gluteraldehyde) has the ability to combine with skin keratin and the reaction is seen as an intense brown stain on the skin surface. The reaction of gluteraldehyde with tissue proteins is complex and irreversible, and it combines with the keratin layer of the walls of the sweat duct to cause closure of the pore and produce anhidrosis. It penetrates the stratum corneum and the verruca tissue, and is reputed to have virucidal activity. Due to the amounts delivered to the tissues in solution, preferably twice daily, its action is relatively superficial. It is non-irritant, easy to apply and does not require any adhesive covering. Removal of the eschar should be carried out every 14–21 days. Mosaic plantar warts do not respond any better to this treatment than to any other.

An environmental dressing has recently been used in the treatment of verrucae, although it has been used in the management of ulcers for several years. Granuflex is a hydrocolloid dressing and produces a moistness in conjunction with a low grade hyperaemia. There has been no scientific evidence to date that this method has particular advantages over any other, but many practitioners advocate its application on mosaic-type verrucae. It is an ideal home treatment on patients who, for any reason, cannot tolerate medicaments, since tissue breakdown will not occur and instances of allergy are minimal. The dressing is changed every 4–5 days and the area need only be reduced monthly.

Podophyllum (syn. Wild Mandrake) is produced from the roots of a perennial herb. It has a cytotoxic action which causes a degeneration of epidermal cells and alters their metabolism. The resin does not penetrate easily and should not be used on verrucae with overlying callus unless it is combined with a keratolytic such as salicylic acid (available as Posalfilin— 20% podophyllum and 25% salicylic acid). Contraindications to its use are pregnancy, broken skin surface and continual use, which may cause dermatitis or severe tissue breakdown. It should only be used under supervision, and if pain or inflammation occurs then the treatment should be discontinued and warm saline footbaths given for their antiphlogistic action. It is dispensed in ointment form and the skin should be protected by means of an aperture plaster to protect the surrounding skin. A minimal amount of the ointment should be applied to the aperture, and it should then be covered with a waterproof plaster. The literature claims that the dressing should be renewed two to three times per week and when the verruca appears soft it should be left open to the atmosphere until it falls off. It is preferable that the coagulum is reduced by the practitioner every 2 weeks.

If any patient, in consultation with the podiatrist, decides on home treatment with a periodic review by the practitioner, an instruction sheet pertinent to that particular treatment should always be given in addition to verbal instructions (see Ch. 6).

Home treatments are usually prolonged and it is possible that natural regression will intervene. This may account for the wide range of self-treatments which are available and the success that is often ascribed to them; however, they are not always satisfactory and may result in more radical methods becoming necessary later.

INFLAMMATORY CONDITIONS
Perniosis (erythema pernio, chilblains)

Chilblains represent one of the conditions in which intervention to control the inflammatory process is necessary in order to prevent additional tissue damage. Theoretically, chilblains can be divided into four stages, but the initial stage, the *cyanotic* stage, often passes unnoticed. The *hyperaemic* stage is noticeable on examination and is symptomatic to the patient. This is followed by the *congestive* stage, after which the lesion may resolve or pass to the *ulcerative* or broken chilblain stage.

In the hyperaemic stage, the areas affected are variously described as red, hot, burning, itchy or painful. At this stage, the patient tends to scratch the area and this can in itself cause a break in the skin. The application of cold compresses is essential to control the symptoms of this stage and to reduce the volume of tissue fluid and blood in the area and diminish the possibility of broken chilblains. Cool evaporating dressings, such as gauze dressings, saturated with witch hazel, are invaluable.

At the congestive stage the principle of treatment is to stimulate the local circulation, and this can be achieved with the use of rubefacients, vasodilator creams or the application of heat. Care must be taken that the peripheral circulation is adequate to cope with the effect of the application of any of the above. Any counter-irritants or heat applied locally will cause an increase in cellular metabolism with a resultant increase in waste products. Cells require an adequate blood supply to deliver oxygen to meet their own increased demands and an adequate drainage system to remove the waste products. The action of a mild rubefacient with gentle massage to the area can be used to stimulate locally when the circulation is impaired, which is the case in many older patients. If appropriate, heat can be applied via the use of an infra-red heat lamp, wax baths or a warm footbath. There are numerous proprietary rubefacients and vasodilators available. If the overlying skin is friable, a solution of weak iodine BP painted on, followed by an application of tincture of benzoin compound, will reinforce the skin and minimise the risk of fissuring.

In elderly patients the risk of tissue breakdown is increased, although this may occur at any age. The most common site for broken chilblains is any area receiving excessive pressure or friction. The dorsum or apices of digits are particularly at risk, as are the medial aspect of the first metatarsal joint in association with hallux abductovalgus and the lateral aspect of a prominent fifth metatarsal head. The objective when this stage is reached is to encourage healing and prevent the entry and spread of infection. The site is extremely tender or painful, and the surrounding tissues are cyanotic due to a generally impaired blood supply in the majority of cases. Where the area has ulcerated in a younger healthy individual, usually as a result of trauma, the surrounding tissues exhibit the signs of an acute inflammation. Healing is achieved by removal of pressure from the area, which should include deflective padding and, if necessary, advice on footwear. Infection is prevented by the application of a topical antiseptic or interactive dressing. Patients who have circulatory or sensation impairment should be monitored very closely and, if deemed necessary, referred to their GP for antibiotic therapy.

Patients who are regularly subject to chilblains should be advised about preventative measures. These should not be limited to the foot but should include advice on keeping the legs warm—trousers and extra thick tights for ladies and 'long johns' for men. If prolonged exposure to cold is unavoidable, the feet should be warmed slowly and not immediately exposed to a source of heat. Warm lined footwear, thick woollen socks (or two pairs of fine socks) should be worn, provided they are not constricting and causing further local areas of ischaemia. Thermal insoles can be manufactured and inserted within the footwear to retain heat. If the footwear or hosiery becomes wet, this should be changed as soon as possible, since damp cold appears to precipitate the formation of chilblains more readily than dry cold conditions. The circulation can be stimulated by rubbing in a cream or ointment specially formulated for the treatment of chilblains, many of which contain an antipruritic agent. Some studies have shown the use of systemic therapy, such as nifedipine, to be of advantage in the treatment of chilblains, and this may prove of benefit to the patient with severe chilling and the complications of ulceration. It should be used only if prescribed by a general medical practitioner.

Ulceration

The management of established ulceration is discussed fully in Chapter 9. There is still much debate concerning the relative values of the various types of wound dressings, but there is overwhelming support from current literature relating to the use of interactive dressings. Regardless of the type of dressing favoured, it is essential to consider the cause and to remove pressure or friction from the ulcerated area. Much of the research into wound dressings has related to the lower limb, but not to the foot which is encased within a shoe and receives continual pressure and stresses when weight-bearing. This must be taken into account in the management; dressings alone will not suffice, and protective or deflective padding must be applied in conjunction with the dressing of choice. Consideration must also be given to footwear and the appropriate advice given—either modifications to existing footwear or, if this is impractical, prescriptive advice on the type of footwear required must be emphasised. In certain cases where there is gross foot deformity, surgical shoes may be necessary.

An additional form is that resulting mainly from sustained trauma as a complication of excessive pressure over areas of corn or callus. This is seen, typically, in conditions such as pes cavus where the foot is rigid and excessive pressure is found under the first and fifth metatarsal heads, and on the dorsum or apices of toes which are clawed, retracted or hammered. Subungual ulceration may be found in patients with peripheral vascular disease or where onychogryphosis or onychauxis is present. Removal of a section of the nail plate is necessary to expose the full extent of the ulceration prior to treatment. Prevention of recurrence can usually be achieved by regular reduction of the nail to a more normal thickness, and if necessary by using an orthotic deflective device. The condition is often aseptic in the early stages when tissue breakdown has occurred under an area of callus or thickened nail plate, but may later become invaded by pathogenic bacteria and display signs of inflammation, including those of cellulitis and lymphangitis if left untreated.

The overlying callus must be completely removed and the area drained of any pus and a swab sent for bacteriological examination. Swabs should always be taken from the sides and base of the ulcer to ensure that all possible bacteria invading the area will be cultured. Superficial swabs may not exhibit all infecting organisms and ineffective antibiotic cover may result. Treatment of an ulcer should be carried out under strict antiseptic conditions, including, inter alia, sterile gloves, sterile blades, dressings and a 'no-touch' technique in order to minimise the risk of cross-infection.

Following exposure and drainage of the ulcer, it should be irrigated with an isotonic sterile saline solution and then thoroughly dried with sterile gauze. Cotton wool should be avoided for this purpose since fibres of this material can be left in the ulcer, acting as a foreign body and delaying healing, causing hypergranulation tissue or trapping bacteria within the wound. The wound should be thoroughly examined and the following details noted: size, edges, state of the base of the ulcer, type and amount of discharge, state of surrounding tissue and any pain factor present. The state of the wound provides an indication of the type of dressing or antiseptic preparation to be applied (see Ch. 9).

The condition should be reviewed within 1–3 days, the deciding factor for return dates being any risk factors as presented by the patient. If extreme inflammation is present, the patient should be seen at short return dates until this has subsided, but any signs of cellulitis require immediate referral to the GP for antibiotic cover. Patients with ulcerative conditions which do not respond to treatment or recur frequently should be referred to their medical practitioner for more extensive investigation.

Sinus formation

Cases of chronic bursitis often result in the tracking of fluid to the surface and the organisation of a sinus which prevents closure and permits the entry of bacteria. Such sinuses may become plugged with hardened fluid and appear cornified, but are of a much softer consistency and are easily enucleated, exposing a clear viscous discharge of synovial fluid if no infection is present. However, as previously stated, this is an ideal portal of entry for bacteria, and closure of the sinus is the obvious objective, although one that is not easily achieved. Bursae are usually found over bony prominences on the dorsal aspect of the digits, the medial aspect of the first metatarsal head and the lateral aspect of the fifth metatarsal head, and easily become inflamed with pressure and friction. This should be minimised with orthoses and footwear modifications. Bursitis is also commonly found on the plantar aspect of the middle metatarsal heads in patients with rheumatoid arthritis affecting the foot, and sinus formation is a frequent complication.

Once the inflammation of the bursa has subsided, the main agents used to close the sinus are liquefied phenol BP, iodi fortis, 95% silver nitrate or 60% ferric chloride solution. Of these, the most effective is phenol, but due to its highly caustic properties it must be used with extreme care. One drop of liquefied phenol should be applied for 2–3 minutes, making sure it is confined to the sinus, which is then washed out with alcohol and covered with a sterile dressing. This should destroy the fibrous walls of the sinus and allow healing, without sinus formation, to take place. Progress of healing should be monitored every 5–7 days, with complete healing in 3–4 weeks. This procedure is unsuitable for any patient who is vascularly or neurologically compromised and should certainly not be used on patients who have rheumatoid arthritis. Iodi fortis or 60% ferric chloride should be applied to the walls of the sinus and the area covered with a sterile dressing; review appointments should be weekly, with reapplication if necessary.

DISORDERS OF THE SWEAT GLANDS

Hyperhidrosis

An hyperhidrotic skin loses its natural elasticity and cannot withstand tensile and shearing stresses, resulting in fissures and blisters. This is an ideal substrate for fungal and bacterial infections to establish themselves, and is a source of embarrassment to the patient.

In the management of hyperhidrosis, it is important to appraise all footwear worn by the patient and also the demands of their occupation. Instances exist where a patient's sensitivity to sweating and foot odour has led to the feet being enclosed in occlusive footwear when the reverse approach was indicated. Occupational factors are less easily controlled, but a willing approach by the patient can often improve the condition, in particular patient compliance with regard to footwear (leather) and hosiery (wool) which will absorb the sweat and prevent it lying on the skin. Various treatment strategies can be adopted for general hyperhidrosis of the feet, depending on the severity of the condition. These range from the application of dusting powders, through swabbing with an astringent lotion, to the administration of footbaths containing an astringent medicament. In cases of general, more severe hyperhidrosis, potassium permanganate crystals dissolved in a footbath are effective, cheap and easily obtained; care should be taken not to make the solution too strong or a brown discolouration of the skin will result. If the hyperhidrosis is severe, daily footbaths with tepid water and a few crystals of potassium permanganate (enough to turn the water pale pink) for 15 minutes over a period of a few weeks should result in a dramatic reduction of sweat symptoms. When the maceration has ceased, the frequency of the footbaths should be reduced to twice weekly. Footbaths containing 3% formalin may also be used, but care must be taken to avoid overuse due to the higher incidence of allergic reactions with this treatment. In less severe cases, contrast footbaths in conjunction with lotions and powders are effective.

The application of spirit-based astringent agents, e.g. 3% salicylic acid, may be applied interdigitally if there is excessive maceration, and the application of dusting powders is advantageous, particularly those which contain an antifungal agent. Interdigital fissuring should be treated rigorously with astringent antiseptics. There are many astringent, antiseptic and antifungal agents available commercially, including insoles which are absorbent and deodorising. The patient should be advised to dispense

with shoes and socks whenever possible, or to wear sandals, to pay particular attention to foot hygiene, to change hosiery daily and to alternate footwear.

This condition is rarely a short-term problem, nor is it one which can be permanently cured by any of the above treatments, but patient compliance to management is easily achieved because of the discomfort. If the excessive sweating of the foot is not an isolated entity, but is more general, help should be sought from a medical practitioner. It may be that the condition cannot be treated, but that underlying factors such as stress and diet can be controlled.

Anhidrosis

Many instances of this condition result from poor peripheral blood supply in the elderly, or in diabetic patients with autonomic neuropathy. Where this is the cause, little more can be done than to apply emollients regularly, preferably daily after washing. The choice of emollient matters little, since the purpose is to prevent moisture loss from the skin. Hydrous lanolin, E45 cream, white soft paraffin, urea-based preparations or proprietary medicaments incorporating lanolin are suitable.

The main complication of anhidrosis is the formation of fissures due to the reduction of epidermal elasticity and applied tensile stress. It can become a considerable problem, causing much pain and disability, as well as being a site for the entry of infection. It is most commonly found on the borders of the heel and is associated with callus formation.

Treatment consists of careful reduction of the callus at the edges of the fissures, application of an antiseptic cream and use of an occlusive dressing for a few days. An alternative to this, provided there is no infection present, is the application of tincture of benzoin to the fissure and approximation of the edges of the fissure with a suitable adhesive such as steri-strip sterile skin closures. This can be painful for the patient immediately on application, and in theory the occlusive qualities of the medicament are contraindicated on an open area, but the treatment is effective.

If the anhidrosis is severe and is associated with thickening of the stratum corneum, a thick layer of emollient occluded with polythene and left in situ overnight is a suitable treatment. Alternatively, 3% salicylic acid in white soft paraffin will have a softening action on the keratin. If fissures are open and infected, antiseptic emollient dressings are indicated until the lesion heals, followed by the regular application of emollients.

FUNGAL INFECTIONS

These are undoubtedly the most common types of infection seen by the podiatrist and are usually caused by *anthropophilic* (human to human) fungi. The source of the dermatophytes can also be *zoophilic* (animal to human) or *geophilic* (soil to human). The superficial fungal infections are most commonly caused by the dermatophytes or ringworm infections and superficial candidosis. The names given to fungal infections are variable and include ringworm, tinea or dermatophytosis. Most dermatophyte infections which involve skin are confined to the stratum corneum and rarely extend beyond the stratum granulosum unless there is hair follicle involvement. When hair follicles are involved, the infection is present in the dermis and there is destruction of the hair follicle. In the dermis, the fungi are surrounded by phagocytes or giant cells. Nail involvement with the superficial mycoses affects the epidermal tissue under the nail plate and causes modification of the epidermal cells and nail dystrophy. The dermatophytes include *Trichophyton*, *Epidermophyton* and *Microsporum*. *Candida albicans* is a normal inhabitant of the mouth, intestine and vaginal mucosa, but established infections may involve skin or nails of the feet. Interdigital infections with *Candida* are more commonly seen in warmer countries or in warmer weather, but onychomycosis due to *Candida* is more commonly seen in colder climates. Most *Candida* infections are endogenous, but under certain circumstances the disease is transmitted from person to person.

The healthy adult has a high level of immunity to fungal infections. This natural resistance is of a non-specific type and depends on genetic factors, age, nutrition and hormone balance. Another determinant is the mechanical barriers of intact skin surface secretions (fungicidal fatty acids in sweat and in sebaceous material). If the skin is degraded in any way—thin and devitalised, hyperhidrotic, fissured, blistered or abraded—then the likelihood of infection becoming established is enhanced. The underlying cause of the fungal infection should be treated, as well as the symptoms. Patients who have diabetes appear to be particularly prone to fungal infection of the feet, especially interdigitally. This is probably due to the increased level of available sugar in the tissues and reduced phagocyte efficiency. Patients on long-term antibiotic therapy are susceptible to fungal infections due to the reduction of the normal skin commensals which compete with the fungi for adherence sites. Immunosuppression through illness, drugs or a congenital condition will also predispose to an increased incidence of infection with either the dermatophyte or *Candida* infections.

Tinea pedis

Tinea pedis is most commonly found in adults; it is relatively uncommon in children. The common causative organisms in this country in order of frequency are: *Trichophyton rubrum*, *T. interdigitale*, *Epidermophyton floccosum*, *Microsporum canis* (cat and dog ringworm), *T. verrucosum* and *T. mentagrophytes*. Less frequently, the following may be isolated: *T. tonsurans*, *erinacei* and *M. gypseum*. *Scopulariopsis brevicaulis* can cause onychomycosis in nails which are already affected by a pathological process such as onychauxis or onychogryphosis, and is most commonly found in the first toenail. Other fungi which can be isolated from dystrophic nails are *Aspergillus*, *Fusarium* and *Pyrenochaeta*. *Candida albicans* can affect skin and nail, particularly at the base of the nail plate under the eponychium, where it is very difficult to eradicate due to its inaccessibility. Interdigitally, *Candida* infections are frequently secondary to dermatophyte infections with associated fissuring. A severe *Candida* infection—*chronic mucocutaneous candidosis*—is a chronic condition, relatively uncommon, which presents in childhood and affects the mouth, skin and nail. In the foot, it is associated with hyperkeratotic areas and dystrophic nails.

The only positive means by which the infecting organism can be identified is by laboratory diagnosis. Superficial mycoses will be identified by direct microscopy and culture. In skin mycosis, the skin scrapings should be taken from the active margin of the skin affected, and if vesicles are present the active fungal cells will be contained in the roof of the blister, which should be removed completely for analysis. Prior to removal of scrapings for mycological examination, the skin should be swabbed with alcohol to remove any medication which may have been applied. Scrapings from nails should be from the undersurface and as far proximally as possible. Fungi in the distal portion of the nail may not be viable if the infection is active proximally, and scrapings taken from that area are frequently negative on culture.

Infection of the host by the fungi is due to penetration of keratinised cells. Fungi are able to enter the keratinised cells by producing enzymes which can degrade or split the keratin, and the fungal hyphae are able to penetrate between the keratinocytes. Consideration of the epidemiological factors involved in dermatophyte infections is relevant when considering the treatment of tinea pedis. The incidence rises in winter with the wearing of occlusive footwear. The main areas where conditions are suitable for transmission of infection are swimming pools, communal changing areas, such as in sports halls and schools, industrial shower rooms used by employees after work, e.g. miners or service-men, or any area where there is liable to be infected skin squames on floors. Dermatophytes can survive for months if not years in desquamated skin cells. If the infection is zoophilic and the infected human has a cat or dog, the infected material is likely to be from the home and the spread can occur directly from the pet or from chairs, floors or floor coverings. An atypical mycosis may have been acquired by a patient who has travelled abroad, particularly outside Europe. This should always be taken into account if an unusual clinical picture is seen.

General issues regarding treatment should be identifying the probable source if possible, and advice on avoidance, foot hygiene and type of footwear. Advice should be given to eliminate barefoot contact with all surfaces which are liable to be contaminated. Personal foot hygiene should be of the highest standard, the feet should be meticulously dried and the shared use of towels or footwear should be avoided. The type of footwear worn by the patient should be considered and, if occlusive footwear cannot be entirely avoided because of the occupation, open sandals should be advised whenever possible to allow free circulation of air. Hosiery should be changed daily and shoes should be regarded as a potential source of reinfection and can be treated with a fumigating agent, e.g. 10% formalin solution. Care must be taken to aerate the shoes prior to use to avoid irritation caused by the formalin. Disinfection of shoes is easily achieved by placing formalin in a shallow container such as a tin lid inside the shoe, placing the shoes inside a plastic bag and leaving for 24 hours. Provided the ambient temperature is about 15°C, the inside of the shoe will be exposed to a high concentration of formalin.

Clinical features

These vary with the severity, site and infecting organism. In its mildest form, tinea pedis may be confused with erythrasma, and the symptoms are negligible. In the more severe form, there is associated inflammation, maceration, fissuring, bleeding, blistering and the possibility of a superimposed bacterial infection. Regardless of severity, similar treatment strategies should be adopted to prevent spread of the fungal infection.

Interdigital areas are most commonly affected in the first instance, particularly the third and fourth web space. The appearance can vary from simple scaling of the skin, with minimal itching, to macerated raw areas with spread of the infection to the undersurface of the toes or to the dorsum of the foot with blistering and

inflammation. There may well be a superimposed bacterial infection with a Gram-negative bacteria. This is commonly of the *Pseudomonas* type. Blistering is usually associated with *T. interdigitale*.

The sole of the foot in the area of the medial longitudinal arch may be affected. The skin in this area tends to be dry, flaky and inflamed, with associated blistering. Differential diagnosis is with pustular psoriasis and eczema. It may spread to the whole of the sole and encroach on the medial and lateral borders of the foot and the dorsum of the toes. In this instance, it is described as a moccasin-type fungal infection due to its typical distribution. Common infecting organisms in this type of dry scaly infection are *T. rubrum* or *E. floccosum*.

Fungal infections associated with hyperkeratosis are commonly found in the heel area, and treatment of this area requires reduction of keratin, either by scalpel and/or with a keratolytic agent, in addition to a fungicidal preparation. The area of the heel appears dry, with fissuring and surrounding inflammation.

Treatment

Fungal infections can spread to any area of the skin or to the nails. It is essential that treatment is effective to prevent spread and reinfection. Treatment should be continued for several months after the clinical signs and symptoms have subsided, in an effort to prevent recurrence. The use of fungicidal powders as a prophylactic measure should be continued indefinitely in patients who are susceptible to infection.

Fungicidal preparations are dispensed in various forms. Topically they can be applied as creams, ointments, lotions, aerosol sprays and powders. These are effective if the infection is not widespread or involves the nails. The time taken to clear the infection is normally about 4 weeks, but the relapse rate is high. This is not surprising if the source of infection has not been identified and eliminated. There is a wide variety of antifungal preparations available without prescription. The choice of base is dependent on the state of the skin. Ointments are normally avoided on moist surfaces because of their occlusive properties; lotions are less occlusive and are indicated interdigitally, on pustular areas and over large areas. Dusting powders must be used in conjunction with either of the above when a fungal infection is present, but may be used alone as a prophylactic measure when infection has cleared. Powders may also be used inside footwear and hosiery. All of the above should be sparingly applied to the affected areas two to three times daily, with regular washing between applications.

In some instances, other actions are required in addition to the use of a fungicide. If inflammation is present, a preparation containing hydrocortisone may be required and is useful in the treatment of eczematous areas which are secondarily infected with fungi. Preparations of this type should be used for a few days only, until the inflammation has subsided, and then a routine fungicidal preparation applied. They should be used with care on children and in pregnancy. Overdosage in topically applied steroid preparations can occur if used long-term on large areas and if absorbed in sufficient amounts to produce systemic effects. If a mild bacterial infection is present, the antifungal agents should be combined with a bactericidal agent, even though some fungicidal agents are effective on some Gram-positive and Gram-negative bacteria. Alternatively, if the bacterial infection is extensive or severe, it should be cleared with antiseptic preparations, or antibiotic therapy if necessary, before commencing treatment with a fungicidal preparation. Keratolytic agents may also be combined with a fungicidal preparation for areas with associated hyperkeratosis.

Some preparations exert a fungistatic/fungicidal action by a variety of mechanisms. Some agents used in the treatment of superficial mycoses may have little or no direct action on the fungi at the concentrations employed, and their beneficial actions are not related to their direct action on fungi, e.g. keratolytics, but they reduce the infection by causing desquamation of the infected keratinised cells.

Antiseptic antifungal preparations tend to have a weak action to both types of infection and they are often messy to apply and can stain the skin, as in the case of brilliant green, Castellani's paint or compound dye. Resorcinol is both bactericidal and fungicidal and also has mild keratolytic properties. It is usually applied in ointment, cream or lotion from between 1% and 10%. Anaflex cream, which contains 10% polynoxylan, is reputed to have an antifungal action. It is an ideal medicament to use initially when there is a coexistent bacterial infection, before changing to a medicament with a more definitive antifungal action. All of the above would be slower in action than drugs which are specifically antifungal.

Keratolytic preparations assist in removing the stratum corneum. The best known example for use on fungal infections is Whitfield's ointment, containing 6% benzoic acid and 3% salicylic acid. It combines the fungistatic action of benzoate and the keratolytic action of salicylic acid. The combination of the two enhances the keratolytic action. Since the dermatophytes reside in the stratum corneum, where keratin is the substrate, desquamation removes the fungus as well as aiding in the penetration of the drug. Since benzoic acid is only fungistatic, eradication of the infection will only occur once the infected stratum corneum has been shed; therefore, continuous application may be required for several months (depending on the extent of the keratin build-up). Long-term application is inadvisable since this is an irritant. This preparation should only be used on hyperkeratotic areas and not interdigitally or on the medial longitudinal arch area where there is no build-up of keratin, as this would result in prominent itching and an undesirable keratolytic action. Mild irritation may occur at the edges of hyperkeratotic areas. The ideal site for the use of this medicament is the heel area. Application is by rubbing in the cream on a twice daily basis, or by a once daily application of a thin layer of cream under an occlusive dressing. Another combination is benzoyl peroxide and potassium hydroxyquinoline sulphate. The combination of the two gives antiseptic, keratolytic and antifungal activity. This is effective against common fungal infections and is available as quinoderm cream and quinoped.

Topical therapy with specific antifungal preparations gives the practitioner and patient a wide selection from which to choose. The following are some of the most commonly used preparations:

Undecenoic acid. This drug is primarily fungistatic, although fungicidal activity may be observed with long exposure to high concentrations of the agent. It is effective against the common pathogens in superficial mycoses of the feet. Concentrations as high as 10% may be applied to the skin. Preparations are not usually irritating, and sensitisation to them is uncommon. It is beneficial in retarding fungal growth in tinea pedis, but the infection frequently persists despite extensive treatment with preparations of the acid and zinc salts. At best, the clinical cure rate is 50%. This is much lower than with tolnaftate and the imidazoles. Preparations containing undecenoic acid are Monphyton, Mycota, Phytocil and Tineafax.

Tolnaftate. This is effective in the treatment of cutaneous mycosis caused by a wide range of the *Trichophyton* species, *E. floccosum* and several of the *Microsporum* species. It is ineffective against *Candida* and less effective in the presence of hyperkeratotic lesions. In tinea pedis the cure rate is around 80%. It is available as Tinaderm and Timoped.

The imidazoles. These have a broad-spectrum antifungal activity and are effective, topically, against nearly all the fungi of clinical interest in podiatry. They are also effective against some bacteria and protozoa. Acquired resistance to imidazoles rarely occurs and has only been seen with *Candida albicans*. The imidazoles are active at the cell wall level of fungi. They inhibit the incorporation of acetate into ergosterol (which is important for the integrity and function of the fungal cell membrane). This causes leakage of cellular contents, and the uptake of essential nutrients is impaired. This explains their selectivity for fungi and the low toxicity to human cells. They are more effective than the undecenoates and tolnaftate in treating superficial skin mycoses. *Candida* fungal infections may also be treated by topical application with the broad-spectrum antifungal preparations 1% clotrimazole (available as Canesten), 1% econazole (available as Ecostatin and Pevaryl) and 2% miconazole (available as Daktarin and Dermonistat).

Any of the above drugs which contain hydrocortisone or nystatin are available only on prescription. Examples of this are Tinaderm M (tolnaftate), Quinoderm cream with 1% hydrocortisone (benzoyl peroxide and potassium hydroxyquinoline sulphate), Daktacort (miconazole) and Econacort (econazole). Others in the azole group are available as topical therapy, but they are prescription-only medicines and include sulconazole (available as Exelderm) and ketoconazole (available as Nizoral).

Without doubt, the most effective topical fungicidal agent to date is terbinafine — available as Lamisil. This is an allylamine antifungal preparation which blocks ergosterol formation in the cell membrane through inhibition of squalene epoxidase. It is effective against the dermatophytes and *Candida*. Unfortunately, at present this is a prescription-only drug. It is also available as an oral preparation and need only be taken for 2 weeks to eradicate skin infections. The reinfection rate with this drug is low, certainly within 6 months of therapy being completed. Other oral therapies include griseofulvin, which is incorporated into keratin and blocks the intracellular microtubules of the fungi, and the azoles, which block ergosterol formation in the cell membrane. All oral therapies are by prescription only.

Onychomycosis (tinea unguium)

Clinical features

In dermatophyte infections of the nail, the clinical appearance is variable, depending on the stage of infection. Initially, only the distal or lateral edges of the nail will be affected, and a white discolouration spreading proximally with some onycholysis will be seen. When the disease is established, the nail will be thickened and crumbly with a yellowish discolouration, and eventually the whole nail plate may be involved. Onychomycosis frequently coexists with skin infection and is often a result of spread from the skin. A vigilant practitioner will be alert to the early signs of infection and early treatment will lead to a higher cure rate with topical applications of a fungicide. Differential diagnosis is with psoriatic nails, onychauxis and onychogryphosis. The commonest cause of onychomycosis is *T. rubrum* and occasionally *T. interdigitale*. There are other dermatophytes of the *Trichophyton* and *Microsporum* species which normally cause scalp infections but which may infect the nails and cause an atypical appearance of pitting, ridging and splitting of the nail plate. *Scopulariopsis brevicaulis* also causes a form of onychomycosis which usually affects the first toenail. It has a brownish appearance and the nail is not crumbly. It infects nails which have previously been traumatised (on rare occasions it can affect the interdigital spaces). Other fungi which may affect dystrophic nails are *Aspergillus*, *Fusarium* and *Pyrenochaeta*.

Treatment

Nail infections are very difficult to eradicate with topical applications of fungicidal preparations, because the infection initially affects the nail on the undersurface and the nail bed is also infected (see Ch. 8). The nail itself acts as a barrier to the absorption of any cream or lotion, and even when the nail is thinned down as far as possible to facilitate this process, it is still an extremely protracted treatment. Creams or lotions should be applied daily and are more effective if the nail plate is occluded, since this enhances penetration of the medicament. This, however, leads to further problems with maceration of the surrounding tissues. Patient compliance often fails due to the time taken to eradicate the infection, which may be anything from 12 to 18 months, if ever. The success rate is extremely low with this method of treatment.

Alternatively, the nail plate may be avulsed with or without phenolisation of the matrix. If the latter method is used, the nail bed must be treated with a fungicidal cream to eliminate the infection from this area or from any modified nail tissue adhering to the nail bed. This must be achieved prior to regrowth of the nail. During the regrowth period, the podiatrist must remove modified callus from the nail bed to ensure that infection is totally eradicated. This is a more effective, although radical, form of treatment than topical preparations only, and is suitable if only one or two nails are affected. When the use of local analgesia is contraindicated, medical avulsion may be attempted with the use of 40% urea cream, and thereafter topical antifungal preparations applied as described above. Although this procedure is painless, success in avulsion is not guaranteed. The surrounding tissues must be protected from the urea cream by the application of an occlusive dressing such as tegaderm or opsite, and this is also applied over the cream to contain it, followed by the application of a tubular gauze dressing. The medicament should be left in situ for 7 days and, frequently, a further application is necessary to achieve complete avulsion.

Systemic treatment of onychomycosis is now probably the treatment of choice in adults. Terbinafine is achieving excellent results with oral therapy, with eradication of the fungus from the nails after only 3 months of treatment, as opposed to a low 40% success rate after 12 months of therapy with griseofulvin.

Any of the creams or lotions mentioned previously for the treatment of tinea pedis may be used in the treatment of onychomycosis. In addition, there are preparations which are specifically for nail infections, such as borotannic complex. This may be used in conjunction with salicylic acid, methyl salicylate and acetic acid. The method of action is that, on application to the nail, the solvents evaporate at body temperature, leaving a clear film over the infected area. Perspiration will dissolve the active complex, which ionises, producing a local area of low pH (about 2.0) that is fungicidal. It is available in a clear straw-coloured paint as Phytex and Onychocil. With both of these preparations, the manufacturers do not recommend occlusive dressings.

Another drug, amorolfine, differs chemically from other antifungals and affects most superficial fungi. It is available as Loceryl, which is a lacquer and is painted over the affected nail plate. Tioconazole is available in solution as Trosyl for use in onychomycosis. It is applied topically to the infected nail. It also contains an undecenoic acid base. The diffusion of tioconazole into human nail tissue is facilitated by long-chain fatty acids and alcohols. Because of the undecenoic acid present in the solution, tioconazole penetrates the nail plate extensively. Unfortunately, success rates are disappointing.

Candidosis

Candida infections can affect both skin and nail (see Ch. 8). The most common sites in the foot to be affected are the interdigital spaces and the nail. In appearance, the web spaces are extremely macerated, with open fissures, and have a distinctive yeast odour. It may be secondary to a dermatophyte infection, and in contrast to the dermatophyte infections it is unlikely to

spread. Paronychia as a result of a *Candida* infection is usually chronic in nature and caused by the *albicans* or *parapsilosis* species. The nail folds and surrounding tissues are grossly inflamed and painful. The affected border of the nail will exhibit onycholysis and there will be a discharge of pus. Staphylococcal and Gram-negative infections may also coexist, and therefore bacteriological identification should also be sought. The nail plate itself may become infected in association with paronychia. The nail plate will not become thickened, but onycholysis and destruction of the distal end of the nail plate may result. This condition is more common when Raynaud's disease, chronic chilblains or Cushing's syndrome are present. It is unusual to find associated skin symptoms elsewhere on the foot.

Most of the superficial *Candida* infections respond to topical applications of the azoles, terbinafine or nystatin. For paronychia, the treatment should be in solution form to enable it to run into the nail folds, and treatment should be continued for 3–4 months. Oral therapy with terbinafine, itraconazole or ketoconazole is necessary when the nail plate is involved.

ACUTE AND CHRONIC INFLAMMATORY CONDITIONS

Inflammatory states arising from trauma may require two methods of treatment that complement each other. The first aims to reduce and control inflammation and swelling by the application of cold when the inflammation is in the acute stage. This is achieved by cold compresses or ice packs. When the inflammation is chronic and congestion of the area is evident, mild heat in the form of ultrasound is recommended. Therapeutic laser and magnetopulse therapy are invaluable to hasten the healing process. A major advantage of magnetopulse is that the padding and strapping need not be removed during treatment. The second method is to support and rest the affected part by the use of padding and strapping.

Padding can be applied directly to the foot or inserted into the patient's footwear as a transitional stage pending the manufacture and fitting of orthoses. Although orthotic therapy is essential in the longer term, immediate relief or reduction of pain is primarily achieved by padding and strapping.

Tension strappings

Figure-of-eight strapping for the foot and ankle (Fig. 12.10)

This strapping may be used for various conditions:

- to support a sprained or weak ankle, either inversion or eversion sprains
- to support a strained foot
- to limit painful movement in the subtalar and midtarsal joints
- to relieve tensile stress on the plantar fascia and its calcaneal attachment.

Depending on which structures require to be supported or rested, this strapping can be applied in order to invert the foot and to support the structures on the medial aspect of the foot and ankle. Medial support is required, with or without the addition of valgus padding or 'D' pads, in cases of sprain of the deltoid ligament, acute or chronic footstrain and plantar fasciitis. Conversely, it may be applied in such a way as to support the structures on the lateral side of the foot and ankle. Lateral support is required, with or without a tarsal platform or 'filler pad', in cases of sprain of the external lateral ligaments of the ankle, and in some cases of pes cavus with associated postural instability. It may also be applied to hold the foot in a neutral position and to reduce tensile stress on the plantar aspect of the foot, and limit the motions in all directions. This is indicated in arthritis of the tarsal region.

The strapping of choice is a 5 cm (2 inches) or 6.25 cm ($2\frac{1}{2}$ inches) elastic adhesive bandage. This is preferable to non-stretch strapping, particularly where oedema is present, as it is less constricting. If hyperhidrosis is present or the patient is allergic to this material, it may be applied over a soft cotton bandage. On the dorsum of the foot, in order to prevent the plaster sticking to hair, cotton wool can be dragged across the sticky surface of the strapping to that area only. There will be some stretch of the material during walking, but if necessary this can be minimised by the addition of two pieces of non-stretch strapping to reinforce and prolong the support given. Of necessity, these strappings are short-term only and should not be reapplied if the skin becomes extremely macerated or signs of allergic dermatitis appear. If reapplication of adhesive plaster is contraindicated but support or limitation of movement is still required, the same strapping may be applied utilising crepe bandage. This will reduce the support which can be achieved and it is also a bulkier form of strapping, which may cause constriction in the footwear, but is a valuable alternative.

Medial support

1. If required, apply a valgus or 'D' pad (Fig. 12.10A).
2. Anchor the first non-stretch strap anteroposteriorly to the lateral side of the foot, and pass it around and behind the calcaneum as low down on the heel as possible. Apply sufficient tension to invert the heel before securing the end of the strap along the medial and dorsal aspects of the first metatarsal, which must be held in plantarflexion. This locks the calcaneum into inversion by supinating the subtalar joint (Fig. 12.10B).
3. From immediately behind the base of the toes on the dorsum of the foot (to prevent swelling occurring here), apply the stretch strapping laterally and obliquely around the forefoot to complete one turn of the metatarsus, then continue round the tarsus with

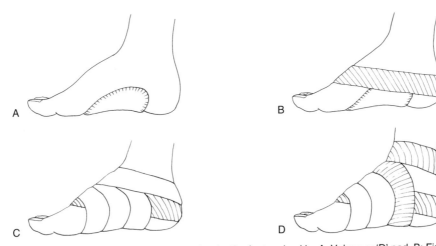

Figure 12.10 Figure-of-eight strapping for the foot and ankle. A: Valgus or 'D' pad. B: First non-stretch tension strap to invert the heel. C: Figure-of-eight elastic strapping. D: Second non-stretch reinforcing strap.

upward tension on the medial border before encircling the ankle and heel as low down as before in order to maintain maximum inversion.

4. Continue across the front of the ankle and once more round the tarsus, from lateral to medial, before again encircling the ankle at a higher level. The second strap should overlap the first by half its width, and should also well cover the malleoli so that it may be finally secured to the leg above the ankle (Fig. 12.10C).

5. Apply the final reinforcing strap of non-stretch strapping to form a 'figure-of-eight' around the tarsus and the malleoli, the lower loop providing a supporting cradle or 'stirrup' while the upper affords a firm attachment to the leg above the ankle (Fig. 12.10D).

The strapping should just avoid the anterior margin of the plantar fatty pad, leaving it free to change shape on weight-bearing, otherwise the edge of the strapping cutting across the fatty pad will cause discomfort.

Depending on the degree of support or correction required, valgus padding may be incorporated into this strapping; it is applied to the foot before the strapping is in place, or alternatively it may be inserted into the shoe. Firm supporting footwear must be worn at all times with this strapping, the unshod foot never being allowed to bear weight. This strapping will give support for up to 10 days before requiring renewal.

Lateral support. The technique is similar to the strapping for medial support but the strapping is applied in the reverse direction, the upward tension being exerted on the lateral side of the foot which is held in eversion. No preliminary reinforcing strap is necessary to evert the foot, but the final reinforcing strap should be applied as previously described but in the reverse direction. Additional lateral support can be provided if necessary by fitting a tarsal platform into the shoe.

Neutral support. The object of this strapping is to restrain painful movement in the tarsal joints. The most comfortable position of the foot should first be established by passive manipulation. No preliminary reinforcing strap is necessary. The flexible bandage is applied as for medial support but without the medial tension. The final reinforcing strap is applied with approximately equal tension on the medial and lateral borders of the foot before being secured to the leg above the ankle. Additional mediolateral support can be provided, if required, by fitting a combined tarsal platform and valgus pad into the shoe—the 'tarsal cradle'.

Care must be taken when applying any restricting strapping to the foot when oedema is present or gravitational swelling occurs towards the end of the day. Advice should be given regarding elevation of the limb, but if the swelling is severe enough to cause discomfort or restrict the circulation to the digits, then the patient should be advised to cut through the strapping on the dorsal aspect up to the level of the base of the metatarsals. This will relieve some of the pressure but will continue to give some support to the foot and ankle. If this is insufficient, then the strapping must be removed or reapplied in the form of a crepe bandage which can be removed by the patient and reapplied the following morning.

Orthotic techniques appropriate as follow-up to figure-of-eight foot and ankle strappings may be any of the following: elastic anklets, corrective or palliative orthoses incorporating valgus, tarsal platform or combined tarsal cradle support, buttressed heels and wedged heels. Unlike the strapping, however, all such devices provide only passive support or correction.

Valgus padding

Valgus padding, so called because it is used in cases of valgus foot, has two separate but related elements, a plantar cushion and a medial flange. The plantar cushion fills the concavity of the longitudinal arch, with the object of affording support to the joints and the muscular and ligamentous attachments which become strained in abnormal pronation. It is essentially palliative in function.

The medial flange extends towards, and if necessary over, the prominences of the sustentaculum tali and the tuberosity of the navicular. Its function is to encourage some degree of inversion of the foot and thereby some correction of abnormal pronation. This is achieved by the pressure of the padding against the firm counter of the shoe. Where such correction is possible, it should be initiated primarily be means of medial heel wedging, but the medial flange is often necessary to supplement the correction.

It follows, therefore, that the design of valgus padding must be varied considerably to meet individual needs. When applied directly to the foot, it is constructed of a compressed felt material of either 5 or 7 mm thickness.

Applications

- As part of a figure-of-eight strapping for footstrain; a thin felt pad having both elements is usually required (Fig. 12.10A)
- As a temporary palliative orthosis or shoe insert; the plantar element alone may be adequate to control symptoms

- As a permanent feature of an accommodative insole for pes planovalgus; both elements are usually required in combination with medial heel wedging. The shape, texture and density of the materials used must be varied to suit the needs of each case and will depend on whether the objective is correction or palliation
- In metatarsalgia and in hallux rigidus, with the addition of metatarsal padding and a shaft pad, respectively.

Valgus padding is contraindicated in the presence of occlusive arterial disease, as it may compress and occlude the plantar arteries and exacerbate or initiate the symptoms of intermittent claudication in the foot. Nor should the plantar element be used alone and continuously as a form of so-called 'arch support'. The degree of compression of the plantar soft tissues required in the attempt to provide direct support to the skeletal arch in that way is likely to produce an unacceptable degree of wasting of the plantar soft tissues. Control of the calcaneal eversion by heel wedging and the medial flange incorporated into an orthotic device is the preferred therapy in chronic abnormal pronation.

Tarsal platform ('filler pad') (Fig. 12.11)

The tarsal platform or 'filler pad' is never applied to the foot except as a short-term measure. It is mainly used as a component of orthoses or as an insert in footwear. Its main function is to bring the lateral border of a highly arched foot into firm contact with the waist of the shoe. By raising the floor level to the foot, it enlarges the weight-bearing area and to that extent relieves the loading on the heel and the metatarsal heads. It also tends to evert the foot, and is useful where there is peroneal strain.

The basic design is that of a platform of firm material extending the full width of the insole, from the anterior margin of the heel seat to just behind the tread (Fig.12.11A). It fills the empty space between the lateral border of a highly arched foot and the waist of the shoe. There is no contact between it and the plantar aspect of the medial longitudinal arch, the bulk of the padding on the medial side serving only to anchor it more firmly to the waist of the shoe. It is the limitation of contact to the lateral border only which tends to evert the foot, thus stabilising the ankle in cases of abnormal inversion. The medial portion of the padding also provides the base for additional valgus padding where this is needed to form a tarsal cradle.

When required, the anterior edge of the platform

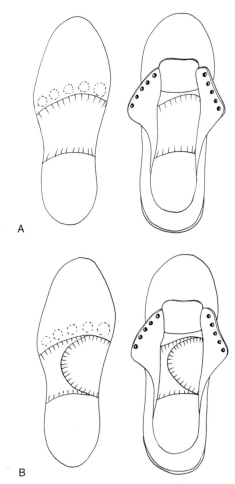

A

B

Figure 12.11 Tarsal platform ('filler pad') and extended to tarsal cradle. A: Tarsal platform on a leatherboard insole. B: Tarsal cradle (combination of platform and valgus or 'D' pad).

may be thickened to form a metatarsal bar, or may be extended under the three middle metatarsal heads to form a 'double-winged' metatarsal pad to protect the first and fifth metatarsal heads; extended as shafts under the first and fifth to protect the middle three; or extended as a shaft under the first alone in hallux rigidus.

Applications

- In *pes cavus*, to redistribute weight from the heel and metatarsal heads
- In *persistent ankle sprain*, to stabilise the foot by obviating forced inversion
- In *painful heel*, in conjunction with a heel cushion.

The combination is more effective than heel cushioning alone and is indicated in all such cases regardless of the height of the longitudinal arch

• In *metatarsalgia* and plantar lesions, in conjunction with suitably shaped metatarsal padding
• In *tarsal arthritis*, in conjunction with valgus padding to form a tarsal cradle.

Tarsal cradle (Fig. 12.11)

This is a combination of a tarsal platform with a valgus support superimposed on it, which provides support for both medial and lateral borders of the foot and restrains the movement of inversion and eversion. Its main application is in tarsal arthritis when it may be used to augment the effect of a neutral figure-of-eight strapping. Like the tarsal platform, it is not applied to the foot but is used as a component of an insole or as an insert in the footwear.

It also has an important application in restraining hypermobility and elongation of the foot in cases of abnormal pronation associated with calcaneocuboid subluxation. The cuboid underlies the front of the calcaneus by a process which extends from its medial, plantar and posterior aspects. Pressure on this process as the calcaneus everts causes some axial rotation of the cuboid and consequential hypermobility of the fourth and fifth metatarsals. In such cases, support to the lateral segment of the foot is necessary, in addition to that provided to the medial segment. The tarsal platform element under the cuboid stabilises the lateral segment much as the valgus element stabilises the medial segment, the entire foot thus being cradled and stabilised much more effectively than by valgus support alone.

Padding and strapping for hallux abductovalgus

The padding and strapping selected for this condition would depend on the cause, mobility and age of the patient. The cause should always be considered, and the application and structure of the padding then related to it. Adhesive padding is always used as a temporary measure prior to the manufacture of orthoses, and the size and shape of the footwear must be given full consideration for both the short- and long-term management of the condition. Strapping may be used on a younger patient with incipient hallux abductovalgus (HAV) to lessen the deviation of the hallux, and thereby relieve strain on the periarticular tissues, and to protect the medial eminence from shoe pressure. In an established case of HAV where correction is impossible, podiatric management consists of protection of the medial eminence by means of a felt crescent or oval cavity pad. The efficacy of this form of deflective padding is dependent on the degree of deformity present. If the degree of deformity is great, then footwear modifications in the form of balloon patches are essential to relieve pressure from the area. Often it is not the medial eminence which is the cause of discomfort but the resultant areas of overloading on the plantar aspect of the foot and the pressure on toe deformities. The most common site of corn/callus on the plantar aspect is on the second, third and fourth metatarsal heads, or any combination of the same. This is due to an incompetent first metatarsal and toe deformities. The padding/orthosis applied should relate to the cause of the overloading. In this instance, a short shaft to the first metatarsal combined with a metatarsal bar should increase the loading through the first metatarsal head and realign the lesser toes if sufficient movement is available.

In a younger patient, where there is still mobility in the joint and passive movement can return the angulation to near normal, it is imperative that a biomechanical assessment is carried out to ascertain if an underlying malalignment, such as forefoot varus, may be responsible for abnormal foot function and the development of the HAV. In this instance, although strapping may be used as suggested above, it is imperative that a functional orthosis is in situ as soon as possible to prevent further deformity occurring. This management strategy should include the use of an exercise regime, night splints if appropriate, correction of any lesser toe deformities associated with the condition (see Silicones, p. 286), and precise footwear advice pertinent to the individual patient. Silicone devices in the form of an orthodigital splint embracing the middle three toes and an interdigital wedge for the first cleft eliminate any possibility of the lesser digits being abducted by the wedge, since they are firmly fixed against the sole of the shoe by superimposed weight. For this reason, the interdigital wedge in this form also exerts better control on the hallux to prevent further lateral deviation.

The strapping of choice is adhesive stockinette or similar, which has one-way stretch only. This is cut into a flask or 'butterfly' shape and the anterior ends are first adhered to the hallux and secured there by a narrow strapping. The non-stretch dimension of this material must lie anteroposteriorly. The main part of the stockinette is then drawn back over the joint with sufficient tension to correct the line of the hallux to the extent required. The 'wings' are then stretched laterally across the dorsal and plantar surfaces of the

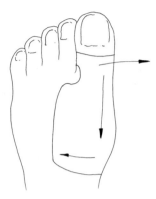

Figure 12.12 Flask strapping to realign hallux abductus. It is first adhered round the hallux; then the hallux is passively moved from its abducted position; after which the strapping is applied with sufficient tension over the prominence and down the medial side of the foot, before being stretched laterally.

metatarsal and adhered, covering any padding which has been applied to the joint. (Fig. 12.12.)

Padding and strapping for hallux limitus/rigidus

The acute form of hallux rigidus is occasionally seen in the younger age group, often associated with a sports injury or repeated minor trauma due to a biomechanical dysfunction, but it is relatively uncommon. It is an extremely painful condition and is associated with inflammation and muscle spasm, traumatic synovitis and subsequent capsular contraction mainly on the plantar surface. Untreated cases, or where there is repeated minor trauma, may display some marginal dorsal osseous lipping and may progress to chronic hallux limitus/rigidus. This often depends on the effectiveness of the treatment at the acute stage and also on the cause. The clinical features are of a rapid onset associated with pain and stiffness in the first metatarsophalangeal joint. The patient has great difficulty in weight-bearing on the area and walks with the foot in a supinated position. Although the joint has inflammatory changes, they are not always obvious superficially. The great toe is frequently held in a plantarflexed position due to muscle spasm.

The treatment of acute hallux rigidus consists of an appropriate physical therapy to reduce the inflammation and pain in the joint and rest. If acutely inflamed, the patient may find contrast footbaths more beneficial initially, prior to the application of heat. In severe cases, rest will consist of total non-weight-bearing and may require a plaster cast, although this is a rare

occurrence. On occasion, hydrocortisone injections into the joint may be required. Normally, padding or strapping to reduce movement and relieve pressure on the first metatarsophalangeal joint on weight-bearing is sufficient. A single-wing metatarsal pad is often the most readily tolerated padding, as it relieves the load on the painful joint, facilitates the inverted position of the foot which is adopted in such cases, and thus helps to minimise dorsiflexion at the joint. As soon as the pain and muscle spasm have been relieved, discontinue the padding and strapping but continue the heat therapy and restore normal movement in the joint by gentle traction and circumduction exercises. It is essential with acute hallux rigidus that the predisposing cause is identified and treated to prevent long-term problems with the joint function.

Chronic hallux limitus/rigidus is a slowly progressive disorder, but may halt at any stage, i.e. it may not become completely fixed. It may or may not be associated with pain in varying degrees. The loss or limitation of movement in the first metatarsophalangeal joint may be associated with pain, especially after walking a distance; however, the pain may be due only to associated lesions. The symptoms of pain will be exacerbated with the wearing of a higher heeled shoe. Because of the lack of movement at the metatarsophalangeal joint, this detracts from the fulcrum action of the great toe. Pain in the first metatarsophalangeal joint may cause the patient to walk on the outer border of the foot and utilise the interphalangeal joint at the propulsive phase of gait when weight is transferred to the medial side of the foot. Secondary problems which may occur in the longer term are as follows:

- due to the foot functioning in a supinated position, there may be the formation of corn and callus on the fifth metatarsal head
- in a foot which adopts a less supinated position, corn and callus may be evident on the second metatarsal head
- the compensatory hyperextension which occurs at the interphalangeal joint leads to callus formation on that area
- there may be strain of the lateral ligaments of the ankle due to the instability of the foot (supination)
- on the dorsal aspect of the first metatarsophalangeal joint, due to dorsal lipping of the metatarsal head, an adventitious bursa may develop from irritation caused by footwear.

These secondary problems must be addressed with appropriate padding and footwear advice.

Pain produced at the first metatarsophalangeal joint on movement can be alleviated by limiting this move-

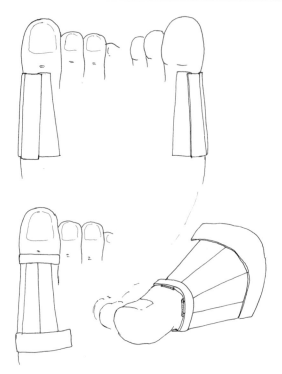

Figure 12.13 Fan strapping for hallux limitus. May be used alone, as illustrated, or in conjunction with a shaft pad.

ment. This can be achieved by means of a long shaft pad applied with rigid 'fan' strapping. If there is insufficient room within the shoe, then the 'fan' strapping may be applied alone. This strapping utilises rigid adhesive strapping of 2.5 cm (1 inch) width (Fig. 12.13). With the first metatarsophalangeal joint held in the neutral position, the strapping is applied from a point just proximal to the interphalangeal joint of the great toe to the base of the first metatarsal. There are five pieces of strapping applied in the following order: the plantar, dorsal and medial aspects of the first ray, and the final two pieces of strapping fill in the spaces between the previous three straps. This is an extremely effective method of limiting the movement in the joint. The strapping is adhered at the distal and proximal margins, as illustrated. Patients obtain great relief from padding and strapping, but at the earliest opportunity long-term orthoses should be prescribed, taking into account the biomechanical abnormality which has led to the pathological changes occurring in the joint. When strapping is contraindicated, the joint can be immobilised by the temporary use of a leatherboard template with a shaft adhered to its undersurface made from either a thin rigid polythene material or other rigid material. The above measures will be inef-

fective unless the appropriate footwear advice is given and adhered to by the patient. There must be sufficient length and depth to the shoes to prevent any impaction of the proximal phalanx on the metatarsal head or pressure on an enlarged joint. The heel height should not be higher than 3 cm and there should be a retaining medium to prevent forward movement and stubbing of the great toe. The sole should be rigid, with an adequate toe spring to assist function at the propulsive phase of the gait cycle. If there is abnormal excessive pronation, the counter of the shoe should be stiff and a patient-specific orthotic may be prescribed to prevent the pronation occurring. Adaptations to footwear, if required, consist of a rocker bar added to the outer soles of the shoe to enable the foot to 'rock' over the fixed joint. A steel stiffener may be inserted between the outer and middle soles to reduce movement and pain in a joint where complete fixation has not yet occurred. These measures can be carried out by a competent shoe repairer or cobbler. Patients who are in occupations which enable them to choose any type of footwear frequently find that clogs are extremely comfortable, and if pain is a factor it is remarkably reduced with this form of footwear. Other measures which may be adopted are stretching or balloon patching to accommodate any joint enlargement, exostosis or bursa formation (see Ch. 14).

Plantar digital neuritis

This condition may be present with or without any obvious structural abnormality and this can make the selection of padding and strapping uncertain. It should be explained to the patient that there are several forms of padding which may alleviate the pain, and when the most appropriate padding has been ascertained it will be manufactured into a long-term orthotic device. A plantar metatarsal pad with a 'U' to the painful area is most often effective when applied with a full metatarsal strapping. Alternatively, a short shaft pad, 2–4 PMP or a metatarsal bar may be the padding of choice. All are commonly used in conjunction with digital splints to realign the toes if necessary. The patient should be reviewed 1 week after the padding is applied, in order to gauge its effectiveness.

Plantar fasciitis

In this condition the main sites of pain are along the medial bands of the plantar fascia and, in addition, there may be localised pain over the medial tubercle of the calcaneum. Pain is felt on initial weight-bearing in the morning or after a period of rest. Prolonged walking gives rise to continuous pain along the medial lon-gitudinal arch of the foot and may be extremely crip-pling. There are various causes for this condition, of which the most common biomechanical condition is excessive abnormal pronation at the subtalar joint. A change of occupation, which involves continuous standing or unaccustomed walking, may be a contribut-ing factor, as may be a sudden excessive weight gain. In addition to the use of therapeutic laser or ultrasound therapy, the application of clinical strapping followed by orthotic therapy is required. As discussed earlier in this chapter, the use of figure-of-eight strapping to invert the calcaneus, either alone or in conjunction with a tarsal platform, is helpful. When the pain is pri-marily along the medial longitudinal arch and there is limited sign of abnormal pronation, the use of *bow* strapping is effective in obtaining short-term relief (Fig. 12.14). This reduces the tensile stress on the fas-cia, and therefore reduces the pain during weight-bearing, and in addition takes up very little room in the shoe. Rigid strapping is used for this purpose in two widths, 2.5 cm (1 inch) for the bands running from the metatarsal head to the heel, and 3.75 cm ($1\frac{1}{2}$ inches) for the strapping across the plantar from the lateral to the medial sides of the foot.

Method of applying strapping

1. Place the foot at right angles to the leg and anchor the first non-stretch strip of 2.5 cm strapping directly over the first metatarsal head. Following the line of the metatarsal, bowstring the strapping along the medial

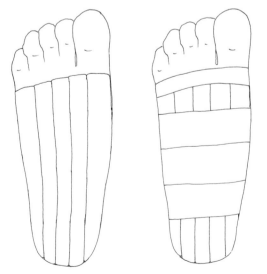

Figure 12.14 Bow strapping for relief of pain in the plantar fascia.

plantar border of the foot and attach it to the medial plantar aspect of the heel; continue round the posterior aspect of the calcaneum by about 2 cm. If the foot to which the strapping is being applied is particularly broad, this first strap may be of 3.75 cm width.

2. This procedure is continued with a further four lengths of strapping, corresponding to the second, third, fourth and fifth metatarsals. Tension must always be maintained when applying the strapping, avoiding any slackness.

3. The first transverse strap is applied just proximal to the metatarsal heads, tension being applied from the lateral to the medial side of the foot. The lateral and medial margins of the strapping are attached on the dorsum of the foot over the fifth and first metatarsal shafts. The second transverse strapping is applied just distal to the medial tubercle of the calcaneum. Two further transverse strappings are required to complete the *filling-in* process.

4. The edges of the strapping are collectively adhered under an edge strapping of 2.5 cm width, which is applied in one length from the fifth metatarsal head on the dorsal aspect of the foot, along the lateral border, round the posterior of the heel, along the medial border and up to the dorsal aspect of the first metatarsal head.

This strapping removes the tensile stress from the plantar fascia on weight-bearing, but as with all other short-term strappings, its use should be limited until an orthotic which is specific to the foot problem has been fitted. It is also essential with painful inflamma-tory conditions to consider the concurrent use of addi-tional therapies.

March fracture

Although this condition requires orthopaedic inter-vention in the form of a walking plaster, relief from pain on weight-bearing can be achieved in the short term by means of a 7 mm plantar metatarsal pad with a deep 'U' cut out over the affected metatarsal.

Freiberg's infraction

Rarely is surgical intervention attempted for this con-dition. Since it requires long-term therapy consisting of removal of pressure from the affected metatarsal head for up to 2 years in order to reduce deformity to a minimum, the optimum therapy is orthotic manage-ment. This should take into account not only removal of pressure from the affected area, but also any biome-chanical malalignments which may be present.

In the short term the padding of choice is a plantar metatarsal pad with a 'U' to the affected metatarsal head, combined with a metatarsal bar to remove as much pressure as possible on weight-bearing. It is important that shoe length is adequate and no back pressure from the phalanx is referred to the metatarsal head. A shoe with a low heel should be advised.

FURTHER READING

On hyperkeratosis
de Launey W E, Land W A 1984 Principles and practice of dermatology. Butterworth, Borough Green
Marks R, Christophers E 1981 The epidermis in disease. MTP Press, Lancaster
Thomson A D, Cotton R E 1983 Lecture notes on pathology, 3rd edn. Blackwell, London

On fungal infection
Emmons C W, Bunford C H, Utz J P, Kwong Chung K J 1977 Medical mycology, 3rd edn. Lea & Febiger, Philadelphia

Frey D, Oldfield R J, Bridger R C 1977 A colour atlas of pathogenic fungi. Wolfe, London

General
Benett R G 1988 Fundamentals of cutaneous surgery. Mosby, St Louis, chs 17, 32
Goodman-Gilman A, Goodman L S 1985 The pharmacological basis of therapeutics, 7th edn. Collier Macmillan, New York

13

Clinical pharmacology

R. M. Morgan

Keywords

Administration of drugs
Dose and frequency of dose
Drugs acting on infections
Drugs acting on the cardiovascular system
Drugs acting on the central nervous system
Drugs acting on the endocrine system
Drugs acting on the gastrointestinal system
Drugs acting on the respiratory system
Drugs used in rheumatic diseases
Excretion
Metabolism
Rate of absorption
Route of administration

Pharmacology is the study of the effects of chemicals on the cells and tissues of the body. These chemicals may be endogenous substances, such as the neurotransmitter noradrenaline, or foreign molecules, such as drugs and poisons. In this chapter, we will consider some of the more commonly used groups of drugs and highlight areas where the podiatrist may need to be vigilant in discussions with patients.

It is important to remember that not only does a drug molecule have an effect on the body, but the body also has an effect on the drug molecule. For example, a drug which is administered for its therapeutic effect may be metabolised by the body to inactive compounds which are then excreted. Thus, pharmacology may be divided into two major areas: *pharmacodynamics*, the study of the effect of the drug on the body; and *pharmacokinetics*, the study of the effects of the body on the drug. We must also consider the possibility that the drug may have effects other than the desired therapeutic effect, and so pharmacodynamics may be further subdivided into the study of the therapeutic effects of a drug, its side-effects and its toxicity.

It is important for the podiatrist to be aware not only

of the range of drugs commonly used in therapeutics, and their effects and side-effects, but also of the possible interactions between drugs, for two reasons. First, many podiatry patients, especially the elderly, receive drug therapy for a number of different conditions. Secondly, the nature of the podiatrist–patient interaction is such that patients may well spend more time talking with their podiatrist than they do talking with their medical practitioner!

Under such circumstances, patients may refer to problems which relate to their drug therapy. Therefore, the podiatrist is in a very good position not only to reassure patients about their problems, but also to identify potential areas for concern, which may be brought to the attention of their GP.

ACTION OF DRUGS

Pharmacology has shown us that drugs may bring about their therapeutic effects in one of three different ways:

1. interaction with receptors
2. interaction with enzymes
3. interaction with transport systems.

Interaction with receptors

Drugs which interact with receptors produce their effects by either augmenting or inhibiting the natural processes of nervous and hormonal control of the body. If a drug produces an effect similar to a naturally occurring compound which interacts with an endogenous receptor, it is called an *agonist*. An example of an agonist drug is salbutamol, which is an agonist at β_2 adrenoceptors in the airways of the lung. If a drug produces an effect whereby a naturally occurring agonist is prevented from acting at its receptor, it is called an *antagonist*. An example of an antagonist drug is propranolol, which prevents the action of noradrenaline on the heart, by blocking β_1 adrenoceptors in cardiac muscle.

Interaction with enzymes

Drugs manifesting their therapeutic effect by an action on an enzyme usually act as *antagonists*, preventing the enzyme from performing its normal metabolic function. An example of a drug which produces its therapeutic effect by antagonising an enzyme is enalapril, which blocks an enzyme called angiotensin-converting enzyme (ACE), so preventing the produc-

tion of angiotensin II and hence producing a fall in blood pressure.

Interaction with transport systems

Drugs which interact with transport systems exert their effects by competing with a natural substrate for the transport system and inhibiting it. An example of this is the diuretic frusemide, which blocks the active transport of chloride ions in the ascending limb of the loop of Henle in the kidney. This causes a decrease in the medullary osmotic pressure gradient and a subsequent diuresis.

ADMINISTRATION OF DRUGS

It should be clear to you at this point that the most important consideration concerning the effect of a drug in the body is the concentration of drug available at the site of action (receptor, enzyme or transport system). If the concentration is too low, there will be little or no therapeutic effect; if the concentration is too high we may get an exaggerated therapeutic effect, or even an unacceptable toxic effect. It must also be remembered that although pharmacologists attempt to target the drug at the required site of action, some drugs may well produce an effect at another site, thus producing a possible range of side-effects. An example of this is seen with salbutamol, which is an agonist at β_2 adrenoceptors in the lung. Although, at normal therapeutic doses, the action of salbutamol is specific to the lung, at higher doses it is possible for this drug to stimulate β_1 adrenoceptors in the heart, causing tachycardia.

A number of factors are important in determining whether or not a drug reaches the desired site of action at a suitable concentration to produce the required therapeutic effect. These are:

- dose and frequency of dose
- route of administration
- rate of absorption
- protein binding and distribution
- metabolism
- excretion.

Dose and frequency of dose

The dose of a drug and the frequency of its administration are of prime importance in determining whether a drug reaches the required concentration in the target tissue. If the dose is too small, or too infrequent, the drug will not reach the required concentration. Conversely, if the dose is too large, or administered too frequently, side-effects or toxic effects may ensue. The actual therapeutic dose used will obviously depend upon the individual drug, as well as on the other factors listed above, but the aim must always be to maintain the concentration of drug at the site of action as closely as possible to the concentration required to produce the desired therapeutic effect.

Route of administration

There are a number of possible routes by which a drug may be administered. By far the most common, and the most convenient for the patient, is the oral route, as this allows patients to administer their own medicine, and continue their normal lives. However, the drug may produce problems of gastrointestinal upset, absorption may be slow and unpredictable or the level of drug metabolism be too high for the drug to be given orally. Some drugs may be administered under the tongue (sublingually), giving rapid absorption and little metabolism. In other cases, drugs may be administered via the rectum in the form of suppositories. This route avoids the possibility of gastrointestinal upset and is used commonly if the patient cannot swallow, or is vomiting.

Administration by inhalation provides a means of delivering the drug directly into the lung. This is of special benefit if the lung is the site of action (as in the treatment of asthma), but also provides for rapid absorption into the blood from the lung mucosa.

Drugs which do not easily cross the wall of the gastrointestinal tract, or for which a rapid therapeutic effect is required, may be given by injection. Drugs administered directly into a vein (intravenous injection) produce an immediate effect, while those administered into muscles (intramuscular injection) may produce either a rapid effect or a slow prolonged effect, according to the type of formulation used. Other routes of injection are subcutaneous (just under the skin) and intrathecal (directly into the cerebrospinal fluid of the spinal cord).

Some drugs may also be administered by direct application to the skin. Whilst this is an obvious way of administering ointments and creams, it is now used for the administration of hormone replacement therapy (HRT), and for the administration of glyceryl trinitrate in the long-term treatment of angina.

Rate of absorption

The rate at which a drug is absorbed into the body is also important in determining the concentration at its site of action. Lipophilic drugs are absorbed rapidly as they are able to cross cell membranes easily. Hydrophilic drugs are absorbed more slowly, unless there is a specific carrier present to promote absorption. Absorption of drugs from the gastrointestinal tract is markedly affected by the presence, or absence, of foodstuffs in the gut at the time of the drug's administration. Some foods will completely alter the absorption pattern of a drug such that it is no longer therapeutically effective. For this reason, patients may be advised to take their medicine on an empty stomach, or to avoid milk or iron preparations whilst taking the medicine.

Protein binding and distribution

The distribution of a drug after it has been absorbed into the bloodstream is also important in determining its action in the body. Many drugs are bound to plasma proteins (especially plasma albumin), and so are unavailable to produce their therapeutic action. In some cases, more than 90% of a drug may be bound up in this way, leaving less than 10% of the administered dose available. It is only the drug which is available free in solution in the plasma which is important in determining the effective plasma concentration.

The distribution of a drug between the various body compartments will depend primarily upon its physical properties. If the drug is highly ionised, or hydrophilic, it will not be able to cross the lipid membranes between the body water compartments, and so will tend to remain in the plasma and not reach its required site of action. Conversely, lipophilic drugs can easily cross these membrane barriers, and so will become distributed throughout the various body compartments.

A major barrier to the passage of drugs into the central nervous system is the blood–brain barrier. This barrier protects the brain and spinal cord, only allowing specific, lipophilic molecules access to the central nervous system. Thus, hydrophilic drugs do not gain access to the central nervous system, whereas lipophilic molecules pass this barrier easily, and can attain relatively high concentrations in the brain.

Metabolism

The metabolism of a drug plays an important role in determining not only whether a drug reaches the required concentration at its site of action, but also the length of time for which that concentration may be maintained. Most drugs are metabolised by the microsomal enzymes of the liver, and are converted to water-soluble metabolites which may be more easily excreted. However, the degree of metabolism varies from almost nothing to almost complete destruction of the drug as it passes through the liver.

Remember that drugs absorbed from the gastrointestinal tract pass directly to the liver via the hepatic portal vein. Therefore, if a drug is highly metabolised during this 'first pass' through the liver, very little of an administered dose may actually reach the systemic circulation at all. It should be borne in mind, however, that metabolic degradation of a drug does not always inactivate the drug, as some metabolites are as active, and possibly more active, than the parent compound.

Excretion

The excretion of drugs takes place mainly via the kidney, although small amounts may be excreted in the faeces, sweat and exhaled air. Therefore, the rate of excretion of a drug or its metabolites will depend upon the rate at which it can enter the nephron tubules of the kidney. Free drug in the plasma, that which is not bound to plasma protein, will enter the nephron by glomerular filtration, but some may be secreted into the proximal convoluted tubules by the acid- or base-secreting pathways. In some cases, these secretory pathways provide a too efficient excretion mechanism and result in only a short duration of action.

In the remainder of this chapter we will look at some of the more commonly prescribed groups of drugs, and summarise their mechanisms of action and possible side-effects.

DRUGS ACTING ON THE GASTROINTESTINAL SYSTEM

Antacids

Antacids are a commonly used group of drugs, often bought over the counter. They can be of benefit for the symptomatic treatment of a number of gastric disorders, such as dyspepsia and reflux oesophagitis. They usually contain aluminium or magnesium salts, or sodium bicarbonate. They should not be taken at the same time as other medicines, as they may impair absorption from the gastrointestinal tract. They should also be used with care, as some preparations, especially those containing magnesium salts, may well cause diarrhoea.

It must always be borne in mind that gastric discomfort may be indicative of underlying gastric disease. Consequently, patients who report frequent use of antacids should be referred to their medical practitioner.

Antispasmodics

Antispasmodics are used to relieve the pain associated with spasm of the smooth muscle of the gastrointestinal tract in diseases such as irritable bowel syndrome and diverticular disease. Most drugs in this group are antimuscarinics, which exert their action by blocking the action of acetylcholine at the muscarinic receptors on the smooth muscle of the gastrointestinal tract. As a consequence, they show typically atropine-like side-effects, such as dry mouth, blurred vision and possible difficulty with the passing of urine. Elderly patients are particularly at risk in developing side-effects with this group of drugs, and in some patients glaucoma may be precipitated. Drugs used in this group are dicyclomine (Merbentyl), alverine (Spasmonal) and mebevarine (Colofac), as well as derivatives of atropine.

Ulcer-healing drugs

The most commonly used group of ulcer-healing drugs are the histamine-H_2 antagonists, cimetidine (Tagamet), ranitidine (Zantac) and famotidine (Pepcid). These drugs are now available over the counter. They act by inhibiting the secretion of hydrochloric acid from the parietal cells of the stomach, and thus allow the ulcer to heal. All three drugs are generally well tolerated, rarely causing rashes, tiredness and mental confusion. However, cimetidine has been reported to produce gynaecomastia (breast development) in males. Cimetidine may well alter the metabolism of other prescribed drugs and so cause either the occurrence of apparent side-effects or loss of therapeutic control.

Other groups of drugs used for the treatment of ulcers in the gastrointestinal tract include pirenzipine (Gastrozepine), a selective antimuscarinic drug, and misoprostol, an analogue of prostaglandin E_1 which inhibits gastric acid secretion. Misoprostol has been reported to produce nausea and diarrhoea, as well as vaginal bleeding in females.

Omeprazole (Losec), which inhibits the proton pump in the parietal cell, has been shown to be effective in the treatment of gastric ulcers resistant to other forms of therapy. However, headache, nausea and skin rashes have been reported following the use of this drug.

Laxatives

The use of laxatives is widespread, especially among the older population, often without medical advice or diagnosis of the need for their use.

Bulk-forming laxatives, such as bran and methylcellulose, exert their effect by increasing the faecal mass and stimulating peristalsis in the lower gut. Stimulant laxatives, such as cascara preparations and bisacodyl, increase gastrointestinal motility, and hence cause evacuation of the bowel. However, they are prone to causing painful abdominal cramps, and their use can result in a period of apparent constipation, resulting in further unnecessary use. Faecal softeners, such as liquid paraffin, are not now recommended for use as laxatives. The prolonged use of liquid paraffin can result in anal seepage of the oil, lipoid pneumonia and interference with the absorption of fat-soluble vitamins.

Osmotic laxatives act by retaining water in the bowel by an osmotic effect, and by changing the pattern of water distribution in the faeces. The most commonly used example is lactulose, a semi-synthetic disaccharide which retains water in the lower bowel and produces a mild laxative effect.

Antidiarrhoeal drugs

Diarrhoea usually occurs as a result of dietary changes, mild food poisoning, emotional disturbances or as a side-effect of other drug therapy. Severe chronic diarrhoea is produced by various infections, ulcerative colitis, thyrotoxicosis and some malabsorption syndromes. Treatment for diarrhoea, is dependent upon the severity of the symptoms and the causative agent. However, in the case of mild, transient diarrhoea, it is usually sufficient to ensure that the electrolyte balance is maintained by the administration of electrolyte solutions. In more severe cases of diarrhoea it is necessary to identify and treat the underlying cause in order to successfully relieve the symptoms. Such cases should always be referred to a medical practitioner.

Antibiotic drugs cause diarrhoea as a result of an upsetting of the balance of the intestinal flora. Drug-induced diarrhoea in other drug groups is usually the result of either gastrointestinal irritation or an upsetting of the balance of sympathetic and parasympathetic activity to the smooth muscle of the gut.

Antidiarrhoeal drugs act either by adsorbing water from the gastrointestinal tract, or by inhibiting gastrointestinal motility. Kaolin is a commonly used adsorbent antidiarrhoeal preparation which can be of some benefit in mild cases, but more severe cases require the use of antimotility drugs such as diphenoxylate (Lomotil) and loperamide (Arret, Imodium). Diphenoxylate is an analogue of morphine and loperamide acts by decreasing gastrointestinal motility, especially the propulsive movement. It has been reported to produce abdominal cramps and some skin rashes; excessive use may precipitate paralytic ileus.

DRUGS ACTING ON THE CARDIOVASCULAR SYSTEM
Cardiac glycosides

Cardiac glycosides, such as digoxin (Lanoxin), are used in the treatment of congestive heart failure and atrial fibrillation (see below). It increases the force of contraction of the failing heart and restores an adequate circulation of blood. The action of digoxin is primarily on the myocardium, restoring the pacemaker potential of the sinu-atrial node and re-establishing sinus rhythm. Side-effects of digoxin include nausea, vomiting and some visual disturbances. The therapeutic efficacy of digoxin is dependent upon the levels of potassium ions in the plasma and so care must be exercised in the use of digoxin in patients also receiving drugs which may cause hypokalaemia, such as the thiazides and loop diuretics.

Diuretics

Diuretics are drugs which bring about an increased urine output by a direct action on the kidneys. They are primarily used for the relief of oedema, but are often used in the treatment of mild to moderate hypertension, because of their ability to increase water loss from the body. There are three groups of commonly prescribed diuretics.

The most common group of diuretics in use are the thiazides. These act to inhibit the reabsorption of sodium ions from the proximal convoluted tubule and the cortical diluting segment of the nephron. Reduction in sodium reabsorption brings about a concomitant reduction in water reabsorption, and hence diuresis. There are a large number of thiazides available, the most common being bendrofluazide, chlorothiazide (Saluric), polythiazide (Nephril), mefruside (Baycaron), cyclopenthiazide (Navidrex) and indapamide (Natrilix).

Thiazide diuretics are essentially well tolerated and produce few side-effects. The most common side-effect, especially in the elderly, is hypokalaemia and occasional skin rashes. The hypokalaemia produced by the thiazides is of special significance if the patient is also being treated with digoxin, as a fall in plasma potassium levels may well precipitate digoxin-related side-effects. Thiazides are often administered together with potassium chloride to offset the hypokalaemic effect.

The second group of diuretics are the so-called

'loop' diuretics. These act by inhibiting the formation of the medullary osmotic pressure gradient in the kidney, by preventing the reabsorption of chloride ions from the ascending limb of the loop of Henle. Frusemide (Lasix) and bumetanide (Burinex) are the commonly used members of this group. The major side-effect with these compounds is hypokalaemia, although gastrointestinal disturbances, tinnitus and deafness have been reported.

The third group of diuretics are the 'potassium-sparing' diuretics, acting upon the sodium/potassium and sodium/hydrogen exchange mechanisms in the distal convoluted tubule. They may be used alone as mild diuretics, but are more commonly used in combination with a thiazide or a loop diuretic to offset the tendency of these drugs to produce hypokalaemia. The commonly used examples in this group are triamterene (Dytac) and amiloride, which act to inhibit the sodium/hydrogen exchange mechanism. Both drugs have been reported to produce skin rashes and some mental confusion.

The aldosterone antagonists, spironolactone (Aldactone) and potassium canrenoate (Spiroctan-M), inhibit the aldosterone-sensitive sodium/potassium exchange mechanism, but can cause nausea and vomiting.

Anti-angina drugs

Angina pectoris is the term applied to the pain experienced when the heart is attempting to function in the absence of an adequate oxygen supply. It is usually associated with a decrease in the effective diameter of the coronary arteries and becomes apparent sometimes under even mild exercise. It may be treated either by the use of coronary vasodilators or by reducing the oxygen demand of the cardiac muscle.

Coronary vasodilators include the nitrates, glyceryl trinitrate, isosorbide mononitrate (Elantan) and isosorbide dinitrate (Isordil, Sorbitrate). Glyceryl trinitrate may be given sublingually or as an inhalation spray for the treatment of acute attacks of angina, and the isosorbide compounds are more often used in the prophylaxis of the condition. All three compounds produce throbbing headache, flushing, dizziness and tachycardia as side-effects.

The calcium channel antagonists, amlodipine (Istin), nifedipine (Adalat), diltiazem (Tildiem) and nicardipine (Cardene) are also used in the prophylactic treatment of angina pectoris as a result of their ability to dilate coronary arteries and increase the oxygen supply to the heart.

The use of beta-blocker drugs in the prophylaxis of angina is dependent upon their ability to reduce the oxygen demand of the heart. Thus, the cardiac muscle is able to produce the required contractile effort, even though the oxygen supply is reduced.

Anti-arrhythmic drugs

Arrhythmias in the heart fall into one of a number of different categories, depending upon their site of origin and their frequency. In general, cardiac arrhythmias result in a decrease in the pumping efficiency of the heart, a fall in blood pressure and a decrease in the efficiency of blood circulation. They may vary in severity from being almost unnoticeable to being life-threatening.

Ectopic beats are occasional extra heartbeats usually initiated within the atria. If they are infrequent in an otherwise normal heart, they rarely require treatment. Atrial flutter and atrial fibrillation are more serious and result from multiple ectopic foci, producing atrial beating rates of 200–300 beats/minute. Ventricular arrhythmias, such as ventricular fibrillation, are extremely dangerous as they result in rapid cardiovascular collapse.

Anti-arrhythmic drugs may be classified into four groups, according to their mechanism of action:

- class I—quinidine, lignocaine, flecainide (Tambocor), disopyramide (Rhythmodan)
- class II—beta-blockers
- class III—amiodarone (Cordarone-X), bretylium, sotalol
- class IV—calcium channel antagonists.

Class I drugs are membrane stabilisers which increase the stability of the cardiac muscle membrane, thus decreasing the incidence of ectopic foci; class II drugs inhibit the effect of the sympathetic nervous system on the heart (see beta-blockers below); class III anti-arrhythmic drugs delay the repolarisation phase of the cardiac action potential; and class IV drugs inhibit the influx of calcium into the cardiac muscle cell, which is a prerequisite of muscle contraction.

All classes of anti-arrhythmic drugs cause a decrease in myocardial excitability, which is essential for their therapeutic action. However, the major side-effect with these drugs is the extension of this myocardial depression into heart failure.

Beta-blockers

Beta-blocking drugs act upon the β_1 adrenoceptors in the heart and vascular circulation. They are of use in the treatment of mild hypertension, angina, myocardial infarction, cardiac arrhythmias and thyrotoxicosis. Unfortunately, although many beta-blockers are relatively specific for the β_1 adrenoceptors in the heart, they may also exert an antagonistic effect on β_2 adrenoceptors in the smooth muscle of the airways in the lung, and thus precipitate bronchoconstriction. For this reason, their use in asthmatics is contraindicated.

The use of beta-blockers as antihypertensive drugs is dependent upon their ability to reduce cardiac output and reset the baroreceptor reflex pathways controlling heart activity. Some also depress the levels of renin in plasma, and so inhibit the production of angiotensin II. Beta-blockers also improve exercise tolerance in the heart, and so relieve the symptoms associated with exercise-induced angina. Their use in the control of cardiac arrhythmias depends upon the fact that some beta-blockers have a membrane-stabilising effect in the heart. Consequently, they allow the sinu-atrial node to re-establish its control of the heartbeat and decrease the incidence of atrial and ventricular extrasystoles.

Beta-blockers are relatively well tolerated by most patients; however, their mode of action on adrenoceptors in the sympathetic nervous system gives rise to a number of side-effects. Most side-effects of beta-blockers are an extension of their therapeutic effects. Thus, they are prone to produce bradycardia, and possibly heart failure in susceptible individuals, bronchospasm and peripheral vasoconstriction, leading to a feeling of coldness in the fingers and toes. Some beta-blockers penetrate the blood–brain barrier and enter the central nervous system. In these cases, side-effects can include sleep disturbances, fatigue and hallucinations. Two beta-blockers, practolol and metipranolol, have been withdrawn as a result of serious side-effects in the eye. Whilst similar effects have not been reported with other beta-blockers, it is prudent to assess any reports of eye problems from patients receiving long-term therapy with beta-blockers.

There are a large number of beta-blockers available, the most common being propranolol (Inderal), acebutalol (Sectral), atenolol (Tenormin), bisoprolol (Monocor), metoprolol (Betaloc, Lopressor) and oxprenolol (Trasicor).

Antihypertensives

Antihypertensive drugs are used to lower the elevated blood pressure of hypertension. Hypertension is a common disease state. Unfortunately, in the majority of hypertensives there is no clinical pointer as to the cause of the elevated blood pressure (primary essential hypertension), although hypertension may also result from identifiable causes such as renal dysfunction, drug therapy and pregnancy. Consequently, in the majority of cases, the treatment of hypertension is often symptomatic, bringing about a fall in blood pressure without treating the underlying cause of the problem. Only in the case of an identifiable cause for the hypertension can treatment attempt to cure the disease.

Blood pressure is generated by the pumping action of the heart pushing the blood through the closed vascular circulation. The resistance to flow of the blood through the arteries produces the pressure. Whilst an adequate blood pressure is essential to ensure a satisfactory circulation of blood through the capillaries, an elevated blood pressure is dangerous because it requires the heart to work harder to pump the blood, and may actually cause breakages in the tiny capillaries of the tissues which cannot withstand elevated pressures. Hypertension may be treated in a number of ways:

- inhibition of the sympathetic drive to the heart
- reduction in the force of cardiac contraction
- dilatation of the blood vessels
- inhibition of the renin–angiotensin system.

Inhibition of the sympathetic drive to the heart

Drugs which inhibit the sympathetic drive to the heart may do so either by reducing the activity of the cardioaccelerator centre in the brain, preventing the activity of the neurohumoral transmitter in the sympathetic ganglia, or by reducing the activity of the neurohumoral transmitter at the junction between the sympathetic nerve and the heart tissue.

The most common drugs used for the initial treatment of mild to moderate hypertension are the beta-blocking drugs, such as atenolol (Tenormin) and propranolol (Inderal). These act by inhibiting the action of noradrenaline on the heart and so bring about a reduction in heart rate (bradycardia) and a fall in blood pressure. The side-effects of beta-blockers have already been discussed.

Another drug, methyldopa (Aldomet), reduces the sympathetic drive to the heart by substituting for dihydroxyphenylalanine (Dopa) in the synthesis of noradrenaline in nerve terminals, resulting in the synthesis of the 'false transmitter', methylnoradrenaline, which is less active than noradrenaline. This action of methyldopa occurs predominantly in the central nervous system to inhibit the cardioaccelerator centre, rather than at the neuroeffector junction in the heart.

Consequently, methyldopa shows some centrally mediated side-effects, such as sedation and depression, as well as failure of ejaculation, skin rashes and fluid retention. Clonidine (Catapres) produces an antihypertensive effect by an action on α_2 adrenoceptors in the medulla oblongata, leading to a decrease in sympathetic drive to the heart, as well as resetting arterial baroreceptors to increase vagal tone to the heart.

Ganglion-blocking agents such as trimetaphan (Arfonad) inhibit sympathetic nerve activity by preventing the action of acetylcholine at the sympathetic ganglia and so reducing the sympathetic drive to the heart. However, ganglion-blocking drugs are not necessarily specific for sympathetic ganglia and also inhibit neurohumoral transmission at parasympathetic ganglia. Consequently, side-effects include tachycardia, dry mouth and visual disturbances.

Adrenergic neurone blocking drugs such as guanethidine (Ismelin) and debrisoquine (Declinax) act by reducing the release of noradrenaline from the postganglionic sympathetic nerve endings. However, because they effectively reduce the amounts of noradrenaline present in the nerve endings, they are likely to produce postural hypotension, resulting in fainting on standing and mild exertion.

Reduction in the force of cardiac contraction

A reduction in the force of the heartbeat may be brought about by inhibiting the influx of calcium ions, which is an essential prerequisite for the initiation of contraction in cardiac muscle. Drugs in this group are called calcium channel antagonists, and they reduce myocardial contractility and alter the conduction of the cardiac action potential across the heart.

Verapamil, which is also an anti-arrhythmic drug, is used in the treatment of angina, hypertension and cardiac arrhythmias, but may precipitate heart failure in susceptible individuals. It should not be used in conjunction with beta-blockers because of the increased risk of bradycardia and heart failure.

Nifedipine (Adalat) and nicardipine (Cardene) reduce the force of cardiac muscle contraction, but do not reduce myocardial contractility. They cause a dilatation of coronary and peripheral arteries and produce side-effects associated with blood vessel dilatation, such as flushing and headache. The vasodilating properties of nifedipine and nicardipine make them both suitable for the treatment of some forms of hypertension; however, these drugs, together with diltiazem, are predominantly used in the treatment of angina (see above).

Dilatation of blood vessels

Directly acting vasodilator drugs produce their therapeutic effect by causing a widening of the diameter of the blood vessels through which the blood is passing, and so reducing the pressure in the arteries. This group of antihypertensives includes hydralazine (Apresoline) and minoxidil (Loniten). The fall in blood pressure produced by these drugs, however, often causes a reflex tachycardia.

Vasodilatation may also be caused by inhibiting the effect of the sympathetic nerve supply to the blood vessels. This may be brought about by the use of α_1 adrenoceptor antagonists, such as doxazosin (Cardura), indoramine (Baratol), prazosin (Hypovase), phenoxybenzamine (Dibenzyline) and phentolamine (Rogitine). The side-effects of this group of drugs are widespread, particularly postural hypotension.

Inhibition of the renin–angiotensin system

Inhibition of the renin–angiotensin system prevents the formation of angiotensin II, which is a powerful vasoconstrictor peptide. Angiotensin II is produced from an inactive precursor, angiotensinogen, by the action of the enzymes renin and angiotensin-converting enzyme (ACE). ACE inhibitors, such as captopril (Capoten), enalapril (Innovace) and lisinopril (Zestril), cause a marked fall in blood pressure by this mechanism. All three drugs cause a rapid fall in blood pressure and so treatment requires initial small doses, followed by a gradual increase in dosage until the desired effect is achieved. Other side-effects include a persistent dry cough, fatigue, weakness, nausea and diarrhoea.

Anticoagulants

Anticoagulants are used to reduce the incidence of unwanted blood clotting in conditions such as deep vein thrombosis. Heparin is a naturally occurring substance, found in basophils, which acts by inhibiting the blood clotting cascade at a number of sites. It may be administered by subcutaneous or intramuscular injection, especially in the management of postoperative thrombosis.

The oral anticoagulants antagonise the effects of vitamin K, and thus produce an inhibition of the blood clotting cascade. The most commonly used oral anticoagulant is warfarin (Marevan), although phenindione (Dindevan) may also be used. Great care must be exercised in the use of warfarin, as it is very strongly bound to plasma proteins. Consequently, the introduction of other drugs into a patient who is stabilised on a particular warfarin dose may result in more warfarin being made available free in the plasma, due to its displacement from protein binding sites. In this situation the patient may experience internal haemorrhage.

Lipid lowering drugs

Lipid lowering drugs are used to decrease the plasma levels of cholesterol and triglycerides, and they are used in patients with severe hyperlipidaemia. Anion exchange resins, such as cholestyramine and colestipol, act by binding to bile acids in the gut, so preventing their reabsorption. This promotes the conversion of cholesterol into bile acids by the liver, and so lowers plasma cholesterol levels. The clofibrate group of drugs, clofibrate (Atromid), bezafibrate (Bezalip), gemfibrozil (Lopid) and fenofibrate (Lipantil), act primarily by decreasing plasma triglyceride levels, although they will also cause a decrease in the circulating amounts of cholesterol. Both groups of lipid lowering drugs have been reported to produce side-effects, including nausea and abdominal discomfort.

A new group of drugs which produce a lowering in plasma lipid levels are the inhibitors of 3-hydroxy-3-methylglutaryl-CoA reductase. Simvastatin (Zocor) and pravastatin (Lipostat) are well tolerated but can cause nausea, constipation and headache.

DRUGS ACTING ON THE RESPIRATORY SYSTEM

Bronchodilators

Bronchodilators are used to increase the diameter of the airways in the lung to assist breathing in clinical situations such as asthma. The diameter of the airways in the lungs is controlled by β_2 adrenoceptors, and so the most effective method of increasing the diameter of airways is by the use of selective β_2 agonists, such as salbutamol (Ventolin), terbutaline (Bricanyl), rimiterol (Pulmadil) and fenoterol (Berotec). However, it must be remembered that these agonists may also cause some stimulation of β_1 adrenoceptors in other parts of the body, especially the heart and skeletal muscle, so tremor and tachycardia may result from their use.

Antimuscarinic drugs also increase the diameter of airway passages, by inhibiting the action of the parasympathetic supply to the lung, so drugs such as ipratropium (Atrovent) may also be used, although these will produce the atropine-like side-effects of dry mouth and blurred vision.

Corticosteroids

Corticosteroids have been used in the treatment of asthma for many years, and nowadays there are a number of aerosol preparations of these drugs. Their mechanism of action is not clearly understood, but they probably reduce the hypersensitivity reactions associated with asthma and hence reduce mucus secretion in the airways. Beclomethasone (Becotide) is the most commonly used drug in this group.

DRUGS ACTING ON THE CENTRAL NERVOUS SYSTEM

Hypnotics and anxiolytics

Hypnotics and anxiolytics are used to sedate the patient. This may be to induce sleep, in the treatment of insomnia, or to relieve a variety of anxiety states. The prescribing of these drugs is widespread, and may well lead to problems of either physical or psychological dependence. The most commonly used group of hypnotics and anxiolytics is the benzodiazepines. Nitrazepam, temazepam, triazolam and lormetazepam are used as hypnotics, and diazepam (Valium), lorazepam and oxazepam are used as anxiolytics. Other hypnotics include chlormethiazole (Heminevrin) and zopiclone (Zimovane), both of which are of particular use in the elderly.

As you would expect with drugs acting as sedatives on the central nervous system, the major side-effects are drowsiness and ataxia (particularly in the elderly). Other, non-benzodiazepine, drugs used for the treatment of anxiety include buspirone (Buspar) and chlormezanone (Trancopal). All hypnotics and anxiolytics have their actions potentiated by alcohol.

Antipsychotic drugs

Antipsychotic drugs (neuroleptics) are used for tranquillising patients without impairing their state of consciousness, in severe anxiety states, schizophrenia and psychoses. They also may exert an antidepressant action. Antipsychotic drugs may be divided into three main groups: group I (chlorpromazine (Largactil)) is characterised by pronounced sedative effects, group II (thioridazine (Melleril)) have moderate sedative effects, and group III (fluphenazine (Modecate) and trifluoperazine (Stelazine)) have few sedative side-effects. All these drugs are likely to cause hypotension and a loss of temperature control in the elderly, and so should be used with care in patients over 70 years of age.

Antidepressants

Antidepressant drugs may be divided into the tricyclic (and related) antidepressants and the monoamine oxidase inhibitors. The tricyclic antidepressants are the drugs of choice in the treatment of the majority of depressive states, because they do not show the potentially dangerous interactions with some foods seen with the monoamine oxidase inhibitors.

Tricyclic antidepressants, such as amitryptyline (Tryptizol), clomipramine (Anafranil), dothiepin (Prothiaden), doxepin (Sinequan) and lofepramine (Gamanil), are most useful in the treatment of endogenous depression associated with psychomotor disturbances. All tricyclic antidepressants produce a range of side-effects—dry mouth, blurred vision and difficulty with micturition—as a result of their antimuscarinic action, and tachycardia, cardiac arrhythmias, postural hypotension, sweating and tremor as a result of their central effects.

Monoamine oxidase inhibitors, such as phenelzine (Nardil), may be used in the treatment of depressive illness which will not respond to the tricyclic group of antidepressants. They are of particular benefit in phobic states and hysteria. However, care must be exercised in their use because of the interaction with some foods. Monoamine oxidase inhibitors prevent the destruction of catecholamines in the body, and so produce a rise in the content of noradrenaline in the body. Some foods, especially cheese, broad beans and meat extracts, contain tyramine which releases noradrenaline, and so patients eating these foods whilst undergoing treatment with a monoamine oxidase inhibitor will experience serious increases in blood pressure, possibly leading to haemorrhage.

Analgesics

Analgesics are drugs used for the control of pain. They may be classified into two groups: non-opioid analgesics, used for the control of pain associated with musculoskeletal disorders, and opioid analgesics, used in the control of pain associated with the viscera.

Non-opioid analgesics include aspirin, paracetamol and ibuprofen (Neurofen), all of which may be purchased over the counter in pharmacies, as well as being prescribed by medical practitioners. In many cases, non-opioid analgesics, such as paracetamol, are prescribed in compound preparations, often with codeine (Co-Codamol) or dextropropoxyphene (Co-Proxamol). The availability of non-opioid analgesics, especially paracetamol, over the counter and by prescription can lead to serious problems of overdose if patients take paracetamol-containing analgesics from both sources. It is of paramount importance to ensure that patients receiving paracetamol-based analgesics do not also take other paracetamol-containing preparations, as this may lead to serious liver damage and death.

Opioid analgesics, such as morphine and diamorphine, are used in the control of severe pain of visceral origin. Most opioid analgesics cause marked respiratory depression and drowsiness, as well as nausea and vomiting in the initial stages of their administration. They may also markedly alter the response to other centrally acting drugs, such as antidepressants.

DRUGS ACTING ON THE ENDOCRINE SYSTEM

Antidiabetic drugs

Two groups of drugs are used for the treatment of diabetes, dependent upon the type of diabetes from which the patient is suffering. In patients where there is no insulin-secreting capacity in the cells of the islets of Langerhans, insulin must be given, usually by intramuscular injection. There are a number of different types of insulin preparation available, varying in the rapidity of onset and duration of action.

In patients where there is still some insulin-secreting capacity, oral hypoglycaemic drugs may be used. There are two groups of oral hypoglycaemic drugs currently in use. The sulphonylureas, such as chlorpropamide and gliclazide (Diamicron) act by increasing insulin secretion from the islets of Langerhans and so return the insulin levels in plasma towards normal. The second group are called biguanides, an example of which is metformin, and these act by decreasing gluconeogenesis and increasing peripheral glucose uptake into cells. These two groups of antidiabetic drugs are of value in non-insulin-dependent patients who do not respond to dietary measures. The sulphonylureas tend to cause gastrointestinal upset, headache and some sensitivity reactions, and the biguanides cause nausea, vomiting and decreased absorption of vitamin B_{12}.

Thyroid drugs

Thyroxine (Eltroxin) is used in a number of clinical situations in which there is a deficiency in thyroid function, such as hypothyroidism. Consequently, it is used in long-term treatment regimes, and a number of side-effects have been reported. These include arrhythmias, anginal pain, tachycardia, headache and skeletal muscle cramps.

DRUGS ACTING ON THE EYE

Anti-glaucoma drugs

Glaucoma is characterised by a rise in the intraocular pressure, producing pain in the eyeball, visual disturbances, eventual damage to the retina and blindness. In nearly all cases, glaucoma is the result of a decrease in the outflow of the aqueous humour from the eye. It may be treated by either reducing the rate of production of the aqueous humour or increasing the drainage rate by opening the drainage channels.

Miotics, such as pilocarpine, may be administered as eye drops and act by causing contraction of the ciliary muscles and a consequent opening of the drainage channel. However, their action on ciliary muscles also causes problems of accommodation and blurred vision.

Beta-blockers act by decreasing the rate of production of the aqueous humour and thus reduce the intraocular pressure. However, there is considerable evidence to suggest that prolonged use of timolol (Timoptol) in the treatment of glaucoma may well lead to the development of systemic side-effects associated with beta-blockers.

Acetazolamide (Diamox), an inhibitor of the enzyme carbonic anhydrase, also causes a decrease in the rate of production of aqueous humour.

DRUGS ACTING ON INFECTIONS

Antibacterials

Antibacterial drugs, commonly called antibiotics, are widely used to treat a range of bacterial infections. They fall broadly into three groups: penicillins, cephalosporins and tetracyclines, plus erythromycin and trimethoprim. The actual drug used in any given situation is dependent upon the type and sensitivity of the infecting organism.

The penicillins are bactericidal and act by inhibiting the synthesis of bacterial cell walls, thus preventing replication of the invading organism. They have a broad spectrum of activity and there is a wide range of penicillin derivatives available, including phenoxymethylpenicillin, amoxicillin, flucloxacillin and ampicillin. All penicillin derivatives cause nausea and diarrhoea, and are liable to produce hypersensitivity reactions, ranging from mild rashes to anaphylactic shock.

Cepahalosporins, such as cephalexin and cefuroxime, are broad-spectrum antibiotics with a mechanism of action similar to that of the penicillins. Their side-effects are similar to those of the penicillins, and patients who show hypersensitivity reactions to penicillins often show similar responses to cephalosporins.

Tetracyclines are broad-spectrum antibiotics, although their use has declined in recent years due to the development of bacterial resistance. However, they are of use in the treatment of some sensitive organisms, such as *Haemophilus influenzae* in chronic bronchitis. Tetracyclines are also used in the treatment of acne and periodontal disease. Tetracyclines are deposited in growing bone and should not be given to children under the age of 12 years or to pregnant women.

Erythromycin has a similar spectrum of antibacterial activity to that of penicillin, but does not cause hypersensitivity reactions. It may, therefore, be used as an alternative, in cases of hypersensitivity, to the penicillins. However, patients who are taking antihistamines such as terfenadine (Triludan) or astemizole (Hismanal) should not take erythromycin as severe cardiac arrhythmias may result.

Trimethoprim is used in the treatment of urinary tract infections and respiratory tract infections which do not respond to antibiotics from other groups.

Antifungals

Antifungal drugs are used in the treatment of a wide range of infections, such as intestinal candidiasis, dermatophyte infections of the skin and thrush. Miconazole is most commonly used for skin infections and thrush, and griseofulvin is used in the treatment of dermatophyte infections of the scalp and nails. Clotrimazole (Canesten) is available over the counter for the treatment of vaginal thrush. Most antifungal drugs, when given systemically, cause nausea, vomiting, diarrhoea and occasional skin rashes.

Antivirals

The most commonly used antiviral drug for systemic infections is aciclovir (Zovirax). This is effective against herpes simplex and herpes zoster infections. Side-effects include skin rashes, gastrointestinal disturbances, headache and fatigue, together with a rise in bilirubin and liver-related enzymes, indicating possible hepatic damage in prolonged use.

Both aciclovir and idoxuridine are used topically in

the treatment of viral infections such as cold sores and shingles. Aciclovir (Zovirax) is available over the counter in pharmacies.

DRUGS USED IN RHEUMATIC DISEASES AND GOUT

Non-steroidal anti-inflammatory drugs

Non-steroidal anti-inflammatory drugs (NSAIDs) are used frequently in the treatment of diseases such as rheumatoid arthritis which produce inflammation and pain in the joints. As such, they are commonly prescribed for elderly patients suffering from rheumatoid diseases. They act by inhibition of the enzyme cyclo-oxygenase, which is responsible for the production of prostaglandins from arachidonic acid. Inhibition of prostaglandin production, in a joint damaged by arthritis, reduces the inflammation and so helps to reduce the pain associated with these diseases.

There are a large number of NSAIDs available on prescription. These include aspirin, indomethacin (Indocid), ibuprofen (Brufen), diclofenac (Voltarol), piroxicam (Feldene) and azapropazone (Rheumox). They are available in a variety of dosage formats, including tablets, capsules, suppositories and skin gels. Furthermore, NSAIDs such as aspirin and ibuprofen (Neurofen, Ibuleve) are available over the counter in pharmacies, where they are marketed for the relief of pain arising from a wide range of causes.

They all commonly produce gastrointestinal upset as a side-effect, and must only be used with great care in patients with a history of gastric ulceration, as their use can lead to severe gastric bleeding and death. These drugs must also be used with care in asthmatic patients, as some people are particularly sensitive to these agents (especially aspirin) and may suffer an asthmatic attack.

One of the major problems with NSAIDs, in the treatment of rheumatoid diseases, is that they often do not completely remove the pain from the joint. Consequently, the patient is left experiencing a certain amount of 'residual pain', for which they will seek a suitable analgesic. The danger lies in the fact that they may then be given another NSAID, leading to a possible overdose.

Pharmacists and their staff are trained to ascertain what other medicines the patient is taking before selling NSAIDs over the counter, but many patients often take advice from other sources. It is important, therefore, to be aware of this potential danger and, if a patient complains of residual pain after taking NSAIDs, to refer them for further professional advice.

Anti-gout drugs

Acute bouts of gout are often treated with high doses of a non-steroidal anti-inflammatory drug, such as azapropazone. However, for long-term control of gout, it is more common to use drugs which decrease the amount of uric acid in the plasma. Allopurinol decreases uric acid formation, but can produce skin rashes, headache and gastrointestinal disorders. Probenecid and sulphinpyrazone increase uric acid excretion by the kidney, but may also produce gastrointestinal disturbances, dizziness and skin rashes.

SUMMARY

We have seen in this chapter that therapeutically administered drugs exert their effects by actions on receptors, enzymes or transport system and that the most important criterion to be considered in determining the effect of a drug is its concentration at the site of action. However, no drug is absolutely specific in its effects on the body and all are capable of giving rise to side-effects and toxic effects ranging in severity from mild to life-threatening.

Whilst it has not been possible to cover every eventuality of side-effect and interaction in the confines of this chapter, it cannot be overemphasised that it is important to listen to patients receiving drug therapy in order to ascertain whether or not they are experiencing adverse effects from their treatment. In most cases, such information will lead to reassurance of the patient that the problem is associated with their drug treatment, but it may also lead to the identification of hitherto unrecorded side-effects of drugs.

14

Orthoses

J. A. Black

Keywords

Casted insoles
Chairside technique
Digital appliances
Elastic anklets and braces
Functional orthoses
Heel orthoses
Hot water plastics
Insoles
Latex technique
Low temperature moulding
Non-casted insoles
Orthoses
Orthotic laboratories
Prostheses
Rapid remoulding
Replaceable pads
Shoe modifications
Silicones
Thermoplastics

It is widely recognised that most foot problems have some mechanical factors involved in their aetiology. Whether arising from some congenital variation in the structure of the foot and leg or acquired as a result of a disease process such as rheumatoid arthritis or one of the neuropathies, the basic philosophy of treatment remains the same. Mechanical foot defects can be controlled only by mechanical means.

This may be achieved by altering the structure by surgical intervention or by actively controlling the biomechanics of the foot and leg with an orthosis. It may be that, with increasing interprofessional awareness and cooperation in the management of patients, combined surgical and orthotic management provides the best treatment plan in many cases. The surgeon may decide that surgery is necessary in order to create an environment where orthotic therapy has a better chance of success in the long term. Similarly, an orthosis may be fitted postoperatively to control or rest the foot, thereby enhancing the healing process.

An appliance which controls or corrects structural abnormality is termed an 'orthosis', (Grk. *orthos*: straight). This term may be applied to all forms of appliances which have a corrective function. Appliances which primarily accommodate and protect deformities without correcting them, e.g. a hallux abductovalgus shield, are termed 'accommodative'. Many appliances combine both corrective and protective functions, depending on the nature of the foot fault, its severity and duration. Appliances which replace missing parts, whether as a result of trauma, disease or surgery, are termed 'prostheses'.

Where correction is possible, even if only partially, the corrective element should always take precedence over the protective element, and this consideration determines the choice of materials. Considerable force is often required to correct even a simple deformity, such as a hammer toe, or to prevent major deformation, such as abnormal pronation, from occurring under load. The more rigid the material, the better its splinting qualities but the lower its tolerance to wear by the patient. It is often necessary in these cases for the patient to become accustomed to the orthosis by gradually increasing the length of time it is worn.

Plastics used in functional orthoses can be simply classified by their ability to resist stress according to their thermoforming temperature. The higher the temperature at which they become malleable, the stronger they are; the lower the temperature, the more likely they are to deform under load. However, the thickness of the plastic is also of considerable importance and there is a direct correlation between rigidity and thickness. More recently, carbon fibre composite materials now offer the practitioner a light, thin and flexible alternative. However, they are difficult to use, requiring a higher forming temperature and a shorter working time, so that the vacuum former must have a rapid action.

Orthoses need to be designed so that they are both tolerable in wear and optimally effective in their therapeutic design. Accommodative appliances, e.g. latex shields, are utilised in established deformities to protect vulnerable tissues from trauma and to some extent to limit painful movement. They may not correct the underlying fault, but they make it tolerable by relieving painful symptoms and controlling secondary lesions. They are more flexible than rigid orthoses and usually can be well tolerated from the beginning. An accommodative device may be desirable for a time before the patient moves to a more corrective one.

Orthoses are worn either on the foot or within the footwear, and however well-designed and accurately fitted they may be, their beneficial effects will be largely nullified if the footwear is unsuitable. Orthoses and footwear must therefore be considered together when treatment is planned. The footwear must be of the correct size and shape, have adequate internal volume in the right places, and be correctly balanced both mediolaterally and anteroposteriorly. Modifications to footwear may be necessary to ensure these points, and those most often required are listed later. It is a sound principle that patients purchase their shoes after the orthosis is fitted. Heel height is of critical importance when fitting a functional orthosis. If the heel height is such that the normal relationship between the forefoot and the rearfoot is disturbed, then the shoe is totally unsuited to wear with the orthosis. The range of stock orthopaedic shoes now available is such that an attractive shoe at a reasonable cost offers the opportunity to provide a comprehensive orthotic and shoe regime for many foot deformities. Stock shoes normally come with an insole system which can be removed and replaced with the prescribed orthosis.

Orthotic technology is constantly developing as new materials and techniques are introduced and a greater understanding of foot mechanics evolves. Only a brief summary of its main aspects is possible here and further reference is recommended to specialist literature on the subject.

MANAGEMENT

It is essential that practitioners develop a sound working knowledge of the materials and techniques available in order to offer their patients a complete service, even if this is to be provided by an orthotics laboratory. At the outset of treatment, a management plan should be explained to the patient, outlining the progress envisaged and explaining its rationale. Patients have a right to know what the practitioner has in mind for their treatment and they should have a clear indication of how long it might take, the extent of potential improvement in the condition and, in the private sector, how much it might cost.

If this is accepted as a reasonable principle of patient management, then it is incumbent on the practitioner to be able to offer the best possible treatment available. If the practitioner is unable to provide this, then the patient should be referred to a clinician with the necessary equipment and skills. Not every patient needs an orthosis, but where this is an integral part of the treatment, patient management and patient awareness of the treatment plan and any possible sequelae must have a higher profile. This is particularly valid with the increasing use of functional orthoses aligned to biomechanical assessment, and the possible medico-legal implications which may arise if the treatment proves to be inappropriate and causes pathology elsewhere in the leg or trunk. If possible complications have not been explained to the patient, then the podiatrist is in a vulnerable position should the patient pursue a claim for negligence.

Before embarking on the treatment plan, certain considerations are important. The physical characteristics of the patient must be assessed, i.e. height, weight and mobility, and also the presence of any physical disability which might preclude the use of certain types of orthoses, e.g. the patient might be blind, rendering the positioning of a replaceable device difficult. In such circumstances, a 'locator' might be necessary to enable the patient to position the orthosis by touch. Should patients have any physical disabilities which prevent them from reaching their feet, orthoses which require careful positioning by them would also be unsuitable.

With such factors taken into account, the type of orthosis and the materials to be used in its manufacture can be considered. Important points are:

• What effect will the material have on the patient's foot? Since the orthosis is going to be in contact with the foot for a long time, will the material be irritant, or likely to cause an allergic reaction? Is it likely to damage the foot? Is the material stable or will it, once placed in the shoe, deteriorate due to the increase in temperature and humidity, and release products which may be irritant or even toxic? These factors are particularly relevant to patients with diminished sensation. An increasing number of patients appear to be becoming allergic to rubber or rubber products and it can prove difficult to find adhesives which do not initiate these allergic reactions.

• What effect will footwear have on the device? The quality or suitability of the patient's footwear may be a major factor in the effectiveness of the orthosis. Unsuitable footwear is probably the most frequent reason for not embarking on some form of appliance therapy and the practitioner frequently has to persuade the patient to invest in new footwear. This is most often experienced when treating adolescent or fashion-conscious women. Often the best compromise is for the patient to wear the orthosis at school or at work and to revert to fashion footwear only at other times. Such an arrangement is not totally satisfactory, as the effectiveness of the treatment may be diminished. This should be explained so that the patient understands clearly where the responsibility lies if the orthosis is not as successful as it might have been.

Replaceable pads

The simplest extensions of padding and strapping to more permanent orthoses are replaceable pads. These devices take many forms and are usually held in place with elasticated bands positioned around the toes or the foot (Fig. 14.1). Before embarking on use of a replaceable pad, the practitioner will usually try the design with clinical padding and assess its potential effectiveness. The role of clinical padding in this form is often undervalued, and substantial biomechanical control can be achieved with the skilful use of clinical padding materials either attached to the foot or positioned in the shoe. Manufacture is straightforward and devices may be made in a variety of materials, depending upon the physical properties required. A device

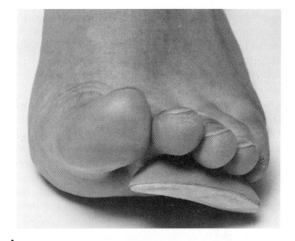

A

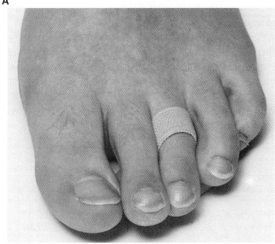

B

Figure 14.1 A, B: Replaceable long prop.

may be required simply to replace fatty padding atrophied by age. Such devices are protective in nature and a material is selected for its ability to resist compression over a long period. Newer viscoelastic forms are much more effective in resisting compressive stress than materials derived from rubber. Table 14.1 lists some materials and illustrates their compressibility and percentage relaxation under compressive stress.

All of the samples in Table 14.1 were 7 mm thick. Tests were carried out for 3 hours on an Instron, a device used to quantify the elasticity of materials. The percentage strain indicates the degree of deformation of the material under stress.

Forces entering the foot can be dissipated in one of two ways: (a) by absorbing the force in such a way that the material decelerates the rate at which forces enter the foot, i.e. shock absorption; (b) by increasing the surface area through which weight is taken. It must be remembered that the orthosis should be placed in a position such that during 'foot-flat' and 'heel-off, the maximum area is in contact with the ground during the gait cycle.

Technological advance in materials has produced a new range of viscoelastic products which provide effective cushioning or dampen ground reaction force. These materials, such as Sorbothane and Viscolas, allow the podiatrist to provided the patient with high quality shock absorption without recourse to cutting, shaping and covering replaceable orthoses. The practitioner should be aware that viscoelastic materials are much heavier than traditional cushioning materials; this could be critical if supplying orthoses to sportspersons or rheumatoid arthritics. Sheets of silicone rubber are now also available in varying thicknesses and have proved most effective in the treatment of plantar keratomas or lesions over pressure areas on the toes.

Replaceable digital orthoses may also be manufactured by the same processes as used for plantar devices. However, practitioners may find that the effectiveness of digital orthoses is governed by their ability to remain in place, and secure anchorage is essential. Figure 14.1 illustrates a long prop; it is important that an assessment of the amount of movement in the interphalangeal and metatarsophalangeal joints has been made before embarking on the manufacture of this type of orthosis. Digital devices may conform to virtually any shape provided the principle has first been assessed with conventional padding.

Figure 14.2 illustrates a variety of replaceable pads.

Elastic anklets and braces

An elastic anklet is useful as an alternative to figure-of-eight strapping when continuing support is required. Commercial varieties are readily available and are usually satisfactory. They may be used with a tarsal platform or a tarsal cradle fitted either into the shoe or onto an insole. A buttressed heel may also be indicated for greater ankle stability.

A metatarsal brace is an elastic bandage encircling the metatarsus, and it usually includes a plantar metatarsal pad. Commercial varieties are usually unsatisfactory because the stereotyped pads attached to them are seldom, if ever, the right shape, size or density for a particular patient. The brace can be easily fabricated from elastic webbing or elastic net. Both materials are available in different widths, and it is advantageous to be able to design both brace and padding according to individual needs. The metatarsal brace may often be combined with a toe-loop or with orthodigital splints where correction and/or protection of the digits is also desired (Fig. 14.3).

There is now a plethora of elasticated supports specifically designed for use in sport. As people are intent on improving their fitness and using sports as a means to better health, sportswear manufacturers have met the demand by producing supports for all the joints which may be stressed during sporting activity. These are usually available from pharmacists or sports shops. The most popular range of supports are those manufactured from neoprene, but need care taken in the fitting of them.

Insoles

Virtually any pathological condition affecting the plantar surfaces can be controlled by appropriate insoles, provided that sufficient depth is made available in the footwear. It is essential that this requirement be specified whenever specially made footwear is ordered. With normal footwear, every effort must be made to save bulk by the choice of material, and by stopping the insole just behind or just in front of the metatarsal heads, depending on the design required

Table 14.1 Percentage strain of a variety of padding materials used in orthotics and prosthetics

Sample	Load (kg)	% strain	Load (kg)	% strain
PPT	20	87.10	40	98.39
Poron	20	75.61	40	87.80
Grey latex foam	20	61.29	40	80.65
NCCR	20	80.39	40	98.04
Clocell	20	70.00	40	78.33

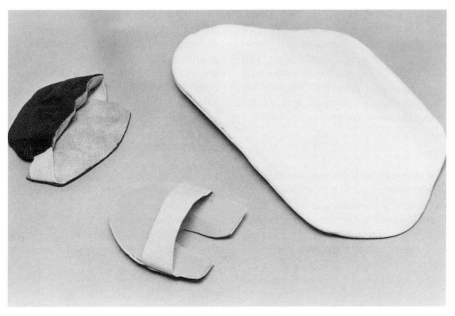

Figure 14.2   Selection of replaceable pads: orthodigital splint; dorsal pad for interphalangeal joint; Hexcelite valgus support covered in latex foam.

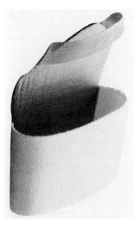

Figure 14.3   Metatarsal brace with toe-loop.

(unless the footwear will accommodate a full-length insole).

There are basically two types:

1. a simple or non-casted insole, which has as its principle the use of the prescribed padding
2. casted insoles made to a cast or model of the foot.

Non-casted insoles

Non-casted insoles are manufactured in such a way that they form part of the shoe. The first prerequisite is the production of a template to the shape and size of the insole of the shoe. From the template, the base material of the insole is then shaped accordingly and placed in the shoe.

The pressure points on the foot may be coloured and the patient allowed to walk for a few minutes until the colour is transferred to the base material. This provides a static impression. Experience will show that if this method is used, the placement of the padding should be moved slightly anteriorly to allow for the elongation of the foot which occurs during locomotion. This adjustment varies from patient to patient, depending upon the elasticity of the foot. For this reason, this method of manufacture is not entirely accurate.

To eliminate error, dynamic impression marks are more valuable. To obtain these, the patient walks for anything up to 2 weeks with the template in the shoe before returning it. Other methods may be used, such as waxing the template. The template is rubbed over with dental wax until a light layer of wax is left on the surface. This gives an accurate impression when walked upon for a few minutes. Whichever method is used, the most important feature is to ensure that the base material fits exactly. Any movement of the insole within the shoe would render it less effective. From the wearmarks provided on the template, appropriate padding is shaped and bevelled to a suitable thickness. This is then adhered to the base material, covered with a fine leather or synthetic covering such as Pampa, and, once trimmed, fitted into the shoe. Figure 14.4 shows the manufacture of a simple insole, without its top cover. It is also possible simply to remove the insole cover from the shoe, incorporate appropriate padding and replace the insole cover.

Casted insoles

Insoles made to a cast may be *accommodative orthoses*, which are designed to support and protect feet which have deformities incapable of correction, or *functional orthoses*, which are designed to correct biomechanical imbalances between the hindfoot and the forefoot, such as forefoot varus or structural malalignment of the foot on the leg, as occurs in hindfoot valgus.

Accommodative orthoses are normally prescribed for conditions where joint pathology renders correction impossible. A large number of acquired and congenital deformities fall into this category. Figure 14.5 shows an accommodative orthosis manufactured for a patient injured in a motorcycle accident. His knee is fused and he presents with an ankle equinus and shortening of one leg by 1.5 inches. The object of the insole is to load the maximum amount of foot surface contact area by filling in the exaggerated arch with a cork/latex compound. Birko cork, latex milk and the varieties of ethyl vinyl acetate foams are excellent materials for this purpose. They provide a flexible support while incorporating forefoot padding to reduce pressure on the first and fifth metatarsal heads. The compound consists of cork, leather dust and fine woodflour to which latex is added until a consistency of porridge is achieved. The mixture is then spread on

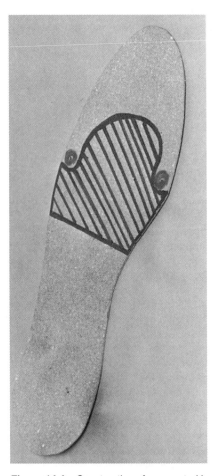 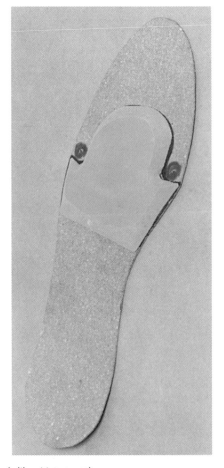

Figure 14.4   Construction of non-casted insole (without top cover).

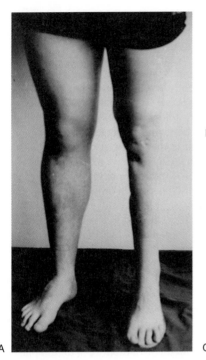

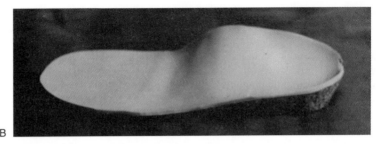

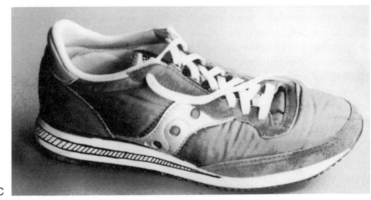

Figure 14.5 Casted insole. A: 1.5 inch shortening of left leg after accident. B: Orthosis in cork/latex compound gives 1 inch heel raise. C: Orthosis is worn in running shoe fitted with additional raise to the midsole (hatched).

the covering of the orthosis, smoothed as evenly as possible and cured or vulcanised for 24 hours. The orthosis may then be finished by grinding, fitting it to the shape of the shoe. In the case illustrated, the orthosis was fitted into a running shoe. Such shoes are excellent for orthoses of this type, because they have all the necessary features one would look for in a good shoe. The midsole has an extra piece added to it to reduce the leg length differential still further.

Ethyl vinyl acetate foams seem to be the material of choice for most accommodative orthoses as they are available in three densities: high, medium and low. They offer the practitioner the ability to provide light, durable, low cost alternatives which may be heat-moulded over a cast or directly onto the patient's foot. The use of these materials is particularly good for rheumatoid arthritics, patients with peripheral vascular disease and in sports orthoses, particularly where a full-length insole is required, as in skiing.

Functional orthoses

Hindfoot/forefoot malalignments underlie many mechanical foot disorders and they are referred to as structural osseous deformities of the foot. The most common frontal plane structural problems which fall into this category are forefoot varus, forefoot valgus and plantarflexed first ray, hindfoot varus and hindfoot valgus. The incidence of these structural deformities is difficult to identify, since little random sampling of the population at large has been carried out; however, one study (Black 1986) identified 44% of those under investigation as having a forefoot/hindfoot abnormality.

Sperryn (1983) highlighted the association between pain in other areas of the musculoskeletal system, such as the knee, hip and back, and biomechanically abnormal feet. Foot pathology is recognised as a major contributory factor in compartment syndromes of the lower limb.

As a general rule, the more severe the structural abnormality, the more rigid the material required to achieve correction, provided the requisite joint motion is available in the foot to allow for realignment. In severe deformities, however, it may be necessary to compromise between what is possible and what is tolerable. It may also be impossible to post the orthosis to the degree required to achieve full correction and still get it into a shoe.

The choice of materials is also subject to other factors outwith the range of joint motion previously mentioned. Factors which have to be taken into account are age, weight, occupation, chronicity of the condition and preferred style of footwear. Furthermore, in the case of the sportsperson, the nature of the event has to be considered, i.e. if it involves running, jumping or contact sport, then the ground/shoe interface has to be considered. Materials range from rigid to flexible. Acrylic resins, such as Rohadur, are rigid plastics and splinting materials. Hexcelite, Aquaplast and the new range of fibreglass fracture splinting materials can provide orthoses which last for many months, as well as the carbon fibre composites previously mentioned. It is possible to manufacture temporary orthoses in situ on the foot using these splinting materials, since their thermoforming temperature can be tolerated by the skin on the sole of the foot. Children normally tolerate semi-rigid or flexible orthoses rather than those of a rigid variety.

Functional orthoses are constructed on plaster models of the patient's foot. The mould or cast is taken with the subtalar joint in its neutral position. The neutral position of the subtalar joint may be determined by one of four methods: palpation, observation, measurement and evaluation. No one method is entirely reliable and the practitioner should always seek to support observation by measurement in determining the position of the subtalar joint neutral position. The neutral position of the subtalar joint occurs twice in the gait cycle, shortly after heel strike and later at the midpoint of midstance, when the foot moves from being a pronating mobile adapter to a supinating rigid lever. This ensures that the contours of the foot accurately reflect the relationship between the forefoot and hindfoot. One procedure is as follows:

1. The patient is placed supine with the feet extending beyond the edge of the leg or plinth in order to secure full muscular relaxation. The patient may lie prone if this is preferred. A pillow or towel is placed under the hip on the same side as the foot to be casted. This brings the foot into a vertical position ideal for neutral casting.

2. The neutral position of the subtalar joint having been previously determined, the foot is held in this position while a slipper cast is taken. Low plaster loss bandage is applied in broad strips two layers thick. The first layer is moulded round the back of the heel and both sides of the foot to just behind the first and fifth metatarsal heads. The upper edge of the bandage is positioned three-quarters of an inch below the malleoli and the lower edge is folded inward to cover the plantar surface. The second layer is placed in simi-

lar fashion around the front of the toes and both sides of the forefoot, and moulded towards the heel so as to overlap the first layer. The lower edge is turned in to meet and overlap the first layer so that the whole plantar aspect of the foot is encased. To facilitate removal, only the tips of the toes are covered. Before the plaster sets, pressure is applied beneath the fourth and fifth metatarsal heads to force the foot into slight dorsiflexion until resistance is met. This ensures that the midtarsal joint is maximally pronated whilst the subtalar joint is held in neutral. All excess water is squeezed from the bandage and the position of the foot is held until the plaster sets and the cast is ready for removal.

3. On removal, it is checked to ensure that it represents exactly the foot which has been casted. Any flaws are made good at this stage while the patient is still present. It is good practice to write an accurate and full description of all the features which are to be incorporated in the orthosis. When fully set, the cast is filled with plaster to make the model on which the orthosis is made.

The cast is best filled with a mixture of dental plaster and stone plaster (Kaffir D), which produces a model of the foot capable of modification and of withstanding heat and the forces created by the vacuum press. Additional plaster should be added to compensate for flattening of soft tissue during weight-bearing, particularly on the lateral plantar aspect of the heel. Similarly, additions must be made to the medial longitudinal arch to accommodate flattening. Failure to make these modifications will result in an orthosis which is not comfortable and which fails to perform its functions. Philps (1990) describes in detail methods of manufacture, uses of materials and means of correction.

Subtalar neutral casts may also be taken with the patient in a supine position, and certain authorities describe the technique with the patient seated. However, irrespective of which method is used, the practitioner must always ensure that the principles are the same. The knee must be fully extended and the foot dorsiflexed to resistance.

Children present particular difficulties when casting. This is especially true of the hypermobile child, and having the child prone makes it less likely that the child will move or interfere with the casting technique. However, establishing where resistance occurs when dorsiflexing the foot can present problems and it is best to dorsiflex the foot to 90°. Children frequently wriggle their toes and their feet if they tend to be 'tickly' when the plaster is being moulded, and every effort should be made to distract the child during the procedure.

Many companies now produce plastics in pre-cut template sizes ready for heating. Once malleable, the plastic is trimmed to its rough shape and moulded either by vacuum-forming or pressure from a rubber sheet until the plastic cools and conforms exactly to the shape and contours of the plantar surface of the foot. Different plastics require heating at different temperatures and for differing lengths of time (Table 14.2). Prior to manufacture, it should be decided whether intrinsic or extrinsic posting is to be used, based on the presenting condition, range of joint movement and the degree of correction required. Posts are best described as platforms added to the plastic shell to provide the correction measured during examination. There is debate as to whether extrinsic or intrinsic posting is more effective. However, it is generally accepted that intrinsic posting is more comfortable while extrinsic posting provides more correction.

Irrespective of which technique is used, the principle is the same. Rigid or high density materials, such as dental acrylic, tensol (liquid plastic), high density polyethylene foam or birko, may be used for posting. These posts or wedges hold the foot in its optimal functioning position under load, restrain it from deforming as it would otherwise do, given the nature of the intrinsic fault, and reconstitute the normal time sequence of events occurring in the foot during the gait cycle. If some accommodation is required, posts may be made of a material which will 'give', such as high density rubber.

A hindfoot post consists of a shaped heel pad placed under the heel of the shell and tapered off on the later-al side to the required angle, varus posting only being used for the hindfoot. This prevents abnormal or excessive subtalar pronation but permits normal pronation to take place. Forefoot posting may be either varus or valgus, as required for inversion or eversion deviations of the forefoot, respectively. A bar of material is placed 0.5–1 cm behind the metatarsal heads, tapering off to the medial or lateral sides to the required angle (Fig. 14.6).

Rigid orthoses thus incorporate all the required correction, yet allow for ease of fitting as they require little room in the footwear. However, complete functional control may not always be tolerated by the patient at first, and the orthosis should be worn for short periods only, increasing daily until the patient becomes accustomed to wearing it all day. Alternative methods of controlling the imbalance in a more tolerable manner are available by the use of laminations of leather or compounds of granulated cork and latex, or by the use of semi-rigid plastics. Forefoot padding may also be added to functional orthoses, if necessary, to make them more comfortable to wear.

A corrected negative mould in modelling clay or Plasticine may also be used to fabricate a rigid orthosis. Moist clay is placed in a tray the size of a shoebox about 25 cm deep. The foot is first wrapped in thin plastic film and then placed on the softened clay and subjected to weight-bearing while the subtalar joint is held in neutral. A block of about 10 cm is placed under the other foot to even up the stance. As the foot sinks into the clay, the sides of the foot are buttressed by pushing extra clay around them to form strong walls about 20 mm high. The foot is withdrawn, leaving an accurate negative impression. The plastic film is unwrapped from the foot and left in the impression. This method avoids any contamination of the clay and possible cross-infection between patients.

Aquaplast is heated until malleable and placed into the negative cast, followed by insertion of the foot. The clay is pushed into the sides of the foot to gain a close contour. The sheet of Aquaplast may need stretching and this can be done to specific areas before placing the foot on top. It is not, however, mandatory that the foot be placed on top, as the Aquaplast can be adequately moulded to the negative. Good accurate results can be achieved by smoothing the Aquaplast into place whilst hot and soft. The device may be trimmed and finished when the patient returns.

It is also possible to manufacture such an orthosis directly onto the patient's foot, should time or circumstances not allow the patient to return later. Low temperature thermoplastics which become malleable in hot water are ideal for moulding straight onto the foot.

Table 14.2 Working temperatures and thermoforming times for plastics in common use

	Temperature (°C)	Time (min)
Hexcelite	72	3
Aquaplast	100	3
Pacton	110	5
Evazote	130	6
Plastazote	140	8
Polythene	140	10
Ortholene	165	14
Polyprophylene	165	15
Rohadur	170	18
TL61 (carbon fibre composite)	180	20

Times are based on the oven being at working temperature. All materials were 3 mm thick. Thicker materials take longer to become malleable.

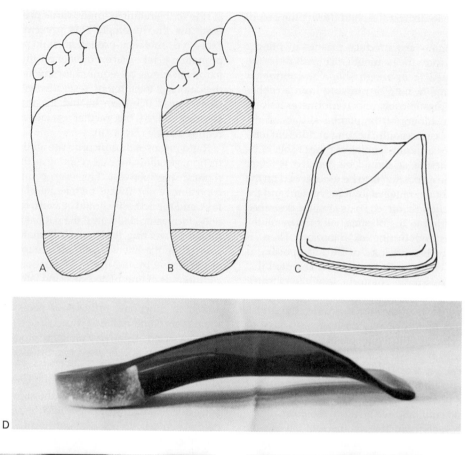

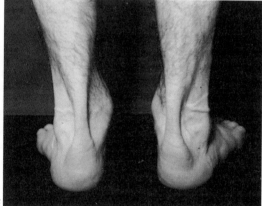
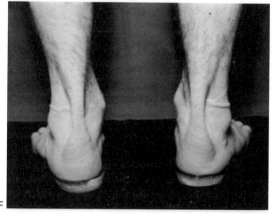

Figure 14.6   Functional orthoses in rigid plastic. A: Relationship to foot and position of hindfoot post. B: Positions of forefoot and hindfoot posts. C: Anterior view of medial (varus) forefoot post. D: Medial view of medial (varus) hindfoot post. E: Pronation associated with hindfoot and forefoot varus. F: Correction of pronation by means of rigid plastic orthoses with medial (varus) hindfoot and forefoot posts.

The only drawback of this method is that two pairs of hands are needed, one to hold the patient's foot in subtalar neutral and the other to place the heated plastic onto the foot. This method may be of particular value in domiciliary visits or where the patient may be unable to attend for a fitting appointment.

One of the more recent introductions is an ever-growing range of commercially made preformed orthoses which may be heated with a hand-held heater, or even a hair dryer, and moulded to the patient's foot for more effective and immediate fitting. For many of them, there are corrective posts which may be applied easily. These add-on posts are usually supplied in 2° or 4° angles and can be applied in multiples for increased correction. These orthoses offer practitioners the potential to provide orthotic therapy without the need for casting and without the need for elaborate manufacturing facilities. There are a number of brands now available, as described below.

Biothotic

This is a preformed orthosis which is available in a variety of sizes. It utilises the principle of the injection of water into an aperture, where it reacts with a resin which swells up to form the medial longitudinal arch of the orthosis and which creates a closely contoured fit. The technique requires the patient to be in a neutral calcaneal stance position on the insole and the foot to be held there until the chemical reaction between the water and the resin is complete. Additional posts can be added and adhered to the orthotic if required.

Australian Orthotics Laboratory (AOL)

This company was founded in 1979 to research biomechanical problems and to develop natural and effective treatments. They have produced a comprehensive range of products, which includes the following standard design features: 4° rearfoot varus wedge, midtarsal joint stabilisation, balanced 4° forefoot wedge, second, third and fourth dorsal metatarsal alignment, and 15 mm heel cup. They are produced in soft, medium and hard density, in four different models and six different sizes, and are manufactured from a composite ethyl vinyl acetate (EVA). This material is commonly found in the midsole of running shoes and is heat-mouldable so that it can be altered to fit each patient.

Cad-cam orthotics

This computer-aided design and manufacturing process is a new method of producing functional orthoses. It is a process developed by an American firm (ADT), which enables practitioners to prescribe and supply devices produced to much finer tolerances than hitherto. It has greater flexibility, with the shell thickness matched to the patient's weight, mathematically correct expansion and posting which allows special accommodations. The orthotic is cut from a block of the material and is not heat-moulded, thus avoiding changes to the molecular structure which could potentially weaken it, and its method of finish allows it to be supplied without covering material, thus requiring less shoe room.

The data for the design of the orthotic are obtained by neutral casts or a scan of the patient's feet using a bioscan developed by ADT, and are stored centrally for repeat manufacture. There is only one licensee operating outside the USA.

Silipos

This company produces a range of insoles manufactured in a cross-linked three-dimensional polymer gel. Its structure reduces shearing stress, while the USP mineral grade oil softens and lubricates the skin. The material is also available in a range of digital pads, which protect a variety of pressure points, and in sheet form for use in the production of chairside appliances.

Heel orthoses

There are a number of orthoses which may be made specifically for conditions affecting the heel. A heel cup may be fabricated on a cast of the heel using plastics already described, or fibreglass. Such devices are well tolerated since they take up little room and can be worn in a wide variety of shoes. Wedges or posts may be incorporated into such devices at the time of manufacture or at a later stage. These devices are corrective in nature. However, palliative heel orthoses may be required for lesions on the plantar aspect of the heel, such as calcaneal bursitis, and for the area around the insertion of the tendo Achilles where the bursae are often subject to irritation from footwear. Skaters are particularly vulnerable to retrocalcaneal bursitis because of the rigidity of the counter surrounding the heel of skating boots. These heel orthoses can be manufactured on casts or made directly onto the heel using silicone. The silicone technique is discussed later.

Painful intractable hyperkeratotic lesions frequently occur on the area of the heel following trauma, or in some cases resulting from harmful X-ray therapy for verrucae. The formation of scar tissue in such cases leaves the practitioner no other course than to rely on palliative orthoses. Most often, these devices are best fabricated in latex for wear on the foot. However, simple heel pads can also be made to fit into the shoe and can be removed for use in other shoes as required.

Latex technique

Deformities of the toes, such as hallux abductovalgus and hammer toes, are often chronic and require protection more or less permanently. In such cases, devices made in latex are often the most effective type of orthosis. Irrespective of the area involved, the principle of manufacture is the same. For the purposes of illustration, the fabrication of a hallux abductovalgus shield is described, but the technique is suitable for digital orthoses as well.

The most important feature is the accuracy of the negative cast. This may be taken in a variety of materials but the most effective are the elastic impression compounds. Dental impression materials are ideal for this purpose and the most cost-effective of these is dental alginate.

Sufficient alginate having been mixed, the gel is spread onto the area to be cast, with a sufficiently wide margin all round. The amount of movement available in the joint dictates whether or not this cast should be taken weight-bearing. If the joint is fixed, a non-weight-bearing cast will suffice, but if it is mobile, the cast is best taken in a weight-bearing position. Before removal of the negative, it is essential to encase the alginate in a light covering of plaster of Paris bandage. This guarantees that there will be no deformation upon removal of the negative. This technique can be adopted for all large alginate casts.

The negative is then filled with plaster, and when this has set the alginate is stripped bit by bit to ensure that the positive remains intact. Any blemishes on the positive are removed with fine sandpaper, and, if necessary, porosities may be filled in with a thin mixture of plaster. The positive is then allowed to dry. Care must be taken not to overheat the cast as this might reverse the chemical process, causing the cast to become crumbly.

The positive is then dipped in latex, each layer being allowed to dry, until several layers have been built up on the cast. At this stage, the correct type of pad is applied according to the therapeutic function required. If an open-cell foam is used, the pad is first covered with adhesive. This seals the pad and prevents latex from permeating into the foam, and it also traps air within the open-cell structure, thereby improving the physical properties of the material. The cast is then dipped twice more to complete the process before being removed from the cast and trimmed. In some cases, it is preferable to cover the cast in a layer of soft leather such as chamois to provide a soft lining for the appliance. If this method is employed, the edges of the leather must be sealed and the appropriate adhesive used, otherwise degradation of the leather may result, due to interaction with the solvents used to stabilise the adhesives.

It is sometimes necessary or convenient to speed up the process for latex orthoses. This may be done either by heating the cast before dipping or by using a hot air blower such as a hair dryer to dry each dip. In this way it is possible to manufacture a latex orthosis from start to finish in 15 minutes. A variety of latex digital shields are shown in Figure 14.7.

Digital appliances for the lesser toes

All necessary designs of digital appliances for the lesser toes can be produced by any of the methods previously outlined for hallux abductovalgus shields. The necessity for negative and positive casting when the latex technique is used, coupled with the smaller size of digital appliances, lends great advantages to the direct moulding techniques utilising silicone rubbers or thermoplastic materials. Silicone rubbers are well proven as the most suitable materials for digital orthoses. They can also be fabricated from orthotic plastic, but it is then usually necessary to line them with softer material for good tissue tolerance. Plastics used for this purpose are designed for finger-splinting, as they are soft and malleable. This combination increases the corrective effect of an appliance whilst maintaining patient tolerance.

The principle of reciprocal dorsoplantar padding is the most effective basis for digital appliances, and this has been previously described (p. 278). When moulded in silicones or thermoplastics, orthodigital splints are infinitely adjustable to individual needs. They may be either full or partial. When full, they completely cover the dorsum of the proximal phalanges and the plantar surfaces of the intermediate and distal phalanges of the middle three toes. When partial, they are reduced in size to fit one or two toes only, or to form a long prop. Maximum effect is thus obtained with minimum bulk. Deformities and lesions of the fifth toe are particularly amenable to well designed partial splints in silicones or thermoplastics.

SILICONES

The use of silicone elastomers in orthotics and prosthetics is probably the most significant advance in this

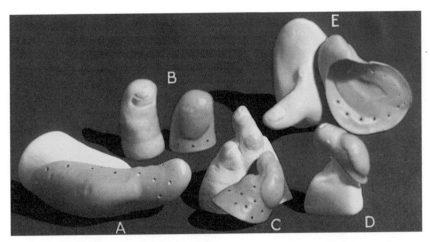

Figure 14.7   Latex digital shields for various sites. A: Hallux valgus. B: Subungual exostosis, when surgery was refused. C: Fourth and fifth dorsal protection. D: Hammer toes. E: Saddle pad for extensor longus hallucis tendon.

field for many years. In the short time since their introduction, rapid progress has resulted in new opportunities of treatment for digital deformity in both the old and the young. Silicones used in podiatry are derivatives of elastomers used in dentistry, although in recent years, specific materials designed for podiatry have become available.

Silicones are presented as a paste or putty to which a catalyst is added. This promotes cross-linking and end-to-end butt-joining of the polysiloxane chains in the paste. After a period, the viscous paste or putty is transformed into a flexible solid. The material, whilst undergoing its change of state, achieves a putty-like consistency which remains for a period ranging from 2 to 8 minutes, depending on the paste/catalyst ratio and the room temperature. This space of time allows the practitioner to fabricate the device. After final setting, the material must be able to withstand repeated functional loading without dimensional change or fracture. There is a wide variety of formulae possible, but the practitioner must be aware of any alterations which he may make as they will directly affect the properties of tension and compression, and setting time, and therefore the subsequent usage of the material. Other external factors also affect the ultimate vulcanisation of the silicone, such as the type of paste, the quantity of catalyst, and room temperature. Silicones set more quickly in high temperatures, whilst cold dramatically delays the onset of chemical change.

Basically, there are two approaches in the use of silicone elastomers. The practitioner may use the material before the phase transition begins. At this stage, the paste is still in a 'flow state' and is best applied by spatula. This technique is best used for manufacturing heel cups, plantar pads and protective forms of digital devices. The practitioner applies the paste and, thereafter, the silicone will flow to cover the proposed dimensions of the orthosis. Initially, this method may be difficult to master because, if the paste is applied too soon after the catalyst is added, it may run out of control. However, it is by far the most effective method of covering large areas evenly, and mastery can be assured after a few attempts.

The other technique involves utilisation of the chemical changes occurring in the paste as the silicone converts from paste to elastic solid. During this phase transition, the material becomes malleable and, provided that the practitioner has included sufficient plasticiser in the formulation and uses liquid paraffin or some similar oil, the silicone can be handled and manipulated like Plasticine.

By far the most rewarding application of this material lies in the correction of congenital digital deformities in children. The same techniques may be used to correct toe deformities in older patients, if sufficient motion is present in the affected joints, and the same methods have been applied to the maintenance of correction following corrective digital surgery. Basically, the splint is fashioned around the toes, and, as the silicone sets, the toes are held in their corrected position until the elastic properties of the material are strong enough to withstand the deforming forces. Figures 14.8 and 14.9 illustrate a variety of basic techniques for correcting the common congenital toe deformities.

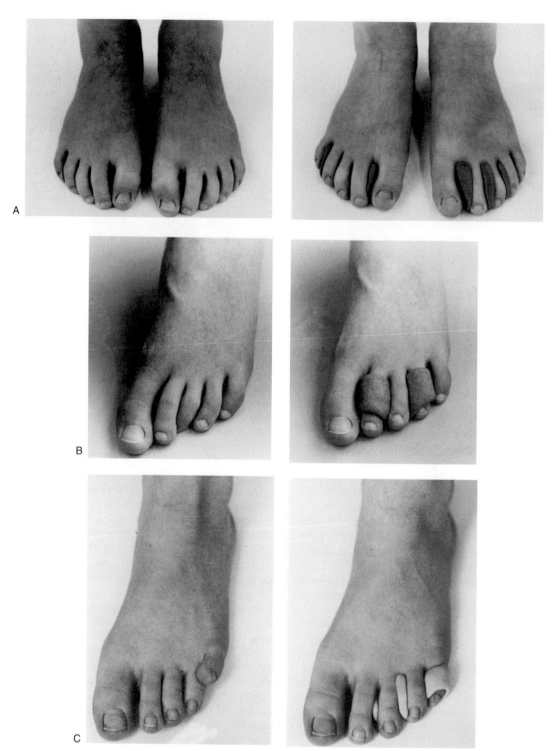

Figure 14.8 Silicone orthoses. A: Multiple prop for congenital curly toes. B: Corrective sling for congenital claw toe. C: Corrective sling for digitus quintus varus.

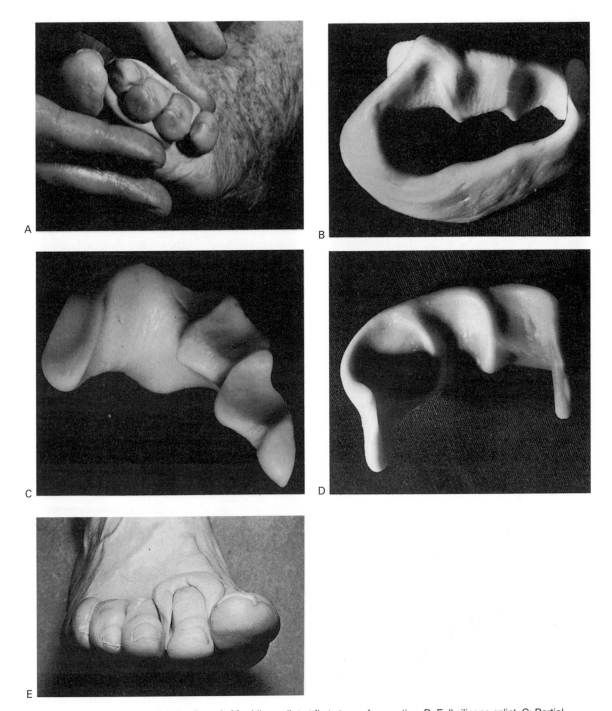

Figure 14.9 Silicone orthodigital splints. A: Moulding splint at first stage of correction. B: Full silicone splint. C: Partial splint with interdigital wedge for first cleft. D: Silicone long prop. E: Single dorsoplantar splint for hammer toe.

When using these materials in the field of postoperative maintenance, one must work in close harmony with the surgeon who has performed the operation. It is essential that the podiatrist has a good knowledge of the surgical techniques which have been employed, so that any splint manufactured for the patient acts as an integral part of the patient's therapy. In Figure 14. 10, a silicone orthosis has been fitted 2 weeks after the patient has undergone a Keller's arthroplasty and capsulotomy of the second and third toes. Assessment of the inherent strength of the lesser digits is important if attempting to manufacture a splint to maintain the position of the hallux in order to avoid moving the lesser digits laterally.

In order to assist the handling properties of the elastomer, 'plasticiser' may be added. The function of a plasticiser is to soften the silicone and make it more flexible. A light grade oil such as baby oil or liquid paraffin may be used, or additives such as 'Atrixo' or 'Siopel'. Plasticisers are able to penetrate between the randomly orientated chains of the polymer and, as a result, the molecules become further apart and the forces between them are lessened. Plasticisers also allow the silicone material to be handled more easily, by preventing the silicone elastomer from sticking to the operator's fingers. The amounts of plasticiser added should not exceed 30% of the bulk used. The more plasticiser that is added, the softer the device and the more liable it will be to deform under load.

Recent innovations on the market are silicone putties. Some have been specially designed for the podiatrist and they achieve their properties by the addition of inert fillers, such as liquid paraffin and zinc oxide, to dimethyl polysiloxane until the material takes on a putty-like consistency. These materials are best catalysed with a cream catalyst.

Modern putties such as Serioro or Podosilk have advanced the quality of putties which allow the practitioner to undertake all techniques including prosthetic manufacture. However, these putties do not have the same life span as traditional paste silicones, but they have the advantages of requiring less effort to mix, and make mastery of the techniques much easier. The same principles apply to all of these materials.

THERMOPLASTICS

Thermoplastic materials are usually products of addition polymerisation. They will soften on heating and harden once cooled without any chemical change taking place. Polymers which are thermoplastic can be moulded to a desired shape when heat and pressure are applied. The most common thermoplastic materials used in podiatry are derivatives of polyethylene, although polypropylene materials are used.

This range of synthetic materials has four main areas of application: (1) firm splinting, (2) impression medium, (3) moulded lining, and (4) modelling and construction.

The firm splinting material is polyethylene sheet, which is not expanded in manufacture and consequently contains no pockets of gas. It is used for direct moulding to positive casts in the production of orthotic shells.

The impression material is the expanded polyethylene which, when inserted into the shoe as a template insole, provides an accurate dynamic impression of pressure areas. The template can then be built up with appropriate padding to produce a permanent insole.

As a lining material, the thermoplastic may be expanded polyethylene or expanded vinyl acetate. After it is heated, moulding is carried out directly on the foot and additional padding and outer layers are added in sequence. This method can be used for hallux abductovalgus shields and similar appliances, e.g. heel cups for bedridden patients to prevent bed sores.

These materials may also be used for taking negative casts. However, if they are to be used for this purpose, care has to be taken to ensure there is no deformation after removal from the foot, and it is sometimes of help to mould a rigid material around the thermoplastic to retain its shape and dimension.

The softer of the two materials is the expanded vinyl acetate (Evazote), which looks identical to expanded polyethylene (Plastozote) but feels much smoother and softer and has a lower tensile strength. Quite com-

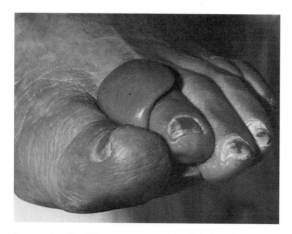

Figure 14.10 Silicone prop and interdigital wedge to maintain position of hallux after Keller's arthroplasty.

plex curvatures can be achieved by moulding these materials, and one of the benefits is that a seamless lining is obtained.

Footwear which conforms accurately to the shape of the foot can be simply constructed by using the various densities and thicknesses of expanded polyethylene. One style is that of the clog with an enclosed front and no heel counter. The sole block is first cut out with a leather knife or on a bandsaw and the foot is placed on top. The upper is then shaped and covered in some appropriate material, e.g. Yampi. This is then moulded round the foot with the foot in place on the sole block and the upper is adhered around the edge of the base. An outer sole can then be added and trimmed. The pair of clogs may weigh no more than 200 g, an important consideration in many cases.

An even lighter style is that of the sandal with a block sole and two or three straps to hold it on to the foot. More complicated styles can also be produced, which, when compared with traditional surgical footwear, are extremely attractive in terms of weight, fitting, style and price.

Almost any shape can be produced by cutting, heating, moulding and buffing thermoplastic materials (Fig. 14.11). To produce a moulded article, the material is heated in an oven at about 130°C until it is soft enough to mould. It cools in a minute or two and retains its moulded shape, at which stage adhesive can be applied. In some cases, the adhesive may be applied before heating, so that the moulding and fixing is done in one stage. Synthetic contact adhesives are suitable for fixing these thermoplastics. Good surface finishing is achieved easily, particularly when this is done on a grinding machine. When heating thermoplastics, it should be remembered that they are all inflammable, giving off strong toxic fumes if allowed to get too hot.

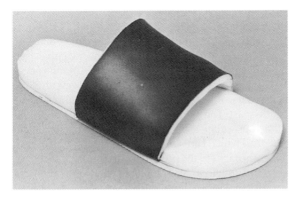

Figure 14.11 Thermoplastic mule made directly onto the foot.

An oven with thermostatic controls is advised and a fire extinguisher should always be at hand.

'Hot water plastics' (Polyform, Aquaplast, Hexcelite)

These orthotic splinting plastics are of particular use when an immediate appliance is required, and this technique is of great value in saving practitioner time. Its essential features are as follows: low temperature moulding; chairside technique; production time of a few minutes; rapid remoulding of part of or the whole device; no waste material, small offcuts being reusable; readily adjustable thickness, as the material can be built up or thinned out as required.

Low temperature moulding. In standard thickness (3 mm), the material can be softened in boiling water for between 1 and 3 minutes to become completely workable and thinned out to an extremely thin layer. At 65–70°C, it becomes workable in about 54–60 seconds, but the moulding characteristics are not as precise as with the 100°C temperature. The plastic will not soften below 60°C.

The material should be dried on a towel before being moulded and it will remain workable for about 3–5 minutes. Fingers should be moistened to maintain a good 'slip' feeling on surface moulding. When moulding, any excess can be trimmed away easily with scissors. Most patients have good tolerance to the hot material directly on the skin, but an intermediate layer of expanded thermoplastic can be included if thought advisable. Cooling can be speeded up by immersing in cold water. If the material is thinned out when moulding, and cooled with ice-water, the hardened state can be expected in about 10–15 seconds.

Chairside technique. The whole device can be produced in as little as 2 minutes but should not normally take more than 10 minutes, allowing for modifications and adjustments.

Rapid remoulding. The advantage of this plastic over silicone rubber is that it can always be remoulded and reshaped by heating part or all of the device. As conditions respond to the orthotic, so the device can be adjusted to correspond to such correction.

No waste. Any small pieces can be reheated and moulded into one new piece. The new material can be flattened into a new sheet of any thickness on a smooth worktop. It will retain its cohesive properties after being heated and dried. Cold material is easily bonded to warm material by using a non-flammable Polyform adhesive. A finished device can be completely remade by placing it back into hot water. If the material has been thinned out while moulding, then in order to obtain the original or greater thickness, it will be necessary to fold over and double the material or to add other sheets.

Complex construction. Where more complex structures are required, and trial and error may be necessary to achieve optimum results, small balls of the plastic may be added, such as under the longitudinal axis of a three-quarter length valgus insole, to gain the desired degree of spring. A valgus insole is very quickly made and can be altered at any time with ease. Heel cups are also easily made and, by careful stretching of the material, can be quickly and accurately produced. Double curvatures are not difficult to make as long as the material is well heated. Combinations of Polyform with silicone rubbers or expanded thermoplastics give good results.

Where a soft appliance lacks strength, Polyform can be added to the original device as a reinforcement or cradle. An analogy is the gumshield worn by boxers, which consists of a strong plastic shell lined with soft material which has been moulded directly to the interior of the mouth. Expanded thermoplastics can be stuck to the Polyform sheet prior to heating and moulding to give an excellent fit when finished. Individual areas of the material can be heated using a hot-air gun, and additional moulding or alterations can be performed.

Hexcelite. This is a remouldable plastic impregnated over soft cotton. The material forms a mesh and, as such, combines features of excellent moulding with ventilation. It is self-bonding, light and has considerable strength. It is a relatively inexpensive material and can be heated in water at 72°C. It sets in 3 minutes and, when malleable, it will bond itself whether wet or dry. It has many uses and the podiatrist need only use imagination to provide a wide array of semi-rigid orthoses. It can be used to manufacture night splints for hallux abductovalgus and it can also be used to splint lesser toes following surgery. By bonding several layers together, functional orthoses can be made in a matter of minutes. These insoles may be made directly on the patient's foot or manufactured on a cast. Posts may be added in the same material. The Hexcelite should be moulded together by rolling with a rolling pin. Any synthetic contact adhesive is suitable for use with Hexcelite.

ORTHOTIC LABORATORIES

The provision and manufacture of orthoses by commercial outlets is steadily increasing. It is now possible to provide patients with traditional types of orthoses, including latex appliances and functional orthoses, for sport and everyday wear. Many outlets produce orthoses on receipt of casts taken by the practitioner. A period of 3 or 4 weeks is about average for this type of service.

Two features are vitally important when using such services. The negative casts have to be accurate and well packed so that there is no damage during transit. The instructions on the prescription form provided must be explicit and detailed. No manufacturer can provide accurate, well-fitting orthoses from badly produced negative casts. It is ultimately the practitioner's responsibility if the orthoses prove to be unsuitable. This method of providing a service is more expensive and, if the practitioner does not have the necessary equipment or expertise, alterations are time-consuming. The practitioner should master the techniques of adjustment, as this not only provides a more effective service, but also enhances the practitioner's professionalism.

PROSTHESES

It is now within the podiatrist's capability to provide patients with life-like prostheses. Digital replacements, whether single or multiple, can be manufactured with silicone elastomers. KE 20 is a white elastomer which can be tinted to a flesh colour by adding a specific colorant provided by the manufacturer or by adding a little Verone RS. The technique is relatively simple and, for a single digit replacement, can be done with the patient present. A negative cast is taken of the digit or digits which are to be used as donor toes. If a fifth toe is to be replaced, a fourth toe may be used. A second toe can be substituted by a third toe, and so on. However, if all toes need to be substituted, then recourse to an individual with similar foot size and configuration is required.

Figure 14.12 illustrates the technique for replacing the fourth and fifth toes. Using dental alginate or one of the dental elastomers other than silicone, a negative cast of the remaining two lesser digits is produced. This is then filled with an appropriately shaded amount of silicone. Exhaust holes must be pierced in the negative cast before commencement of the procedure. After the negative cast has been filled, the operator must wait until the paste has become a flexible rubber before removing the negative cast. The resultant mould is trimmed or drilled to the appropriate size and then bonded to a small silicone prop which runs under the remaining toes to provide anchorage for the prosthesis. These are particularly successful devices and patients find the cosmetic improvement exceedingly satisfactory.

For total replacement of all toes, a positive cast of the remaining stump is necessary to provide a base to

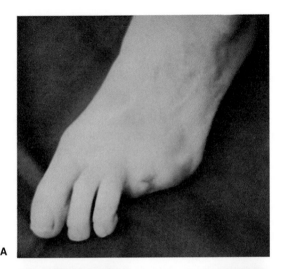

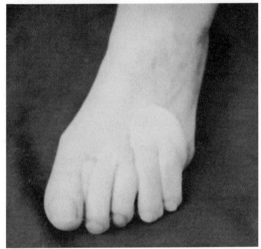

Figure 14.12 A, B: Silicone prosthesis for fourth and fifth toes.

which the donor toes are bonded with silicone. When using this technique, an adequate amount of shaded elastomer with the correct proportions of added plasticiser must be premixed so as to ensure that there will be no possibility of producing a two-tone prosthesis.

Where larger portions of the foot are lost, traditional methods of incorporating open-cell foams in latex are still considered effective. Attempts to provide life-like prostheses for these feet with silicone prove to be both too costly and too heavy to be effective, because of the large amount of silicone required. Until flesh-like foaming elastomers are produced which can withstand the destructive forces of weight-bearing, traditional methods prove more satisfactory.

SHOE MODIFICATIONS

Heels

Thomas heel

The heel is built out anteriorly under the instep to give solid support to the waist of the shoe, in order to prevent it giving way under excessive pressure. Normally, an extension half the width of the heel is sufficient for this purpose, and this saves additional weight. It ends either as it meets the sole or shorter than this as may be required. It is usually applied to the medial side in some forms of pes planovalgus, to provide medial support, but can equally well be of value when applied laterally ('reverse Thomas heel') to give lateral support where required in pes cavus or talipes varus. The extension may be combined with wedging if necessary ('crooked and elongate heel').

Buttressed heel (flared heel, floated heel)

The heel is built out laterally or medially as required to provide additional lateral or medial support, and also, if necessary, to restrict abnormal inversion or eversion, respectively. The lower the heel, the more effective is the additional support.

Heel wedges

Heel wedges may be applied internally to the heel seat or externally to the shoe heel. Internally, they are used to correct or stabilise excessive eversion of the calcaneus within the shoe and hence abnormal pronation of the foot. Externally applied, they tilt the heel seat into an inverted position. Either form may therefore be of value in the management of different forms of pes planovalgus.

Internally, cork sections tapering from medial to lateral are shaped to conform to the size and shape of the heel seat, tapered off anteriorly and inserted under the heel sock. The degree of corrective wedging must be individually assessed. The cork sections are slightly cupped in the centre to ensure a close fit to the heel of the foot.

Externally, a leather or rubber wedge is inserted between the lifts of a leather heel or added to a solid heel as close as possible to the heel seat. If necessary, both forms may have to be applied, the internal wedging often constituting a main feature of a permanent insole. Additional measures such as a Thomas heel or valgus support may also be necessary. Wedging on the lateral side of the heel may occasionally be required with a reverse Thomas heel to control talipes equinovarus.

Excavated heel

The heel seat is hollowed out and filled with shock-absorbent material in cases of painful heel, but this is possible only in well-built or specially made surgical footwear. It is indicated particularly where it is desired to lower the heel of the foot in relation to the heel quarters and counter of the shoe, as in posterior calcaneal lesions (posterior tuberosity, retrocalcaneal bursitis). For painful plantar lesions of the heel and for normal footwear, a tarsal platform with a heel cushion is simpler and may well suffice.

Shank stiffener

Firm, splinting material (stiff leather, glass fibre) is inserted in the shoe between the heel seat and the tread of the shoe to prevent the waist buckling. It may be combined with a Thomas heel.

Heel height adjustments

The height of the shoe heel is designed to accord with the 'pitch' (forward slope) of the shoe and the 'toe-spring' (upward tilt of sole) to ensure that the shoe is properly balanced anteroposteriorly. With any given shoe, the heel height should not therefore be greatly varied, except as a temporary measure pending the provision of new shoes with the correct heel height. Heels may be raised temporarily to compensate for a short tendo Achilles, or to relieve pain in a strained calf muscle.

Soles

Sole wedges

Sole wedges are used to tilt the plane of the sole medially or laterally. They are only of value if worn over long periods and they should therefore not be fixed to the underside of the sole, where they would quickly wear away and require frequent replacement. Instead, they should be placed between the insole and the outer sole. Although this is possible with specially made shoes and the superior kind of mass-produced shoes designed with separate insole and outer sole, it is not possible with many modern styles of shoe. Sole wedges therefore have a very limited application and the desired effect is usually better achieved by an appropriate design of orthotic insole.

A medial sole wedge may be indicated in conjunction with a medial heel wedge to stabilise a hindfoot varus. A lateral sole wedge is sometimes used in conjunction with a medial heel wedge (contralateral wedging). The intention is to invert the hindfoot and evert the forefoot in cases of supinated forefoot in children. The effectiveness of the lateral sole wedge depends both upon the degree of corrective pronation which can be obtained at the midtarsal joint and upon this being maintained throughout the midstance and propulsive phases of the walking cycle. These effects are difficult to ensure, and for this reason, together with the impracticability of sole wedges in many modern types of children's shoes, it is usually preferable to rely on over-correction of the calcaneus by medial heel wedging, leaving the pronation of the forefoot to be maintained by the shift of body weight to the lateral border of the forefoot as it bears weight. An appropriate orthotic insole is indicated, eliminating the need for sole wedges.

Metatarsal bar

As with sole wedges, this transverse bar should also be placed between the insole and outer sole of the shoe to avoid excessive wearing and the danger of tripping. It is similarly unsuitable for many modern footwear styles and so has a limited application, the desired effects being more readily and precisely achieved by the design of individual insoles.

Rocker sole

This is an effective means of providing a relatively pain-free first metatarsophalangeal joint in cases of hallux rigidus. The shoe is built up with an additional outer sole which has its greatest thickness under the metatarsophalangeal joints and tapers away at its distal and proximal edges. The heel is also raised to a similar maximum thickness to maintain the balance of the shoe, but it is tapered off at the back. The effect when in use, as the name suggests, is to enable the foot to rock forward instead of bending at the metatarsophalangeal joints. The same principle applies to some designs of platform soles. Some, but by no means all, provide for toe-spring and are quite easy to walk in, and many so-called health sandals employ the same geometry in their solid wooden footwear.

The fitting of a rocker sole is best carried out by a reliable shoe repairer, although test additions can be made from cork sheets of 8–10 mm thickness as a temporary trial before committing the shoe to a permanent alteration. Both shoes need the same modification, regardless of whether the condition is unilateral or bilateral.

Uppers

Modern shoe manufacturing techniques, particularly those with moulded soles, make shoe modifications much more difficult, if not impossible. This applies particularly to modification to the uppers.

Simple stretching

This can be achieved with a swan-neck shoe stretcher or by using a mechanical stretching machine with a variety of expandable lasts. The aim is to provide a pocket in the upper or an overall increase in accommodation. The shoe is worn by the patient and the area of protuberance is carefully delineated by applying an accurately sized piece of adhesive tape over the area. The bulge of the instrument used to stretch the upper must coincide exactly with the area of tape. A softening solution can be applied to the upper, particularly if it is leather, to allow easier stretching. In many cases this is all that is required to alleviate a hammer toe or enlarged joint.

Slit release

This involves cutting through the layers of material of the upper to allow more accommodation for the forefoot. The cuts are made longitudinally and there should be several, spaced closely together, to achieve the best effect. If placed low down on the sides of the upper adjacent to the sole, they are more discreet.

While appearing to be a drastic method, it is sometimes the only expedient pending the provision of more suitable footwear, and it is very suitable for footwear worn only indoors and for housebound patients.

Balloon patching

This is a method of providing an even greater pocket in the upper. A piece of soft leather is inserted into an oversized hole that has been cut in the upper. When stitched or stuck into place, it effectively provides extra space. It is a skilled job for the shoe repairer.

Extra eyelets

This is a simple technique to provide an extension of the lacing section towards the front of the shoe so that it can be opened up more widely to allow a deformed foot to enter more easily. If the extra eyelets are provided at the proximal end of the laced section, the girth of the shoe will be increased to provide extra space for a swollen foot or ankle.

Vamp replacement

In certain cases of severe digital deformity, and also in the case of misfits in surgical footwear, it may be necessary to remove the entire vamp and replace it with another to give more depth.

FURTHER READING

Black J A 1986 The influence of the subtalar joint on running injuries of the lower limb. Sport and Medicine
Cavanagh P R 1980 Symposium on the foot and leg in running sports. Mosby, St Louis
Coates T T 1983 Practical orthotics for chiropodists. Actinic Press, London
D'Ambrosia R D, Drez D 1988 Prevention and treatment of running injuries. Slack, New York

Philps J W 1990 The functional foot orthosis. Churchill Livingstone, Edinburgh
Sperryn P N 1983 Sport and medicine. Butterworth, London
Sperryn P N, Restan L 1983 Podiatry and the sports physician – an evaluation of orthoses. British Journal of Sports Medicine 17(4)
Vixie D E 1980 Symposium on the foot and leg in running sports. Mosby, St Louis

15

Physical therapy

A. Williams

Keywords

Active movement
Cold therapy
Effleurage
Faradism
Friction
Gait
Heat therapy
Interferential
Isometric exercise—dynamic
Isometric exercise—static
Manipulation
Massage
Mobilisation
Passive movement
Passive stretching
Pettrisage
Tapotement
Ultrasound

Physiotherapy is a systematic method of assessing musculoskeletal, cardiovascular, respiratory and neurological disorders of function, including pain, and of dealing with or preventing those problems by natural methods, including massage, manual therapy, exercises, heat and cold therapy and a range of electrotherapies.

Physical therapy is that part of physiotherapy which, using natural methods, deals with the various conditions associated with podiatry.

Massage has been used by humans as a form of treatment since the early civilisations. It was certainly used in China and India, and in ancient Rome and Greece it was used both for the treatment of sports injuries and for pre-sport fitness. Although massage was in decline earlier this century, it has now regained popularity. The classical massage techniques are used for conventional treatments, i.e. sports massage, aromatherapy and manual lymphatic drainage. Other techniques such as *connective tissue massage*, *shiatsu* and *acupressure* are also used. The classical massage techniques are *effleurage*, *pettrisage*, *frictions* and *tapotement*.

Effleurage (stroking) can be either a deep or superficial stroking movement using the palm of the hand to conform to the contours of the part being treated. The movement is always in the direction of venous or lymphatic flow, i.e. towards the heart. If used softly, slowly and superficially, it promotes relaxation of both the patient and muscle tissue. Used fast and deeply, it will stimulate blood flow and increase muscle tone before sporting activity. Used slowly and deeply, it will increase venous and lymphatic flow, reducing oedema.

Pettrisage (kneading) uses the palm and the fingers at different depths and speeds. There are also different techniques: *picking up*, i.e. lifting and squeezing the muscle; *wringing*, i.e. lifting, squeezing and wringing the muscle in opposite directions; *skin rolling*, i.e. skin and subcutaneous tissue grasped and rolled between the fingers.

It is used to mobilise the skin and fibrous tissue, reduce muscle tone and increase venous and lymphatic flow.

Frictions (finger kneading) are circular or transverse movements using one or two fingers with gradually increasing pressure. They are used to mobilise deep or superficial structures, i.e. ligaments, tendons or tendon sheaths after trauma. They also reduce haematoma formation and can produce temporary analgesia.

Tapotement (tapping) can be either a light or deep fast tapping with alternate hands to produce an erythema of the skin, or to stimulate muscle activity. The other method is *clapping* with relaxed cupped hands to mobilise chest secretions, or it can be used as a sports warm-up. Before massage, patients should be warm and comfortable.

Contraindications. Patients with thrombosis, tumour, tuberculosis, infection or poor skin condition should not receive massage treatment. Care should be taken over bony prominences and with patients who have damage to the nervous system.

MANUAL THERAPY

Manual therapy is the passive movement of joints. This can be defined as *manipulation*, a sudden movement or thrust at the end of the joint range that is beyond the patient's control, or *mobilisation*, a passive movement performed within the control of the patient.

Manipulation can be used with or without anaesthetic. It is used to improve the joint range of stiff peripheral and spinal joints, or to relocate dislocated joints.

Mobilisations are oscillatory movements of peripheral or spinal joints in either the physiological or accessory range of the joint. The movements can be performed with the joint held in its mid-position or held in compression or distraction. The oscillations are usually at the rate of two to three per second. They can be small movements at the end of the range to improve joint movement, or larger movements in the mid-range to increase the blood supply and also to aid the relief of pain.

Mobilisations can be used to loosen adhesions after trauma, such as the medial or lateral ankle ligaments after a sprain, or joints stiffened by a period of immobilisation, or to mobilise joints where the movement is inhibited by pain, as in arthritic conditions. It is a very useful technique for restoring movement and reducing pain in such conditions as hallux rigidus and hallux abductovalgus.

EXERCISE THERAPY
Passive movements

This is when the therapist or patient moves the part without any active muscle activity. Passive movements are used to maintain or gain a range of movement. This can be by using mobilising techniques for joints, as in manual therapy, or by passive stretching of soft tissues.

Passive stretching

The technique is to hold and maintain the proximal part firmly in the correct anatomical position, and then hold more distally to stretch out the tight structures to the limit of the pain-free range. Hold for 20 seconds and then release slowly. This should be repeated three or four times. The patient or a family member can be instructed in the technique so it can be continued at home.

When sufficient range has been gained and the patient is happy to bear weight, more dynamic stretching can be attempted. Where there has been limitation of dorsiflexion, double leg calf stretches can be tried. With the arms outstretched at shoulder level, the patient leans forward to take support against a wall, and walks the legs backwards, keeping the heels down on the floor at each step, until a pull is felt in the calf. The position is held for 20 seconds.

When the patient is ready to return to sporting activity, stretching should be part of both the warm-up and warm-down routines and should be used for strengthening (see also Ch. 11).

Active exercises

These are used:
- to increase strength of muscles
- to restore or increase the range of joint movement
- to improve joint stability, to improve balance, to improve coordination and to improve gait to as near normal as possible.

Isometric (static) exercise

The muscle is actively contracted against resistance but there is no joint movement, for example:

1. in sitting, with hips and knees and ankles at right angles, press the soles of the feet hard into the floor
2. in sitting, put one foot on top of the other, press down with the upper foot and up with the lower foot, balancing the muscle work so there is no movement.

Isotonic (dynamic) exercise (see also Ch. 11)

On contraction, there is elongation or contraction of the muscle, causing joint movement, which can be free or resisted, for example:

1. sitting with one leg crossed over the other, plantarflexion, dorsiflexion, inversion, eversion and circling movements can be performed with the free ankle
2. sitting with both feet flat on the floor, spread the toes
3. sitting with one foot on a paper towel, keep the heel still and try and draw the paper under the medial longitudinal arch by flexing the metatarsophalangeal joints.

Non-weight-bearing exercises can be resisted with the help of a crepe bandage or a length of commercial exercise rubber. Weight-bearing exercise should always be attempted first using both feet, for example:

1. standing, with hand support if necessary, go up onto the balls of the feet and then rock back onto the heels
2. walking on the inner and outer borders of the foot
3. walking backwards, sideways and in small circles, etc., should all be tried before going on to running, jumping and hopping.

To improve joint proprioception, which is often disturbed after trauma, immobility or pain:

1. stand on the uninjured leg and raise the other off the ground and hold for 10 seconds, and then change legs
2. as above, but with the eyes closed.

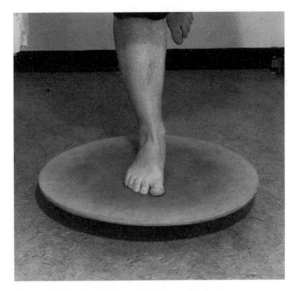

Figure 15.1 Use of the wobble board to improve balance.

To improve balance and coordination a wobble board is ideal (Fig. 15.1). This is usually a circular board with a rocker or hemisphere attached underneath. The patient stands with both feet on the board, with arm support if necessary, and transfers the weight backwards and forwards and side to side. This can be progressed to standing on one foot in the centre of the board, and balancing, and then further progression to weight transference as before.

The use of isotonic exercise for sportspersons is discussed further in Chapter 11. Isokinetic exercise is also described in Chapter 11. This involves the use of expensive exercise machines and is thus mainly employed in rehabilitation departments or sports centres.

Gait

In assessing gait it is very important to look at the patient as a whole. Normal gait requires mobility of lumbar spine, hips and knees, as well as of the ankles and feet. There must be correct leg lengths, good muscle power, balance and coordination. The stride length and stride timing have to be equal. A full-length mirror is important so that the patient can see the problem and see the correct way to improve.

Gaining the cooperation of the patient and letting him/her know that you both have the same goals is the keystone to good rehabilitation.

COLD THERAPY

When ice is applied to the skin, heat is conducted from the skin to the ice in order to melt it. To change its state, ice requires considerable energy. To raise the temperature of 1 g of ice at 0° to 1 g of water at 37°C requires 491 joules (J) of energy.

The initial response of the skin to cooling is local vasoconstriction to preserve heat; this is followed by vasodilation. Thereafter, there is alternate constriction and dilation. The cold decreases the blood flow and slows down tissue metabolism. In trauma, this limits the invasion of blood into the tissues and decreases acute inflammation.

Reduction of pain is probably due to the stimulation of the cold receptors. This is a temporary effect, but active movements can be attempted during the relief of pain.

Spasm and spasticity can also be reduced, temporarily allowing more active rehabilitation.

Application

Ice packs. Crushed or flaked ice is placed inside a dampened terry towel bag or dampened folded towel and placed over the area for 10–20 minutes. The limb is never rested on the pack, as the uneven pressure could cause an ice burn.

Ice towels. This is useful for larger areas. Immerse two terry towels in a bucket containing two parts of flaked ice to one part of water. Wring out one towel, leaving ice clinging to it, and apply to the area. Change the towels every 1–2 minutes. A swollen limb can be treated this way whilst it is in elevation.

Immersion. In a suitable container filled with 50% ice and 50% water, immerse the limb for 5–10 minutes. Care must be taken as this can cause severe pain.

Ice cube massage. This is used for small areas. Hold the ice cube in a cone of dry towel and apply the ice directly onto the skin; massage in small circles for 5 minutes. It can be used on the muscle belly, tendons, ligaments or trigger points.

Commercial flexible ice packs. These contain a gel that does not go solid when frozen, so the pack can be moulded to the part. They come in different shapes and sizes, and can be kept in the freezer of a domestic fridge.

In all applications care must be taken not to produce an ice burn. This can be prevented by oiling the skin first.

Contraindications

- Any patients with impaired circulation, i.e. Raynaud's disease and peripheral vascular disease
- Cold sensitivity syndromes
- Hypertension or other cardiac problems
- Peripheral nerve injuries.

HEAT
Physiological effects

- *Hyperaemia*—dilation of local blood and lymph vessels. Increased flow of blood leads to increase in oxygen and nutrients. Congestion is relieved; the increased circulation promotes tissue repair.
- *Relief of pain*—there is a sedative effect on nerve endings.
- *Increased metabolism*—the increased arterial flow causes the walls of the smaller arteries to relax and the vessels to dilate, whilst the increased venous flow carries away waste products and toxins.

Indirect effects

- Speed of skeletal muscle contraction increases
- Muscle tension decreases
- Muscle spasm is reduced
- Joint stiffness is decreased
- Extensibility of collagen tissue increases.

SUPERFICIAL HEAT – HOT PADS, WAX BATHS, INFRARED LAMPS

DEEP HEAT – ULTRASOUND, SHORT-WAVE DIATHERMY

PARAFFIN WAX

Paraffin wax has the capacity to hold heat. It is used for treatment of sprains, strains and arthritic conditions of the feet or hands. The paraffin wax bath consists of an outer casing which holds the electric heater and an inner chamber which contains the wax. The bath is thermostatically controlled and wax is melted to a temperature of 40–44°C.

Technique

The wax is applied by either immersing the patient's hand or foot in the wax and immediately removing it or pouring the wax over the limb. This is repeated six to eight times, forming a glove or sock. This is covered with wax paper and then a towel, and the patient rests for 20–30 minutes.

At the end of the treatment the wax peels off easily, leaving the skin pink and sweating, and ready for mobilisation or exercises.

The temperature of the wax must be checked before treatment.

ULTRASOUND

This is produced when a high frequency alternating current is passed through a crystal (usually quartz). The crystal is attached to a metal diaphragm, which forms the face of the treatment head. Changes of shape of the crystal cause the diaphragm to vibrate and produce the ultrasound waves.

The waves produced are longitudinal and cause compression and rarefaction in the cells in their path, up to a depth of 5 cm. The human ear detects sound at the frequency of 20 000–30 000 Hz. The frequency used in treatment is usually between 1 and 3 MHz.

Physiological effects

- **Thermal**—the local rise in temperature produced in the tissues increases the rate of tissue repair. It also increases the extensibility of collagen tissue which helps in releasing adhesions and scar tissue. The heat will also help to relieve pain and muscle spasm.
- **Non-thermal**—the variation in pressure on the cells caused by the alternate compression and rarefaction increases the cell's permeability and tissue fluid exchange. This helps to disperse oedema and also helps to reduce pain.

Technique

Set the machine for frequency and depth. A couplant of either gel or water is essential to stop transmission of sound waves back into the air.

Gel. The manufacturer's own (not KY jelly, which is too thick for the transmission of the sound waves) is applied to the part. The treatment head is put in contact and the intensity turned up. The treatment head is moved in a circular or figure-of-eight motion over the surface, maintaining an even pressure (Fig. 15.2).

Water bath. This is useful for irregular surfaces like the metatarsals. The foot is placed in a bowl (not metal) in which there is enough water to cover the foot and half an inch of the treatment head. The head is moved parallel to the part, in a circular motion at a distance of quarter of an inch from the skin.

Treatment dosage

This is dependent on the diagnosis and the area to be treated:

- Frequency
  - 1 MHz for deep structures, 3 MHz for superficial structures
- Continuous
  - for a thermal effect
  - chronic conditions
- Pulsed
  - for a non-thermal effect
  - acute conditions

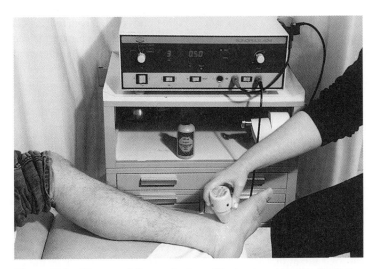

Figure 15.2 Ultrasound: the application of the treatment head to the foot.

- Intensity
  — lower intensity for acute symptoms: 0.25–0.5 W/cm; higher intensity for chronic symptoms: 0.8 W/cm upwards.

Uses

- Soft tissue injuries
- Inflammatory conditions
- Rheumatic and arthritic problems
- Scar tissue.

This makes it a very useful treatment modality for many foot conditions such as plantar fasciitis, metatarsalgia, small joint problems and tendon and ligament problems of the foot and ankle.

Contraindications

These include conditions of the blood vessels which render them unable to meet demand for additional blood supply, sepsis, tumours and after radiotherapy.

Short-wave diathermy is discussed in Chapter 11.

NON-THERMAL ELECTROTHERAPY

Faradism—muscle stimulation

Faradism involves the use of a low frequency current, 50–100 Hz. It is a faradic type interrupted direct current with a pulse rate of 0.1–1 ms. This would produce a tetanic muscle contraction, which would be very uncomfortable, so the current is surged to produce an alternative contraction and relaxation of the muscles similar to the normal muscle contraction of muscles with a normal nerve supply.

It is used to facilitate muscle contraction when the patient finds it difficult to produce effective muscle action. This may be because of inhibition due to pain after injury, postoperatively or arthritis. It may be used to re-educate a muscle action. This could be after prolonged disuse, as in flat foot, or incorrect use, as in abductor hallucis in hallux abductovalgus. It is also used to stretch and loosen adhesions and to improve venous and lymphatic drainage.

Faradism can be produced by large multifunction machines, but the most useful are small portable, battery-operated machines with automatic surging.

Technique

1. To help contract the calf muscle, possibly after trauma or immobilisation, two metal or rubber electrodes are placed, one above each other, over the mus-

cle belly and held in place by straps or bandage. Patients are warned that first they will feel a prickling sensation and then the muscle will contract and the foot will plantarflex and they will not be able to do anything to stop it. Patients are asked to contract with the machine as they get used to it, and the power is turned gently down so that they are contracting on their own.

2. To stimulate the intrinsic muscles a foot bath with half an inch of water is used. One electrode is placed under the heel and the other under the metatarsal heads. The patient is instructed in the same way. To stimulate abductor hallucis using the bath, one electrode is placed under the medial side of the heel and a button electrode is used on the motor point of abductor hallucis (Fig. 15.3).

Electrodes

1. Metal plates—often made from pure tin (for high conductivity) on layers of soaked lint
2. Rubber electrodes—impregnated with graphite for conduction
3. A disc or button electrode covered with lint for individual muscle stimulation.

Faradism is a passive exercise but can cause muscle fatigue, so 5 minutes' treatment is the average to start with.

Interferential

Two medium frequency alternating currents of differing frequencies from 400 Hz to 4250 Hz are applied to the body. Where they cross, they 'interfere' with each other and set up a beat frequency. This is a low frequency current. The two currents can be varied between 0 and 250 Hz to produce different physiological effects.

Relief of pain

There may be an effect on the pain gate by the short duration pulses at 80 Hz.

Endorphin release can be activated by 2.5 or 130 Hz.

The pumping action on the blood vessels speeds up the metabolic rate and the removal of metabolites (0–100 Hz or 0–250 Hz).

Motor stimulation

There will be contraction of muscle between 0 and 100 Hz. This is deeper in the tissues than is the case with Faradism, although 0–50 Hz can be effective for

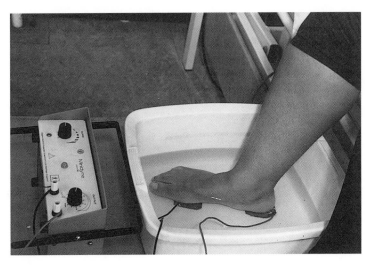

Figure 15.3 Faradism: the electrodes are placed to stimulate the intrinsic muscles of the foot.

the more superficial layers, but the patient cannot contract with it.

The pumping action is very effective for the absorption of exudate.

Technique

The site for treatment is assessed. Two pairs of electrodes with colour-coded leads are placed diagonally opposite each other, making sure the part to be treated is where the two currents cross. Damp sponge pads are placed on the skin under the electrodes so there is no chance of an electrical burn. The electrodes and pads are held in place with straps or bandages.

The power is turned up with the patient telling the therapist as soon as a tingling is felt. It must be comfortable. The treatment time is 10–20 minutes.

Contraindications

These include patients with thrombosis or pacemakers, and care should be taken with patients with heart conditions and tumours.

Interferential is a useful therapeutic tool for the treatment of many foot conditions, including sports injuries, trauma, arthritic problems and soft tissue problems such as plantar fasciitis.

FURTHER READING

Corrigan B, Maitland G 1974 Musculoskeletal and sports injuries. Butterworth, Oxford

Donatelli R, Wooden M J 1993 Orthopaedic physiotherapy, 2nd edn. Churchill Livingstone, New York

Forster A, Palastanga N 1988 Clayton's electrotherapy: theory and practice, 9th edn. Ballière Tindall, London

Gardiner D M 1981 The principles of exercise therapy, 4th edn. Bell and Hyman, London

Grisogono V 1989 Sports injuries – a self help guide. John Murray, London

Hollis M 1989 Practical exercise therapy, 3rd edn. Blackwell Scientific, Oxford

Kahn J 1991 Principles and practice of electrotherapy, 2nd edn. Churchill Livingstone, New York

Kisner C, Colby L A 1990 Therapeutic exercise foundations and techniques, 2nd edn. F. A. Davies, Philadelphia

Low J, Reed A 1990 Electrotherapy explained. Butterworth-Heinemann, Oxford

Low J, Reed A 1994 Physical principles explained. Butterworth-Heinemann, Oxford

Norris C M 1994 Flexibility principles and practice. A & C Black, London

Thomson A, Skinner A, Piercy J 1991 Tidy's physiotherapy, 12th edn. Butterworth-Heinemann, Oxford

Wells P E, Frampton V, Bowsher D 1994 Pain management by physiotherapy, 2nd edn. Butterworth-Heinemann, Oxford

16

Principles of infection control

J. C. McDermott

Keywords

Carriers
Chief sources and reservoirs of infection
Cleaning
Colonisation
Cross-infection
Direct contact transmission
Disinfection
Disruption of transmission routes
Elimination of sources
Endogenous sources
Exogenous sources
HBV and HIV: implications for podiatrists
Infection
Infection control: strategies and methods
Infection control: terminology and concepts
Infective dose
Normal body microflora
Pathogens
Portals of entry
Portals of exit
Sources and vehicles of infection
Sterilisation
Transmission of infection

The prevention of all treatment-associated infection, both in their patients and in staff themselves, is an integral part of the professional responsibilities of podiatrists. An increased awareness of hepatitis B and AIDS has heightened the concern of health care personnel over risks of infection. While concern over infections caused by hepatitis B virus (HBV) and human immunodeficiency viruses (HIV) has focused attention on danger in clinical practice, they must be viewed in the context of infection control in general.

The basic principles and terminology of infection and its control are considered here, but because initial training, professional experience and working circumstances vary greatly, it is impossible to dictate a single infection control regime suitable for all practitioners.

However, equipped with a sound knowledge of the principles involved, individuals can select and implement measures most appropriate to their own practice.

INFECTION

Terminology

The fields of infection and infection control have evolved specialised terminology but, unfortunately, universally agreed definitions of all terms are not available, some variation in usage being demonstrated in published literature. However, there is agreement on the essential concepts, and these are the basis of the following summary of terminology and associated information.

Pathogen

Pathogenicity is the ability of a microorganism to invade a host and cause disease; hence organisms which do so are termed pathogens. However, it is important to realise that the original concept of there being pathogens and non-pathogens must be modified in the light of modern knowledge. While only true (virulent) pathogens may cause infection in a completely healthy host, there are many others which can cause infection if the body is weakened in some way. These *opportunistic* pathogens demonstrate that infection is but one outcome of a complex relationship between the body and microorganisms, infection occurring when the balance of circumstances favours a potential pathogen. Given appropriate circumstances, virtually all microorganisms are potential pathogens.

Infection

Infection is the multiplication of microorganisms in or on body tissues, with an accompanying response by the body's immune system. Products of this immune response, e.g. antibodies against the organism, can be used to detect/diagnose infection or to monitor progress of an infection. Note that this differs from *contamination*, which merely implies the presence of microorganisms which may or may not become established.

Importantly, not all infections result in clinical infection, i.e. visible disease symptoms. Lower level infections occur in which microorganisms become established and there is immune response but no clinical symptoms become apparent, i.e. subclinical infection is present. Even infections which eventually become overt will not show clinical symptoms in the early stages.

Infective dose

The number of cells/particles of a microorganism which are required to establish infection is referred to as the infective dose. Pathogens differ in infective dose, some requiring smaller numbers for successful invasion than others. More importantly, for any infectious agent, the greater the number contacting the body, the more probable it is that infection will become established. It follows that practical measures taken to reduce the number of microorganisms reaching the patient's tissue will reduce the likelihood of infection.

It is not possible to achieve the complete absence of microorganisms in the proximity of a patient. However, for minor non-invasive procedures, appropriate cleaning or disinfection will reduce the probability of microorganisms reaching the body in sufficient numbers to cause infection. When the body is more susceptible to invasion, e.g. due to surgery or other tissue damage, more stringent efforts must be made, by the use of sterile instruments and aseptic techniques, to minimise the numbers of microorganisms entering tissue.

Colonisation

This differs from infection, in that, in colonisation, an organism becomes established in or on the body but neither symptoms nor a significant immune response occur. However, colonisation may progress to infection should circumstances subsequently favour the microorganism.

Carriers

Carriers are people colonised or subclinically infected with a pathogen who show no clear symptoms but who are nevertheless infectious. The carrier state may be preceded by clinical infection, but not necessarily. Carrier states may be temporary or long-term, even permanent. Relevant pathogens include *Staphylococcus aureus*, HBV and HIV.

Sources of infection

A source is a site where potential pathogens can grow and multiply. A similar but more variable term is *reservoir of infection*, which has been used for sites where survival rather than growth occurs, as an alternative to *source*, or to describe a particular category of source. It will be used here for sites where survival or accumulation rather than growth is to be expected.

Vehicles of infection

Many movable objects can become contaminated and transfer microorganisms to a susceptible person or body site. Some are naturally mobile because of their lightness, e.g. minute skin scales or respiratory droplets, while others are deliberately moved, e.g. instruments. Such objects are vehicles of infection, capable of transmitting an infective dose but not usually of supporting microbial growth. Viruses, in particular, cannot multiply outside host cells, but transmission can occur via contaminated instruments, e.g. wart viruses, HBV and HIV.

The preceding points have important implications for infection control. While it is relatively straightforward to identify high risk vehicles (e.g. instruments) and to render them safe by appropriate techniques, individual sources of infection are less easily identified. In particular, staff or patients colonised or in a symptomless stage of infection are sources, but they will not exhibit convenient symptoms warning of a possible infection risk. Continual awareness of the potential threat from sources, even unidentified ones, is required, and safe working practices which minimise the risk of infection from such sources must be implemented.

Cross-infection

The term cross-infection is used specifically in clinical contexts to describe the spread of infections to patients from staff or other patients. It often involves staff–patient contact or transfer of organisms via clinical equipment. Cross-infection is a significant risk to patients and many control procedures are aimed at its prevention.

Portals of entry

These are sites by which microorganisms gain access to the body, most pathogens having one usual portal, although some are more versatile. Once established, organisms may remain near the entry site, causing localised infection, or spread internally to involve other areas of the body. The respiratory, gastrointestinal and genitourinary tracts are common portals of entry, but microorganisms rarely penetrate intact healthy skin.

Entry through skin is usually via damaged areas, including minute abrasions, sites damaged by pressure, venous ulcers and areas weakened by excessive exposure to moisture. Deliberate penetration occurs in surgery but damage may also result from other proce-

dures, e.g. nail reduction or treatment of keratoses and verrucae. As the skin is an important defence of the body, every effort should be made to avoid unnecessary damage and accidental penetration during procedures. Furthermore, any article penetrating skin or contacting damaged tissue is a potential vehicle of infection and must be free of microorganisms which it could transport across the integument barrier.

Portals of exit

These are sites from which pathogens exit the body and from where they are spread to other people, or other sites on the same body. Portals of entry and exit are often one and the same, e.g. infected wounds exuding pus, but pathogens causing systemic infections may exit from different sites. HBV and HIV may exit from any site where bleeding is caused by deliberate or accidental penetration of skin. Pathogens infecting superficial tissues (e.g. dermatophyte fungi, wart viruses, *Streptococcus pyogenes*) will be shed in skin particles or lesion exudates, while other pathogens whose primary target is not skin may, particularly in advanced cases, cause skin lesions containing the infectious agent, e.g. tuberculosis.

The spread of infectious material from exit sites must be minimised by, for example, use of adequate dressings on infected lesions, safe disposal of contaminated dressings and decontamination of instruments.

Normal flora of the body

Every human body is colonised by a large number of commensal microorganisms—the 'normal flora' of the body. Many species, mainly but not exclusively bacterial, occur amongst the flora, and different body sites support mixed populations of organisms suited to the particular conditions. The skin, mouth, upper respiratory tract and the large intestine are important sites of body flora.

The skin not only has a resident flora which is permanently present (e.g. *Staph. epidermidis*) but it is also frequently contaminated with flora from other body sites. These do not usually become established permanently on skin but are so often present that they may be considered as transient normal flora. Above the waist, organisms from the respiratory tract often occur, e.g. *Staph. aureus*, while below the waist intestinal species may be present, e.g. *Pseudomonas* spp. At any time, additional transient contaminants acquired from the environment and other people may occur on the skin.

In health, the normal body flora is harmless or even

beneficial, presenting competition to the establishment of incoming pathogens. However, it includes species which, while usually harmless in their normal sites, can be serious pathogens in wounds or damaged skin, e.g. *Staph. aureus* and *Strep. pyogenes*. In circumstances when local conditions allow excessive growth of a commensal species (e.g. erythrasma), or contamination of wounds occurs, or the body is weakened by systemic disease (e.g. venous ulcers in diabetics), many other commensal species act as opportunistic pathogens of skin tissue.

Chief sources and reservoirs of infection

The chief sources of infection may be categorised as:

* *endogenous*—sites of flora or infection on a person's own body
* *exogenous*—infected or colonised people; infected or colonised animals; environmental sources.

Endogenous sources

Infections of wounds and damaged skin are most commonly caused by organisms from the patient's own body which gain access to vulnerable areas on the foot. Examples include:

* *Staph. aureus* from nasal flora or, in some people, from colonised skin sites; this organism is commonly involved in external wound infections
* *Strep. pyogenes* from the throat or mouth
* *Corynebacterium minutissimum* from skin flora
* *Candida albicans*, a fungal opportunist, e.g. from skin or mouth
* Various intestinal bacteria
  — *Escherichia coli*
  — *Pseudomonas aeruginosa*
  — *Klebsiella* spp.
  — *Proteus* spp.
  — *Clostridium perfringens* (previously *C. welchii*).

In addition to sites of body flora, any existing infected area (e.g. boils, ulcers) is a dangerous potential source from which pathogens can be transferred to damaged tissue. The importance of endogenous sources in potential wound infections means that local flora must be reduced before invasive procedures, and transmission of organisms from other body sites must be prevented.

Exogenous sources

Infected or colonised people. In clinical situations, important and obvious sources of cross-infection are staff or patients with clinical infections of the skin or other accessible sites, e.g. the respiratory tract. However, it is worth reiterating that human sources of various pathogens, including HBV or HIV, are often in symptomless states.

Commoner sources of cross-infection are sites of flora on staff or other patients which, while harmlessly colonising those people, can cause infection if transferred to vulnerable foot tissue, e.g. approximately 30% of patients and staff will be nasal and/or skin carriers of *Staph. aureus*.

Infected or colonised animals. Animals can be colonised or infected by microorganisms which can cause human infections. Patients attending for treatment may have been infected from domestic animals, e.g. by zoophilic dermatophytes such as *Microsporum canis*. Infestation of clinical premises by mice, cockroaches or Pharoah's ants may occur (Pharoah's ants are a minute, inconspicuous species sometimes encountered in warm hospital environments). Such vermin and pests can harbour pathogens, including species acquired from clinical and human waste.

Environmental sources and reservoirs. Survival or growth of microorganisms outside the body is determined by their requirements and the environmental conditions. Many microorganisms associated with the human body are unlikely to grow in the environment as they have specific requirements which would be absent, e.g. for complex nutrients or living host cells. All organisms need moisture for growth, and therefore even less demanding species are prevented from multiplying by the dryness of most clinical areas. However, wet sites in clinical areas are potential sources or reservoirs, allowing growth of some organisms and aiding survival of others. Any body of standing water supports growth of bacteria, particularly Gram-negative bacilli which need minimal nutrients. Wet sites such as soap receptacles, leaks or spillages from pipes or equipment, and residual water in stored utensils are potential risks. Even aqueous solutions of chemicals, including disinfectants, especially if overdiluted or aged, will allow survival and even growth of microorganisms.

Dry sites are reservoirs of viable microorganisms surviving in dirt and dust. In general, Gram-negative bacteria survive poorly in dry conditions, whereas Gram-positive bacteria and fungi survive rather better. The resistance of bacterial spores to desiccation and even disinfection is well established. Protection by materials of bodily origin aids survival, e.g. dried blood, exudate and skin particles. Reduction in numbers due to cleaning procedures is counterbalanced by day to day contamination shed from staff and patients, by clinical waste (e.g. skin and nail debris), and by dirt or dust from clothing and footwear. Therefore, continual effort is required to restrict contamination to acceptable levels.

Transmission of infection

For infection to occur, microorganisms from an exogenous or endogenous source must be transmitted by some means to a new host or host site. Details of transmission routes vary widely in individual instances but may be generally categorised as follows.

Direct contact transmission

This involves direct physical contact with, or close proximity to, a human source or reservoir. It includes close-range transmission of pathogens in droplets or skin particles shed from the body which fall immediately onto surfaces within 1–2 m, i.e. they do not become truly airborne. Those most likely to transmit exogenous infection to patients are staff who are themselves infected or colonised or whose hands and clothing are contaminated from other patients. Staff involvement in direct contact transmission, especially via hands, is of *major importance* in clinically acquired infections.

This category could also include endogenous infection involving transmission from own-body sites, e.g. wound infections caused by organisms from skin or other sites via hands or clothing. Some pathogens usually spread by direct sexual contact, e.g. HBV and HIV, may also be transmitted by clinical contact if blood contaminates skin or mucous membranes. Measures to prevent contact transmission include hand/skin disinfection, protective clothing and 'no-touch' techniques.

Indirect transmission routes

These usually involve intermediate vehicles which transfer microorganisms from an animate or inanimate source or reservoir to a vulnerable host site. If the pathogens originate from a human source, this is often termed indirect contact.

Transmission by clinical items. Any contaminated article coming into proximity or contact with vulnerable tissue is capable of transmitting infection. Background items, e.g. furniture, are relatively low risk while articles in direct patient contact are high risk. Potential vehicles include scalpels, burrs, handpieces and other instruments, swabs, dressings and drapes, antiseptics, syringes and injected solutions. Re-usable

instruments and multi-use containers of pharmaceuticals are more likely to become contaminated than single-use items. Surfaces including trolley tops may contaminate items placed on them. Adjustable lamps used during procedures may transfer contaminants to and from hands. Surfaces allowed direct contact with a patient's skin, e.g. foot rests if not protected by a sheet, can transfer organisms between patients.

Airborne transmission. True airborne transmission, commonly associated with respiratory infections, should have little significance in chiropody procedures. Apart from close-range contamination near the body, previously noted, airborne contamination appears to be significant only when tissue is exposed for prolonged periods, e.g. during extensive surgery (Ayliffe & Lowbury 1982, Meers 1983).

However, clinic dust is a reservoir of infection and may contain remnants of skin, nail, blood, pus and lesion exudates. Various activities may render it airborne, and thus able to settle afterwards on exposed surfaces. Dry sweeping of skin and nail debris, vigorous movement of curtain screens, overcrowding and unnecessary human activity all increase airborne contamination. While this risk is difficult to quantify, these activities are undesirable near clinical procedures or unprotected sterile items.

Transmission by animals. Vermin and insects may shed contaminants when feeding or defaecating. They may also act simply as vehicles, transferring contamination on their body surfaces from dirty areas, such as drains and disposed wastes. Either way, contamination of the clinical environment, surfaces and unprotected materials may occur.

Faecal transmission. Faecal–oral transmission is of major importance in food- and water-borne infections. While this has no direct relevance to podiatry, note that hands and skin are often contaminated with faecal organisms, including potential wound pathogens, after toilet use, and dispersion of such contamination is more likely if diarrhoea is present.

HBV and HIV infections

In view of current concern over HBV and HIV infections, a brief overview of these infections is given here, drawing on the concepts established above.

Hepatitis B virus

HBV is one of several viruses which can cause hepatitis, i.e. inflammation and necrosis of liver tissue. The combination of HBV infection and the body's immunological response follows a complicated course which may result in a range of consequences, e.g.:

- *subclinical infection*—this is the commonest form of infection in adults and is usually undiagnosed.
- *acute infection*—after a long incubation period (1–6 months) the clinical phase usually lasts for up to a month, after which most patients slowly but fully recover; in rare cases infection leads rapidly to liver failure and death.
- *chronic hepatitis (carrier state)*—develops from the above forms of infection in a minority of cases. These carriers may be symptomless or may undergo progressive liver damage which is eventually fatal. Either carrier state may result ultimately in primary liver cancer.

As with other viruses, the components of HBV are antigenic and some of these antigens, together with the antibodies formed against them, may be present in blood and are used to monitor the infection and to indicate the carrier state. HBsAg is the viral surface antigen which, though not infectious itself, indicates that the person is infected and infectious. This disappears as recovery progresses but its persistence longer than 6 months after infection indicates a chronic carrier state. Components of the virus inner core are also antigenic, e.g. HBeAg, the presence of which in the blood of carriers indicates that the person is highly infectious.

Human immunodeficiency viruses

The main cellular target of HIV infection is a type of T-lymphocyte, known as T4 (helper) cells. These cells play a vital part in the body's response to infection by stimulating the activity of other T-lymphocytes, B-lymphocytes and phagocytic cells. Any reduction in number or function of T4 cells leads to impaired humoral and cell-mediated immunity, with a consequent vulnerability to infection.

Initial infection by HIV causes little or no discernible illness (although the infected person is infectious) and within several weeks *seroconversion* occurs, i.e. production of anti-HIV antibodies. However, while presence of these antibodies is useful as the basis of detection tests for HIV infection, within the individual they are ineffective in terms of eradicating the virus. After seroconversion has occurred, the infected individual remains seropositive and potentially infectious.

Individuals who are positive for anti-HIV antibody present differing states of health, reflecting progressive stages (of very variable duration) of the infection:

- many remain symptomless carriers for prolonged

periods, e.g. several years; others, although otherwise symptomless, have persistent generalised lymphadenopathy (PGL)
- variable states of ill health short of fully expressed AIDS which may involve PGL, weight loss, diarrhoea and other symptoms, such as minor opportunistic infections (including tinea infections); such states may be referred to as AIDS-related states (ARC)
- acquired immune deficiency syndrome (AIDS): drastic reduction in immune defence results in severe opportunistic infections, even by weak opportunists, and unusual cancers
- nervous system involvement may also occur which can result, e.g. in pre-senile dementia and peripheral neuropathy.

The proportion of HIV infections which will result in symptoms is unknown; to date, most anti-HIV antibody positives have developed some form of ill health up to and including AIDS, and it is likely that all will develop some degree of illness eventually.

Implications for podiatrists

Both viruses are blood-borne but are also present in other body fluids, including semen and vaginal secretions—hence their association with entry of blood through mucous membranes or damaged skin, and with sexual transmission. Both infections have an increased incidence in certain groups, e.g. illegal drug injectors, homosexual/bisexual males and heterosexuals with multiple sexual partners; but in this context it is much more relevant that these infections are *not* confined to such high risk groups. Both HBV and HIV infections are currently on the increase, both have potentially serious consequences and there is no cure for either; therefore, prevention of infection is the only effective strategy.

A podiatrist is unlikely to know whether or not a patient belongs to a high risk group and, in any case, other patients not in these categories could still be infected. Therefore practitioners must treat all invasive procedures, contacts with blood/tissue fluids, and blood/tissue fluid contamination of instruments as dangerous, however unlikely it seems that the patient constitutes a risk. All sharps used in procedures *must* be sterile. HBV is more infectious and rather hardier than HIV, but this distinction is irrelevant in most circumstances as effective prevention must take into account the possible presence of either virus.

No vaccine is currently available against HIV infection, and although an effective HBV vaccine is now available, only a small minority of the population will be protected by this in the foreseeable future. As health care workers with direct patient contact, podiatrists are an at-risk group and should seek HBV vaccination. In no way does staff vaccination reduce the necessity for other infection control measures, which are essential to protect patients from both these, and other, infections.

INFECTION CONTROL

The modern term, infection control, reflects the realistic objective of reducing infection to the practicable minimum, rather than claiming the ideal of total prevention. Infection has always been of major concern to professionals involved in the surgery and treatment of wounds. Much is now known about prevention of infection generally and wound infections in particular. If the established principles and practices of infection control are implemented, infection following podiatric procedures should be uncommon, especially as many procedures are relatively minor in terms of tissue invasion. Infection control in clinics must encompass measures to prevent patient infections from both endogenous and exogenous sources, and also to protect staff from becoming infected from patients.

Knowledge of infection control in clinical situations stems largely from efforts to prevent infections in hospitals, and comprehensive texts on these aspects have been produced (e.g. Lowbury et al 1981, Bennett & Brachman 1986, Ayliffe et al 1990). In addition, the Society of Chiropodists (Anon 1987) has indicated to its members recommended procedures for particular aspects of routine practice. The following section will summarise the underlying principles of infection control in the context of podiatry and indicate how they provide a rational basis for safe procedures.

Terminology

Sterilisation

This is a process which renders an item free from all living microorganisms, i.e. it becomes sterile (BS 5283 1986). There are no degrees of sterilisation; all microorganisms, including bacterial spores, must be killed or removed. Any process which does not achieve this is a disinfection and not a sterilisation process. Sterilants are chemical agents capable of sterilising, but few can achieve this in routine podiatric circumstances.

Disinfection

Disinfection is a process by which microorganisms are reduced to a level harmless to health. In contrast to sterilisation, there are degrees of disinfection, the level of microbial reduction considered necessary being dependent on the item to be disinfected and the infection risk it presents. Bacterial spores are often little affected. Disinfection, unlike sterilisation, can be applied to living tissue, e.g. skin, as well as to inanimate articles.

Disinfection methods, particularly chemical disinfectants, often demonstrate a particular spectrum of antimicrobial activity, varying in effectiveness against different types of microorganisms. The terms *bactericidal* and *fungicidal* indicate capability of killing bacteria and fungi, respectively. Similarly, *sporicidal* and *virucidal* indicate ability to kill spores and to inactivate viruses, respectively. These properties are determined under laboratory test conditions and such terms should *not* be taken to mean that disinfection so described or labelled will kill all of the specified type of microorganism under conditions of ordinary use. A term such as *germicide*, while implying antimicrobial activity, is too vague and should not be used.

Antisepsis

Antisepsis is the destruction or inhibition of microorganisms on living tissues, having the effect of limiting or preventing the harmful results of infection (BS 5283 1986). Antiseptics are chemical agents used to achieve antisepsis; they are usually unsuitable for general use on inanimate articles, for reasons of either lower antimicrobial action or cost-effectiveness. Some antiseptics inhibit rather than kill microorganisms, this capability being described by terms such as *bacteriostatic* or *fungistatic*.

Asepsis

The term asepsis means an absence of contamination or, perhaps more realistically, absence of infection (sepsis) resulting from contamination. This should be the objective underlying all clinical procedures. Aseptic techniques are safe methods of working on patients by which contamination is minimised and thus infection prevented—in this context, largely by the prevention of cross-infection and the protection from contamination of damaged foot tissue. As appropriate, both sterilisation and disinfection are employed to achieve asepsis.

Strategies and methods of control

As microorganisms may be transmitted by so many

routes, a similarly wide range of measures must be employed in infection control. All individual control measures stem from the three basic strategies of infection control (Ayton 1981, Lowbury et al 1981):

1. elimination of sources and reservoirs of infection
2. disruption of transmission routes
3. increasing or restoring host resistance to infection.

In any particular circumstances, which will vary for individual practitioners, these strategies provide a framework for a sensible choice of suitable control measures. Strategies 1 and 2 above are especially relevant to practical podiatry and are discussed in the following sections.

Elimination of sources and reservoirs

Important sources of infection are patients with existing clinical infections, e.g. septic lesions, fungal infections, verrucae. Successful treatment not only benefits that patient but also eliminates him as a source of cross-infection. During a course of treatment, dressings minimise exit of pathogens from such sources. Endogenous infected sites must be covered by dressings before invasive techniques or exposing nearby tissue.

Less commonly, podiatrists providing hospital ward services may encounter *source isolation*. Some patients with serious infections are isolated by a variety of measures to prevent cross-infection from them to others. Essentially, both the patient and his immediate environment are considered to be contaminated, and measures are enforced to prevent transfer of pathogens from these by either personnel or equipment. Appropriate protective clothing must be donned and, after patient care, must be discarded within the isolation area. Instruments may require special arrangements for decontamination before re-use and thorough hand cleansing after patient contact is most important. Practitioners treating such patients should familiarise themselves with, and adhere to, the isolation procedures in force at that time.

Podiatrists with clinical infections are clearly a risk to patients. Particularly relevant are infections on the hands or other exposed areas of skin, e.g. furuncles, infected cuts or paronychia. Covering small lesions by waterproof plasters and wearing gloves reduces risk to patients, but such measures may not suffice to eliminate the risk, especially in procedures where glove puncture is possible. Where there is any doubt, direct contact with patients should be avoided until the infection is resolved. Infections of other parts of the body also constitute a significant risk, e.g. streptococ-

cal sore throat. Skin affected by chronic skin conditions such as eczema or psoriasis may become colonised with *Staph. aureus* and lead to profuse shedding of the organism. Practitioners who become carriers of HBV and HIV are very unlikely to transmit such infection to patients. As infection and circumstances vary greatly, practitioners should seek medical advice if in any doubt of the advisability of contact with patients, particularly with regard to invasive procedures. Other possible sources amongst staff include symptomless carriers of wound pathogens such as *Staph. aureus* and *Strep. pyogenes*. Routine screening of staff for such carriage is not justified but may be necessary in certain circumstances, e.g. to investigate an outbreak of wound infections.

Accumulations of dirt anywhere in the clinical environment are reservoirs of infection which should be eliminated by cleaning, with additional disinfection if necessary. Clinical waste must not be allowed to contaminate the area and should be disposed of hygienically. Collection of patient debris at source using a disposal bag, partially inserted underneath the sheet protecting the foot rest and anchored by the foot (Paterson 1985), is a sensible measure. Wet sites resulting from faulty equipment or plumbing can be eliminated by repair or replacement. Other wet sites need a common-sense approach to alteration of working procedures or choice of materials. Examples include disinfecting and drying cleaning utensils before storage, and replacing bars of soap lying in a wet dish by cleaner draining storage or, better still, by a suitable detergent/disinfectant dispenser.

Prevention of animal pest infestations is aided by maintenance of building structure (to inhibit access) and high standards of general cleanliness throughout the premises to deny them food, water and breeding sites. Should infestation occur, eradication can be difficult and professional pest control operatives should be contacted. If the source of a patient's infection is found to be a family pet (e.g. *M. canis*), then successful treatment of the person may require veterinary treatment of the animal to prevent reinfection.

Disruption of transmission routes

Essentially, this is achieved by effective decontamination of inanimate vehicles and by procedures designed to exclude contamination at the point of patient contact, the latter including hand/skin disinfection and other aspects of aseptic technique.

Decontamination of inanimate articles is based on cleaning, disinfection and sterilisation. These techniques represent increasing degrees of decontamination and are employed according to the infection hazard posed by particular articles or circumstances. As a general rule, the closer an article approaches susceptible tissue or vulnerable items such as sterile instruments, the more thorough the decontamination required. Cleaning is usually adequate for most general items, such as furniture, utensils and laundry. Disinfection is necessary when a specific infection risk is known to exist, e.g. articles in the vicinity of treatment procedures, blood spillages, and for articles which are unsuited to sterilisation but require more thorough decontamination than cleaning. Sterilisation is necessary for all items penetrating the body or contacting exposed tissues.

Cleaning

The clinical environment should present a high standard of general cleanliness. Inadequately cleaned clinics will not only contain unnecessary reservoirs of microorganisms but will also reduce patients' confidence and staff morale. Cleaning should not be dismissed as a background chore that has little to do with the professional staff, but should be part of an integrated programme of clinical decontamination. In this context, it implies thorough cleaning at sufficiently frequent intervals using effective agents and appropriate, well maintained equipment. Such cleaning is a surprisingly efficient method of decontamination and is all that is usually necessary for routine surfaces and equipment such as floors, furniture, sinks, toilet facilities and similar items. Disinfection of these is unnecessary, firstly because such items normally present an insignificant infection risk, and secondly, because recontamination is inevitable and reaches a similar equilibrium level whether or not disinfectants are used. However, disinfection is justified for such items on specific occasions of known increased risk, e.g. blood spillage.

In addition to preventing excessive accumulations of contaminated dirt, cleaning should not itself increase any risk of infection. Both the methods and materials employed must themselves be hygienic. There are two main dangers here: the distribution of dust-borne contamination and the growth of bacteria on wet cleaning utensils. Dry dusting or sweeping, including the sweeping up of debris after patient treatment, is not acceptable in clinical areas, and suitable vacuum cleaners (BS 5415) or dust-attracting mops should be used instead. Vacuum cleaners should incorporate efficient filters, regularly checked and replaced as necessary, and inner disposable paper bags which retain debris and microorganisms. Dust-

attracting mops must themselves be cleaned as soon as they are visibly dirty or at least every 1–2 days.

Wet cleaning should be done with clean water and a detergent, changed frequently to maintain effectiveness. Cloths, preferably disposable, for damp-dusting surfaces and 'string mops' for cleaning floors are more suitable than sponge utensils, which are less easy to decontaminate after use. Utensils for wet cleaning are known to support the growth of bacteria, particularly Gram-negatives, if they are not effectively decontaminated after use. Ideally, such items as re-usable cloths, mopheads, buckets and wet parts of cleaning machines should be cleaned after use, heat-disinfected if possible, and then stored dry. Unless serviced by a centralised hospital cleaning service, practitioners may consider this an unattainable standard, but serious efforts should be made to avoid heavy contamination of wet utensils which in turn would contaminate the very items they are supposed to clean. Utensils should at least be cleaned in fresh hot water and detergent, and then rinsed and dried. Storage of all ancillary equipment, including cleaning materials, should, of course, be separate from the area used for patient treatment. Routine cleaning activities, even if done well, carry a risk of dust disturbance or splashing and should be completed as long as possible (ideally at least an hour) before treatment of patients, to allow airborne contamination to finish settling.

Floors, toilet facilities and furniture should be washed or damp-dusted daily as appropriate. Sinks also require thorough cleaning daily, and additional cleaning if soiled during use, with either detergent or mild abrasive cleaning products. Sites which could harbour stagnant water, e.g. soap ledges, must be dried. Walls in good repair are of little significance in infection and, unless soiled, require infrequent cleaning; every few months should suffice. In contrast, adjustable lamps positioned immediately above the patient and which are frequently handled should be cleaned daily, and disinfection between patients could be recommended.

Some exceptions to daily cleaning of floors and furniture may be necessary. If floor areas on which patients walk barefoot exist, there is the risk of cross-infection, and careful organisation of patient movements or use of overshoes could eradicate this. As some foot conditions will render patients vulnerable to infections, while other patients may have existing infections, it is difficult to justify contact with a floor that is not at least cleaned between patients. Similarly, furniture or surfaces in the immediate vicinity of treatment procedures justify extra cleaning and even disinfection between patients, especially before invasive procedures.

Re-usable instruments should be cleaned after use before further decontamination and re-use. After a rinse in cold water, they may be cleaned manually using a brush and mild detergent. Rubber gloves should be worn, as thick as is consistent with dexterity, and every care taken to avoid accidental injury while cleaning, rinsing and drying sharps, because of the risk of HBV and HIV infections. Used instrument brushes should be cleaned and disinfected, preferably sterilised, and not simply left by the sink. Instruments and other utensils should not be cleaned in the same sink used for clinical handwashing, but if this is completely unavoidable, the sink should be cleaned and disinfected after use for instruments.

Alternatively, ultrasonic cleaning in detergent solution can be employed for instruments, in which case the manufacturer's instructions on method and suitable agents should be followed. Note that ultrasonic baths are a cleaning aid only and do not kill microorganisms—they may even disperse aerosols of microorganisms if lids are not tightly fitted. Furthermore, they should not be allowed to retain water or stagnant cleaning solution, which could support the accumulation of bacteria. For further details of cleaning methods and agents, the reader is referred to comprehensive texts on clinical hygiene (e.g. Maurer 1985).

Disinfection

Many agents have been employed for disinfection in clinical situations, including steam, hot water, chemical vapours, chemical solutions and ultraviolet radiation. The agents most relevant to podiatric clinics generally are hot water and chemical disinfectants. Hot water has the advantage of being effective against all types of microorganisms except bacterial spores; it needs little expertise, leaves no residues and is inexpensive. However, it is unsuitable for very heat-labile items, cannot be used on living tissue, and is not practicable for larger items. Chemical disinfectants can be used on surfaces and furniture, and some are suitable for skin disinfection. Unfortunately, as a group they have many disadvantages, including possible toxicity, corrosiveness, variable antimicrobial effectiveness, inactivation by many materials, undesirable odours or residues, limited in-use life, and a general requirement for skilled use to be effective.

Despite the widespread use of chemical disinfectants in the past, it is now accepted that they should be used only when there is a clear need for disinfection additional to thorough cleaning, and when no practical alternative is available. If possible, hot water should be used instead, particularly as items too sensitive for heat sterilisation often withstand the lower temperatures used for disinfection.

In summary, heat disinfection is the preferred method for inanimate items of suitable size for immersion, whereas chemicals are employed for larger items and surfaces, for skin disinfection, and when heat is not practicable.

Disinfection by hot water. Articles should be cleaned first, then fully immersed in hot water, ensuring parts are not protected by trapped air. Temperatures of at least 65°C are necessary; higher temperatures decrease the time required for effective disinfection. For routine use, the values in Table 16.1 are applicable.

Such treatments are recommended to kill vegetative bacteria on items such as heat-labile instruments (Central Sterilising Club 1986). Thermostatically controlled washer/disinfectors with timed cycles, and washing machines incorporating a disinfecting hot water rinse, are available. Heat-resistant instruments should be immersed in boiling water for at least 5 minutes (BMA 1989). 'Instrument boilers' need careful use as they usually lack time-controlled cycles and can also pose problems of operator safety. It must be emphasised that disinfection, even at high temperatures, is not sterilisation and it should not be used when sterility is required.

Disinfection by chemicals. Despite their disadvantages, chemical disinfectants are required for certain tasks and are effective when used correctly. However, users should be aware of various factors which influence the efficiency of disinfectants.

Concentration of disinfectant solutions is important in determining efficiency and the recommendations of manufacturers or suppliers must be followed. For this reason solutions should never be 'topped up' by the addition of more water, with or without additional disinfectant. Once prepared, in-use solutions deteriorate, resulting eventually in a lower actual concentration which is ineffective. If possible, make up fresh solutions daily; this need not be wasteful if appropriate quantities are prepared. Otherwise, it is essential to note shelf-life information and to prepare fresh solutions when required, marking the date prepared and

Table 16.1 Disinfection by hot water

Temperature (°C)	Minimum time
65	10 min
70	2 min
90	1 s

use-by date as appropriate. Remember that disinfectant solutions can act as sources or reservoirs of pathogens.

All disinfectants can be inactivated to some extent by various natural or synthetic materials, such as hard water, detergents, soaps, tissue or other body material, cork, cellulose (e.g. cotton wool) and plastics. This is potentially serious, as many articles used to contain or apply the disinfectants, and items for disinfection themselves, may reduce the effectiveness of the process. If required, the manufacturer's advice should be sought on these aspects.

Dirt, especially dried organic materials, may inhibit disinfectants by inactivation and by presenting a physical barrier to penetration of the solution. The level of initial microbial contamination also influences the number of microorganisms surviving after a given treatment. Therefore, if possible, articles should be cleaned to remove dirt and reduce contamination before disinfection.

Disinfection is not instantaneous and adequate contact time must be allowed. This varies from seconds to prolonged soaking, depending on the agent and the item involved.

An important and very variable factor in chemical disinfection is the user, and many studies have shown human ignorance or error to be responsible for ineffective clinical disinfection. The number of different chemical agents should be kept to a minimum and clear instructions must be available on preparation, circumstances for use, method of use and acceptable in-use life.

Types of chemical disinfectants. Many categories of chemicals have been used in disinfection, but relatively few are suitable for clinical use. Others, while effective, have been superseded by more modern agents. Properties of the chief types in current use are summarised here.

Phenolic compounds. These are widely effective against bacteria and fungi but have a poorer action against viruses. Organic matter has little inactivating effect, and therefore they are suitable for use in dirty conditions or on soiled items, but not when there is contamination by blood. In-use concentration is usually 1% or 2% v/v for clean or dirty conditions, respectively.

Combination with a suitable detergent (anionic or non-ionic) aids penetration of dirt, but they are inactivated by cationic detergents. Clear soluble phenolics (e.g. Stericol, Clearsol and similar products) are preferable to cruder coal tar derivatives and are used for environmental disinfection in hospitals, e.g. for contaminated areas and floors, and for operating rooms. 'Pine' type products, though chemically related, are often poor disinfectants and are too easily inactivated to be generally accepted for clinical use.

Chlorine compounds. These are very effective against most microorganisms, including viruses. They are usually the agent of choice when there is risk of viral infection, including blood spillages. However, they are more easily inactivated by organic matter than are phenolics, and therefore items must be cleaned first, or sufficiently high concentrations must be used to compensate for the loss. It is important to ensure adequate activity of the in-use solution, usually expressed in terms of percentage or ppm (parts per million) of available chlorine. Solutions for routine clinical use should contain 1000 ppm (0.1%) and strong solutions (e.g. for blood spillage) should contain 10 000 ppm (1%) available chlorine. Products may be purchased as liquid concentrates, powders or tablets which are diluted or dissolved in water. Typical chlorine-releasing agents employed as ingredients include hypochlorites and dichloroisocyanurates (NaDCC). Product information must enable accurate calculation of available chlorine concentration.

- Sample calculation. Thickened liquid concentrates (e.g. Domestos) typically contain 10% (100 000 ppm) available chlorine. If diluted in water, a 1% v/v solution (1 volume disinfectant to 99 volumes water) would contain 100 000/100 = 1000 ppm (0.1%) available chlorine. A cautionary note on liquid concentrates: concentration varies between brands and degeneration can occur in storage (Coates 1988).

Dichloroisocyanurate tablets are available, which have the advantages of long storage stability and simplicity of preparing in-use dilutions (Coates 1985).

Iodine compounds. Alcoholic solutions of iodine are effective disinfectants but cause tissue irritation and staining. Improved alternatives are available. Iodophors, which are organic complexes containing iodine (e.g. povidone-iodine), are less irritant and less likely to stain. Iodophors have a wide spectrum of activity against bacteria, fungi, viruses and, unusually, bacterial spores on prolonged contact. Iodophor preparations are used for skin and hand disinfection, and wound antisepsis.

Alcohols. Ethyl and isopropyl alcohols have a wide and rapid antibacterial action, but a poorer action against some viruses. They are most effective in aqueous solution, typical concentrations being ethanol at 70% and isopropanol at 60–70%, although higher concentrations are sometimes used. They may be used for rapid disinfection of clean skin, hands and hard surfaces, and for combination with other antimicrobial agents. Ready-to-use disposable wipes containing isopropanol are available.

Biguanide compounds. The most widely used is chlorhexidine (Hibitane), which is effective against Gram-positive and Gram-negative bacteria but poor against viruses. Combination with alcohol increases its effectiveness and accelerates disinfection. It is inactivated by many materials, including soaps and anionic detergents, and cannot be recommended for general environmental use. However, it is widely used for skin and hand disinfection, showing very little toxicity and having both immediate and residual action. It is available as both aqueous and alcoholic preparations (e.g. Hibiscrub, Hibisol).

Triclosan (2,4,4'-trichlor-2'-hydroxydiphenylether). This is effective against Gram-positive and Gram-negative bacteria with little reported toxicity, and is available as both aqueous and alcoholic preparations (e.g. Aquasept, Manusept). Several have been reported to be effective in hand disinfection, but generally chlorhexidine preparations are better.

Quaternary ammonium compounds. These form a group of chemicals which have both surfactive and disinfectant properties, to varying degrees. Although active against Gram-positive bacteria, they are poor against other microorganisms and are too easily inactivated for clinical use. However, cetrimide is one which, in combination with chlorhexidine, provides effective wound-cleansing agents (Savlon-type products).

Glutaraldehyde. This has been used widely for cold 'sterilisation' in podiatry, although probably only disinfection was achieved in normal practice. It is a widely effective disinfectant, with good antiviral action, and is sporicidal in certain conditions. Thorough disinfection requires 20–30 minutes' immersion (sterilisation requires 3–10 hours). As it is an irritant, disinfected items should be rinsed in sterile water. Glutaraldehyde (e.g. Cidex) still has restricted specialised use in hospitals, but its routine use in podiatry cannot be recommended. Alternative disinfection, or sterilisation by heat, should be used for items previously treated by glutaraldehyde.

Hexachlorophane. This once-popular compound is effective against Gram-positive bacteria but poor against other microorganisms. Chlorhexidine and povidone-iodine products are more generally effective after single or repeated applications, and therefore are to be preferred.

Disinfection of specific items. Items suitable for heat disinfection include cleaning utensils (especially if used in operating rooms or on contaminated areas), routine laundry, instrument brushes, reagent bottles before refilling, containers for antiseptics, general purpose bowls and containers for non-sterile cotton balls, etc. Sterilisation of some of these may preferable, e.g.

instrument brushes. In the absence of sophisticated disinfection facilities, cloths and mops may be cleaned, then placed in a container to which boiling water is added and kept immersed for at least 10 minutes before drying and storing dry. Alternatively, after cleaning they can be immersed in a 1% phenolic or chlorine-based disinfectant for 30 minutes, then rinsed and stored dry. Note that some materials, e.g. plastics, may inactivate disinfectants and that utensils should be stored dry, and not in disinfectant. Clinical laundry can be cleaned in an ordinary automatic using a prewash followed by a wash at the highest temperature setting, unless known contamination by HBV is present.

Floors and surfaces contaminated with tissue other than blood should be cleaned then disinfected with 1% phenolic or 0.1% chlorine-releasing agent. Ideally, blood spillages should be disinfected before cleaning to counter any risk of HBV and HIV; disposable gloves should be donned and the spillage covered with paper towels or other absorbent disposable material. Chlorine-releasing agent (10 000 ppm available chlorine) is then poured on and left for at least 10 minutes. The area is then cleaned, again using disposable materials. All items (gloves, towels, etc) are then disposed of as contaminated waste. Alternatively, purpose-made packs of granular NaDCC or other antiviral agents are available for wet spillage treatment, in which case the manufacturer's instructions should be followed. Hands should always be washed after dealing with spillages.

Small areas of clean impervious surfaces, e.g. trolley tops, foot rests, adjustable lamps, and other hand-contact surfaces in the chair's vicinity, can be disinfected with agents that are unsuitable or uneconomic for wider environmental use. Although 1% phenolics could be used, alcohols or alcoholic chlorhexidine, as wipes or sprays, are faster-acting/drying and likely to be more convenient for use between patients (e.g. Azowipes, Hibispray and Dispray type products). Cartridges of local anaesthetic should be wiped with alcohol before use. Handpieces are potential vehicles of infection between patients via the operator's hands, and ideally should be sterilised. If disinfection is used, manufacturers may advise on appropriate methods; alternatively, clean thoroughly then disinfect with alcoholic chlorhexidine.

Skin disinfection. Hands of staff and skin of patients both require adequate decontamination, the degree necessary being dictated by the circumstances. Whatever method is used, effectiveness depends largely on the care and thoroughness of the operator. Handwashing facilities vary, but taps operated without hand contact (e.g. foot operated) are best, and if ordinary taps are fitted they should be turned off using a paper towel.

Hands. The main purpose of routine handwashing is to remove transients acquired from previous contacts, particularly patients. Although loosely adhering transients can be removed by washing with ordinary soaps, detergent/disinfectant preparations containing chlorhexidine, povidone-iodine or Triclosan are more effective, and on repeated use, they also progressively reduce the more accessible flora. Intervening washes with ordinary products eliminate this residual benefit, and therefore, as daily case loads may include treatments which require hand disinfection, it is sensible to use disinfectant preparations for all clinic handwashing. However, choice of agent is less important than thoroughness of application (Ayliffe et al 1990). If hands are visibly clean, rapid and highly effective disinfection between patients or during procedures can be achieved with alcoholic disinfectant preparations. Handwashing with non-disinfectant products is not adequate for surgery, invasive techniques, treatment of damaged tissue or dressing changes.

Further reduction of skin contamination is required for some procedures, e.g. nail surgery. The aim is to reduce flora as much as possible on hands and on forearms from where organisms may also be shed. Initially, the hands and forearms are subjected to prolonged double washing with detergent/disinfectant preparations (as above), attention also being paid to cleaning nails and nail folds. If brushing is employed to remove loose skin squames, it should only be done at the start of a clinical session. Use of an alcoholic disinfectant preparation after washing will increase the degree of this initial disinfection. For subsequent cases, these alcoholic preparations alone, well rubbed in, are very effective, although washing is necessary if hands are soiled. Note that hand disinfection is not an alternative but an addition to wearing gloves for aseptic procedures.

Hand cream may be employed to offset the drying effects of disinfectant products, but it should be one which is compatible as commercial products often inhibit disinfection; pharmacists can advise on suitable products.

Patients' skin. Intact skin should be cleaned before disinfection if possible. As immediate, effective disinfection is required, alcoholic skin disinfectants are the agents of choice. Chlorhexidine is less likely to cause any reaction, although povidone-iodine has wider antimicrobial action; normally either is suitable. Friction is an important factor in skin disinfection; rubbing the site thoroughly with the agent (subject to patient comfort) is more effective than merely wiping

or spraying. Combined detergents/disinfectants (e.g. Savlon) may be used for damaged skin which requires cleaning. Injections (e.g. local anaesthetic) present little danger of infection but skin is usually prepared by swabbing with alcohol.

Sterilisation. Of the many methods of sterilisation available, only steam at increased pressure and dry heat are likely to be used directly by the podiatrist.

Steam at increased pressure. This is generally recommended for use on clinical materials whenever possible (British Pharmacopoeia 1983). Steam hot enough to sterilise necessitates pressure vessels, termed sterilisers or *autoclaves*. Saturated steam sterilises articles it contacts, the time required depending on the temperature. Minimum treatments required are:

- 15 min at 121°C
- 10 min at 126°C
- 3 min at 134°C.

Additional time must be allowed for heating to sterilisation temperature and for cooling after sterilisation. Saturated steam can be obtained only in the absence of air. In sophisticated equipment, air is evacuated, enabling penetration of steam even into wrapped/porous materials (e.g. dressings), and evacuation after sterilisation facilitates drying of such items. The basic types affordable by practitioners rely on simple displacement of air by steam generated within the steriliser. Removal of air, steam penetration and subsequent drying are therefore not as efficient in these models. Although wrapped/porous items may be sterilised, they are usually too wet for clinical use. However, these small sterilisers are very suitable for rapid sterilisation of unwrapped instruments. When removed, instruments must be covered immediately to prevent contamination. A sterile cloth may be used but, alternatively, a lid sterilised separately in the same cycle could be clipped onto the instrument tray.

Dry heat. An electrical, fan-assisted hot-air oven should be used. Microorganisms are more resistant to dry heat than to steam, and therefore higher temperatures, usually 160–180°C, are required for sterilisation within a practicable time, e.g. 20–30 minutes at 180°C (British Pharmacopoeia 1983). All items must reach sterilisation temperature before holding time commences. As heating time varies with the load, it is often underestimated, especially for items wrapped or in containers, e.g. individually wrapped small instruments require about 15 minutes' initial heat penetration time. Dry heat has the advantage that instruments can be packaged and is suitable for non-stainless steel, but the longer cycle time is a disadvantage.

Whichever method is chosen, sterilisers must be of a

suitable design (BMA 1989) and should be regularly serviced and tested. On a more frequent basis, chemical indicators which change colour when exposed to specific temperatures for sufficient time (available from medical equipment suppliers) are useful to detect failure to achieve sterilising conditions, although they are not an absolute guarantee of sterility. Types are available for steam and dry heat and these are to be recommended, particularly for hot-air sterilisers where it is very difficult to predict the time required for packaged items.

Items which should be sterilised include scalpels, files, burrs, forceps, probes, nail clippers, tissue nippers, drill handpieces (if suitable), scissors, cryosurgical probes and instrument brushes. For other materials obtained pre-sterilised, e.g. dressing packs, it is important to check the integrity of packaging and sterility indicator if present, discarding any that are suspect.

Glass bead sterilisers. These units reach very high temperatures (e.g. 235–250°C) and very short process times are suggested by manufacturers. A report on such a unit stated that such temperatures, given adequate time and with certain precautions, 'should be sufficient for the purpose of sterilizing chiropody instruments' (Corner 1987). Further to this provisional acceptance, note that only part of an instrument is treated, use must be immediate and sterilising conditions cannot be checked directly by indicators. For some practitioners, such units may represent an improvement on previous instrument treatment, but, overall, their use cannot be recommended in a modern fully effective sterilisation programme.

Further microbiological aspects of clinical work

Protective clothing

Any serious attempt at aseptic technique precludes contact of the practitioner's bare hands with damaged skin or exposed tissue, i.e. 'no-touch' techniques should be used. The wearing of sterile gloves for such procedures should be more widely adopted, and any claimed reduction in tactile sensitivity can be solved by careful choice of glove size and material. Apart from patient protection, there is the risk of contamination of podiatrists' skin by HBV or HIV, and gloves should always be worn for giving injections, changing dressings, cleaning wounds and for any invasive procedure. Cuts or abrasions on the hands should be covered by waterproof plasters even when gloves are worn. Hands require washing after a gloved procedure, as not all gloves are structurally perfect.

The wearing of masks is unnecessary for minor procedures, including routine dressing changes. Situations requiring masks include nail drilling for the podiatrist's protection and nail surgery, where effective masks to filter/deflect organisms from the mouth away from the operation site are necessary. Masks must be discarded after each use and not worn around the neck to be donned at intervals. Note that drilling of mycotic nails is unwise; not all debris is removed by the drill vacuum and significant amounts escape to contaminate the clinical environment and the practitioner.

The usual clinical coat is satisfactory for many procedures but needs protection when significant debris is expected, particularly from any infected patient, to prevent cross-infection occurring via the coat. A gown, plastic apron or adequately sized impermeable paper sheet or drape would serve the purpose. Purpose-made gowns or suits of appropriate material should be used for surgical procedures, and hair should be completely covered by a surgical cap. If surgical footwear is fitted, avoid contamination of previously disinfected hands.

Aseptic technique

Initial disinfection of the patient's skin should be followed by the use of sterile instruments whenever skin is penetrated, accidental breach is likely or previously wounded tissue is being treated. Other materials used on or near such vulnerable areas, e.g. dressings, must also be sterile. Single-use sachets of antiseptics, etc., are preferable but, if communal ones are used, individual quantities should be dispensed without contaminating the remainder. For example, small quantities can be poured from bottles into sterile pots, taking care not to touch the pot with the outside of the bottle, or solutions can be transferred by bulb pipettes, which should be disposable or cleaned and disinfected before re-use.

Sterile fields. A sterile field is an area in which contamination is kept to an absolute minimum, although unlikely to be sterile in the full microbiological sense. Such a field may be established by starting with a sterile surface and thereafter taking every care to avoid contamination of that area. The surface must not be touched by bare hands, and any necessary items are transferred aseptically onto it. The initial surface may be formed by a sterile drape/towel, or the unfolded inner (sterile) wrapping of a dressing pack, placed on a disinfected trolley top. If pack wrapping is used it must be unfolded by the corners, taking care not to reach over the contents as they are uncovered because contaminants are shed from skin and clothing. Additional items may be slid gently from their sterile wrapping onto the sterile field, or transferred by sterile forceps. Outer wrappings are always contaminated and should not be opened near the sterile field.

Sterile instruments should be arranged in the field conveniently within reach. After use (i.e. when they are contaminated), they should be placed elsewhere for disposal, or on a separate secondary field (e.g. clearly to one side) for possible re-use, but not back amongst sterile items. (Note that re-use on a patient may be contraindicated, e.g. if an infected or dirty lesion is being treated an instrument used earlier may reintroduce contamination into cleaned tissue.) It may prove convenient to use a sterile, empty steriliser tray as a secondary field which can be used later to transport used instruments. Contaminated disposable items, e.g. swabs, should be disposed of immediately and should not re-enter the sterile field. Overall, there should be a one-way movement from sterility to patient to disposal or secondary field.

Dressing changes. Hand disinfection is necessary before commencing, after removal of the old dressing and after completion of the treatment, and at any time during the procedure should hands become contaminated. The old dressing is removed using disposable gloves (or forceps) which, with the dressing, are immediately disposed of carefully. After hand disinfection, sterile gloves are donned for the remainder of the treatment.

Microbiologically clean wounds should need no further cleaning, but practice varies. Sterile saline may be used, or antiseptic preparations for contaminated areas as considered necessary. After treatment, all used and unused materials from dressing packs should be disposed of, as they are no longer sterile.

Waste disposal

Clinical waste should be placed carefully in bags and sealed before removal to prevent contamination of the area. Bags should be colour-coded to distinguish ordinary from contaminated waste (e.g. used dressings). There is no universal code, though yellow is used in the UK to denote contaminated waste for incineration, and practitioners should check local policy. Bags should not be overfilled and must be removed from the clinical area frequently, at least daily. They should be stored safely and protected from damage, until removed by disposal personnel.

Re-usable instruments should be bagged or containerised for return to a central sterile supplies unit, or cleaned before return, or cleaned and re-sterilised in-house, depending on individual arrangements. Disposal of sharps requires great care to protect the practitioner and others from the risk of HBV and HIV infection; they must be discarded into an approved rigid container (e.g. meeting DHSS specification TSS/S/330.015) and sent for incineration.

Operating rooms

The design of operating facilities has evolved essentially for the needs of hospital surgery. Such facilities with positive pressure, high efficiency filtered ventilation systems and various ancillary support areas may sometimes be available to hospital practitioners, and indeed access to these may be necessary for treatment of high risk patients. However, infection rates associated with minor surgery and ambulatory care services are low, and such complex facilities should not always be necessary.

In general surgery, airborne contamination appears to have little responsibility for postoperative sepsis (Ayliffe & Lowbury 1982), and during minor operations of short duration, true airborne contamination is unlikely. The greatest risk will be from staff and the standards of their aseptic techniques but, nevertheless, adequate ventilation is important to reduce contamination dispersed from personnel while minimising entry of airborne contamination from outside. If extraction alone is used, there is a risk that extracted air will be replaced by contaminated air from surrounding areas, i.e. there is an inflow of 'dirty' air towards the operation area. A compromise would be extraction to the outside in combination with sufficient filtered air inlets at selected sites to replace the extracted air. Practitioners intending to expand significantly into surgery should seek expert advice on their particular facilities to ensure that adequate safe ventilation is provided.

Operating rooms should be clearly separated from the general clinic and access restricted to essential personnel. They must be large enough to allow unimpeded movement without contact contamination from other people, furniture and surfaces. Only essential equipment and surgical supplies should be stored in the room and their use should be restricted to surgery and associated procedures, such as immediate instrument sterilisation. Initial interview and preparation of the patient should take place elsewhere, and adequate facilities for scrubbing up and dressing of surgical staff must be provided.

Thorough cleaning of general surfaces should be carried out daily and the floor cleaned after each session; routine disinfection of floors should not be necessary. Known occurrences of contamination, especially by tissue or blood, do require disinfection. Overcrowding and vigorous movements should be avoided in operating rooms, as they increase airborne contamination. Clinical waste must be removed carefully to avoid contamination of the room or associated clean facilities.

Laboratory specimens

Podiatrists could make more use of the expertise of microbiology laboratories. Laboratory investigation of samples from skin, nails or infected wounds can confirm infection and/or identify the pathogen, thus aiding choice of the most effective patient management. In fungal infections, where symptoms are often insufficiently specific, definitive diagnosis can only be achieved by microscopy and culture techniques.

If possible, samples should be taken before commencing antimicrobial treatment, as this may inhibit the isolation of pathogens. The receiving laboratory will advise on containers, and packaging for samples. Usually, swabs from wounds are collected into capped containers while skin scrapings and nail clippings may be collected in paper sachets which maintain dry conditions and prevent overgrowth by saprophytes. As much material as possible should be collected to increase the probability of isolating the pathogen. Specimens must be taken carefully, avoiding contamination of self, the clinical surroundings and the outside of the container. As much clinical information as possible should be provided to aid investigation.

Infection control policies

Any practice, large or small, should have a written control policy. This should include instructions on sterilisation of various items, use and concentrations of disinfectants or antiseptics, waste disposal, treatment of spillages, etc. For the individual practitioner this will serve as a useful *aide memoire*, while in larger units all staff should be able to consult it for information on agreed procedures. Health service and hospital podiatrists should ensure compliance with the local health authority or hospital policy on infection control. In units with several staff, there should be a designated person with responsibility for implementation and monitoring of control measures.

Cleaning staff must be given clear instructions on methods required and adequate facilities, and they should be given time to discharge their duties effectively.

Elaborate infection surveillance systems are not necessary, in view of the low risk associated with well-run ambulatory care facilities. Full note should be taken of any infections which apparently result from podiatric treatment, and overall incidence of these should be reviewed periodically. Undue incidence should alert staff to review control measures, seeking expert advice if necessary.

Infection control personnel are employed by health authorities and hospitals and these local sources are the best initial points of contact for any practitioner. Much published information is also available, including material from public health laboratories and government departments, and is continually being augmented.

REFERENCES

Anon 1987 Control of cross infection. Journal of the Society of Chiropodists 42: 115
Ayliffe G A J, Lowbury E J L 1982 Airborne infection in hospital. Journal of Hospital Infection 3: 217
Ayliffe G A J, Collins B J, Taylor L J 1990 Hospital-acquired infection: principles and prevention, 2nd edn. Butterworth, Sevenoaks
Ayton M 1981 National surveillance of communicable diseases. Nursing 1: 1248
Bennett J V, Brachman P S (eds) 1986 Hospital infections, 2nd edn. Little Brown, Boston
British Medical Association 1989 A code of practice for sterilisation of instruments and control of cross infection. BMA, London
British Pharmacopoeia 1980 Addendum 1983 Sterilisation. A56 Appendix XVIIIA. HMSO, London
British Standard 5283 1986 British Standards glossary of terms relating to disinfectants. British Standards Institute, London

Central Sterilising Club 1986 Sterilisation and disinfection of heat-labile equipment. CSC, Birmingham
Coates D 1985 A comparison of sodium hypochlorite and sodium dichloroisocyanurate products. Journal of Hospital Infection 6: 31
Coates D 1988 Household bleaches and HIV. Journal of Hospital Infection 11: 95
Corner G A 1987 An assessment of the performance of a glass bead steriliser. Journal of Hospital Infection 10: 308
Lowbury E J L, Ayliffe G A J, Geddes A M, Williams J D (eds) 1981 Control of hospital infection – a practical handbook, 2nd edn. Chapman and Hall, London
Maurer I M 1985 Hospital hygiene, 3rd edn. Edward Arnold, London
Meers P D 1983 Ventilation in operating rooms. British Medical Journal 286: 244
Paterson R S 1985 In: Neale D, Adams I (eds) Common foot disorders, ch. 13, 2nd edn. Churchill Livingstone, Edinburgh

FURTHER READING

Adler M W (ed) 1993 ABC of AIDS, 3rd edn. BMJ Publishing, London

Ayliffe G A J, Lowbury E J L, Geddes A M, Williams J D (eds) 1992 Control of hospital infection – a practical handbook, 3rd edn. Chapman and Hall, London

Gardner J F, Peel M M 1991 Introduction to sterilisation, disinfection and infection control, 2nd edn. Churchill Livingstone, Melbourne

Pratt R J 1988 AIDS: a strategy for nursing care, 2nd edn. Edward Arnold, London

Royal College of Nursing 1987 Introduction to hepatitis B and nursing guidelines for infection control. RCN, London

Russell A D, Hugo W B, Ayliffe G A J (eds) 1992 Principles and practice of disinfection, preservation and sterilisation, 2nd edn. Blackwell Scientific, Oxford

17

Local anaesthesia

D. L. Lorimer

Keywords

Choice of anaesthetic
Digital nerve trunk blocks
Field block anaesthesia
Local infiltration
Nerve trunk blocks
Techniques of administration
Tibial nerve
Toxicity
Safety considerations

The ability to perform procedures which are in themselves painful makes it essential for podiatrists to be able to anaesthetise selected areas of the foot. The methods employed range from local infiltration of the anaesthetic agent at the site, to nerve block techniques, which will prevent sensory stimulus from a predictable area of the foot. The choice of method and site of injection must be based on factors which are in the best interests of the patient and which use the lowest dosage of anaesthetic agent.

A single site on the weight-bearing plantar surface will generally involve blocking the tibial nerve, whereas a single site on the dorsum can be anaesthetised by local infiltration. Multiple sites on the dorsum may be better anaesthetised by a block of the nerve which supplies the area, which could be the sural, saphenous, deep or superficial peroneal. If both of the latter are to be blocked, it is better practice to block the common peroneal nerve, but it should be remembered that this can also affect motor function in the leg until the effects of the anaesthetic agent on the nerve have stopped.

The most frequently used sites for the administration of anaesthetics in the foot are the digital nerves, predominately those of the hallux. The nerve supply to each digit is by four nerve trunks, two of which are on the dorsum and two on the plantar aspect. Textbooks of anatomy identify these as having a predictable location, but in many instances the nerve trunk can be shown to have subdivided before entry to the toes (Bruce 1989). This is usually accompanied by a similar subdivision of the small blood vessels, which will increase the vascularity of the area into which the injection is to be made.

As a general consideration, before giving an injection to produce analgesia, the operator should have a clear understanding of the anatomical structures together with possible variations (Wildsmith & Armitage 1987). In addition, the following objectives should be observed:

1. The anaesthetic agent to be injected should be deposited accurately to ensure effective contact with the nerve trunk, so that the concentration of the local anaesthetic agent perfusing into the nerve trunk is sufficient to ensure the blocking of its central core fibres. This is particularly important in the case of the thicker nerve trunks, such as the tibial nerve (Fink 1989). If there are any suspected anomalies, such as early bifurcation of the nerve, the deposition of the fluid should be wider. To prevent incomplete blockade of nerve conduction, it is suggested that 8 mm of the length of the nerve must be bathed in anaesthetic solution (de Jong 1994).

2. Inadvertent intravascular injection should be avoided to minimise the risk of systemic toxic reactions, particularly when administrating the fluid in highly vascularised sites. The essence of good practice is in the use of minimum dosage, and therefore excessive quantities should be avoided.

Local anaesthetic agents in current use are very safe, but this safety is dependent upon an accurate assessment of the patient's physical and clinical states and the site, as well as the type and the composition of the anaesthetic solution (Covino & Vassallo 1976). Before administering a local anaesthetic, the patient's medical history should be elicited and, if there are any doubts, the opinion of the patient's physician sought. However, it should be stressed that allergy or adverse reactions to amide anaesthetics are extremely rare and, if reactions do occur, they are usually the result of systemic toxicity, overdose or patient anxiety. The procedures which should be followed in assessing the patient's health state are discussed in Chapter 2, but particular attention should be paid to the following points:

1. Interaction with systemic drug therapy relates mainly to the drugs which impair aspects of the liver's ability to detoxify the anaesthetic agents. There are two groups of drugs which have this effect, namely the monoamine oxidase inhibitors (MAOIs) and the procarbazine drugs. MAOIs are used to control acute anxiety states in patients and the procarbazines are anti-tumour drugs used mainly in the control of Hodgkin's disease. These drugs inhibit the action of the hepatic microsomes, in particular the microsomal cytochrome P450 enzymes responsible for the biotransformation of local anaesthetics to simpler chemical structures (Vickers et al 1984).

Patients being treated with benzodiazapines should also be treated with special care, for although this is not a drug interaction these tranquillising drugs can act as anticonvulsant drugs and mask the early signs of toxicity. If an adverse reaction does occur to the local anaesthetic, the patient may become suddenly and deeply unconscious (Wildsmith & Armitage 1987). Other drugs which can cause problems in association with local anaesthetics are the antihypertensive drugs, such as diuretics. Again, this is not a drug interaction, but postural hypotension may be experienced with risks of fainting when the patient resumes an upright position after treatment.

2. Patients on steroid therapy are more easily put under stress and have lower resistance to infection. Such patients will have a card identifying the details of the drug therapy. Patients who are receiving anticoagulant therapy will have a similar card; they will need special consideration in the control of bleeding. This precaution also applies to those who are haemophiliacs or have other haemorrhagic diseases and to patients with leukaemia who have a lowered resistance to infection.

3. The use of local anaesthesia in pregnancy should be limited to emergency situations and its use during the first trimester should be avoided if possible, although this may be a difficult stage to ascertain. Of greater importance is the choice of anaesthetic agents and the dosage levels applied to the patient, because of the effects on the fetus via transplacental transfer. The longer-lasting local anaesthetics, particularly, may not be metabolised so easily, due to lack of development of the enzyme systems in the fetal liver. The agent which crosses the placenta most easily is prilocaine (de Jong 1977) and its use should be avoided if possible in such patients.

4. Patients who suffer from impaired liver function, from such causes as infective hepatitis or cirrhosis, may have a reduced or negative ability to metabolise amide-type anaesthetic agents, although current opinion suggests that it would only be in extreme cases that the liver's metabolic reserve would be compromised (de Jong 1994). Care should be taken in the initial assessment of the patient to establish the

possibility of liver disease or alcohol drinking patterns, which have potentially harmful effects. Systemic reactions have been noted in patients with severe hepatic disease (Seldon & Sashara 1967). A consideration associated with liver function occurs in the metabolism of prilocaine. One of its main metabolites is a substance called o-toluidine, which can induce methaemoglobinaemia in humans (Covino & Vassallo 1976). For this reason, it is advisable to avoid high dosage levels of this agent.

5. A consideration of renal function is also necessary, although it is not as important as liver function (de Jong 1994). The kidneys excrete up to 10% of lignocaine and mepivacaine, and up to 16% of bupivacaine, in unaltered form, but only 3–6 hours after ingestion; therefore impaired renal function could be a contraindication to the use of local anaesthetics (Wildsmith & Armitage 1987).

6. Patients with hypertensive cardiovascular disease should not have anaesthetic agents containing adrenaline administered to them, as there is an increased risk of cardiotoxicity (de Jong 1994). Similarly, patients with peripheral vasospastic conditions, such as Raynaud's phenomenon, should not receive anaesthetics with added vasoconstrictors, and the tourniquet effect of the fluid with plain solutions of an anaesthetic on the digit should be avoided.

7. Local sepsis at the proposed site of injection precludes the administration of the anaesthetic agent, as this could facilitate the spread of sepsis. Around the site of sepsis the tissue pH is usually more acidic, and this will inhibit the action of the anaesthetic agent and may encourage the operator to administer higher doses as tissue acidosis reduces the quantity of local anaesthetic base that can be mobilised (de Jong 1994). Where an anaesthetic agent has to be used to facilitate the treatment of a septic condition, the site for the nerve block should be well clear of the sepsis.

8. A number of patients may have a lowered resistance to secondary infections. This group could be particularly at risk from infection introduced at the site of the injection. The general conditions which may cause this lowered resistance are nephritis, the anaemias, uncontrolled diabetes and, of course, patients on steroid therapy. Controlled diabetics should not be in danger from the use of plain solutions of anaesthetic.

9. Epileptics not well stabilised by drug therapy could be influenced by the stimulation of the central nervous system which may result from the administration of local anaesthetics.

10. The administration of local anaesthetics requires good patient compliance. Its use in certain groups may require additional justification as the only means of effecting treatment. It may not be suitable for use with the very old or young, the very nervous or hysterical, the mentally impaired and the insane. In all cases where local anaesthetics are used, the patient should have the process clearly explained so that a rapport is built up between the patient and the practitioner. The administration of local anaesthetics does not require the elaborate range of preparations which are associated with general anaesthetics, but the patient should be advised to have a light meal about 4 hours before the procedure. The patient's normal medication can be taken, provided it does not interact with the anaesthetic agent.

Immediately prior to the administration of the local anaesthetic it is good practice to encourage the patient to empty the bladder. The administration of premedication is not usually considered necessary but nervous patients may be given a dose of a benzodiazapine such as temazepam. Even without the administration of such agents, the patient should be advised not to drive for about 1 hour (Reynolds 1993).

TOXICITY

Toxic effects from the administration of local anaesthetics can be considered to fall into three categories: allergy, systemic toxicity and local tissue toxicity (Covino & Vassallo 1976).

Allergy

A number of reports of suspected allergy tend to appear from time to time, but these were mainly associated with the ester type of anaesthetics derived from para-aminobenzoic acid. Most researchers suggest that allergy to amide-type local anaesthetics is extremely rare (Covino & Vassallo 1976). Additives are used in local anaesthetic agents which may be the cause of allergy, but this too is extremely rare. Examples of such additives include agents to alter the pH of the solution or preservatives in solutions stored in multidose bottles.

Systemic toxicity

The toxicity of an anaesthetic agent of the amide type is dependent on its chemical structure and on the ability of the liver enzymes to metabolise it. Prilocaine, which is metabolised at a much faster rate than lignocaine, is considerably less toxic. As a result, the choice of agent and the subsequent dosage require careful consideration.

The ability of local anaesthetic agents to affect the

central nervous system (CNS) produces a range of progressive symptoms. At normal dosage levels, accurately administered, the patient may display the early signs of CNS stimulation, becoming excited, talkative and euphoric. Another symptom is numbness of the tongue and also of the tissues around the mouth, but this may be ascribed to the highly vascular nature of these areas, which provide a focus for a purely local reaction.

The first real sign of CNS toxicity is light-headedness and dizziness, soon to be followed by difficulty in focusing the eyes and tinnitus. There may be slurred speech, shivering and light muscle twitch in the face and sometimes in the extremities (Covino & Vassallo 1976). The patient may appear drowsy, disorientated or even become fleetingly unconscious. Should the toxic reaction continue, the patient will become convulsive with generalised tonic–clonic state. Following this, depression of the CNS activity ensues with respiratory depression and arrest of function (Stricharz 1987).

The effects on the cardiovascular system at toxic levels result in decreased myocardial activity and cardiac output, which, combined with peripheral vascular vasodilation, produces circulatory collapse. Toxic reactions resulting from the maladministration of local anaesthetics are usually due to intravascular injection, excessive dosage or careless administration on vascular sites. The treatment of such reactions consists of adequate ventilation of the lungs, and anticonvulsant agents such as diazepam. Vasopressor drugs, such as adrenaline, may be used to support circulation, or physical methods may be used if necessary. Physical methods of life support are discussed in Appendix 3. Practitioners intending to employ the use of local anaesthetics should become familiar with the procedures for resuscitation of patients, but it is good practice to remember that careful monitoring of the patient's reactions during the process of administration will ensure that any adverse reaction is halted at an early stage.

Local tissue toxicity

Studies have been carried out to investigate the effects of local anaesthetic agents on certain body tissues to determine their potential for irritation (Covino & Vassallo 1976). In high concentrations, local anaesthetics can cause haemolysis of red blood cells, but this is at concentrations much higher than are used generally in the UK. The significance of these tests has not been defined, but it is advisable to remember that if blood is drawn back into the syringe during aspiration, it is

prudent to discard the remaining anaesthetic and replace it.

It has been noted in studies that local anaesthetic agents, again at high concentrations, have caused damage to the sciatic nerves of frogs. It has also been noted that the preservatives sometimes used in local anaesthetics have caused neurotoxicity, with some loss of ability to detect sensation. There are a few reports of some loss of sensation after the application of local anaesthetics, but in all cases observed by the author this has been short-lived, with full sensation restored after 3–4 months at the latest.

CHOOSING AN ANAESTHETIC AGENT

The first factor in the sequence is determined by the procedure to be performed, its length and possible postoperative pain. Procedures of short duration and little postoperative pain can be adequately covered using lignocaine or, if a higher dosage is required, prilocaine, which has a lower level of toxicity. Procedures of longer duration, or those which are perceived to produce unacceptable levels of postoperative pain, may require bupivacaine or etidocaine. With both of these, clear instructions for postoperative management is necessary as there is prolonged loss of sensation and proprioception.

Procedures where bleeding needs to be controlled, or where prolonged action is necessary without the toxic potential of bupivacaine, may require the use of an added vasoconstrictor.

Procaine

This was the first of the synthesised local anaesthetic agents, which was used extensively until lignocaine and the other amide compounds were introduced. Procaine is an ester-type substance which is metabolised, predominantly, by the plasma pseudo-cholinesterases to para-aminobenzoic acid. It has about one-quarter of the systemic toxicity of cocaine, which it largely supplanted. The duration of action of procaine is short (20–30 minutes) and its chemical structure unstable, particularly in relation to heat, compared with the amide substances by which it was largely replaced. It is little used clinically, but reference is made to its toxicity relative to other local anaesthetic substances.

Lignocaine

This drug is normally prepared as a hydrochloride salt and is one-and-a-half times more toxic than procaine. Its rate of onset is rapid and its effect is more intense and lasts longer than procaine, with effective anaesthesia of up to 3 hours but normally accepted as 1.5 hours (Reynolds 1993). The maximum safe dose (MSD) in the UK for an adult male weighing 70 kg is 200 mg in plain solution and 500 mg with added vasoconstrictors (see Table 17.1).

Vasoconstrictor additives are used to prolong its action unless contraindicated by the site of the injection or the patient's state of health. Lignocaine is an amino-acyl-amide and, as such, is detoxified in the liver, with small amounts being excreted unchanged by the kidneys (less than 10%) and in the bile (less than 7%) (Dripps et al 1988).

Its use in podiatry is as a surface anaesthetic for very nervous patients (EMLA cream), for local infiltration or nerve trunk block. It is mainly used by podiatrists in 1% and 2% plain solutions.

Bupivacaine

Like lignocaine, this is prepared as a hydrochloride salt. It is four times as toxic as lignocaine, but when used for specific nerve blocks it has a duration of action of up to 6 hours. The MSD in the UK is 150 mg and it is generally used in concentrations of 0.25% or 0.5% in plain solution (see Table 17.1).

Bupivacaine is used when a longer-lasting analgesic effect is required after techniques which produce some postoperative pain. Its rate of onset is very slow and

Table 17.1 Maximum safe dosage (MSD) (after Reynolds 1993)

	MSD, plain solution (mg)	MSD with vasoconstrictor (mg)	Dose per kg of body weight
Lignocaine	200	500	3 mg
Bupivacaine	150	150	2 mg
Etidocaine	300	–	4 mg
Mepivacaine	400	–	6 mg
Prilocaine	400	600	6 mg

The information in this table is in mg of the agent for a 24-hour period and the MSD in column 1 is calculated on the average body weight of 70 kg, based on information applicable to the usage of local anaesthetics in the UK. Variations may be found in other national formularies. The MSD with added vasoconstrictors is also shown where appropriate. For the purposes of administering doses of local anaesthetic, a more accurate method is to relate the dosage in mg of the agent to kg of the patient's body weight. This takes account of variations in the size of patients and should be a principal consideration when assessing patients of small physique.

allowance should be made for this when using it. Like lignocaine, it is detoxified in the liver.

Etidocaine

This substance (not currently available in the UK) is also a longer-lasting agent, with effective analgesia of up to 4 hours' duration. Although its duration of action is shorter than that of bupivacaine, its rate of onset is faster than that of lignocaine, which increases patient confidence in the effectiveness of the anaesthetic agent and thus in the operator. It is capable of producing intense motor blockade, and because of its high plasma-binding property has the lowest transplacental transfer ratio (Reynolds 1993).

It is prepared as a hydrochloride salt and is normally used in 1% concentration in plain solutions. The MSD is 300 mg in the UK.

Mepivacaine

This drug has properties similar to lignocaine and is prepared and detoxified in the same way. It has a similar duration of action to lignocaine but the maximum safe dosage is twice as high (400 mg) and its rate of onset is faster. In ankle block techniques, the higher maximum safe dosage level of mepivacaine is particularly useful in permitting the use of higher volumes when required.

Prilocaine

Prilocaine has properties similar to lignocaine but is only half as toxic. Its effects on the central nervous system and the cardiovascular system is less pronounced than those of lignocaine, but one of the main metabolites of prilocaine is o-toluidine, which is considered to be responsible for the production of methaemoglobin in humans; however, to produce such an effect it would be necessary to administer in the region of 600 mg, which is far in excess of the MSD. This may limit its use in podiatry, where pregnancy may not be acknowledged by patients in its earlier stages. It is detoxified in the liver. The MSD is 400 mg for the average male of 70 kg body weight.

TECHNIQUES OF ADMINISTRATION

In podiatric practice, two techniques of administration of local anaesthetic agents are used—local infiltration and nerve trunk block. Infiltration is used to raise an intradermal, or subdermal, weal around a superficial lesion, usually on a non-weight-bearing surface, to produce anaesthesia. It may also be used in nerve block techniques to facilitate painless access to deeper nerves. Nerve trunk blocks are most commonly used either to single nerves or in digital blocks.

The risk of the patient fainting can be reduced by having the patient supine. Some elderly patients, obese patients or those with breathing difficulty may find it preferable to be semi-recumbent. In addition, this allows patients to be more relaxed and to be able to divert their gaze away from the operating area. Local skin preparation is important to reduce the risks of bacterial entry through the site of injection. The point of entry and the adjacent skin should be prepared with a suitable antiseptic skin cleanser, which may be preceded with a soap and water wash if necessary. The operator's hands should be scrubbed thoroughly and barrier gloves worn. The site of the injection should be further cleansed with a swab impregnated with isopropyl alcohol and allowed to dry immediately prior to the administration of the anaesthetic agent (Wildsmith & Armitage 1987).

The selection of hypodermic needles is important, as the finest needles, 25 or 27 gauge, produce the least pain, but when it is necessary to advance to a more deeply placed nerve trunk, it may be advisable to use a more rigid needle. The use of blunt needles, i.e. needles produced without the sharp bevelled point or with a bevel at a much steeper angle, in reaching deeply placed nerves such as the tibial nerve reduces significantly the danger of nerve damage and inadvertent entry into blood vessels. The use of these needles makes entry through the skin more difficult and makes the use of an intradermal weal essential. In some cases, operators use electric stimulating needles to locate the site of deep nerve trunks, but these seem to be of value only to the less experienced practitioners and they sometimes cause the patient some discomfort.

The use of plain solutions of local anaesthetic agents avoids unnecessary impairment of tissue nutrition due to local vasoconstriction when agents with added vasoconstrictors are used. Local anaesthetic agents with added vasoconstrictors, such as adrenaline, should not be used in sites where the blood supply is via end arteries, such as in the digits. Accurate location of the site and minimising the dosage used, coupled with aspiration before injecting, will ensure minimal risks of toxic reactions (Bruce 1989).

Local infiltration

This technique of administration starts with the raising of an intradermal weal at a suitably selected site. This is done by inserting the needle at an angle of 45° to the skin with the bevel uppermost. When the bevel is covered, pressure should be applied to the plunger so that fluid is expelled, sufficient to raise a small bleb or pool of fluid under the skin, which will show white against the surrounding skin. The needle should then be passed through the skin and directed under the lesion, depositing fluid. In order to ensure a complete area of anaesthesia around the lesion, the needle may have to be withdrawn to the point of entry and directed in other directions under the lesion, in a fan-shaped pattern. Local infiltration is seldom possible on weight-bearing areas of the foot, when the subdermal structures will resist the passage of the fluid and the needle.

NERVE TRUNK BLOCKS
Digital nerve block

The most commonly used form of nerve block in podiatry is the digital block which, because of the nature of the nerve supply, requires separate consideration. As discussed earlier, the nerve supply to a digit is by way of four small nerves, two on the dorsum and two on the plantar aspect, which may have subdivided before entering the septal planes of the digit. The techniques discussed assume that the anatomical norm applies; premature subdivision would be dealt with by small compensatory deposits, the site of which could be identified by the areas remaining unaffected by the anaesthetic agent.

The digit should be examined to select two sites on the dorsum, so that the medial dorsal and plantar nerves can be reached from one point of entry and the lateral dorsal and plantar nerves can be reached from the other (Fig. 17.1). At the same time, it is useful, mentally, to subdivide the proximal phalanx into thirds, so that the site of injection will be over the proximal end of the medial third at this point; the narrowest part of the phalanx will allow the easiest access to the plantar nerve trunk with the least possibility of striking the phalanx with the needle and possibly causing damage to the periosteum (Fig. 17.1).

The intradermal weal should be raised in the manner described previously. The amount of fluid required for this stage is unlikely to exceed 0.25 ml on each site. The needle should then be directed towards the point of entry for the weal at a steeper angle (closer to 90°) and towards the dorsal nerve trunk. Approximately 0.5 ml of fluid should be deposited slowly and steadily after having aspirated the syringe to ensure it is not inserted into a blood vessel. Upon

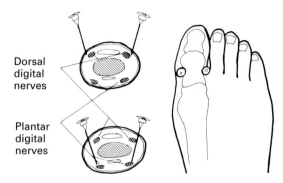

Figure 17.1 Location of dorsal and plantar digital nerves and sites for intradermal weals.

completion of this, the needle should be withdrawn. Aspiration should be carried out before each deposition of anaesthetic agent. If, on aspiration, blood is seen to enter the barrel of the syringe, no further use of that fluid and syringe should be made. This precaution is to protect against the remote possibility of re-entry into another blood vessel and the consequent deposition of damaged blood cells into the circulation.

The needle should be inserted through the original point of entry and advanced towards the plantar (Fig. 17.1) until it is located over the nerve, and up to 0.5 ml should be deposited around each nerve trunk. Satisfactory anaesthesia should be possible with up to 2.5 ml of a 2% anaesthetic agent. It is important in digital anaesthesia to avoid depositing excessive amounts of fluid or encircling the digit with a subdermal ring of fluid and producing a tourniquet effect, with a risk of restricting circulation. This two-point entry technique is a modification of the Stockholm technique. The lesser digits seem to allow further modification of this technique to a single entry on the dorsum, but unless the toe is very narrow it is a modification capable of producing internal damage and it is better to retain two points of entry.

Upon completion of the injection procedures, it is better to delay testing for loss of sensation until a digital hyperaemia appears, as this indicates the blockade of the sympathetic fibres and the onset of sensory loss. The patient may describe the toe as having a numb or tingling sensation. Delaying testing for sensation until the outcome is more predictable will ensure greater patient confidence in the whole process.

Specific nerve block

Anaesthesia of all or part of the foot may be obtained by selective nerve trunk blocks. The sensory supply from the larger nerve trunks, although more predictable, is more absolute, and areas on the margin may be served by more than one nerve trunk, making careful testing of the anaesthetic effect essential; however, their larger size allows them to be located accurately by palpation, and digital pressure will produce distal paraesthesia.

This precision in locating the nerves reduces the necessity to use large quantities of solution, by enabling it to be deposited accurately, as well as minimising the risk of failure of the blockade. The increased size of the blood vessels which often accompany the nerve trunks necessitates exact location of the hypodermic needle to avoid intravascular injection (Fig. 17.2).

The raising of an intradermal weal is not always seen as essential but it allows pain-free relocation of the needle should this be necessary. Deposition of the fluid at the site should be slow, in order to minimise discomfort from the disruption of the fascial planes. The volume employed can be reduced to about 0.5 ml, but it is advisable to use higher concentrations to ensure an adequate length of blockade. Where suitable, the use of an added vasoconstrictor will allow a lower concentration of the agent. The nerves which can be blocked are as follows:

- tibial
- sural

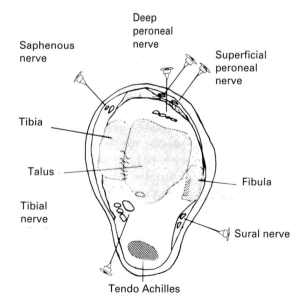

Figure 17.2 Location of the nerve trunks at a transverse plane through the ankle joint.

- saphenous
- deep peroneal
- superficial peroneal (before or after subdivision)
- common peroneal.

The tibial nerve (Fig. 17.3)

At the ankle, the tibial nerve passes behind the medial malleoleus, lying laterally to the posterior tibial artery. As it passes behind the flexor retinaculum, divisions start to take place into its three terminal branches (calcaneal, medial and lateral plantar nerves). Examination of cadavers shows that this bifurcation can take place proximally to the flexor retinaculum in a significant number of cases, indicating that the best clinical practice is to locate the nerve slightly proximally to the medial malleolus (approximately 2.5 cm from the central point of the medial malleolus towards the shaft of the tibia). On most patients, it is possible to elicit paraesthesia using digital pressure, thus confirming the location for injecting the anaesthetic agent. Some practitioners use low voltage stimulating apparatus to locate the nerve trunk, as described earlier, and this can be useful in the early stages for less experienced practitioners.

The best site to locate the block is as the nerve passes behind the medial malleolus or just a little proximal to it. The raising of an intradermal weal at the point of entry assists the operator in locating the needle accurately and allows it to be advanced slowly. The use of the blunt (non-sharp) needles allows the nerve to be located by eliciting paraesthesia, while the risk of penetrating the artery or damaging the nerve trunk is much reduced. Once the patient has felt paraesthesia, the syringe can be aspirated, an essential safeguard in this site (Zenz et al 1988). Blockade of this nerve can be effected using 2 ml of a 2% solution of lignocaine, but sometimes it is helpful, where accurate location cannot

be assured, to use a 1% solution, which allows greater volume to be deposited. It is also helpful to use local anaesthetics with added adrenaline, which can also reduce the necessary volume.

The sural nerve (Fig. 17.4)

This nerve is located on a line between the lateral aspect of the tendo Achilles and the lateral malloleus. It is closely associated with the course of the short saphenous vein. Its sensory supply is to the lateral aspect of the foot, the fifth toe and, in a significant number of instances, a small portion of the lateral aspects of the calcaneal area. It may have subdivided into a number of its terminal branches, and this, combined with its passage over relatively well covered areas, makes palpation difficult but not impossible. In most instances, it can be located and blocked using small amounts of anaesthesia, but occasionally, due to early bifurcation, it is necessary to lay a 'track' of fluid between the lateral malloleus and the lateral aspect of the tendo Achilles (Fig. 17.4). Even this latter can be accomplished using a 0.5 ml 2% solution. It is generally better to initiate the process with an intradermal weal.

The saphenous nerve (Fig. 17.5)

This terminal branch of the femoral nerve supplies the medial aspect of the dorsum of the foot, occasionally extending to include the surface over the medial side of the metatarsophalangeal joint. It is found on entering the foot on the anterior aspect of the medial malleolus closely associated with the great saphenous vein (Bruce 1989). It is not easily located, but it is possible to produce paraesthesia and thus locate the nerve by applying pressure at a site close to the vein on the anterior aspect of the medial malleolus.

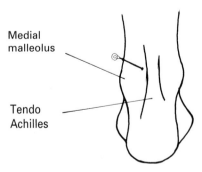

Figure 17.3   Site of injection for the tibial nerve.

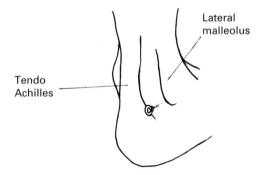

Figure 17.4   Site of injection for the sural nerve.

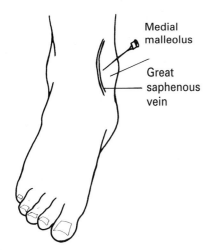

Figure 17.5   Site of injection for the saphenous nerve.

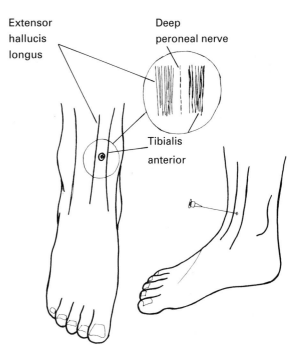

Figure 17.6   Site of injection for the deep peroneal nerve.

The raising of a weal on the surface midway between the tendon of the tibialis anterior and the great saphenous vein (Fig. 17.5) allows the needle to be advanced towards the medial malleolus, where, after aspirating, the local anaesthetic should be deposited close to the vein. Effective blockade of the nerve is possible with 0.5 ml of a 2% solution; however, it may be necessary to use up to 1.5 ml of the solution.

The deep peroneal nerve (Fig. 17.6)

This nerve is located lying deep to the anterior tibial artery, positioned between the tendons of the tibialis anterior and the extensor hallucis longus. This nerve, which is a terminal branch of the common peroneal nerve, has a very limited range of sensory distribution, usually supplying the opposing sides of the hallux and the second toe.

The artery may be located easily by palpation or by using Doppler apparatus. An intradermal weal should be raised over the site (Fig. 17.6), which will allow the needle to be advanced to one side of the artery. At this point it is possible to detect the force of the flow of the blood through the expansion of the artery, and soon the patient should experience paraesthesia. In some instances, paraesthesia is not felt and the needle should be advanced steadily until resistance is felt from the tibia. With either resistance or paraesthesia, the needle should be withdrawn slightly (about 1 mm).

Holding the point of the needle steady in this position, the syringe should be aspirated, and if this is clear, a suitable dose of the fluid deposited. This is usually about 1 ml of a 2% solution. There may be some resistance to the fluid being deposited because of the closeness of the septal planes.

The superficial peroneal nerve (Fig. 17.7)

This nerve, also a terminal branch of the common peroneal nerve, becomes subdermal at the proximal end of the lower one-third of the leg on the anterolateral surface. At this site, it is possible to produce paraesthesia by applying firm pressure. On becoming superficial the nerve quickly divides into medial and lateral branches and is responsible for the sensory supply to the lower anterior surface of the leg, as well as to most of the dorsal aspect of the foot.

As the nerves pass into the foot, the medial branch lies immediately lateral to the tendon of the extensor hallucis longus. The lateral branch lies lateral to these structures at the same level.

The branches may be anaesthetised using small quantities of fluid (about 1 ml of a 2% solution) at either of the sites described or where the nerve becomes superficial in the lower part of the leg.

The common peroneal nerve (Fig. 17.8)

This nerve, arising from the popliteal fossa, passes over the neck of the fibula before dividing to become

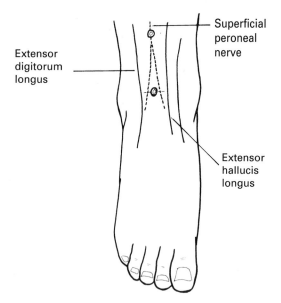

Figure 17.7 Site of injection for the superficial peroneal nerve.

the deep and superficial peroneal nerves. Where the nerve curves around the neck of the fibula, it can be palpated easily, and access to it is simple, as it is in a situation not complicated by the presence of major blood vessels. Raising an intradermal weal allows the needle to be advanced slowly towards the nerve, the site of which can be indicated by a finger palpating the nerve (Fig. 17.8). Satisfactory anaesthesia can be obtained with 1 or 2 ml of a 2% solution. Using the common peroneal nerve reduces the number of injections when both the deep and superficial nerves have to be blocked, and reduces significantly the total dosage of anaesthetic agent required.

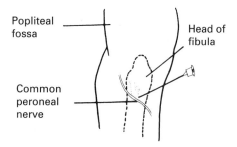

Figure 17.8 Site of injection for the common peroneal nerve.

FIELD BLOCK ANAESTHESIA

This involves the blocking of nerve conduction to a whole segment of the forefoot, usually from the level of the base of the metatarsals. It is sometimes referred to as Mayo block or ray block. The location of the nerves at these sites is more predictable but is complicated by the close association of the nerves and the blood vessels and by the necessity of having to pass through the dorsal and plantar interosseous muscles as well as the plantar intrinsic muscles. Variations in location may make it necessary to lay a 'track' of anaesthetic fluid, so it is essential that the needle is withdrawn along the same line as it was advanced, due consideration being given to the vascularity of the site. Variations in the location of the plantar nerve may make it necessary to supplement with a block to the tibial nerve.

The most commonly used field block in the foot is that to the first metatarsal segment. Blockade of the fifth metatarsal segment is less common, as is that to the other metatarsal segments, but all of these are described as they have minor variations in technique.

The dosage of anaesthetic substance may be quite high, with 6–8 ml of 2% lignocaine being normal for a profound blockade of a metatarsal segment. It may be necessary to use an anaesthetic agent with an added vasoconstrictor, as the vascularity of the area reduces the effective time for anaesthesia. Patients who have a lower body weight may necessitate the use of lower percentage concentrations to avoid breaching the maximum safe dosage of the anaesthetic.

Anaesthetic block of the metatarsal segments involves the passage of hypodermic needles between the shafts of the metatarsals close to their base, and thus it is necessary to establish clear clinical guidelines to determine the optimum passage between the bones. A simple guide is to locate a point on the medial aspect of the first metatarsal about 1 cm distal to its base, and a point on the lateral aspect of the fifth metatarsal, 2.5 cm distal to its base (Fig. 17.9). A line drawn between these two points will ensure clear passage between the shafts.

First ray or Mayo block

The nerve supply to the first metatarsal segment is from one of the terminal branches of the deep peroneal nerve (dorsolateral), with the other terminal branch supplying the dorsomedial aspect of the second metatarsal segment. The dorsomedial aspect of the first segment is supplied by the medial terminal branches of the superficial peroneal and in some cases terminal

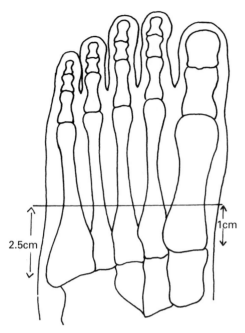

Figure 17.9 Guideline to intermetatarsal route.

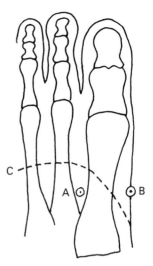

Figure 17.10 Site of injection for first ray block. 'A' and 'B' show the positions of the intradermal weals and the dotted line 'C' is the line of the venous arch.

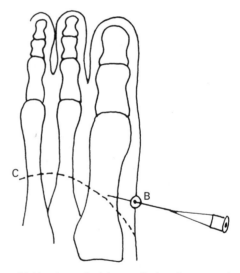

Figure 17.11 Anaesthetising mediodorsal nerve trunks.

branches of the saphenous nerve. The plantar aspects of the first segment are supplied by the terminal branches of the tibial nerve.

The nerve supply to the medial plantar aspect of the segment is superficial at the base of the first metatarsal and medial to the plantar aponeurosis. The nerve supply to the lateral plantar aspect of the segment lies deep to the plantar aponeurosis at the level of the base of the first metatarsal and is the second terminal branch of the medial plantar nerve.

The venous arch over the dorsum of the foot provides a good visual guide to locate the various nerves when used in conjunction with the osseous landmarks of the base of the first metatarsal. Using these two features, it is possible to identify the two optimum sites of entry on the dorsum between the first and second metatarsals (Fig. 17.10, position A), and on the medial aspect of the first metatarsal shaft (Fig. 17.10, position B) where intradermal weals, to facilitate entry, can be raised. The dotted line (C) represents the line of the venous arch.

To anaesthetise the dorsomedial branches of the first metatarsal segment, the hypodermic needle should be passed through the intradermal weal (B) and directed towards the point where the venous arch crosses over the tendon of the extensor digitorum longus, where the major trunk will be located. After aspirating, deposit up to 1 ml of the anaesthetic agent and then

withdraw the needle steadily and unhurriedly, leaving a 'track' of fluid all the way up to the point of entry (Fig. 17.11). This will ensure that any small irregular branches are anaesthetised.

Using the same point of entry, the needle should now be advanced laterally over the plantar surface of the metatarsal to a point in line with the lateral aspect of its base. This should be close to the medial edge of the plantar aponeurosis (Fig. 17.12). Aspiration should not be necessary at this site and about 1–1.5 ml of anaesthetic fluid should be deposited. As the needle is

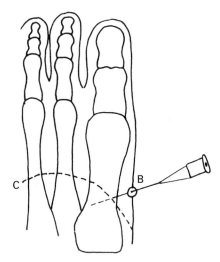

Figure 17.12 Injection site for medioplantar nerve supply to the first ray.

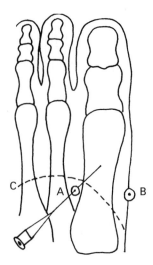

Figure 17.13 Direction of the needle for terminal branches of the superficial peroneal nerve (dorsolateral nerve supply).

withdrawn, continue to deposit the fluid, leaving a track to deal with any irregular branches of either the medial plantar nerve or the saphenous nerve which may be found at that level. This process will complete the blockade of the plantar medial aspect of the segment.

Small terminal branches of the superficial peroneal nerve often supply the dorsolateral aspect of the first metatarsal segment, and it is necessary to ensure that these are also blocked. To accomplish this, the needle is passed through the intradermal weal (A) and is directed medially over the surface of the metatarsal shaft towards the point where the venous arch crosses the tendon of extensor hallucis longus. At this point, about 0.5 ml of the anaesthetic agent should be deposited after aspirating and the needle withdrawn, keeping positive pressure on the plunger so that a 'track' of fluid is left to catch any irregular nerve supply which may be present (Fig. 17.13).

To complete the dorsal block, it is now necessary to pass the needle through the intradermal weal (A) and direct it towards the base of the first metatarsal shaft (Fig. 17.14). It is necessary to ensure that the numerous vessels are avoided and that aspiration is carried out before depositing usually about 1 ml of the anaesthetic. On withdrawal of the needle, it is essential that a 'track' of fluid is not deposited, in case of inadvertent intravenous injection in this vascular region.

The remaining nerve trunk serving the first metatarsal segment is the second terminal branch of the medial plantar nerve, which also serves the medial

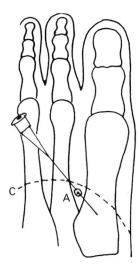

Figure 17.14 Injection to anaesthetise the deep peroneal nerve (dorsolateral nerve supply).

aspect of the second ray segment. The best palpable indicator of its position is the tendon of the flexor hallucis longus, to which it runs parallel at a distance of 8–10 mm.

Entry should be made through the intradermal weal (A) and the needle directed in an anteromedial direction towards the plantar surface of the foot between the metatarsal shafts. The target area is the lateral aspect of the distal one-third of the metatarsal shaft (Fig. 17.15) and it will be necessary to pass through the

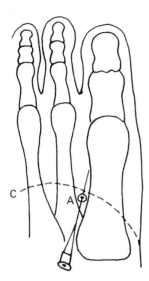

Figure 17.15   Injection to anaesthetise the second terminal branch of the medial plantar nerve.

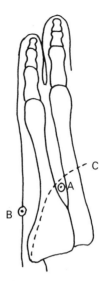

Figure 17.16   Sites for intradermal weals in the fifth ray block.

muscle of the flexor digitorum brevis. Once the needle is considered to be in position, then up to 2 ml of the anaesthetic should be deposited slowly. On withdrawal of the needle, the plunger of the syringe should not be depressed in case of inadvertent intravascular injection.

Fifth ray block

This segment is supplied by nerves from three sources. The lateral branch of the superficial peroneal nerve supplies the medial dorsal aspect. The terminal branches of the sural nerve supply the lateral, the dorsal and, in some cases, the lateral plantar aspect. The plantar and, in most cases, the lateral plantar aspects of the segments are supplied by the lateral branch of the lateral plantar nerve, which lies superficial to the plantar aponeurosis, parallel to the line of the flexor digitorum brevis. The medial plantar aspect of the segment is supplied by the medial terminal branch of the lateral plantar nerve, which also supplies the lateral plantar aspect of the fourth metatarsal segment.

Two intradermal weals are necessary (Fig. 17.16), with the first site placed proximally to the venous arch (C) over the space between the two metatarsal shafts, where it will give access to the terminal branch of the superficial peroneal nerve as it lies superficially and medially to the tendon of the extensor digitorum longus (Fig. 17.17). It also allows access to the medial branch of the lateral plantar nerve by passing between the fouth and fifth metatarsal shafts and through the

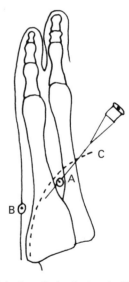

Figure 17.17   Injection site for the terminal branch of the superficial peroneal nerve.

dorsal and plantar interossei muscles (Fig. 17.18). Because of the vascularity of the of the area, it is necessary to aspirate before depositing the agent. Approximately 1 ml of the fluid should be adequate for anaesthesia and, again, as a result of the vascularity, fluid should not be expelled on withdrawal of the needle.

The terminal branches of the sural nerve are blocked

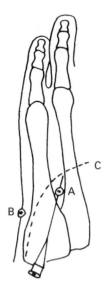

Figure 17.18 Injection towards the medial branch of the lateral plantar nerve.

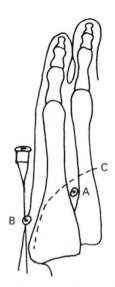

Figure 17.19 Injection towards the terminal branches of the sural nerve.

by inserting the needle through the intradermal weal (B) and advancing it posterodorsally towards the lateral side of the venous arch, avoiding penetration of the vessel. After depositing approximately 1 ml of the anaesthetic, the needle should be withdrawn slowly leaving a large 'track' of the fluid to block any irregular branches (Fig. 17.19).

The lateral branch of the lateral plantar nerve is also reached through the same intradermal weal (B). The needle should be advanced anteromedially towards the line of the flexor digitorum longus. Once on site, about 1 ml of the fluid can be deposited without aspiration and the needle withdrawn, leaving a 'track' of fluid as before up to the point of entry. This should ensure that any small irregular nerves are blocked (Fig. 17.20).

Middle ray blocks

To block the second, third and fourth metatarsal segments only minor modification of the techniques described is required. The third and fourth segments are usually supplied, dorsally, on the medial and lateral borders, respectively, by the medial terminating branch of the lateral branch of the superficial peroneal nerve, which normally passes superficially to the venous arch. The plantar supply is from the lateral branch of the medial plantar nerve but may also be supplied from the lateral plantar nerve.

Both the dorsal and the plantar nerves may be

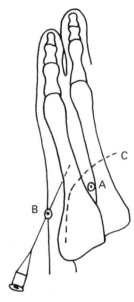

Figure 17.20 Injection site for the lateral plantar nerve.

reached from the intradermal weal sites 'A' and 'B' in Figure 17.21. The line indicated by 'C' in the same diagram is the approximate line of the venous arch. On the plantar sites, the nerves are accompanied by a number of blood vessels, making aspiration essential; similarly fluid should not be expelled from the needle as it passes through the tissues. The plantar nerves are placed deeply to the plantar aponeurosis, and the

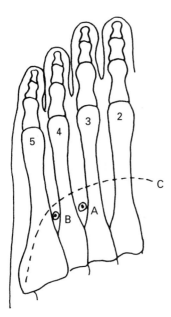

Figure 17.21   Sites of intradermal weals for the fourth ray block.

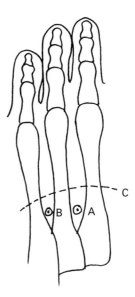

Figure 17.22   Sites of intradermal weals for the third ray block.

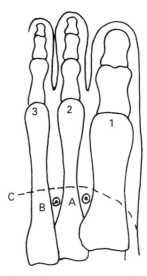

Figure 17.23   Sites of intradermal weals for the second ray block.

dosage of approximately 1 ml of anaesthetic should be delivered slowly to minimise disruption of the tissues and discomfort to the patient.

Anaesthesia of the third metatarsal segment can be accomplished by raising intradermal weals at the sites indicated in Figure 17.22 and following the same general directions as above. The second metatarsal segment can be anaesthetised by raising intradermal weals at the points indicated in Figure 17.23. The technique described in the first ray procedure for the deep peroneal nerve also needs to be applied.

A general consideration which applies to all the procedures described for ray blocks concerning the location of the nerve supply deriving from the medial and plantar nerves is the proximity of the site of the injection to a very well vascularised area. In addition to this, there is the need to pass needles through muscle tissue to reach the sites. One way to minimise this risk is to block the tibial nerve as it passes behind the medial malleolus. At this site the nerve is more easily accessible and generally it is possible to administer a low dosage of the agent. Ultimately, the site chosen must reflect the clinical needs of the patient and the limitations imposed by the procedure.

POSTOPERATIVE SUPERVISION

It is important to ensure that the patient is properly advised of all of the outcomes of the procedure which has been employed, and although the possibility of adverse outcomes from the anaesthetic are rare, it is wise to ensure that the patient has clear instructions in both verbal and written form regarding the steps to be taken, in case of problems arising (see Ch. 6).

SAFETY CONSIDERATIONS

The administration of local anaesthetics using syringes

and needles imposes the obligation on the operator to apply stringent safety precautions to prevent the possibility of needle-stick injuries to the operator or the patient. Opinion changes on the methodology for containing the dangers and every effort should be made to ensure that the latest local and national regulations are known and applied.

All sharps should be discarded in the approved way in designated sharp disposal containers, which should ensure that they do not pose a risk to cleaning staff and others who are concerned with the control of the surgery. Syringes should not be held in the hand, apart from when being used or transported to their container. The sheathing of needles after use is considered to constitute a risk of needle-stick injury to the operator, and the use of needle holders is recommended.

REFERENCES

Bruce S D 1989 Techniques of regional anaesthesia. Appleton & Lange Mediglobe, Warwalk, Connecticut
Covino B G, Vassallo H G 1976 Local anesthetics. Grune & Stratton, New York
de Jong R H 1994 Local anesthetics, Mosby, St Louis
de Jong R H 1977 Local anesthetics. Charles C Thomas, Springfield, Illinois
Dripps R D, Eckenhoff J E, Vandam L D 1988 Introduction to anesthesia, 7th edn. WB Saunders, Philadelphia
Fink B R 1989 Mechanisms of differential blockade in epidural and subarachnoid anesthesia. Anesthesiology 70: 851–858
Reynolds E F (ed) 1993 Martindale, the extra pharmacopoeia, 29th edn. Pharmaceutical Press, London
Seldon R, Sashara A A 1967 Journal of the American Medical Association
Stricharz G R (ed) 1987 Local anesthetics. Springer Verlag, Berlin
Vickers M D, Schieden H, Wood-Smith F G 1984 Drugs in anesthetic practice, 6th edn. Butterworth, London
Wildsmith J A W, Armitage E N 1987 Principles and practice of regional anaesthesia. Churchill Livingstone, Edinburgh
Zenz M, Panhans C, Niesel H C, Kreuscher H 1988 Regional anesthesia. Wolfe Medical Publications, London

18

General principles of surgical practice

A. J. Clark

Keywords

Absorbable sutures
Aftercare
Atrophy complications
Choice of dressing
Drains
Dressings
Epidermoid cyst
Equipment
Exsanguination
Fibroma
Haematoma
Haemostatic control
Infection
Keloid
Medication
Neurological complications
Non-absorbable sutures
Oedema
Osseous surgery
Postoperative care
Postoperative instructions
Pressure neuritis
Removal of sutures
Seroma
Surgical wound
Suturing
Suturing equipment
Techniques of application
Tissue viability
Vascular complications
Wound dehiscence

Surgery may fail for several reasons, amongst which are inadequate pre-operative assessment and patient selection, insufficient preparation and organisation, inappropriate techniques and poorly planned postoperative care. Before elective surgery is undertaken, the most essential question to be considered is whether the surgery is necessary. To answer this properly it is essential to establish a clear picture of the patient's condition, which must include their life style and their expectations of the surgery, in conjunction with a thorough investigation of their suitability for ambulatory surgery.

Major factors in this process are the duration and severity of the symptoms. Any previous treatments which have been undertaken must be identified, as must the prognosis of the condition if left untreated. While the patient's medical status must be fully assessed, the patient's expectations and the level of compliance are also very important in aiding a full and rapid recovery. In establishing a comprehensive assessment, the patient's attitude towards the condition is a crucial factor. Patient compliance may be indicated from their record of previous treatments and the number of cancelled or missed appointments. It may be that the general practitioner is able to advise on the patient's compliance with other therapies which may have been initiated. The demands of the patient may affect their availability for treatment, as may their domestic circumstances. If the patient is living alone, it is important to establish the level of support available from friends and family. Poor patient compliance will complicate the pre- and postoperative stages of a surgical procedure, which will affect the healing time as well as its quality.

The patient should have a realistic expectation of the process and outcomes of surgery (Ch. 6). The procedure could be traumatic to the patient if they are unprepared for surgery, and it is important to discuss the procedure and evaluate their response. Only when they understand what will occur can they give informed consent for the surgery.

Different patient groups present particular problems. The use of premedication to relieve anxiety in a very nervous patient may be of benefit. Diazepam 5–10 mg orally, 2 hours before surgery is often employed. The age of the patient must also be considered, as elderly patients carry a greater surgical risk due to the ageing process, and this must be viewed in conjunction with a detailed medical history. If necessary, a risk index (i.e. physical status classification) can be carried out to assess their suitability for surgery (Keats 1978, Culver et al 1991).

The very young patient also presents special problems; the level of anxiety and a lack of compliance during the procedure are factors to be considered, and again the use of a pre-operative sedative may be advisable. During the assessment process, it must be remembered that the podiatrist is a part of the health care team, and discussion with the general practitioner, the hospital consultant or any other member of the team involved with the patient will strengthen the practitioner's understanding of the patient's health and circumstances. Cooperation is important in improving the quality of information received during the history-taking and examination of the patient (see Ch. 2). The podiatrist can then call on other professions for support in premedication or in the postoperative care of the patient.

The practitioner must discuss the advantages and disadvantages of surgery compared with those of conservative treatment. This is necessary in order to establish 'informed consent', which is a legal requirement. The patient should fully understand what is causing the condition and what can be done to treat it, including all possible outcomes and complications. This must be achieved using words which the patient understands.

Healing by second intention, as after nail surgery, is dependent upon a number of variable factors. In trying to predict the healing time, the important factors are the depth of the wound, its surface area, the degree of stress exerted on the site, the degree of operative trauma and the amount of tissue loss. The clinical implications of any systemic disease must also be considered in assessing patient suitability for surgery, as this can greatly affect the healing time (Zederfeldt et al 1986).

TISSUE VIABILITY

In planning the most suitable approach for any procedure, it is essential to visualise the position and identify all of the structures in the operative field. This review must include the position of any sensory nerves emerging through the deep fascia, the position of the neurovascular bundles, the tendons passing over or inserting into the area, and the underlying bones and joints. It is also necessary when choosing the site of an incision to consider how suturing and scar formation may affect the patient, and it is important to consider the direction of the cleavage lines of the skin. These were first described by Langer, but more recent authors advocate the use of the skin creases as a definition of the lines of stress and therefore a more accurate guide to the most suitable direction of incision (Borges 1984). This minimises any tension on the wound and allows the scar to blend with the existing skin creases.

After reduction of a deformity is completed, the operator may have to consider the amount of overlying tissue and remove any which is redundant, to accommodate the change in position. Elliptical incisions allow the removal of excess tissue and, in the case of digital surgery, often result in the removal of all or part of the associated corn or callus. The direction of the incision may also be used as a method of correction for the deformity and this is clearly seen in Chapter 20 in the description of correction of an adductovarus deformity of the fifth toe. In all surgical cases, it is important that sufficient tissue is removed to produce good cosmesis; however, removal of too much tissue will produce excessive wound tension, leading to postoperative complications such as wound dehiscence. If insufficient tissue is removed, the remaining excess may result in the development of a dead space lesion and fluid aggregation which will retard healing.

The technique of dissection uses the line between the tissue planes to develop tissue cleavage, which minimises tissue disruption, reduces the amount of cell damage and limits the inflammatory response. This technique also allows for the orderly closure of each layer where necessary. The tissue planes can be divided at specific histological barriers. It is important to remember that the dermis and epidermis gain blood supply from vessels passing through the superficial fascia, and separation of the junction can adversely affect the superficial tissues, causing sloughing.

The success of surgery can be affected by many factors. Surgery can be restricted by poor haemostatic control obliterating the field; good visibility is essential and if haemostasis is proving difficult to maintain then regular swabbing is required to allow a successful outcome. Another problem facing the podiatrist is the displacement of structures as a result of deformity, and it is important that there is sufficient visibility to allow the podiatrist to identify the position of all structures within the surgical field. Working through a very small incision may make recognition of structures difficult and the procedure more complicated. Keeping the size of the wound small may be counterproductive to both the podiatrist and the patient by making the procedure more difficult, and if tissue has to be removed then the incision must be sufficiently large to allow this to be achieved. The excised tissue should be sent for histological examination and pathological report to identify the cell types and to ascertain whether or not it is benign.

During the procedure, it is important to irrigate the wound regularly with sterile saline solution, which will allow clearer visibility. This may be mixed with Betadine solution which will act as an antiseptic to reduce any possible infection. Irrigation prevents the tissues from drying out due to excessive exposure, and sterile saline solution can also be used to flush debris from the wound after osteotripsy or rasping of bone. Irrigation is carried out using a syringe to create sufficient pressure to clear the debris from the area without damaging the tissues or lodging debris in the wound margins. Any excessive force used during the procedure will be reflected in the amount of tissue loss occurring postoperatively. This is most relevant when osseous deformity has displaced structures.

SURGICAL WOUND

The surgical wound should allow the podiatrist a clear and unrestricted visual field, enabling accurate and precise correction of a deformity, but it also carries with it some problems. The sutured wound offers many advantages to the practitioner, as the opposing surfaces will limit the introduction of bacteria into the wound and will reduce its surface area. Any tissue loss, which would normally be replaced over a period of weeks, is now replaced in a much shorter timescale. In the initial stages of wound healing, when the wound is becoming organised, the sutures act to support and maintain the integrity of the clot and the healing tissues, improving healing times, while the proximity of the wound edges limits the area of entry for bacteria. Over areas of high stress, the sutures also act to limit distortion of the tissues and therefore reduce healing times. The use of sutures is discussed under a separate heading. There are a number of other methods of closure, the simplest being the use of Steristrips (3-M), which give good wound closure and will give support to the tissues. The adhesive strips come in a variety of sizes, which will accommodate most wounds; they are simple to apply and can be used to reinforce sutures where necessary. Some of the more common problems which occur will be discussed under 'postoperative complications'.

EQUIPMENT AND TECHNIQUES OF APPLICATION

There is a large range of instruments available to the practitioner, but the podiatric surgical set should be sufficient for a variety of techniques. It is most important to make sure that there is more than one set available at all times in case of accident where the instruments become contaminated.

The number of each type of instrument will depend upon the range of surgery undertaken, and the set does not include any consumable items or any power equipment. Most hospital sterile supply departments carry lists of surgical packs which they make up for different departments and it is probably easier to customise one of the existing packs with extra podiatry instruments. Alternatively, the podiatrists can create their own specialised pack. It should include a number of scalpel handles, as they may be required at various points in the procedure.

Once the wound is established, it is important to identify the structures, and this is achieved by the use of retractors. The tissues should be displaced with the minimum of damage and the procedure can continue using either blunt or sharp dissection. Sharp dissection using scalpels or scissors is necessary to deepen a wound or to release structures, while blunt dissection using forceps or dissector can be used to increase the size of the wound. At all stages, the tissues should be handled with the greatest of care to minimise trauma to the area.

The scalpel has a variety of uses and this is reflected in the range of associated techniques (Anderson & Romfh 1980). The type of scalpel grip will vary depending on which of the particular features the practitioner considers most important at each stage in the procedure. The fingertip grip is often used for making the initial incision and allows the maximum cutting edge to be in contact with the skin for greater control, particularly in longer incisions. The palm grip can be used where greater pressure is required as it offers more stability while pressure is being exerted. A pencil grip can be used throughout the procedure, varying the angle of the blade. This allows great precision and control of the scalpel, facilitating the accurate initial incision, with only a minimum of the blade in contact with the patient.

A vertical placement of the blade will give a small incision which can be enlarged. With this angle, known as a 'press cutting' technique, the incision is highly controlled in length and direction. Sliding the blade over the tissues under pressure produces an accurate continuous incision which will vary in depth depending upon the degree of pressure. It is important that the area is stabilised to avoid excessive skin movement which can result in a jagged wound or an alteration in the direction of the incision. The operator must apply sufficient tension to the wound to allow an accurate incision of the area (Fig. 18.1) and it is important that the scalpel is kept vertical to the patient to avoid an oblique incision of the tissues. The scalpel should be changed after the first incision, to reduce the possibility of wound infection. It is best to incise the superficial fascia with short strokes, as this will allow more haemostatic control and clearer visibility of the tissues. The superficial fascia has a limited cosmetic importance and has a different structure from the underlying tissues. The initial incision should completely cut the skin, leaving vertical wound edges for apposition on completion of the procedure. Repeated

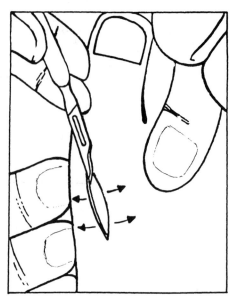

Figure 18.1 Initial incision using a press cutting technique, with the assistant creating suitable skin tension.

incisions increase the probability of irregular wound edges giving rise to greater tissue damage which may retard wound healing. Skin tension on the area will give greater separation, control and accuracy to the operator. Skin hooks allow tissue to be handled with minimum trauma and also aid in wound closure. They are used to hold the subcutaneous tissues and epidermis during closure, producing minimal tissue damage.

There are many types of retractor available and it is best to include retractors of different sizes, both small- and wide-headed. The choice is related to the size and position of the wound, as the retractors allow much clearer visibility of the wound and can protect soft tissue structures from damage. The practitioner can also use a self-retaining retractor, which allows the assistant much greater freedom, but this increases the possibility of tissue damage, due to the constant pressure it exerts. It is the role of the assistant to retract the tissues and protect the surrounding structures, increasing the size of the window through which the operator can work.

The importance of a good assistant cannot be over emphasised, as most forefoot surgery occurs through relatively small incisions requiring good teamwork.

Dissecting forceps allow small amounts of tissue to be handled firmly and accurately with the minimum of trauma. There are a number of types: the Adsons forceps with wide arms and small jaws give secure and accurate tissue handling, and the straight dissecting forceps are used to hold the wound margins during suturing.

The MacDonalds dissector can be used to elevate or protect structures and can separate tissue by blunt dissection. Backhaus towel clamps can also be used during procedures, to aid in the removal of sections of bone. Their jaws can pierce the section, giving the operator greater control during the process of excision.

There are two distinct groups of instruments used for cutting bone. The first group, the *rongeurs*, have 'spoon-like' jaws for 'nibbling' bone and are used to remove osteophytes or to reshape bone. The second group includes the bone cutters of varying types. They have a variety of jaw shapes and can be single- or double-action. The double-action type will give greater accuracy and mechanical advantage, reducing the strain necessary to cut through the bone.

Power equipment offers greater accuracy and is essential if more complex surgery is undertaken. The oscillating bone saw is used most effectively on larger bones, e.g. the first metatarsal. It offers the advantage of minimal bone fragmentation, giving smoother edges which need less rasping. This reduces the possibility of any bone fragments being included in the wound. When using power equipment, care must be taken to protect the surrounding tissues. The bone can be damaged by a tearing action if the saw blade is blunt, and excessive heat is produced which burns the bone and leads to necrosis. Shortening of the bone should be taken into account when planning surgery and its results (Butterworth & Dockery 1992).

The surgical drill is often used to reduce irregular bony surfaces and an alternative is the power rasp, used in osteotripsy. Most pneumatic equipment allows the interchanging of handpieces, which facilitates the use of all three types of equipment. The use of the drill or rasp is common in minimal incision surgery, but it is important that the resulting debris is removed from the area by flushing the wound with sterile saline solution (Hymes 1977).

Artery forceps are another multipurpose tool which can be used to separate and clamp tissue, and to secure a tourniquet. It is important to have sufficient forceps to deal with any problem that may occur. In podiatry, fine-jawed forceps give much greater control than the standard jaw and are of more use.

Contamination of a set of instruments must not interfere with a procedure and, to cover all contingencies, it is important to have more than the required number of sets of instruments sterilised. It is best to use a standard pack of instruments, as this offers the operator continuity. Instruments can be packed individually to supplement the sets as required.

HAEMOSTATIC CONTROL

This has to be considered throughout the three phases of surgical practice, pre-operatively, during the operation and postoperatively. Pre-operatively, it is important to investigate thoroughly any history of bleeding, e.g. prolonged bleeding after tooth extraction or any earlier surgery, history of anaemia or recurrent infection, and medication which may prolong clotting time. For patients who describe periods of excessive bleeding after minor injury, it is prudent to establish formally the patient's clotting time and bleeding time. These factors do not preclude patients from undergoing surgery, but they should be considered as part of the decision-making process concerning the patient's suitability. There may be a physical problem which affects the patient, e.g. a history of back or lower limb problems may exclude elevation of the lower limb in the process of exsanguination.

Elevation of the limb pre-operatively for approximately 3 minutes reduces the vascularity of the area, and exsanguination using a pressure bandage further reduces the blood in the limb. For some procedures, surgery may be carried out with the limb in an elevated position without the use of a tourniquet, and although there may be some bleeding, it will not interfere with the operation. If the procedure involves only the nail or distal interphalangeal joint, then a digital tourniquet can be used and this must be released after 20 minutes to avoid any tissue damage due to anoxia.

The use of a pneumatic cuff placed at the lower third of the calf and inflated to approximately 250 mm mercury (Hg) gives constant haemostasis. The use of a mid-thigh tourniquet inflated to 400 mmHg has the advantage of increasing the tourniquet time to 2 hours, whereas an ankle tourniquet can only be used for 1 hour. A thigh tourniquet is preferable because there is less danger of compressing the neurovascular structures against the underlying bone. The tourniquet site should be wrapped with gauze to protect the area and underlying structures. The cuff is normally inflated only after the limb has been elevated for 3 minutes to reduce the vascularity of the limb. The application of a tourniquet can produce discomfort.

Pre-operative measures include the choice of a local anaesthetic agent, preferably one with added adrenaline which does not cause vasodilation, although plain solutions of local anaesthetics, most often used in podiatry, which produce local vasodilation need not be precluded. The action of local anaesthetics on the vaso nervosum leads to a loss of vasomotor tone, allowing the hydrostatic pressure to produce vasodilation which is apparent in varying degrees in most patients.

The use of 1:200 000 added adrenaline offers a much longer period of anaesthesia, but the resultant vasoconstriction precludes its use on the lesser toes, although several studies (Scarlet et al 1978) have concluded that it produces a negligible effect on the vascular flow when used with lignocaine, due to the vasodilatory action of the latter. The use of added adrenaline in ankle block anaesthesia is well documented and offers a great reduction in the blood supply to the plantar surface on the foot, as well as prolonged anaesthesia, even with lower doses of anaesthetic.

During the procedure, any vessel which is bleeding can be ligated using an absorbable suture material, e.g. Dexon, thus improving visibility in the field. Another method of haemostatic control is electocautery, which is available in a number of forms, including disposable units (Aaron Medical Industries USA, Cardiokinetics Ltd UK). It is important that the tip is at the optimum temperature; if it is not hot enough it will adhere to the tissues, and if too hot, it will burn through the vessel instead of sealing it. The use of chemical haemostatics is to be avoided, as they may produce increased tissue necrosis and thus a higher risk of postoperative infection.

Postoperative bleeding is less of a problem in an incised wound, as there should have been haemostatic control throughout the procedure. If the surgery was undertaken using a tourniquet then there may be some bleeding on its removal. Postoperatively, a variety of agents are available to control bleeding. Absorbable agents such as the gelatin or calcium alginate sponges help control bleeding by magnifying the surface area in the clot and absorbing several times their own weight of blood. These substances are absorbed over a 4–6 week period, are non-irritant and do not elicit a tissue reaction. They are useful in wounds which will heal by secondary intention. Oxygen-regenerated cellulose is an agent which acts by absorbing blood, and it is bactericidal against a wide range of organisms. Bone wax can also be applied to control haemorrhage from cut sections of bone, although both bone wax and oxygen-regenerated cellulose may affect bone healing.

OSSEOUS SURGERY

Working to correct deformity by the removal of bone or correction by repositioning bone is a considerable challenge to the podiatrist. The use of X-rays to give a clear understanding of the position and quality of bone is essential before commencing surgery (see Chs 2 and 3). The X-ray can also be used to allow the podiatrist to plan the procedure, deciding where any bone will be cut and at what angle. This is of great importance when using closing wedge procedures, to allow the podiatrist to evaluate the surgery in advance and plan the most appropriate angles and positions to gain correction.

As part of the evaluation of the surgery, the practitioner will consider how the corrected position can be maintained. The use of an external dressing or bandage may be sufficient to control the position of the joint, but in many cases a more stable fixation is required and the fixation technique will depend on the procedure undertaken. Stainless steel wire is commonly used for internal fixation to close an osteotomy, giving stability and strength, but it can produce severe compression at the site of the insertion, with a risk of necrosis of the bone. Kirschner wires are used to give some compression and stability in digital arthrodesis, the gauge of the wire determining its strength. Often a number of Kirschner wires may be used to give maximum control of the corrected post-operative position. The Kirschner wire should normally be removed after 3 weeks, although this has the disadvantage that it can create a tract for the entry of infection. Staples and clips offer permanent internal fixation but are more difficult to use because of the equipment needed and the variability in the amount of compression they produce, which may be due to the positioning of the clip and the irregularity of the bone surfaces.

Screws produce stability and can be used to aid fusion, but the positioning of the screw can also act to distort the alignment, and care should be taken to consider its position relative to the direction of the two sections. The screw can act to displace the two sections of bone, and its application is a skilled exercise involving a large amount of specialised equipment. The use of an external supporting or controlling cast will also maintain the correct position. This can be constructed from plaster of Paris bandage, or more light-weight synthetic materials. The elderly patient will benefit from the increased mobility that a light-weight cast allows. An advantage of synthetic casts is that they achieve their maximum strength in a much shorter period of time, but they cost considerably more than the equivalent plaster of Paris cast and the material also has a limited shelf-life.

SUTURING

Sutures hold the wound edges in apposition, encouraging the healing process. This depends upon accurate coaption and the minimum of tissue trauma. It is important that the wound edges are either slightly everted or level, but not inverted as this retards healing and can lead to the development of elevated and unsightly scars. It is also important that the stitches are not too tight as this may lead to avascularity of the wound edges and, in conjunction with postoperative oedema, may produce a localised tissue necrosis. The tension of the suture is also important as it must allow for postoperative oedema. Excessive tension may lead to rupture of the suture. Sutures should coapt throughout the full depth of the wound, not only the superficial tissue, thus avoiding the development of a dead space area which could retard healing and act as a possible focus of infection (Fig. 18.2).

There are several different forms of sutures, each with a particular function (Brown 1986). The most common form is the single interrupted suture; it holds the wound edges in apposition and using a surgeon's knot of three throws followed by two throws, it avoids slippage and is therefore very secure (Fig. 18.3). The

stitches may be placed in close proximity or used in conjunction with horizontal mattress sutures, which will coapt a larger section of the wound.

An alternative type of suture is the vertical mattress suture, which gives deep and superficial levels of wound coaption, passing through the tissues at two depths. Another method is the half-buried mattress suture, which is excellent at holding wound margins together after tissue excision. This type of suture passes from the surface of one wound margin into the deeper tissues in the opposite wound margin and then superficially back to the initial wound margin, leaving the suture visible only at the first wound margin (Fig. 18.4).

Continuous sutures, such as the simple running suture, can be advantageous to the practitioner, as they avoid repetitive knot tying, and offer continuous wound coaption. They are also used in closing subcutaneous tissues. On completion of a suture, the practitioner should check the position of the knot, which should lie to one side of the incision. It should not lie over the incision as it may act as an irritant to the wound and become trapped in the clot formed by postoperative bleeding.

Drains serve to reduce the accumulation of fluid at the site of the wound. This reduces the possibility of seroma and haematoma formation, and reduces pain and the possibility of tissue necrosis due to swelling, thereby increasing the rate of healing. The drain is normally kept in place for 48–72 hours, but it may act as

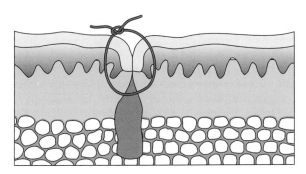

Figure 18.2 Poor suturing technique, showing inversion of the wound edges and dead space in the tissues.

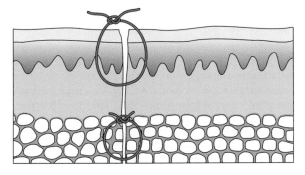

Figure 18.3 Interrupted suture (non-absorbable) and buried subcutaneous suture (absorbable).

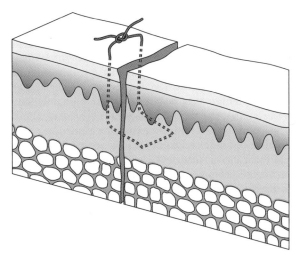

Figure 18.4 Half-buried horizontal mattress suture—used to give deep and superficial closure and greater wound stability.

an irritant and a route of infection, and can also produce discomfort or pressure ischaemia on the tissues. The simplest type of drain is a sterile rubber tube inserted into the wound with a small section protruding from the wound. This is often known as a 'Penrose drain' and it depends upon the position of the limb to maximise drainage. To reduce the possibility of infection, a closed suction drain can be used. This has a sealed container which can collect only a fixed amount of fluid. It is often used to reduce any accumulation of fluid after wound infection.

Suturing equipment

The following list of instruments is sufficient for most minor procedures:

- 2 pairs of Kilner needle holders
- 2 pairs of 5 inch toothed dissecting forceps
- 2 pairs of suture removal scissors
- dressing scissors and forceps.

There are two groups of suturing material: non-absorbable and absorbable sutures. In each group there is a variety of different structures, monofilament or multifilament, and a number of different materials, natural and synthetic, with a range of needle shapes and suture lengths. The practitioner must consider the particular qualities required from any suture material, including its tensile strength, its elasticity and plasticity, and the strength of the knot. Braided or multifilament sutures allow greater tracking of body fluids along the material. Natural fibres elicit a greater tissue reaction than synthetic materials. All suture materials elicit some tissue reaction which lasts for between 5 and 10 days.

After this period, most non-absorbable sutures will be removed. Monofilament nylon and polypropylene produce the least tissue reaction. In ascending order of their tensile strengths, braided nylon, braided polyester or stainless steel may be used, although polyester and stainless steel both produce more tissue reaction. The stainless steel suture can also produce some discomfort but it gives good skin closure and a very stable wound scar. Stainless steel wire is even stronger and is used commonly as skin closure clips, but its use is not favoured for minor surgery.

Non-absorbable sutures

The most common suture material used is braided silk. It is dyed black to make the suture clearly visible in the wound. Silk is not a particularly strong material and, as a natural fibre, elicits a slightly greater tissue reaction. Its advantages are that it moulds well onto the surfaces of the wound and is an easy material to tie, offering small secure knots with the minimum distance between sutures if necessary. Silk is described as non-absorbable, but if left in the tissues over a long period of time, it initially loses its tensile strength and then degrades. This is unlikely to occur in the types of procedures carried out by podiatrists, and any subcutaneous sutures can be of the absorbable type. Synthetic materials which can be used as an alternative to silk include Dermalon and Novafil (Davis and Geck). Dermalon is a monofilament nylon material which is non-capillary and elicits a minimal tissue response due to its structure. This is also true for Novafil, a monofilament polybutester which has similar properties. If necessary, braided nylon, braided polyester and stainless steel may be used in ascending order of their tensile strengths (Yu & Cavaliere 1983).

Absorbable sutures

As mentioned in the previous section, there is a range of natural and synthetic suture materials. The natural materials are commonly labelled as either chromic or plain catgut, which consists of processed sheep intestine. As a 'foreign' protein, this type of suture elicits a high tissue response and is not recommended for wound closure as it attracts a higher level of bacterial infection than many other materials, especially when compared to the alternative synthetic materials such as Dexon, which is a coated polyglyolic acid having similar properties to catgut and producing a minimal tissue reaction. It can be used for wound closure, as well as subcutaneously, since it does not lead to scarring.

Removal of sutures

The time-scale for the removal of sutures depends on the site of the sutures, the wound strength, the healing rate and the type and number of sutures involved. Generally, sutures are removed after approximately 5–10 days and, if over a joint, after 6–12 days. It is important to ensure that all sutures are removed in order to avoid the possibilities of infection tracking along the course of the suture, or of any tissue reaction caused by the suture in the wound. Removal of the sutures should be carried out with the minimum of tissue trauma, by cutting the suture so as to avoid pulling the knot through the tissues. After removal of the sutures, it is important to protect the wound from trauma which will disrupt the healing process.

POSTOPERATIVE CARE

After surgery, it is important to establish the highest level of asepsis possible while undertaking postoperative care. The wound must be protected from contamination and trauma, particularly any mechanical irritation between wound and dressing. Ambulatory surgery, as its name suggests, encourages patient mobility, and with this comes the increased possibility of trauma. To combat this, there is a range of options open to the practitioner.

Choice of dressing

This must relate to its function and to the properties which are considered essential. The ideal wound dressing must be impermeable to microorganisms and must be able to meet the following criteria:

- to absorb any wound discharge
- to maintain a suitable environment for wound healing
- to minimise the shedding of fibres which could interfere with the healing process
- to be removed without causing trauma to the wound.

Medication

Systemic medication for pain control during the first 48–72 hour period is often advisable and is best undertaken in consultation with the patient's general practitioner. It is important to ensure that the patient takes the prescribed medication before cessation of the effects of the local anaesthetic, as this will give the patient greater comfort by ensuring that the pain transmission channels in the nerve remain blocked for longer.

Dressings

There are many types of wound dressings available, e.g. semi-permeable films such as Opsite (Smith & Nephew), which can be sprayed over the wound, and also hydrocolloids, e.g. Granuflex wafers or granules (Squibb Surgicare). Another wound dressing is Debrisan (Pharmacia), a dextranomer which absorbs wound exudate. It is produced as a paste and a powder.

The dressing must be able to absorb any discharge from the wound without compromising its function. It should not act as a mechanical irritant by being too large or too loose. If the dressing absorbs any blood, it may become rigid and adhere to the wound, acting as an irritant, promoting entry of microorganisms and thus failing to maintain a suitable environment for healing. Some dressings are applied with the knowledge that they will harden, e.g. a dressing soaked with povidone-iodine will harden to act as a splint and can be used to aid in the maintenance of a corrected position. If this rigid dressing is used, it is first necessary to apply a non-adherent layer, and this is followed by a covering of sterile gauze to protect the wound. This will also act as an absorbent for discharge. The dressing is completed securely and neatly by using a Kling bandage applied with some tension to prevent displacement. Where the dressing encircles the toe, it should not compress the tissues excessively or it may cause pressure necrosis of the wound.

Aftercare

The postoperative care of the patient can influence the cosmesis and healing time. Prior to surgery, the patient should have been advised that, to maximise postoperative care, they must be available to attend for treatment should the need arise. It is equally important that the practitioner is also available and that there is sufficient time in the schedule for such a contingency.

The practitioner should give the patient clear instructions to follow (Box 18.1). The use of written instructions is advised and they should be discussed with the patient before leaving the surgery. It is important that the patient has unambiguous instructions giving a clear indication of the stages of the process, the most immediate of which is postoperative bleeding, followed by postoperative pain.

The patient should remain in the surgery for approximately 45 minutes after the procedure to allow the practitioner to monitor any bleeding which may occur. Should there be marked haemorrhage at a later stage, the patient should return to the surgery for investigation. The degree of postoperative pain is individual to each patient and each procedure. Prior advice should minimise this, and recourse to suitable painkillers is also helpful. If it is thought necessary, a mild sedative may be prescribed, but this would be for a 48–72 hour period only.

The foot should be protected from trauma and rested during this period, and the elevation of the limb will reduce some of the postoperative oedema and the associated throbbing sensation. Ice packs (see Ch. 15) will also aid the reduction of the postoperative swelling. The patient must keep the dressing dry, because if it becomes moist, the number of bacteria present will increase. It is impossible to stop the spread of skin flora

---

Box 18.1 Postoperative instructions

The following instructions are for your benefit and will help to reduce any swelling or pain and encourage healing. Please follow them.

1. Please go directly home. Do not drive yourself if you are so advised. If your journey will take more than 15 minutes, elevate your feet.
2. To encourage a quick and uneventful recovery, **do not** sit with your feet down or with your legs crossed for any length of time as this may cause swelling and pain.
3. Some bruising and swelling is to be expected and there is no cause for alarm.
4. Whenever possible sit with your feet elevated at least as high as your hips.
5. Keep the bandages dry and clean. Do not remove them to inspect the wound. A small amount of bleeding is normal and may mark the bandage.
6. Ice packs will reduce any discomfort and swelling but make sure the pack is sealed to avoid wetting the dressing. (A simple ice pack can be made by soaking a kitchen towel in cold water, squeezing out excess water; then put the towel inside two plastic bags and place in the freezer for 30 minutes. It can then be draped over the foot.)
7. Do not get the dressing wet. Cover the foot with a plastic bag and place on the side of the bath. Do not use the shower as the water will penetrate the bag and dressing.
8. Exercise your legs frequently by bending your knees and ankles to stimulate the circulation and healing.
9. Protect your foot at night to avoid any pressure from the bedclothes.
10. Reduce your smoking and consumption of alcohol.
11. Drink plenty of fluids.
12. Call the podiatrist on the number supplied if:
    a. your dressing becomes soaked with blood or if it becomes tight and your toes tingle or feel numb
    b. discomfort is not reduced by your medication
    c. you knock or injure the foot
    d. you develop a high temperature.

---

into the area of the dressing, but with suitable changes of dressings the possibility of infection is minimised.

Mobilisation of the patient as soon as possible is important to avoid postoperative complications, notably deep vein thrombosis. Mobilisation will aid the reduction of postoperative oedema and encourage patient morale. The use of a trauma shoe to minimise compression of the wound during the postoperative period will benefit the patient (Fig. 18.5). There is a variety of types, which all protect the foot and allow mobility with little restriction. It could also be an appropriate stage to give advice on footwear for the future, designed to prevent a recurrence of the defor-

mity. The practitioner may advise the patient to obtain shoes which will allow the insertion of orthoses, if that is necessary. The use of exercises as part of the postoperative process can improve the range of mobility and prevent muscle wastage. This is an important factor in maintaining correction and avoiding any delay in osseous development.

In most cases of conservative surgery, the procedure will not correct any underlying biomechanical deformity, and while the surgery may improve the cosmesis of the foot, the condition may recur unless the range of motion is controlled by orthoses. This is another area which must be discussed as part of the patient evaluation for surgery. Once the wound has healed and a suitable orthosis is in place, the patient should be monitored as part of the follow-up process. This will give maximum benefit from surgery and will give the practitioner invaluable information about the audit of procedures.

POSTOPERATIVE COMPLICATIONS

Pain

Pain is the first and most common postoperative experience that the patient is likely to meet and it is important that the strategies are in place to deal with this before the surgery is undertaken. It is suggested that between 20% and 75% of patients may suffer from the failure of postoperative pain control (Spence 1990). The use of systemic medication in conjunction with good patient preparation and compliance will do much to alleviate this problem. The pain may be due to an overtight dressing rather than the surgical procedure and it is important that this problem is not trivialised or ignored. Pain is recognised as having depressive effects which may further hinder patient/practitioner relationships. Support from the general practitioner in the prescription of non-steroidal anti-inflammatory drugs (NSAIDs) may help to alleviate these symptoms, particularly if the medication is initiated while the anaesthesia is still functioning.

Infection

The tissue planes discussed earlier normally restrict the spread of infection, acting as anatomical barriers. Deep fascia is the most important of these, sealing the deeper structures and compartmentalising them. However, in most surgery this barrier is breached, allowing the entry of bacteria into the deeper structures.

Infection may occur as a result of defective surgical

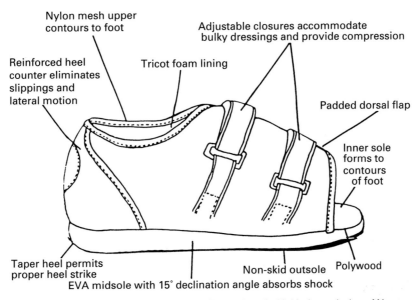

Nylon mesh upper
contours to foot

Adjustable closures accommodate
bulky dressings and provide compression

Reinforced heel
counter eliminates
slippings and
lateral motion

Tricot foam lining

Padded dorsal flap

Inner sole
forms to
contours
of foot

Taper heel permits
proper heel strike

EVA midsole with 15° declination angle absorbs shock

Non-skid outsole   Polywood

Figure 18.5   Postoperative trauma shoe. (Reproduced with kind permission of Nova Instruments Ltd.)

technique or inadequate postoperative care. The area may be red, hot, swollen and tender as a natural sequel to surgery, and there may be some postoperative bleeding. These should subside during the first 72 hours, but if the area becomes more inflamed and painful, it is essential the practitioner examines the wound.

Any serious discharge from the wound is a cause for concern and a swab should be taken and sent for examination. The tension of the wound should be examined for any abscess formation and, if there is any doubt, it is wise to commence antibiotic therapy. This can be adjusted after the results of the swab become available. The infection may occur as a result of a dead space lesion, allowing either haematoma or seroma formation, and the infection may form an abscess in the tissue space.

It is important to drain the abscess to avoid encouraging bacterial growth, leading to increased tension, which in turn can lead to necrosis of the overlying tissues. In order to avoid disturbing the wound unnecessarily, particularly during the first 72 hours, it is important to establish whether any clinical signs which may present are of systematic origin or are due to local infection.

Wound dehiscence

Wound dehiscence or the splitting of a wound is a possible outcome during the postoperative period. It is important to consider the sequelae to wound closure that can lead to postoperative infection or poor wound healing. The suture should produce wound apposition without producing tension and restricting the postoperative oedema which occurs as part of the healing process.

Haematoma

Haematoma formation within the wound can be caused by poor haemostasis, i.e. the failure to coagulate or ligate a vessel. In some cases a haematoma can occur despite good haemostatic control, and if untreated it can cause distension, which may lead to marked postoperative swelling. This could lead to rupture of the wound or to the development of superficial gangrene of the overlying tissues. Should this occur, the wound should be opened, the coagulum removed and the edges re-sutured.

Seroma

Distension may also occur as a result of seroma formation. A seroma is an accumulation of lymph and tissue fluid produced when the skin and subcutaneous fascia have been separated from the underlying fascia, allowing fluid to collect. The fluid can be drawn off using a syringe, with the puncture site distant from the wound. This distended area can act as a focus for infection and produce a dead space within the wound. If this area becomes infected, the bacterial toxins can produce cellular necrosis and microvascular thrombosis, which will delay tissue replacement and epidermal migration, resulting in tissue necrosis of the wound edges. The infection will impair the function of the fibroblasts which produce wound collagen and this will further weaken the wound. The availability of oxygen in the tissues is essential for wound healing, and any reduction in that level due to infection or any other factor will also impair the healing process.

Oedema

Marked postoperative oedema may also lead to deformation of the tissues, which may distort wound apposition and affect the healing process. Weight-bearing sites or joints can produce greater wound tension and this extra stress may lead to wound dehiscence.

Drains

The use of drains in small surgical wounds is often undesirable, as they may act as routes for infection and there should be sufficient drainage through the apposed wound. Loss of apposition by the use of drains leads to healing by secondary intention, increasing healing time and leading to an irregular and pronounced scar. The wound may heal but produce a hypertrophic scar which is elevated, and it may itch and appear red. It is commonly very sensitive to touch and pressure. The scar can be treated with antihistamine creams or infiltrated with hydrocortisone or by ultrasonic therapy. If the scar fails to resolve, its excision should be considered, although early excision carries a high incidence of recurrence.

Keloid

Another type of hypertrophic scar is a keloid, in which the hypertrophy extends beyond the wound margins into the surrounding normal skin. There is a higher incidence of keloid formation in children, adolescents and the Afro-Caribbean population. This hypertrophy can lead to recurrent ulceration, corn and callus formation, and thus higher levels of discomfort. If the scar becomes fixed to the underlying tissues, such as deep fascia or tendon, this may restrict mobility and negate the purpose of the operation.

Any displacement of the underlying superficial fascia can lead to irregular continuity of the tissues. Should the superficial fascia become involved with the wound closure, this can retard healing and lead to the development of a cyst or fibroma.

Epidermoid cyst

If a portion of the epidermis becomes inverted and becomes buried with the subcutaneous tissues during closure, this may lead to the development of an epidermoid cyst. This normally appears as a circumscribed fluctuant swelling lying on or close to the scar. It will cause little discomfort unless over an area subject to stress, but it is often cosmetically unacceptable. It can be excised and the wound closed.

Fibroma

The development of a fibroma may result from the introduction of starch from the practitioner's gloves into the wound, which will act as an irritant, producing a foreign body reaction. After wound closure the irritant will be trapped in the tissues and gradually become established. It appears as a fairly rigid swelling which has symptoms similar to the epidermoid cyst and would be treated accordingly.

Neurological complications

Neuropraxia, causalgia and hyperaesthesia

Neuropraxia, or transient sensory loss, can be the result of compression of the sensory nerves by the tourniquet, or trauma due to poor tissue handling. There is no actual damage to the nerve and the recovery of the tissue can take place over a period from a few hours to about 7 days. More serious nerve damage could result in a considerably longer period of recovery and may produce causalgia. This is most commonly seen in the lower limb, involving the tibial nerve. It may produce a burning or itching sensation, which can give great discomfort or long-standing acute disabling pain. Hyperaesthesia of the sensory nerves is another possible sequel, and in this, the patient cannot tolerate any contact with the area involved. The discomfort can be particularly severe at night and there appears to be some link with impaired vasomotor tone, anaemia and B_{12} deficiency.

Pressure neuritis and nerve entrapment

Pressure neuritis, due to contraction of deep fascia, can produce paraesthesia in the area. This may also be associated with the amount of postoperative oedema present, and only after a 5–14 day postoperative period is this identifiable. If the fascia or retinaculae become thickened, this can produce a nerve entrapment. Any lesion can compress the nerve to cause entrapment, producing motor and sensory impairment and leading to paralysis and tingling or itching. Ultimately, trophic changes will occur in the skin. The position and distribution of the symptoms will indicate the nerve involved, and palpation at the site of the entrapment will produce pain both proximal and distal to the site (*Valleix phenomenon*).

In a small number of cases, there may be residual chronic intractable pain due to nerve damage. The use of corticosteroid injections, with or without local anaesthetic, can help to alleviate the symptoms. If medication fails to alleviate the problem, exploratory surgery may be necessary to identify the cause of the condition.

Again, in a small number of cases, a sensory nerve may be severed, giving a permanent sensory loss. This *neurotmesis* may cause the patient concern and it is important that the practitioner is supportive and clearly explains this outcome.

Vasomotor disturbance can lead to trophic changes, producing great pain and tenderness. This affects bone and soft tissues, presenting symptoms of swelling, discolouration, hyperhidrosis and temperature change and hyperaesthesia. Should these symptoms present, early treatment is essential, as the longer the condition exists, the less good the prognosis.

Vascular complications

The history-taking and examination of the patient (Ch. 3) should have established any conditions present which may impair the vascular response. However, any surgery carries the risk of some local or systematic reaction which can compromise or impair the success of the procedure. The causes may be pre-existing systemic disease, the surgery, or the postoperative care. Any abnormality in clotting time can affect the postoperative management, and the excessive use of ice packs can produce vasodilation, complicating postoperative care.

Ill-considered placement of a tourniquet can also lead to vascular complications by compressing the vessels against underlying bone, leading to inflammation and damage. This can lead to phlebitis and thrombophlebitis, which can also occur as a result of venous stasis induced during surgery. The patient will then have the added risk of possible pulmonary embolism. Local thrombosis formation is another sequel which may be caused by poor tissue handling; here the area will be cold, pale and tender. This is often a precursor

to gangrene, when there is limited collateral circulation, but the involved vessels may recanalise.

Excessive tourniquet time can lead to an increase in clotting time, and the metabolites which are normally controlled by the body's buffering systems alter the pH of these tissues, giving tissue acidosis. The ischaemia also leads to tissue destruction and muscle fatigue, which increase healing time and may lead to the formation of splinter haemorrhages appearing in the affected area. The tissues with the highest metabolic rates are the first to become damaged. Nerve tissue will progressively lose its conductive ability and muscle will gradually swell, increasing the tension in the area. Skin and superficial tissues can survive 6–8 hours before irreparable damage occurs.

Atrophy complications

Immobilisation of the foot may lead to atrophy of the tissues which can affect the postoperative recovery of the patient. Part of the foot can be compressed within a cast, thereby restricting tissue nutrition. In the early stages of wound healing, compression may lead to ischaemia of part of the wound and surrounding tissues, leading to ulceration of the overlying skin and underlying tissues. If untreated, this ulceration may progress to involve bone, leading to osteomyelitis.

This immobilisation of any part of the limb will affect muscle bulk and strength due to lack of muscular activity, and, over several weeks, may produce fibrotic changes leading to increased healing time and osteoporosis, which may extend the period of external support, thereby creating a spiral of events. The muscle atrophy will restrict ambulation and in the elderly patient may be a permanent feature. It is therefore important to establish a programme of physical therapy to exercise the musculature to avoid any loss of motion. This will also stimulate blood supply to the area, which will encourage healing and muscle strength, which in turn will promote healing of the bone. If the area is immobilised, a gradual disuse atrophy can ensue, producing osteoporosis, retarding the callus development and delaying fusion. Normally in younger patients, the removal of the cast and subsequent ambulation will lead to the rehabilitation of the muscle. However, in some patients a generalised osteoporosis in the foot can lead to stress fractures after the cast is removed, which will interfere with mobilisation of the patient.

These changes are often most evident around the calcaneum where scarring may be evident, with a marked reduction in the quantity of superficial fascia and in the quality of the tissues in general.

REFERENCES

Anderson R, Romfh R 1980 Techniques in the use of surgical tools. Appleton Century Crofts, New York, ch 1, p 1–11

Borges A F 1984 Relaxed skin tension lines (RSTL) versus other skin lines. Plast. Reconstruct. Surg. 73: 114–150

Brown J 1986 Minor surgery. Chapman and Hall, London, ch 9, p 48–51

Butterworth R, Dockery G L 1992 Forefoot surgery. Wolfe Publishing, London, p 242

Hymes L 1977 Forefoot minimum incision surgery in podiatric medicine. Futura Publishing, New York, p 32–38

Keats A S 1978 American Society of Anesthesiology, Classification of physical status – a recapitulation. Anestheseliogy 49: 233

Lawton J, Carrel, Sokoloff T 1992 Complications in foot and ankle surgery. Williams & Wilkins, Baltimore, ch 14, p 363

Scarlet J H, Walter J H Jr, Bachmann R J 1978 Digital blood perfusion following injections of plain lidocaine and lidocaine with epinephrine, a comparison. Journal of the American Podiatric Association 68(5)

Spence A 1990 Chairman, Commission on the provision of surgical services, pain after surgery, working party report. p 5, Table 1

Yu G, Cavaliere R 1983 Suture materials. Journal of American Podiatry Association 73(2): 57–64

Zederfeldt B, Jacobson S, Ahonon J 1986 Wounds and wound healing. Wolfe Medical Press, London, p 12–13

FURTHER READING

Epstein E, Epstein E Jr 1979 Techniques in skin surgery. Lea & Febiger, Philadelphia

Gerbert J, Sokoloff T 1981 Textbook of bunion surgery. Futura Publishing, New York

Hara B, Locke R, Lowe W 1976 Complications in foot surgery. Williams & Wilkins, Baltimore

Irvin T 1981 Wound healing. Principles & practice. Chapman and Hall, London

McGlamry E 1987 Fundamentals of foot surgery. Williams & Wilkins, Baltimore

Mercado O A 1979 An atlas of foot surgery, vol 1. Carolando Press, Baltimore

Passmore R, Robson J 1976 Companion to medical studies, vol 1, 2nd edn. Oxford University Press, Oxford

Saleh M, Sodera V 1988 Illustrated handbook of minor surgery and operative technique. Heinmann Medical

Smith C, Aitkenhead 1985 Textbook of anaesthesia. Churchill Livingstone, Edinburgh

Surgical wound infection rates by wound class, operative procedure and patient risk index. American Journal of Medicine 91 (suppl. 3B): 152–158

Weinstein F Principles and practice of podiatry. Lea & Febiger

Wood Jones F 1948 The structure and function as seen in the foot. Ballière Tindall & Cox, London

Yale J F 1987 Podiatric medicine, 3rd edn. Williams & Wilkins, Baltimore

19

Nail surgery

A. S. Banks
E. D. McGlamry
D. L. Lorimer

Keywords

Frost's root resection
Partial nail avulsion
Phenolisation
Subungual exostosis
Total nail avulsion
Winograd's operation
Zadik's operation

Nail surgery performed by podiatrists has been developed to a high level of sophistication using phenolisation techniques, and with the very low regrowth rates—at 1.3% (Cooper 1965), 1.5% (Gallocher 1977), 2.3% (Livingston 1990) and 4.5% (Ashcroft et al 1979)—obtained as a result, this method of treatment now dominates the radical treatment of painful nail conditions. If the conservative treatment of onychocryptosis or severe involution fails to provide long-term relief, or if it is considered inappropriate in cases of long term maintenance of onychauxis or onychogryphosis, then recourse to nail surgery is likely to achieve that objective. In cases of onychocryptosis or involution, two procedures are available: total or partial removal of the nail plate with destruction of the matrix. In cases of onychauxis or onychogryphosis, the only procedure usually possible is total avulsion with destruction of the matrix.

In the case of onychomycosis, it is possible to consider total avulsion with or without destruction of the matrix. The decision depends on the ability of nail to regrow. The administration of systemic or topical antifungal agents is indicated when the matrix is not destroyed and nail regrowth is considered possible (Ch. 8). In such cases, it is possible to consider the use of a 40% urea cream applied topically and held in place by an occlusive dressing (Port & Sanicola 1980). Although the phenolisation of the matrix has become dominant, the cold steel techniques are also described, and these are also being used in conditions where it is not desirable to retard the rate of healing of the tissues with the use of phenol.

AVULSION

Partial nail avulsion

The foot must be prepared using the measures described in Chapter 18, to minimise the risk of infection, and a local analgesic administered (see Digital nerve block, Ch. 17) to operate without causing pain. To allow the procedure to be carried out in a bloodless field, an Esmarch bandage should be applied to the digit.

The Esmarch bandage is applied from distal to proximal so that the toe is gradually exsanguinated. Once the bandage is applied, it should be secured at the base of the digit in as broad a form as possible to ensure that the underlying structures are not injured. The toe should be swabbed again and the foot draped.

The instruments chosen for this procedure should include MacDonald dissectors in two sizes, small, medium and large artery forceps, Thwaite's nippers, a range of instruments for dressings and, if required, nail chisels. Using a fine dissector, the nail plate is freed from the sulcus and the eponychium (Fig. 19.1A). Any debris should be removed at this stage. The object of a partial avulsion is to remove a section of nail sufficiently large to leave the remaining surface of the nail plate flat. This is done by using the Thwaite's nippers to make a clean straight cut along the nail plate to the level of the eponychium.

At this stage opinions vary, with some operators easing the Thwaite's nippers below the eponychium and completing the separation to the level of the matrix (Fig. 19.1B). Alternatively, the cut can be completed using a nail chisel. Either method is acceptable but it should be remembered that when using a chisel, the instrument should be held steady to avoid damage to the surrounding soft tissues, and the movement continued in the same direction as the first part of the cut.

The cut section of nail is then removed using a suitably sized pair of artery forceps locked onto it (Fig. 19.1C). The section is then rotated so that the lateral margin rolls upwards and inwards. Part of the nail matrix may become detached with removal of the section of nail, but the nail should be examined to check for the *frond* effect at the base. Presence of the frond indicates the satisfactory separation of the nail from the matrix.

The sulcus must be cleared of all debris and hyperplasic tissue (Fig. 19.1D). At this stage, as at all other

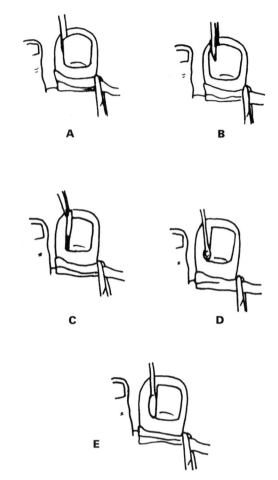

Figure 19.1 A: Separation of the nail plate from the nail bed using a MacDonald dissector. B: Cutting a section of the nail using Thwaite's nippers. C: Removal of the section of nail using artery forceps. D: Removal of debris and hyperplastic tissue with a Volkmann spoon. E: Phenolisation using a cotton wool bud.

stages, the area should be thoroughly cleansed and dried. It is now necessary to destroy the area of matrix from which the section has been taken. Several methods may be used: chemical (phenolisation, trichloroacetic acid, sodium hydroxide) or using specialised apparatus (cryotherapy, electrosurgery or galvanism).

Phenolisation

This is the method most commonly used and is acknowledged to have the highest success rate (Morkane et al 1984). Liquefied phenol BP is applied to the area to be treated and worked thoroughly using a metal instrument or a fine sterile cotton wool bud. The phenol should be applied for a minimum of 2 minutes, but often 3 minutes may be needed. Care should be taken to limit the application of the phenol only to the area to be destroyed, and the field of application should be dry. If cotton wool buds are used, they should be changed every 30 seconds (Fig. 19.1E).

Alternatively, the phenol can be applied for up to 2 minutes, the area dried out with a fine sterile cotton wool bud and the process repeated for the same length of time. Whichever method is used, the most important factor is to apply the phenol so that it is well worked in to the tissue to be destroyed. It is also important to check before using the phenol that it has not become contaminated or had its effectiveness impaired in any way, and to this end its condition should be strictly monitored. Some practitioners use phenol in crystalline form as a method of avoiding the risk of its contamination. After this application, the area should be irrigated with alcohol to wash out the phenol and terminate its action. The area should then be dried.

Finally, the Esmarch bandage is removed and the digit observed for the return of arterial blood. This is usually rapid but its return must be observed and recorded. The entire area should be covered with a sterile dressing, which may include a broad-spectrum antiseptic. After treatment, a short waiting time, usually 15 minutes, before returning home is useful in case bleeding is excessive.

Trichloroacetic acid

This may be used in the same way as liquefied phenol BP, but the time of application usually needs to be extended slightly (by about 1 minute).

Sodium hydroxide

This may be used as a 10% solution instead of liquefied phenol; its effect is more rapid. It is usually applied until the tissue blanches thoroughly. The area is then dried with a sterile cotton wool bud and carefully washed out with 5% acetic acid to neutralise the sodium hydroxide (Greenwald & Robbins 1981). Normally, one application in the manner described for liquefied phenol will be found adequate, provided that it is applied to a completely dry field. Appropriate sterile dressings should be used with follow-up care as described previously.

Total nail avulsion

The foot should be prepared in the manner described previously. The nail sulci and eponychium are freed carefully from the nail plate and all debris removed. An elevator is then inserted under the free edge of the nail and the plate separated. When this stage has been reached, locking forceps are attached to the edge of the nail so that the lateral margin of the nail rolls upwards and inwards. The procedure is then repeated on the other border and the nail is eased away from any remaining attachments. Finally, all epidermal materials should be removed and the area thoroughly cleansed using sterile cotton wool buds.

The matrix should be destroyed by one of the methods described for partial nail avulsion, but since the area to be treated is larger, it may be necessary to extend the time of application a little to ensure complete destruction. It is also essential to ensure that the agent being used is introduced to all areas of the matrix.

Postoperative care

Following nail surgery, it is essential to give the patient clear and concise advice concerning any immediate postoperative problem which might arise. It is prudent to give the patient an advice sheet similar to that based on the principles described in Chapter 6.

The return date will vary depending on the particular circumstances of each case but should be within 3–7 days following the procedure. At this visit the original dressing should be removed, the condition reviewed and another dressing applied. Strict antiseptic precautions should be observed using sterile dressings and a 'no-touch' technique employed.

After removal of the original dressing the area should be irrigated and swabbed with a sterile solution which may or may not contain an antiseptic agent. The area should be clean and show some granulation tissue; there may be some serous exudate. Any pain which may still be experienced by the patient may be a result of the trauma to the area, but it usually disappears after the first redressing. On rare occasions the patient may experience *phenol flare*, an acute inflammatory response to the application of phenol. It is a rare phenomenon, and largely unexplained, which usually settles after 4 or 5 days and will call for extra reassurance and support for the patient from the podiatrist. It responds well to the foot being immersed twice daily in a warm hypertonic footbath (40°C) of magnesium sulphate. It should be remembered that the use of phenol is not without risks and it can slow down the rate of healing, making it essential that the patient has easy access to support from the podiatrist (Greene 1964).

If the area appears healthy and free from infection, a sterile dressing with or without an antiseptic agent should be applied and held in place with tubular gauze dressing. It is advisable to give explicit instructions regarding the avoidance of trauma and keeping the area dry in the early stages. These procedures should be carried out weekly until healing is complete. At this stage, further advice on prophylactic care should be given, to underline that given at the time the procedure was decided upon. Later, provided progress to resolution is uneventful, the patient can assume responsibility for bathing and redressing the area, always assuming the patient's compliance (see Ch. 6).

ALTERNATIVE TECHNIQUES

There are several alternative incisional methods which are now increasingly employed to give long-term relief to persistent onychocryptosis and involution.

Winograd's operation

This procedure is carried out by means of a double incision (Winograd 1929). The first begins at the distal edge of the nail plate on the affected side and extends longitudinally down to bone under the eponychium and through the matrix. The second incision starts in the same place and is carried in a slight curve through the paronychia soft tissue to meet the proximal end of the first. The entire elliptical wedge of nail plate, matrix and granulation tissue present is then underscored and removed down to bone in one piece. The sides of the incision are brought together and then sutured (Fig. 19.2).

Frost's root resection

In this procedure an L-shaped incision is made from the distal tip of the nail plate into the eponychium on the dorsum and then laterally (Fig. 19.3). The flap of tissue is reflected, the entire section of nail plate, bed and matrix is excised in one piece, and the flap is replaced. Sutures are not normally required but may sometimes be indicated.

Zadik's operation

The nail plate (or a section of nail plate if only one side requires treatment) is removed, a longitudinal incision is made on each side of the base of the nail and the resulting flap of eponychium is turned back. The nail matrix is then excised and the flap realigned and then sutured (Fig. 19.4).

It cannot be stressed too strongly that skilled aftercare is as essential a part of nail surgery as the operation itself. Unskilled treatment and lack of competent postoperative supervision could well give rise to questions as to the efficacy of nail surgery, but when properly performed, adequately followed up and when careful attention is paid to the elimination of the

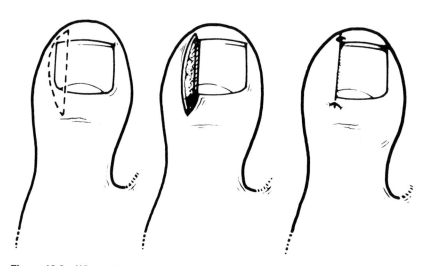

Figure 19.2 Winograd partial matrixectomy procedure for relief of ingrown toenail. (From McGlamry 1987, with permission.)

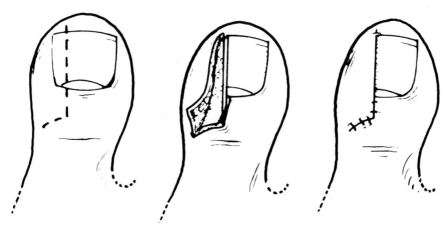

Figure 19.3   Frost's partial matrixectomy procedure for relief of ingrown toenail. (From McGlamry 1987, with permission.)

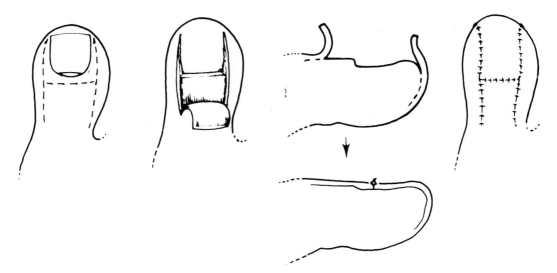

Figure 19.4   Zadik's total matrixectomy procedure. (From McGlamry 1987, with permission.)

causative factors, the surgical techniques outlined certainly give excellent results and favourable prognoses.

SUBUNGUAL EXOSTOSIS

A subungual exostosis is a small outgrowth of bone under the nail plate or near its free edge (Fig. 19.5). Most frequently, it occurs on the hallux as a result of trauma and is a source of considerable pain. As the outgrowth increases, the toenail adheres closely to it and undergoes some displacement from the nail bed

(see Ch. 8). The epidermis covering the exostosis becomes stretched and thinned and takes on a bright red colour. This will blanch on the application of pressure. The protuberance offers a hard resistance to pressure and there is usually a clear line of demarcation around the area. This, combined with the bright colour, readily distinguishes the exostosis from a subungual heloma. When the exostosis occurs distal to the nail plate, the bright red gives way to a yellowish grey colour. Accurate diagnosis of this condition requires X-ray examination (see Ch. 4).

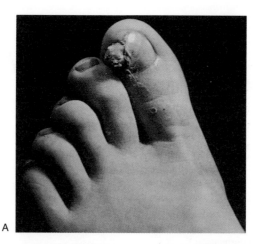

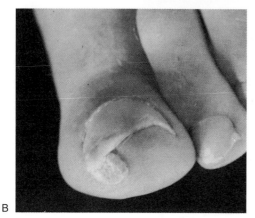

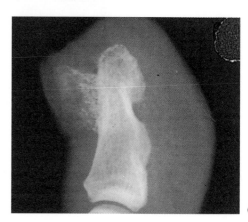

Figure 19.5 A, B: Subungual exostoses. C: X-ray shows elevation of nail plate by exostosis.

Aetiology

It may occur from a single sudden trauma such as stubbing, although this is rare, or may be due to a repeated trauma such as continual, though perhaps slight, trauma from shoes which are either too short or excessively high-heeled.

Pathology

Following injury to the periosteum of the distal phalanx, periostitis occurs. Initially, there is an outgrowth of cartilage which later ossifies.

Treatment

Temporary relief may be given by means of protective padding and supervision of footwear, but surgical excision is always the most satisfactory treatment. After the nail plate has been avulsed, a horizontal linear incision is made around the medial and lateral aspect of the phalanx. The nail bed is then carefully elevated and reflected. The exostosis can now be resected. The area is then smoothed flush with the phalanx and the nail bed is replaced and sutured.

REFERENCES

Ashcroft D J, Lavis G J, Russell L H 1979 Retrospective analysis of partial nail avulsion. Chiropodist 4: 100–109

Cooper C T 1965 Phenol-alcohol nail procedure: postoperative care, a comparative study. Journal of the American Podiatry Association 55: 661–663

Gallocher J 1977 The phenol alcohol method of nail matrix sterilisation. New Zealand Medical Journal 86: 140–141

Greene A A 1964 The application of the phenol-alcohol technique for toenail correction. Current Podiatry 13: 20–23

Greenwald L, Robbins H M 1981 The chemical matricectomy. Journal of the American Podiatry Association 71: 388–389

Livingston L 1990 An evaluation of nail surgery carried out in the chiropody department, Darlington Health Authority between 1979 and 1987. BSc Honours project, Sunderland Polytechnic

McGlamry E D (ed) 1987 Comprehensive textbook of foot surgery. Williams & Wilkins, Baltimore

Morkane A J, Robertson R W, Inglis G S 1984 Segmental phenolisation of ingrowing toenails: a randomized controlled study. British Journal of Surgery 71: 526–527

Port M, Sanicola K F 1980 Nonsurgical removal of dystrophic nails utilizing urea ointment occlusion. Journal of the American Podiatry Association 70: 521–523

Winograd A M 1929 A modification in the technic of operation for ingrown toe-nail. JAMA, January: 19

20

Digital surgery

A. S. Banks
E. D. McGlamry

Keywords

Arthrodesis
Arthroplasty
Extensor hood resection
Extensor substitution
Extensor tendon lengthening
Fifth digit
Flexor stabilisation
Flexor substitution
Heloma molle
Metatarsophalangeal joint capsulotomy
Neuroma
Plantar capsule release
Sequential approach to digital surgery
Surgical correction
Tenotomy

Digital deformities provide a source of complaint for many patients. Fortunately, most of these can be corrected surgically. Selection of the appropriate procedure rests upon an understanding of the type of deformity and its aetiology (Jimenez et al 1987).

APPLIED ANATOMY

Normal digital function and stability are achieved by smooth coordinated muscle function. The primary muscles involved in maintaining digital stability are the dorsal and plantar interossei and the lumbricales. They act to stabilise the proximal phalanges firmly against the metatarsal heads, thereby ensuring a rectus digital alignment and firm contact of the digital phalanges with the supporting surface. With this function effectively executed, the subsequent contraction of the leg muscles will not alter the rectus digital alignment. If a stable proximal phalanx is not present upon contraction of the more powerful longus muscles then the toe will buckle. Such functional imbalance will lead to the development of hammer toe deformity (Jarret et al 1980).

Flexor stabilisation

In the normal foot, sufficient stability exists within the osseous structures to adequately support the body. However, when the foot pronates excessively much of this normal intrinsic stability is lost (Fig. 20.1). In such instances other structures will be required to render the necessary support for adequate function. Most often, the flexor digitorum longus, tibialis posterior and flexor hallucis longus muscles will need to begin function earlier, and maintain contraction longer than is normal.

This results in the flexor digitorum longus contracting before the intrinsic muscles have been able to stabilise the proximal changes. The digits buckle, the proximal phalanges are dorsiflexed and hammer toe deformities are thus initiated (Jarret et al 1980). When such instability is present in gait, the lesser digits will be seen to grasp the weight-bearing surface during midstance and the propulsion phase.

Extensor substitution

As previously discussed, the lumbricales function in concert with the interosseous muscles to stabilise the proximal phalanges of the lesser digits during the stance phase of gait (Fig. 20.2). However, the lumbri-

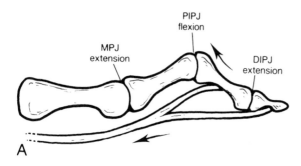

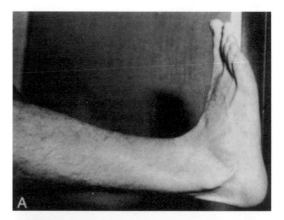

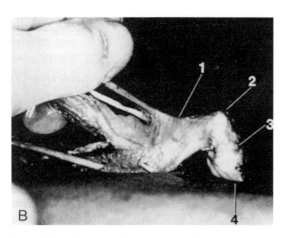

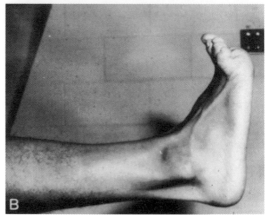

Figure 20.1 Flexor stabilisation. In weight-bearing, the phalanges cannot be plantarflexed through the ground. In such instances, plantarflexory force is retrograded proximally, creating dorsiflexion at the metatarsophalangeal joint (MPJ). A: When flexor digitorum brevis is the primary force, the proximal interphalangeal joint (PIPJ) is plantarflexed. B: When flexor digitorum longus is the primary plantarflexory force, the distal (DIPJ) and proximal interphalangeal joints are both plantarflexed.
1, MPJ extension; 2, PIP flexion; 3, DIP flexion; 4, ground reactive force. (From McGlamry 1987, with permission.)

Figure 20.2 Extensor substitution. A: Clinical demonstration of normal digital extension with foot dorsiflexed. B: Extensor substitution with excessive dorsiflexion of digits. Notice that the retrograde force of the toes is transmitted to the metatarsal head, accentuating plantar protrusion of the metatarsals. (From McGlamry 1987, with permission.)

cales have a dual action. These muscles are also active during the swing phase of gait against the metatarsal head. When subsequent contraction of the extensor digitorum longus occurs, the digit is maintained in a rectus alignment. In such proper circumstances, the extensor digitorum longus will exert most of its power in assisting dorsiflexion of the ankle joint during the swing phase of gait.

However, if the extensor digitorum longus has to contract prior to the lumbricales, or if the intrinsic muscle function is impaired, the lesser digits will be seen to assume a hyperextended position during the swing phase of gait. This is referred to as extensor substitution and it results in retraction of the toes. It should be noted that toe purchase of the ground is delayed (Jimenez et al 1987).

Some of the causes of extensor substitution are neuromuscular diseases, other forms of weakness of the tibialis anterior and ankle joint equinus. In certain neuromuscular diseases (i.e. Charcot–Marie–Tooth), intrinsic muscle function is lost and allows the long extensors to pull the digits into a dorsiflexed position. Any condition which leads to the weakness of the tibialis anterior will result in prolonged contraction of the long extensor muscles—a true extensor substitution (Green et al 1976). Patients with limited dorsiflexory motion at the ankle will also over-exert

the long extensors in an attempt to achieve more dorsiflexion.

This type of digital contraction may also be noted in the cavus foot which is not afflicted with neuromuscular disease (Whitney & Green 1982; Fig. 20.3). When the cavus foot assumes a plantarflexed position at rest, increased tension is placed upon the long extensor tendons. This tension is, in turn, transmitted to the extensor hood apparatus surrounding the metatarsophalangeal joint, pulling the digit into a more dorsiflexed position. Eventually, adaptive contracture occurs dorsally at the metatarsophalangeal joint and is followed by a loss of efficient intrinsic muscle function. The flexor digitorum resists this dorsal pull and thus contributes to the buckling of the digits at the interphalangeal joints and hence the clawing of the toes.

Flexor substitution

Flexor substitution is the least common cause of hammer toe deformity (Jimenez et al 1987). It is seen where there is extensive weakness of the triceps surae, and the remainder of the posterior leg muscles must supply the force necessary for propulsion. The flexor digitorum longus is included in this overactivity, which will result in rather abrupt accentuation of the hammer toe as the

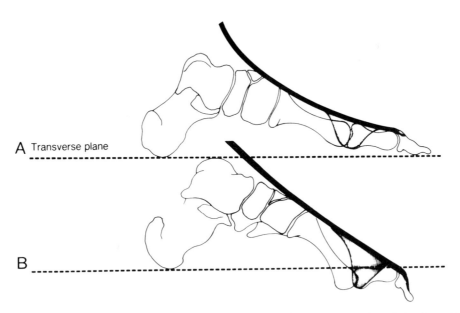

A Transverse plane

B

Figure 20.3 A: Relationship of extensor tendons and hood apparatus in normal foot. B: In a foot with anterior cavus deformity, the forefoot at rest drops into plantarflexed attitude. This places tendons under increased tension, resulting in buckling of the toes at the metatarsophalangeal joints. (From McGlamry 1987, with permission.)

patient propels forward. A marked supinatory twist of the foot may be seen to occur concomitantly.

SURGICAL CORRECTION

Surgery should be aimed at relieving the immediate symptoms of the patient, as well as providing a long-lasting correction of deformity. Procedures may consist of soft tissue releases and/or osseous approaches. In general, soft tissue procedures alone fail to maintain adequate correction of deformity over the long term (Jimenez et al 1987). However, several of these techniques when combined with osseous procedures may produce a successful outcome. Ultimately, the choice depends upon the severity of deformity, which digits are affected, the ambulatory status of the patient and the aetiology of the contracture.

The first concern with osseous surgery is to determine which procedure is indicated: arthroplasty or arthrodesis. Arthrodesis is rarely performed upon the fifth digit, as it creates a very rigid toe which is not readily accommodated by shoes. In more severe contractures, arthrodesis may be preferred, as the correction tends to be better maintained. Patients suffering from extensor substitution generally require arthrodesing techniques, as the function of the lumbricales may be irretrievably lost (especially in the presence of neuro-muscular diseases). Mild or moderate hammer toe deformities due to flexor stabilisation may benefit from either type of surgery and have equally good results. However, if an arthroplasty is performed then the excessive pronation must be adequately controlled postoperatively to reduce the risk of the return of the hammer toe deformity (Jimenez et al 1987).

Arthroplasty (Fig. 20.4; also Plate 1)

A 2.5–3 cm longitudinal skin incision is made over the dorsal aspect of the digit, taking care to avoid completely penetrating through the skin. With medial and lateral tension being applied to the margins of the incision, dissection is deepened to the level of the superficial fascia. This layer may be distinguished as the skin margins are retracted and the vascular structures become visible. The superficial fascia is then incised parallel to the skin incision and vessels are identified and coagulated. Once the extensor tendon can be seen, the deep fascia has been reached (Post 1982, Jimenez et al 1987).

By using a brushing stroke with the scalpel, the superficial fascia is separated from the underlying deep fascia, extensor hood and the joint apparatus. All major vessels will be contained within the superficial fascia and it is possible to proceed with the proposed procedure without fear of inflicting neurovascular compromise.

The digit is now flexed and medial and lateral vertical incisions are made at the joint level to sever the collateral ligaments. A transverse incision is then completed to transect the extensor tendon at the level of the proximal interphalangeal joint. The joint surfaces should be readily apparent upon flexion of the toe. Further dissection is usually required to sever the collateral ligaments totally and to free the head of the proximal phalanx. The same medial and lateral vertical incisions are repeated at the joint level, this time with the blade entering the joint itself. If ligamentous attachment is still present then the blade is introduced into the joint from within and advanced medially and laterally around each of the condyles of the phalangeal head. The head of the proximal phalanx should be totally freed at this point.

A power instrument or bone-cutting forceps may then be used to remove the head of the proximal phalanx. The remaining bony stump should be rasped smooth to discourage future irritation. The extensor tendon is then reapproximated using a 3–0 or 4–0 absorbable suture. The subcutaneous tissue is closed using a 4–0 or a 5–0 absorbable suture. The skin may be closed.

Postoperative care

The toe is typically maintained in some type of a surgical dressing for at least 10–14 days. Non-absorbable sutures may be removed at this point. Afterwards, dressings may be removed and bathing allowed, although the toe may require further dressings or some type of splintage to maintain alignment and discourage tenderness or excessive swelling.

During the initial postoperative period, a surgical shoe is probably best suited for walking. Once dressings have been removed, the patient may still prefer to use the surgical shoe, as it is common for the digits to remain tender if placed in a closed shoe at this point. After several weeks the patient will probably tolerate a tennis shoe or a depth Oxford. Ladies may have difficulty wearing a dress shoe comfortably for several months following surgery, as it is not unusual for some induration to remain within the toe until most of the scar tissue has remodelled.

Arthrodesis

The dissection sequence for arthrodesis of the proximal interphalangeal joint is the same as that for an

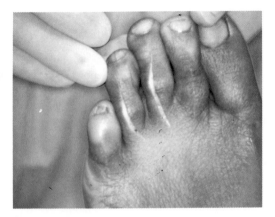

A

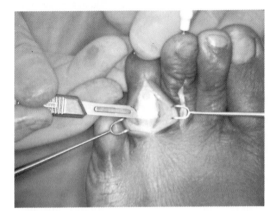

B

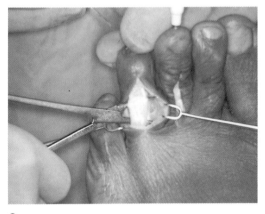

C

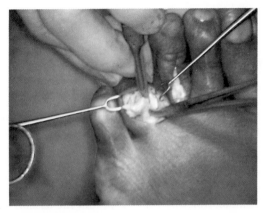

D

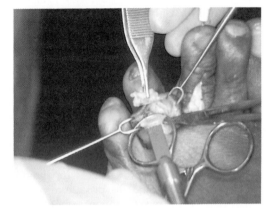

E

Figure 20.4   Arthroplasty. A: Midline dorsal longitudinal skin incision affords excellent exposure of the toe while avoiding neurovascular structures. (From McGlamry 1987, with permission.) B, C, D: An alternative technique to transecting the tendon is demonstrated, with undermining and retraction. Collateral ligaments are then cut to deliver the phalangeal head. E: Bone is resected with either a power saw or bone forceps.

arthroplasty. Surgery takes on a different approach once the head of the proximal phalanx is freed.

End-to-end arthrodesis (Fig. 20.5)

The cartilaginous surfaces of the proximal phalangeal head and the base of the middle phalanx are removed. This may be performed by either power or hand instruments. However, hand instruments tend to provide a better 'raw' bone surface, which is thought to encourage earlier osseous fusion. If powered instruments are used then further dissection may be required to free the attachments of the extensor tendon from the dorsal aspect of the base of the middle phalanx to allow access for the saw (Soule 1910).

A 0.045 inch Kirschner wire (K-wire) is then introduced into the central position of the proximal phalanx to identify the medullary canal. This will allow for smooth passage of the wire later in the procedure. The K-wire is then loaded into the wire driver. The distal aspect of the toe is then grasped medially and laterally with two fingers, with a third finger being placed plantarly to effect hyperextension of the distal interphalangeal joint. The K-wire is then introduced into the base of the middle phalanx centrally, and advanced distally through the tip of the toe. If the position is not satisfactory then the wire should be completely withdrawn and the procedure repeated. One may find that the second attempt is more difficult,

as the wire tends to follow the path of the canal created initially by the wire. Increasing the speed of the wire driver may help to overcome this problem.

Once a suitable position is attained, the K-wire is guided distally until only a small portion is visible at the base of the proximal phalanx. At this point an assistant will stabilise the proximal phalanx with a forceps while the operator drives the wire from distal to proximal into the previously opened medullary canal of the proximal phalanx. If the wire is driven slowly, one may feel the faint resistance of the subchondral bone plate at the base of the proximal phalanx and stop the wire driver. Another uncut wire lined up with the tip of this wire may be used to gauge depth position to ensure that one has not crossed into the metatarsophalangeal joint. Next, the arthrodesis site is examined to ensure that adequate apposition has been attained. The wound is then closed in the standard manner.

Peg-in-hole arthrodesis (Fig. 20.6; also Plate 2)

Once the head of the proximal phalanx has been exposed, the medial, lateral and plantar condyles of the head are resected. The remaining cartilaginous distal cap is also resected, taking care to preserve the integrity of the dorsal cortex. The 'peg' is smoothed with a burr on its corners and a hole is fashioned in the base of the middle phalanx. One should start the drill

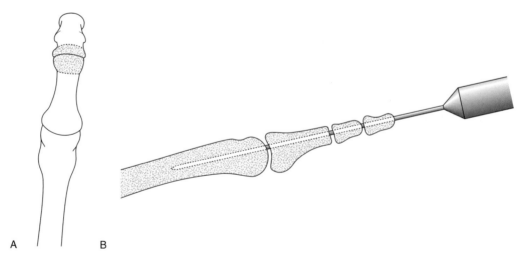

A B

Figure 20.5 Arthrodesis. A: Articular ends of apposing bones must be resected, exposing raw cancellous bone, to ensure rapid arthrodesis. B: Internal fixation with Kirschner wire eliminates motion at the joint and assists in early union. Where metatarsophalangeal joint release has been effected, the wire may be extended across the joint to maintain alignment during early healing.

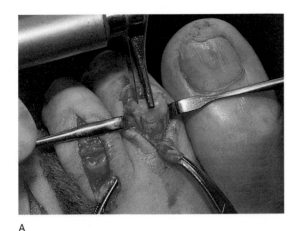

A

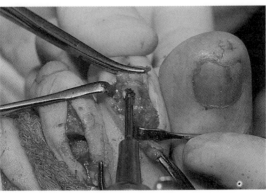

B

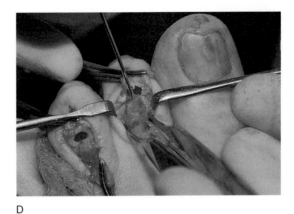

D

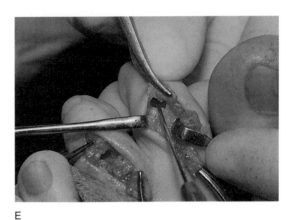

E

C

Figure 20.6   Peg-in-hole arthrodesis. A: The medial, lateral and plantar condyles are resected, as well as the distal articular cartilage. The dorsal cortex is carefully preserved. B: A ball burr is then used to contour the phalanx into a suitable peg. C: Starting with a very small ball burr or a side cutting burr, the initial hole is made in the base of the middle phalanx. Progressively larger ball burrs are used to ream the middle phalanx into a satisfactory receptacle. D: A hand-held Kirschner wire is used to identify the medullary canal of the proximal phalanx. Note the fully developed hole in the middle of the phalanx. E: The Kirschner wire is then introduced into the middle phalanx and directed distally through the tip of the toe. The surgeon holds the distal aspect of the toe rectus or in slight hyperextension. The wire driver is then moved to the end of the toes and the wire is retrograded across the arthrodesis site into the proximal phalanx. Fixation of the peg-in-hole arthrodesis is not mandatory, but enhances the overall stability.

hole with a fairly small drill and gradually increase its diameter using progressively larger burrs until the hole approximates the size of the proximal peg. A trial seating of the arthrodesis is performed, with a forceps being used to guide the proximal peg while the other hand firmly stabilises the middle phalanx (Young 1938).

Once seating has been accomplished, the forceps should be used to grasp the proximal phalanx at its juncture with the middle. With the forceps held in this position and the joint thence unseated, it will be possible to estimate how much of the peg was actually seated.

If the fit is secure then wire stabilisation is not necessarily required, although the security of such fixation is generally preferred. Where deemed appropriate, a 0.045 inch Kirschner wire may be used for stabilisation as previously described.

Follow-up care

As mentioned previously, K-wires are not essential for peg-in-hole arthrodeses, provided a good snug fit has been achieved. If wires are used, they should remain in place for 4–6 weeks before removal. For end-to-end arthrodeses, the wire should preferably remain in place for at least 6 weeks. Some type of external splintage of the digits (i.e. toe crests) may still be helpful for a few additional weeks. A closed shoe may be used once the wires have been retracted, although ladies may not be able to wear dress shoes comfortably for 1–2 months after this point (Jimenez et al 1987).

THE SEQUENTIAL APPROACH TO DIGITAL SURGERY (Fig. 20.7)

One quandary which may be encountered when repairing hammer toe deformities is how far to go before adequate correction is obtained and can be reasonably maintained. A sequential approach to digital surgery has been devised which provides the operator with a reliable means to assess intra-operatively the efficacy of the procedure. After each manoeuvre, if adequate correction has not been obtained then it is best to proceed in a logical fashion to the next step. The sequence is described below (Jimenez et al 1987).

Pre-operative evaluation

The first step is to evaluate the degree of deformity prior to surgery in order to ascertain which, if any,

osseous procedures are indicated. One may also sense the steps which may be required to release the contracture completely, by examining the digit while a loading force has been applied to the forefoot. Loading the forefoot stimulates the weight-bearing attitude and allows one to note the relationship of the proximal phalanx to the metatarsal. If the proximal phalanx returns to a rectus alignment, then more elaborate intervention may not be needed. However, if the phalanx remains dorsiflexed relative to the metatarsal, or if there is a transverse plane deviation, then several steps will most likely be required.

In performing an arthroplasty, the head of the proximal phalanx is initially removed. The amount of bone removed is that which is required to relieve soft tissue tension while maintaining the length of the toe in relation to its neighbouring digits. This will eliminate the osseous prominence and in a milder deformity may provide enough relaxation of the soft tissue structures to provide good correction.

If an arthrodesis is to be performed, then the head of the phalanx is free. Dorsiflexory pressure should once again be applied to the forefoot. If the proximal phalanx returns to a rectus alignment without resistance, then this may be all the release that is necessary. However, if resistance is met, then one needs to proceed to the next step.

Extensor hood resection

Although the extensor digitorum longus tendon has its terminal insertion at the distal phalanx of each digit, the tendon slips richly invest the metatarsophalangeal joint area by fibrous expansions, forming what is known as the extensor hood. The primary force of the extensor tendons at the digital level is applied not within the toe itself, but more proximally at the hood apparatus. After digital deformity has been present for a sufficient time, the extensor hood adapts and assists in maintaining the deformity. At times, these hood fibres will need to be released to allow adequate repositioning of the toe (Jimenez et al 1987).

To accomplish this, one lifts the extensor tendon distally and slightly dorsally to place tension on the hood fibres. The scalpel is then placed parallel to the tendon at its medial edge. The blade is rotated 90° and the medial expansions are severed. The same manoeuvre is performed laterally. The tendon should then be lifted free of its underlying attachments to the phalanx. The butt end of the scalpel handle should be able to pass beneath the tendon to the level of the metatarsal neck and beyond. If resistance is met then

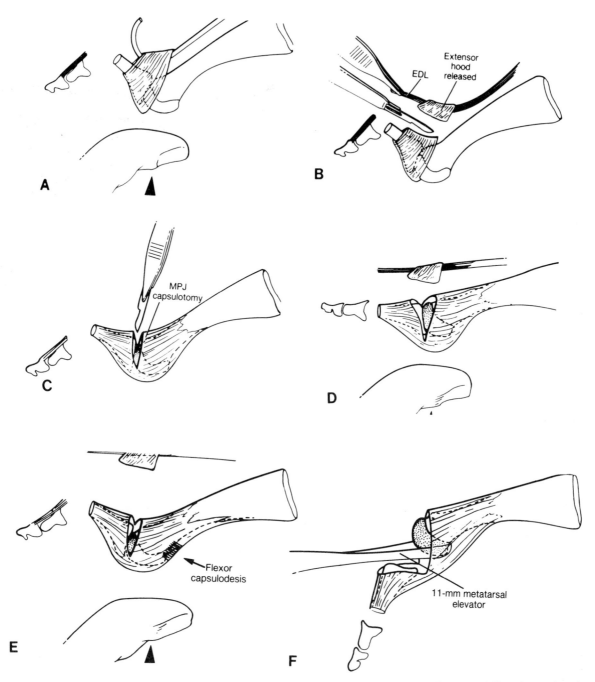

Figure 20.7   Sequential approach. A: Following phalangeal head resection, the push-up test is repeated. Note the continued dorsiflexed position of the proximal phalanx. The next sequential step is indicated. B: Extensor hood release is performed and the push-up test repeated. Unless the metatarsophalangeal joint realigns easily, the next step is performed. C: Capsulotomy of dorsal, medial and lateral aspects is effected. D: Push-up test shows realignment of the joint, indicating adequate correction of the digit. E: Failure to realign indicates capsulodesis of flexor apparatus to the metatarsal neck. F: The metatarsal elevator is used to release the flexor capsule from the metatarsal neck. (From McGlamry 1987, with permission.)

the above procedure is repeated. Once the hood has been thoroughly released, the push-up test is again effected.

Metatarsophalangeal joint capsulotomy

If the extensor hood resection failed to relieve the contracture adequately, then it becomes necessary to incise the dorsal, medial and lateral capsule of the metatarsophalangeal joint. Using a forceps to grasp the proximal phalanx, distal distraction is applied. This causes a dimple to form dorsally in the joint capsule. The blade is introduced dorsally at that point and and passed medially and laterally. Should contracture remain following the push-up test then further surgery will be necessary (from 16 mm film, *Approaches to Digital Surgery*, Podiatry Institute, Tucker, GA, 1973).

Plantar capsular release

With long-standing deformities, the flexor plate, which is normally supported beneath the central plantar aspect of the metatarsal head and neck, may be displaced medially or laterally or may be fibrosed to the metatarsal neck just proximal to the plantar cartilage. Such capsulodesis will prevent plantarflexion of the toe when the forefoot is loaded. If the flexor cap is displaced medially or laterally, it will draw the toe medially or laterally as the forefoot is loaded. Such displacement is almost always the cause of digits exhibiting medial or lateral deviation at the metatarsophalangeal joint. Plantar capsular release will be required in such instances and this is greatly facilitated by the use of the McGlamry metatarsal elevator. Having completed release of the flexor plate, the toe should easily return to a rectus position when the foot is loaded (from 16 mm film, *Approaches to Digital Surgery*, Podiatry Institute, Tucker, GA, 1973).

Extensor tendon lengthening

When a moderate to severe contracture is present, one should anticipate the need for an extensor tendon lengthening. This is performed just prior to and in conjunction with the extensor hood resection. A longitudinal incision is made along the medial or lateral margin of the tendon and a haemostat is introduced beneath the extensor tendon, and opened. The tendon is then incised longitudinally at its midpoint so that it is split into two equal parts. At the proximal aspect of the incision, the lateral one-half of the tendon is severed. This is then retracted distally and the more medial half of the tendon incised distally at the proximal interphalangeal

joint level (Jimenez et al 1987; Fig. 20.8). At closure, the tendon is repaired in an appropriately lengthened position.

Additional notes

If the metatarsophalangeal joint capsule requires release, the operator may elect to use a Kirschner wire to maintain the digit in the corrected position while the capsular structures heal. This is highly recommended if the plantar capsule has been released. Once the wire has been retrograded through the digit to the base of the proximal phalanx, the metatarsophalangeal joint is repositioned and the wire is driven into the metatarsal several centimetres.

Postoperatively it will be necessary to protect the wire from bending forces to prevent breakage or a pin tract infection (Fig. 20.9). This protection is best achieved by using a Darco-type trauma shoe with a built-up insole of one-quarter inch or one-half inch felt all the way forward to the area beneath the sulcus (1, in Fig. 20.9C). This allows the toes to be relieved of any weight-bearing stresses.

If the flexor plate has been released, then the wire should remain across the metatarsophalangeal joint for only 3–3.5 weeks. At this point the wire should be retracted across the joint into the proximal phalanx, so that the motion at the metatarsophalangeal joint may be limited if the wire is left in position for a longer period of time. By retracting the wire into the toe at 3.5 weeks, the joint may still require splinting to help maintain alignment for several more weeks, but a passive range of motion exercises must be initiated.

Primary contractures of the distal interphalangeal joint may result in mallet toe deformities which require surgical intervention (Fig. 20.10). The procedure of choice in most cases is arthroplasty of the distal interphalangeal joint (Jimenez et al 1987). The preferred approach is usually two transverse semi-elliptical incisions at the level of the joint. The corresponding skin wedge is excised and the head of the middle phalanx exposed in a manner similar to a hammer toe correction. The head of the middle phalanx is then resected and the wound closed as previously mentioned. Subcutaneous sutures are not usually necessary. The excised wedge of skin removes redundant tissue and effectively tightens the skin to retain the straightened alignment once the phalangeal head has been removed.

Follow-up care

Postoperative care is essentially the same as that outlined previously for hammer toe repair.

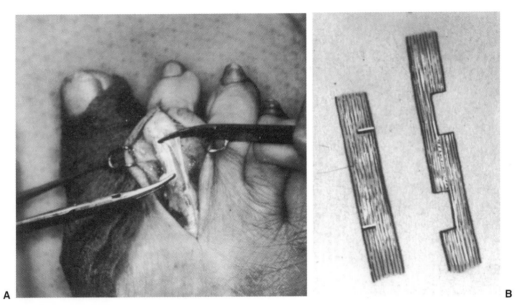

Figure 20.8 Z-plasty lengthening of the extensor tendon. A: Tendon is split longitudinally into two equal parts. B: The lateral and medial incisions enable retraction distally to the new length required.

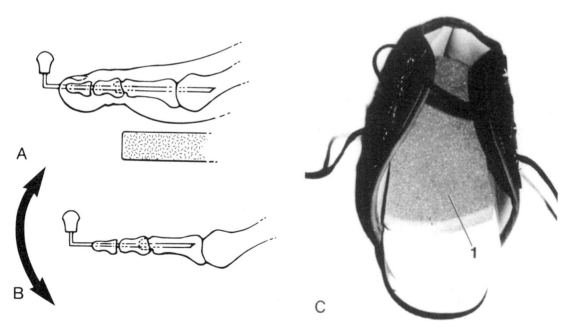

Figure 20.9 Kirschner wires are protected from bending forces to avoid metal fatigue and breakage, and to prevent tissue irritation resulting in pin tract infection. A: Built-up insole removes pressure from the underside of the toe. B: Pin which does not cross the metatarsophalangeal joint allows bending of the toe without strain to the wire. C: Darco trauma shoe is built up with cork or with heavy felt forward to sulcus under the toes. The toes are allowed to float over the end of the insole. (From McGlamry 1987, with permission.)

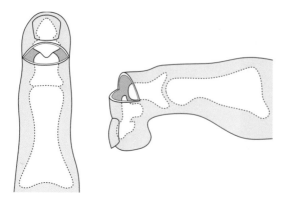

Figure 20.10 Incisional approach for the correction of mallet toe.

THE FIFTH DIGIT

The fifth digit is often considered separately because it presents special requirements for accommodation in shoes (Korn 1980) (from 16 mm film *Approaches to Digital Surgery*, Podiatry Institute, Tucker, GA, 1973). The fifth digit is rarely arthrodesed as this creates a rigid member which is easily irritated by most shoes. However, arthroplasty alone is often insufficient to provide an asymptomatic toe.

Synostosis of the middle and distal phalanges (Fig. 20.11)

This hereditary condition results in loss of much of the flexibility of the toe, and following the removal of the head of the proximal phalanx, the hyperkeratotic skin lesion may at times shift distally over the middle phalanx. This transfer may be prevented in most instances by performing a hemiphalangectomy of the middle and distal phalanges in conjunction with the original arthroplasty (Jimenez et al 1987).

The surgery is approached through a lazy-S incision over the fifth digit. Arthroplasty is performed at the proximal interphalangeal joint. Further distally, the soft tissues are dissected free from the lateral aspect of the synostosis comprising the middle and distal phalanges. Dissection is carried slightly dorsally and plantarly onto the phalanx with careful preservation of the tendinous attachments. This should expose the osseous structures and the lateral one-quarter of the phalanges should be removed with bone-cutting forceps. The remainder of the surface is then smoothed with a rotary burr.

Adductovarus deformity (Fig. 20.12)

In some patients, the fifth toe may be seen to underlap the fourth digit, assuming an adductovarus attitude.

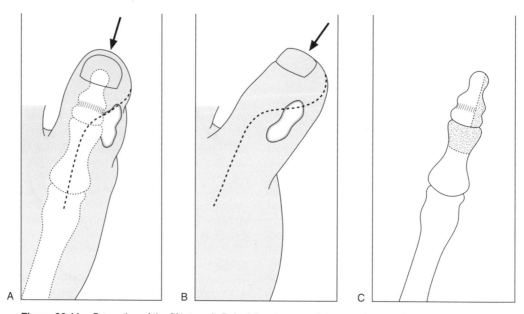

Figure 20.11 Correction of the fifth toe. A, B: Incisional approach in exposing proximal interphalangeal joint and lateral aspect of middle and distal synostosis. C: Represents a typical bony resection, in which appropriate bone is resected from the proximal phalangeal head, and the lateral aspect of the middle–distal synostosis is resected and smoothed.

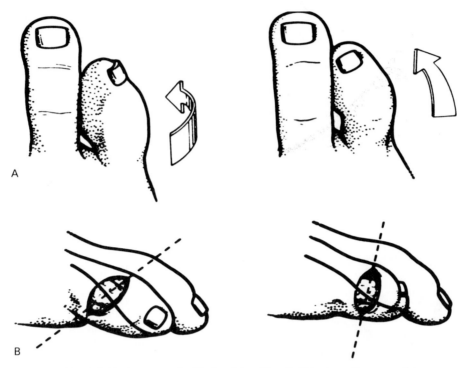

Figure 20.12   A: Adductovarus and adductus deformities. B: This shows the appropriate placement of axes to effect correction of adductovarus and adductus deformities of the fifth toe.

This position may lead to the presence of a heloma at the lateral nail groove. The excessive pressure against the nail may also lead to onychauxis.

Adductovarus deformity may be corrected non-comitantly by incorporating an elliptical skin wedge excision to aid in derotating the toe (Mahan 1987).

Heloma molle

A common condition seen by any foot specialist is the heloma molle, which forms in the fourth web space. This is the result of shearing forces between the head of the proximal phalanx of the fifth toe and the base of the proximal phalanx of the fourth toe. Satisfactory resolution of the lesion may be provided by arthroplasty of the fifth toe. Generally speaking, additional procedures are not required on the adjacent fourth digit for this problem.

THE HALLUX

Occasionally the hallux itself may require surgery, apart from hallux abductovalgus repair. One common condition which may manifest is the interphalangeal sesamoid (Fig. 20.13; also Plate 3). This accessory bone will lie intra-articularly within the more dorsal aspect of the flexor hallucis longus tendon. Often the ossicle will serve as the genesis of a hyperkeratotic plantar lesion. Surgical excision is at the level of the interphalangeal joint, slightly more dorsal than plantar. The capsule of the joint is incised in a longitudinal fashion along with the periosteum as a single layer. The sesamoid may then be palpated with an instrument and excised. The dissection may be facilitated by maintaining the interphalangeal joint in a flexed position. Alternatively, a transverse incision on the plantar aspect of the hallux or an 'S' incision may be used for exposure.

One may also see hyperkeratotic lesions on the plantar medial aspect of the hallux. Typically, these 'pinch calluses' will be due to biomechanical imbalances. However, there may also be hypertrophy of the condyles of the head of the proximal or base of the distal phalanx. Surgical reduction of these osseous prominences may be accomplished through the medial incision described above.

Follow-up care

Postoperative care for the hallux is essentially the

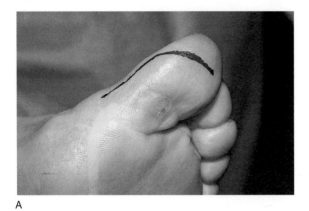

A

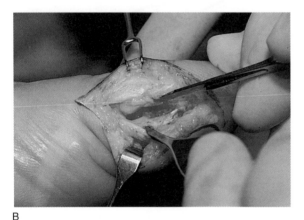

B

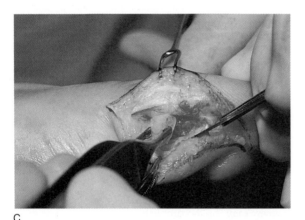

C

Figure 20.13 A: Skin incision for access to the medial and plantar aspects of the hallux interphalangeal joint. Note the lesion plantar to the location of the interphalangeal joint. B: Capsule opened and flexor tendon retracted plantarly, exposing sesamoid. C: Note the thickness of the sesamoid.

same as that for lesser digits. Walking may be allowed immediately and dressings maintained until sufficient healing has occurred, but very restricted activity should be anticipated for the first week or 10 days. A return to wearing shoes is allowed as symptoms permit, usually 3 weeks postoperatively.

Tenotomy

Occasionally one may encounter an older patient with a reasonably flexible contracture of the toe and an associated heloma. If the patient is fairly appropulsive then an isolated tenotomy may be used to help alleviate the condition (Jimenez et al 1987). The surgical technique involves making a small puncture incision at a level where the tendon is readily accessible. Using a number 11 blade, the tendon may be placed on tension and 'snapped'. Closure usually requires only one suture.

It is very important to initiate early splintage or a digital traction device to prevent the tendon from fibrosing with the toe in a contracted position. One must also be aware of the risk involved with isolated tenotomies, especially the accentuation of deformity in the other digits. Once the tendon has been cut, the load

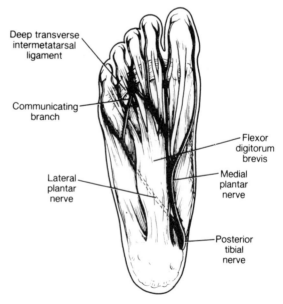

Figure 20.14 Neuroma. Illustration of involved anatomy from the plantar approach. (From McGlamry 1987, with permission.)

from that tendon will be dispersed to the remaining intact slips and may increase any deforming influence to the other toes.

NEUROMA (Figs 20.14 and 20.15)

Surgical incision of Morton's neuroma may be required in patients who have failed to obtain relief from conservative measures. Excision may be accomplished through either a dorsal or plantar incision (Miller 1981, 1987). The authors' preference is a dorsal incision beginning at the base of the third web space and extending proximally over the third intermetatarsal space for 2 or 3 cm. Dissection is carried through the fascia and loose connective tissue to the floor of the intermetatarsal space. Attention is directed distally where the digital branches of the nerve are identified, isolated from the surrounding tissues and transected.

Using Metzenbaum scissors, the neuroma is dissected proximally from its soft tissue attachments and cut at the most proximal to the transverse metatarsal ligament. Closure is accomplished with either 3–0 or 4–0 suture for the subcutaneous tissue. The skin is closed according to preference.

Postoperatively, a compression bandage is maintained for 2 weeks, followed by some type of elastic compression for several additional weeks.

A transverse plantar incision may be just proximal to the interphalangeal sulcus to affect flexor tenotomy and capsulotomy where needed. A linear plantar incision is sometimes used, although the authors prefer the transverse approach as a finer scar usually results.

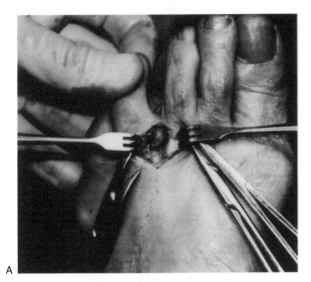

A

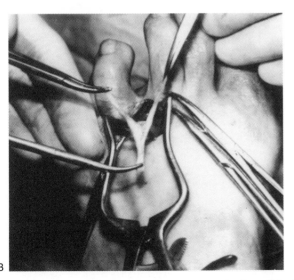

B

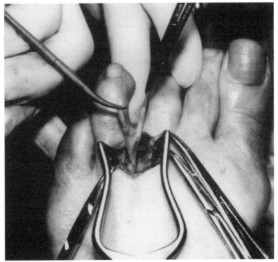

C

Figure 20.15   A: Neuroma shown exposed in the floor of the interspace. B: Distal branches of the neuroma have been resected and the nerve traced proximally. C: Nerve resected proximal to the transverse metatarsal ligament.

REFERENCES

Green D R, Ruch J A, McGlamry E D 1976 Correction of equinus related forefoot deformities. Journal of the American Podiatry Association 66: 768–779

Jarret B A, Manzi J A, Green D R 1980 Interossei and lumbricales muscles of the foot – an anatomical and function study. Journal of the American Podiatry Association 70: 1–13

Jimenez A L, McGlamry E D, Green D R 1987 Lesser ray deformities. In: McGlamry E D (ed) Comprehensive textbook of foot surgery. Williams & Wilkins, Baltimore, p 57–113

Korn S H 1980 The lazy approach for correction of painful underlapping fifth digit. Journal of the American Podiatry Association 70: 30–33

McGlamry E D (ed) 1987 Comprehensive textbook of foot surgery. Williams & Wilkins, Baltimore

Mahan K T 1987 Plastic surgery and skin grafting. In: McGlamry E D (ed) Comprehensive textbook of foot surgery. Williams & Wilkins, Baltimore, p 685–713

Miller S J 1981 Surgical technique for resection of Morton's neuroma. Journal of the American Podiatry Association 77: 181–188

Miller S J 1987 Morton's neuroma syndrome. In: McGlamry E D (ed) Comprehensive textbook of foot surgery. Williams & Wilkins, Baltimore, p 38–56

Post A C 1982 Hallux valgus with displacement of the smaller toes. Medical Record 11: 120–121

Soule R E 1910 Operation for the correction of hammer toe. New York Medical Journal: 648–650

Whitney A K, Green D R 1982 Pseudoequinis. Journal of the American Podiatry Association 72: 365–371

Young C S 1938 An operation for the correction of hammer toe and claw toe. Journal of Bone and Joint Surgery 20: 715–719

21

Podiatric surgery

P. Milsom

Keywords

Digital amputation
    Metatarsophalangeal level
    Middle phalanx level
    Proximal phalanx level
Excision arthroplasties
    Keller's
    Valanti
First metatarsal osteotomy
    Akin
    Austin
    Reverdin
    Reverdin–Green
    Wilson
Ganglion
Lesser metatarsal osteotomies
    Chevron
    Dorsiflexory wedge osteotomy (DWO)
    Helal's
    Metatarsal base DWO
    Metatarsal head resection
    Plantar metatarsal condylectomy
Myxoid cyst
Plantar fibromatosis

Podiatric surgery is an aspect of day care surgery which has become established within a number of units in the UK, although the discipline is already well established in the USA. It is a service which will become established in more centres in the UK, mainly driven by the quality and cost savings it represents to the National Health Service (NHS), but also due to the easier access for patients combined with increased demand because of the high rate of patient satisfaction it produces. The number of practitioners needed to meet the patient's demand is also increasing, through postregistration courses to educate podiatrists towards a nationally accepted surgical qualification.

With this form of surgery, the patients are treated using local anaesthesia and with a low pressure ankle tourniquet to achieve haemostasis. The procedures described in this chapter are examples of the techniques performed by podiatrists in addition to those described in Chapters 19 and 20, and together represent the development and refinement of surgical procedures to treat a large range of painful conditions which, when resolved, greatly improve the quality of life for the patient.

FIRST METATARSAL OSTEOTOMY

Wilson

This technique, which was first described in 1963, relies upon a 45° cut across the neck of the first metatarsal (Fig. 21.1). Once accomplished, this allows the metatarsal head to slide laterally and posteriorly and thus to be moved into a better position. A modified procedure which is often utilised involves angulation in the sagittal plane to allow the plantar displacement of the distal segment (Fig. 21.2). The head is then compressed onto the first metatarsal shaft in a corrected alignment, and crossed or parallel Kirschner (K) wires placed across the osteotomy site to stabilise the union (Fig. 21.3).

The Wilson's procedure is particularly useful for reducing the length of first metatarsals which are too long or which have a small amount of degenerative

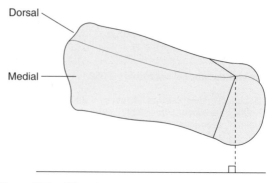

Figure 21.2 Wilson's osteotomy, modified to avoid movement to a dorsiflexed position.

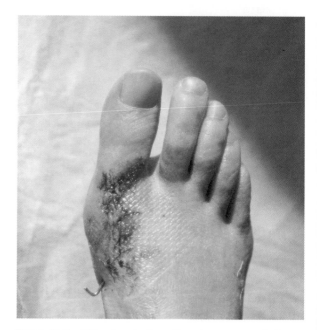

Figure 21.3 Wilson's osteotomy 2 weeks postoperatively.

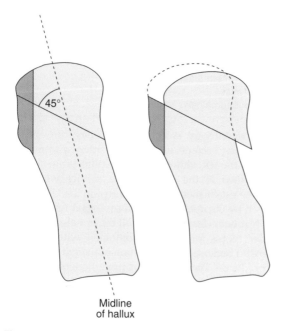

Figure 21.1 Wilson's osteotomy (A/P view).

change at the first metatarsophalangeal joint, as seen using clinical and radiological methods of examination (Fig. 21.4).

Weight-bearing must not be allowed for 2 weeks, to allow most of the resultant oedema to diminish (Fig. 21.5). Stability is maintained with a slipper, or below-knee synthetic fibre cast, fashioned around the hallux to splint it into a good alignment. The cast is removed at 6 weeks postoperatively, and radiographs are taken to confirm osseous healing has taken place (Fig. 21.6). Physiotherapy treatment should be recommended using passive mobility to restore or retain movement as soon as possible.

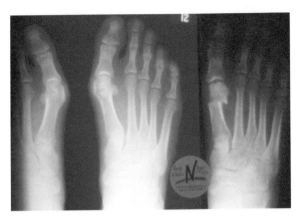

Figure 21.4 Wilson's osteotomy. X-rays pre- and postoperatively.

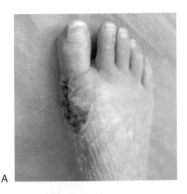

A

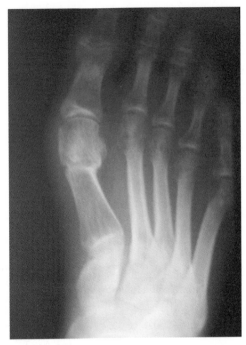

Figure 21.6 Wilson's osteotomy. X-ray showing union.

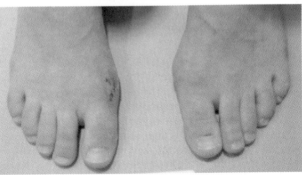

B

Figure 21.5 Wilson's osteotomy, showing correction attained. A: 3 weeks after operation. B: 11 weeks after operation.

Austin

This procedure is one which is most frequently undertaken for the correction of hallux abductovalgus in podiatric surgery. It was first performed in 1981 by D.W. Austin and is a transverse 'V-shaped' osteotomy of the first metatarsal head with lateral displacement and soft tissue release.

Procedure

A 4–5 cm curvilinear incision is made, centred over the first metatarsophalangeal joint between the medial pseudo-exostosis and the extensor hallucis longus (EHL) tendon. The incision is deepened, the nerve and blood vessels are protected via retraction and the vessels are clamped and ligated where necessary. Capsular exposure allows a linear, T- or U-shaped capsulotomy.

The osseous hypertrophy is exposed and resected, remodelling the medial and dorsal surfaces of the metatarsal head. A linear longitudinal lateral capsulotomy and lateral sesamoid release with adductor tenotomy are performed and then a 60° transverse osteotomy is made within the metatarsal head and neck (Fig. 21.7). The head is then displaced laterally and compacted onto the metatarsal shaft, reducing the distance between the first and second metatarsal heads, and realigning the hallux. Angular rotation and relative length of the first metatarsal can be altered by varying the osteotomy angle.

The remaining ledge on the medial metatarsal shaft is remodelled using a drill and burr. Crossed K wires (or screw fixation) are used to provide stability across

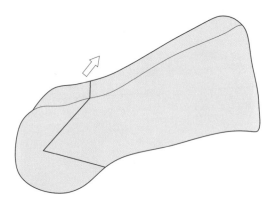

Figure 21.7 Austin osteotomy. Medial view showing 60°
cut.

the osteotomy site. Capsular closure suturing further
reinforces the corrected hallux position.

Postoperative care

This consists of 48 hours' bed rest with the limb elevated. Hip, knee and foot exercises should be carried out
at regular intervals to prevent thrombotic and embolic
incidence. Non-weight-bearing exercise and movement of the first metatarsophalangeal joint are to be
encouraged at an early stage to prevent postoperative
stiffness. Re-dressings should normally be carried out
after 1 week, and the sutures removed after 11–14 days
have elapsed. Kirschner wires should be removed after
4–6 weeks and weight-bearing gradually resumed,
provided there is satisfactory osseous healing.
Functional orthoses should be prescribed at this stage
if indicated.

Reverdin

The Reverdin osteotomy involves the removal of a
wedge-shaped section of bone from the first metatarsal
head, leaving a lateral cortical hinge (Fig. 21.8). The
osteotomy is closed, thereby effectively reducing the
proximal articular set angle (PASA—Fig. 21.9) and
realigning the hallux on the first metatarsal in a rectus
position.

The intermetatarsal angle (IMA) is also decreased by
the retrograde force of the hallux on the metatarsal
head. The pre-operative IMA must be reducible by lateral intermetatarsal compression and mobility noted
or observed at the metatarsocuneiform joint; the
sesamoids are freed from adherence and relocated
beneath the metatarsal head.

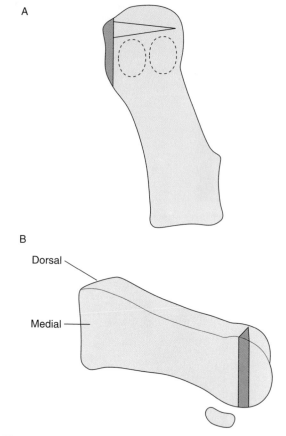

Figure 21.8 Reverdin osteotomy. A: A/P view. B: Medial
dorsal view. Note the intact cortical hinge.

Procedure

An inverted 'L' capsulotomy is performed and the
capsule is reflected from the dorsal and medial aspects
of the metatarsal head. The sesamoids are protected
from the saw blade, minimising the risk of postoperative sesamoid degenerative arthritis. A medial transverse wedge of bone is then resected. The distal cut is
made 2–3 mm posterior to, and parallel with, the articular surface and the osteotomy is closed; the cuts converge before reaching the lateral cortex, leaving a
hinge (Fig. 21.8).

Fixation is not necessary, as the retrograde lever
force involved is sufficient to stabilise the osteotomy.
Immediate weight-bearing can be permitted with the
patient wearing postoperative shoes. A postoperative
night splint may be incorporated, to maintain the
operative correction.

Postoperative hallux limitus is usually caused by
derangement of the sesamoid apparatus and poor

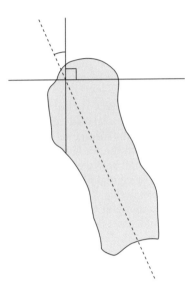

Figure 21.9   Proximal/articular set angle (PASA)—first metatarsal head.

remobilisation. Sesamoiditis can be avoided if the osteotomy is performed superior to the sesamoids. The Reverdin–Green modification (Fig. 21.10) attempts to prevent these complications, by avoiding the sesamoid apparatus and increasing bone to bone contact, thereby providing a larger area of osseous healing.

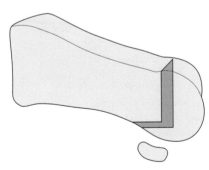

Figure 21.10   Reverdin–Green modification (medial dorsal view).

Akin

This procedure realigns the hallux but does not decompress the first metatarsophalangeal joint (MPJ). If the patient's symptoms lie within the MPJ, this procedure is contraindicated, especially in the presence of degenerative changes (osteoarthritis).

A small wedge of bone is resected from the proximal phalanx in a position selected to redress the abducted alignment of the hallux. A lateral cortical hinge is preserved and the closing wedge osteotomy (CWO) performed (Fig. 21.11).

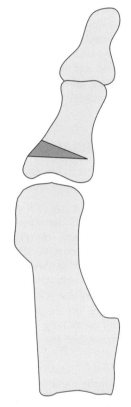

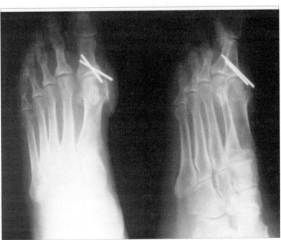

Figure 21.11   Akin closing wedge osteotomy.

Procedure

A 3.5 cm dorsomedial incision is made over the proximal phalanx of the affected hallux, extending from the metatarsal neck distally to slightly anterior to the interphalangeal joint. Pre-operative stencils using the radiographs are useful in determining the amount of bone to be resected. The converging osteotomy cuts converge within the phalanx, allowing the osteotomy to close without loss of stability. The osteotomy site is supported with crossed Kirschner wires or a stainless steel wire suture; the tied tails of the latter are buried into the bone to avoid soft tissue irritation.

Full osseous healing takes between 6 and 8 weeks, and the Kirschner wires are removed at between 4 and 6 weeks.

LESSER METATARSAL OSTEOTOMY

There are many different techniques but the most frequently performed procedures are as follows:

1. *Chevron osteotomy*, in which a V-shaped osteotomy is made in the dorsal metatarsal neck, allowing sagittal plane dorsal displacement (Fig. 21.12). Altering the angle of the osteotomy allows shortening, dorsiflexion, plantarflexion or transverse plane angulation at the metatarsal neck. The angulation of the osteotomy in the sagittal plane is between 15° and 20° to the vertical, depending on the individual metatarsal concerned. The aim is to raise the metatarsal head sufficiently to decrease, but not eliminate, its weight-bearing role.

2. *Dorsiflexory wedge osteotomy (DFWO)*. This osteotomy tilts the entire metatarsal head dorsally. Its use is confined to metatarsals which are excessively long, enlarged plantar condyles, and individual plantar grade metatarsals.

The osteotomy is made through the metaphysis at the surgical neck, leaving a plantar cortical hinge (Fig. 21.13). A burr should not be used as it leaves a U-shaped gap at the apex of the osteotomy cut. Pressure applied from the plantar aspect allows the osteotomy site to close, establishing a corrected transverse metatarsal alignment.

3. *Metatarsal base DFWO*. A closing wedge osteotomy 1cm distal to the metatarsal cuneiform joint provides dorsiflexion of the metatarsal (Fig. 21.13). With a longer lever arm than the wedge made at the head of the metatarsal, a small base wedge resection produces a greater amount of sagittal plane correction.

4. *Helal's osteotomy* (Fig. 21.14). A 15° sagittal plane osteotomy cut is made at the metatarsal neck. Early movement should be encouraged postoperatively; transfer lesions are a known complication (the author estimates a 10% overall complication rate).

5. *Plantar metatarsal condylectomy*. First described by DuVries, dislocation of the metatarsophalangeal joint allows resection of the plantar aspect of the metatarsal (Fig. 21.15). A common complication is iatrogenic postsurgical arthritis.

6. *Metatarsal head resection*. This has a limited application and is only used in elderly patients with marked arthritic degenerative changes of the metatarsophalangeal joints.

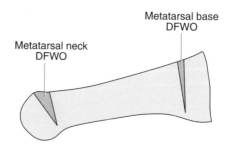

Figure 21.13   Lateral view of metatarsal neck and base dorsiflexory wedge osteotomy (DFWO).

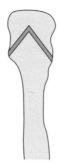

Figure 21.12   Lesser metatarsal osteotomy—chevron (dorsoplantar view).

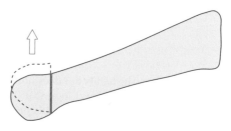

Figure 21.14   Helal's osteotomy (lateral view).

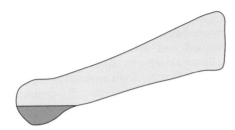

Figure 21.15   DuVries condylectomy (lateral view).

7. *Reverse Wilson's osteotomy*. This is the reduction of a tailor's bunion (fifth MPJ bunionette) via a transverse sliding/osteotomy of the surgical neck of the fifth metatarsal, allowing medial displacement of the metatarsal head and thereby reducing the width of the forefoot and aligning the fifth ray.

Various closing wedge osteotomies are performed along the length of the fifth metatarsal, depending on the apex of the deformity.

EXCISION ARTHROPLASTIES—FIRST RAY

There are two commonly performed excision arthroplasties, the Keller and Valanti procedures. The indications for both procedures are specific to elderly (i.e. 65 years plus), inactive or minimally active patients with pain and deformity at the first metatarsophalangeal joint associated with degenerative change.

Keller's excisional arthroplasty

Surgical technique

Once a profound local anaesthetic Mayo block is achieved, the foot is prepared and draped in the appropriate manner (Ch. 18). A 3.5–4.5 cm dorsal linear incision is made from the hallux interphalangeal joint to the first metatarsal neck. Conventionally, the curved linear incision is placed along the medial aspect of the extensor hallucis longus tendon and care is taken to avoid the medial branch of the superficial peroneal nerve. The wound is deepened to the deep fascia and joint capsule, and the joint osteophytic lipping is exposed via a linear or 'T-shaped' capsulotomy. Hypertrophy of bone is resected using an oscillating saw and/or drill and burr. The joint surface is examined, and the degenerative change over the articular surface is assessed. If the joint is beyond surgical repair, further dissection is performed to expose the base of the proximal phalanx.

The flexor tendons are protected throughout this dissection by retraction and the judicious use of bone levers. The base of the proximal phalanx is then resected, along with one-third of the proximal phalangeal shaft. Alignment is then assessed and the relative range of plantar and dorsiflexion considered. The cut surface of bone is 'saucerised' to provide an increased/smoother range of motion. The wound is irrigated with buffered saline solution and a Kirschner wire placed in a retrograde fashion to maintain alignment. The capsule is closed in a 'purse string' fashion to eliminate dead space within the wound. Superficial closure of the wound is a matter of individual choice for the operator and what is appropriate for the patient. The foot is dressed with absorbent and compressive layers of gauze, Velband and bandaging. A postoperative shoe is fitted and the patient returns home following a suitable period for recovery.

The wound is re-dressed at 5–7 days after the procedure, and sutures are removed at 11–14 days. The wire remains in place for 4 weeks.

Valanti procedure

Originally advocated for younger active patients with degenerative change, experience suggests that the indications for surgery are the same as for Keller's procedure discussed above. The dissection to the level of the joint capsule is similar to Keller's procedure; angled resections of bone are made into the first metatarsal head and base of the proximal phalanx at 40° and 60°, respectively (the precise angle varies depending on the biomechanics and the extent of degenerative change of the joint).

The plantar aspect of the base of the proximal phalanx is contoured and a non-absorbable suture placed through the metatarsal and the proximal phalanx to maintain alignment. The wound is then closed.

DIGITAL AMPUTATION
Considerations in digital amputations

Even with the painful symptoms which often accompany digital deformity, patients are reluctant to accept amputation, which should only be considered as an option after all other treatments are deemed to have failed. Patients are concerned about postoperative 'loss of balance', but in reality the major complication in the digital amputee is not a loss of balance; rather, it is the drift of the adjoining digits into the large interdigital space created. This tendency to drift begins immediately following surgery and can be minimised, initially with dressings and later with a silicone interdigital wedge as a spacer.

Creating a buttress amputation stump by preserving the metatarsophalangeal joint and the base of the proximal phalanx decreases the risk of digital deformity. Following amputation, regenerative attempts within digital nerve branches result in short-term paraesthesia, which usually resolves without the need for active treatment.

Total amputation may be indicated in unsalvageable digits or where insufficient interdigital space exists to satisfactorily realign the affected toe. The level of amputation is determined by the lesions or the symptoms.

Distal partial amputation

Distal pathologies such as mallet toes with onychogryphosis are classic indications for a partial distal amputation. A half oval incision is made to incorporate the nail and periungual tissues. The incision is deepened into the distal interphalangeal joint and the collateral ligaments severed. The distal phalanx is separated from the plantar soft tissues via sharp dissection, and a plantar flap is raised. The dorsal and plantar flaps are approximated.

'Dog ears' are reduced via an elliptical excision over the 'dog ear', or a 60° wedge-shaped plantar skin section is excised.

Middle phalanx amputation

The digit is disarticulated at the proximal interphalangeal joint or an osteotomy is made across the middle phalanx. Care should be taken not to produce tension across the skin edges.

Proximal phalangeal amputation

A circumferential double racket handled incision centred over the midshaft of the proximal phalanx provides access to the proximal one-third of the shaft of the proximal phalanx. The toe is amputated at this level and the cut surface of bone smoothed with a rongeur and Bell's rasp. The small stump provides a cosmetically acceptable result and an effective buttress which limits digital drift into the amputation space.

Digital amputation at metatarsophalangeal joint level

A pear-shaped skin incision is placed over the metatarsal head and the digit to be disarticulated at the metatar-sophalangeal joint. The incision is deepened to the metatarsophalangeal joint capsule, and digital nerves are identified and severed proximally within the wound. Blood vessels are identified and diathermy is used where necessary. A circumferential capsulotomy is made and the digit is amputated. It is preferable that the wound is closed in layers with absorbable and non-absorbable sutures.

GANGLION

This is joint capsule or tendon sheath herniation, commonly situated over the dorsal aspect of midtarsal joints or the first metatarsophalangeal joint.

Conservative treatment includes intralesional infiltration with hyaluronidase, with compressive dressing. Simple aspiration occasionally resolves the lesion; however the majority of ganglia require excision in toto with compressive dressing postoperatively.

MYXOID CYST

Lesions are commonly located at the lesser toe distal interphalangeal joints. A myxoid cyst is a slowly forming cyst of mixed tissue origin prone to recurrence. Chronic myxoid cysts rupture and reform without treatment, but most require surgical excision.

PLANTAR FIBROMATOSIS

This is soft tissue mass arising within the plantar medial longitudinal arch of the foot. Plantar fibromatosis is a benign fibrous tumour involving plantar fascia, non-encapsulated and remaining as isolated nodes or multiple nodules merging together. Macroscopically there is no distinct differentiation from normal fibrous tissue. The plantar fascia comprises three bands (medial, lateral and central). Most plantar fibromatoses are identified within the central band of the plantar fascia. The medial band is commonly involved, but involvement of the lateral band is rare.

There is a known association with palmar fibromatosis (Dupuytren contracture), epilepsy and Peyronie's disease. There is a greater prevalence in males than females (2:1). The presence of knuckle pads over the finger proximal interphalangeal joints is a common finding. There is also an association with fibrous tissue, Keloid scars, endocrine diseases, (e.g. diabetes, thyroid and parathyroid) and alcoholism.

Dorsiflexion of the toes allows better visibility of the soft tissue mass. Palpation of the area shows that the skin and subcutaneous tissue are not adhering to each other, a useful differential diagnosis between adnexal growths and skin tumours, e.g. dermatofibroma which is manipulated with the skin. The differential diagnosis should also include fibrosarcoma, rheumatoid nodule, neurofibroma, ganglion, cyst or foreign body. The microscopic histopathology observations are pathognomic (readers are referred to histological texts). The surgical approach is to excise the lesion with a 5 mm border of 'normal fascia'. There is a high incidence of recurrence.

22

Fluid silicone implantation of the foot

S. W. Balkin

Keywords

Fluid migration
Fluid silicone implantation technique
Histopathology
Local anaesthesia
Silicones as biomaterials
Silicone elastomers as medical devices
Silicone fluid
Silicone fluid and the foot

Historically, heloma (corns) and calluses have been treated with myriad palliative measures, and more recently by surgical intervention. Since 4 April 1964, an independent study has focused on a fundamental mechanism associated with pressure-related foot disorders—loss of fatty tissue. An injection procedure has been developed by which silicone fluid is implanted to form a stable subdermal cushion between skin and weight-bearing bone. The internal pad eliminates or reduces pain and frequency of care for most patients treated, and, in insensitive feet, reduces the incidence of pressure ulcers. This chapter summarises a 32-year clinical experience and presents background information on medical silicone devices.

HISTORICAL PERSPECTIVE

Frederick Stanley Kipping, born in Manchester, England, in 1863, is the recognised father of silicone chemistry (Fig. 22.1). He published 54 papers between 1899 and 1944 that laid down the foundation for this research. Seeing no immediate value for materials he labelled silicones, and termed 'uninviting glues', he lamented that 'the prospect of advances in this section of organic chemistry does not seem very hopeful'. Professor Kipping died in Criccieth, Wales, in 1949, unaware that his pioneering work would give rise to a variety of commercial and medical products common-

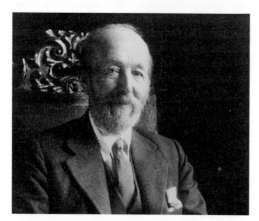

Figure 22.1 Frederick Stanley Kipping (1863–1949).

ly called organosilicon polymers.

Silicone products combine the fields of both inorganic and organic chemistry. Inorganic silicon and oxygen provide inertness and stability, while carbon and hydrogen impart softness and plasticity found in the organic world of living things. They can be made as watery liquids, oils, viscous fluids, gels or elastomers almost indistinguishable from natural rubber (Braley 1965).

Silicones as biomaterials

A biomaterial is any material, natural or man-made, that can be used in contact with living tissue to augment or replace natural functions. It cannot be metabolised or induce a chemical reaction. The properties for ideal biomaterials have been established (Scales 1953) and are as follows:

- chemically inert
- non-carcinogenic
- capable of sterilisation
- no inflammatory or foreign body reaction
- not physically modified by soft tissue
- producing no state of allergy or hypersensitivity
- capable of resisting mechanical strains
- capable of fabrication in the form desired.

Silicone polymers meet these demands and are among the most versatile biomaterials, having a wide range of medical application (Frisch 1983).

Silicone elastomers as medical devices

The first major medical device to use silicone chemistry was the Holter hydrocephalus shunt. Made of sil-

icone rubber, this life-saving product remains in place for a person's lifetime and has been implanted in hundreds of thousands of people to drain excess fluid from the brain to the heart (Nulsen & Spitz 1952). Other such life-saving devices are heart pacemakers and heart valves. Additional elastomeric silicone products for surgical implantation include the following:

- hand and foot implants for joint reconstruction
- catheters, drains and tubing
- penile implants for male erectile dysfunction
- testicular implants for poorly developed or diseased testes
- artificial urethra
- implants for paralysed vocal cords
- implants for cosmetic facial repair
- silicone intraocular lenses following cataract removal
- birth control implants.

Chemically related to rubbery silicone elastomers are silicone gel-filled breast implants, available since 1962 and implanted in 1–2 million women. A total of 80% were for cosmetic mammary enlargement, and 20% for reconstruction following mastectomy. After 30 years, anecdotal reports claimed the implants could cause immune-related or connective-tissue disorders, such as systemic lupus erythematosis, scleroderma, rheumatoid arthritis or polymyositis. Patient complaints included chronic fatigue, muscle pain, joint pain and swollen lymph nodes. This issue received unprecedented media and medical attention; however epidemiological studies in the United States concluded that there is no scientific evidence correlating breast implants and connective tissue disease (Gabriel et al 1994, Sanchez-Guerrero et al 1995). The United Kingdom Department of Health arranged for their own Medical Devices Agency and an independent Expert Advisory Group to assess the literature for those alleged disorders. A total of 270 papers were reviewed and conclusions similarly found no scientific evidence linking silicone gel-filled breast implants with any risk of connective tissue disease (Gott & Tinkler 1995). The speculative controversy continues.

Silicone fluid

The United States Food and Drug Administration and the United Kingdom Medical Devices Agency include fluid silicone in the class of implantable medical devices. One of the first medical applications of silicone oil was its use 45 years ago to lubricate needles and syringes. Coating the exterior of single-use disposable needles reduces the pain of needle entry, while lubricating the syringe interior facilitates plunger movement. Virtually every injection leaves a trace of silicone oil at the injected site. People with insulin-dependent diabetes who require one to four insulin injections daily for a lifetime accumulate the fluid in their bodies; however, exact amounts cannot be ascertained. No known reactions indicate excellent biocompatibility. A similarly safe application is the lubrication of surgical suture needles, which allows for easier passage through tissue.

Silicone fluid and breast enhancement

From the late 1950s to the 1970s, thousands of women worldwide received unauthorised silicone injections to enlarge breasts and contour body parts for cosmetic purposes. Between 750 and 2000 ml per patient was injected (Kagan 1963). These massive amounts of unknown, impure or adulterated fluid silicone caused major infections, tissue necrosis, and in some, loss of breasts. In a few reported instances, intravascular injections were followed by death. This procedure, which was never approved and is now discredited, persists, as do complications (Chen 1995).

Silicone fluid for facial defects

The commonly used unit for viscosity of fluids is the centistoke (cs), with water having a centistoke value of 1. Silicone fluid used to replace soft tissue has a viscosity of 350 cs and can easily be injected using a 25–27 gauge needle and a standard syringe. Two authorised studies that investigated silicone fluid facially as a soft tissue substitute were conducted between 1964 and 1981. The first was for wrinkles and facial atrophy and the second for facial atrophy only. Hemifacial atrophy, known as Romberg's disease, is a neurological disorder causing severe cosmetic deformity. It is characterised by a progressive wasting of skin, facial fat, muscle and bone. The amount used in one such officially studied patient totalled 97 ml (Franz et al 1988).

Silicone fluid and the eye

The first approved injection of silicone fluid in the USA was granted in 1994 for treatment of complicated detached retina. Injected silicone serves as a tamponade to mechanically hold the retina in place until it reattaches. Vitreal–retinal surgeons rate the procedure as 60–75% successful and as the standard care for this problem that can cause blindness. The viscosity of silicone oil used in the eye is 5000 cs, or 15 times more viscous than the fluid injected for soft tissue defects. It requires a power injector, 19 gauge needle and special tubing and syringes to inject the 4.5–6.0 ml of silicone needed to fill an eye (Scott 1989).

Silicone fluid for the foot

The rationale for considering injectable silicone in the foot is that, regardless of causes leading to increased digital or plantar pressure, there is an associated loss of subcutaneous fatty tissue (Ctercteko et al 1981, Delbridge et al 1985, Boulton 1986). Development of essentially inert silicone fluids provided the possibility of augmenting the body's own soft tissue by injection.

THE STUDY

During a 32-year period (1964–1996), medical grade silicone fluid of 350 cs viscosity was studied as a soft tissue substitute for relief of pressure-related foot disorders. A total of 1362 private patients received subdermal injections at several thousand digital or plantar sites (Fig. 22.2).

In most cases the fluid was an attempt to relieve shoe or weight-bearing pain. For those with insensitive neuropathy, pressure ulcer prevention was the goal. Thirty-eight of 116 people with diabetes had moderate to profound sensory loss as determined by light touch, pin-prick or Semmes–Weinstein monofilaments.

Prospective candidates met two essential criteria: the problem area, whether painful or not, had to be pressure-related and it had to be localised. Foot disorders in this category are corns, calluses, scars, fat pad

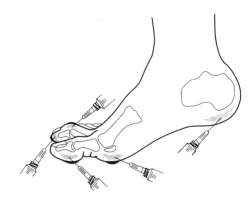

Figure 22.2 Typical digital and plantar pressure sites that injectable silicone may benefit.

depletion and healed insensitive digital or plantar ulcers. Previous care in all instances had been inadequate and included trimming of keratoses, off-loading pads, in-shoe devices or special shoes. Approximately 10% received silicone injections following surgical failure to relieve pain, or when bone surgery created new sites of abnormal pressure.

After 1 year of study, during which no inflammation or adverse responses were seen in non-diabetic feet, patients with diabetes or impaired arterial vascularity were similarly treated for localised pressure disorders. All were informed that silicone fluid was not approved for the foot, but that it was suggested as an alternative to control pain, reduce frequency of care or prevent surgery. In painless feet, the objective was ulcer prevention. Each was advised that traditional methods of treating these conditions, whether conservative or surgical, involved pressure reduction, and that injected silicone, when effective, achieved the same result, often long-term.

Treatment failure was discussed with the patients, as was the possible need for future booster injections, potential skin discolouration, and more importantly, rare discomfort that might require surgical silicone removal due to fluid migration. Advice was given that any foreign or implanted material can cause infection, rejection, allergic or systemic reaction, although none of these has been observed following over 20 000 recorded silicone foot injections. Patients were allowed an immediate post-implantation return to regular activities, wearing shoes of personal choice. No other methods of pressure reduction were used in conjunction with silicone implantation.

Local anaesthesia

Obtaining plantar anaesthesia with minimal pain can be a challenge. The first and fifth metatarsal heads are readily anaesthetised medially and laterally from non-weight-bearing areas, but central sites 2, 3 and 4 require special attention.

Posterior tibial nerve blocks, which remove all plantar sensation, are unnecessary, as only small localised pressure areas need be prepared prior to silicone implantation. Rapid induction techniques requiring less anaesthetic agent have been effective. A Cook–Waite dental syringe with a 1.8 ml 3% mepivacaine cartridge and attached 27 gauge 22 mm ($\frac{7}{8}$ inch) double-ended needle have been the materials of choice for both digital and plantar anaesthesia.

The skin is prepared with 70% isopropyl alcohol and a sterile gauze wipe. At the end of 2–3 seconds of freeze spray with a fluorocarbon-based skin refrigerant such

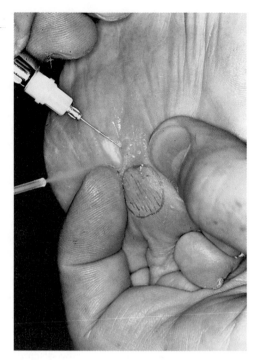

Figure 22.3 Three-second fluorocarbon refrigerant spray reduces skin temperature to between 5°C and −10°C, allowing for 'near painless' injection.

as Fluro Ethyl (Gebauer USA) or Frigiderm (Delasco USA), also used during dermabrasion, a 'dart-like' needle entry is made 1.5–2.0 cm proximal to the central point of pressure (Fig. 22.3). One or multiple digital or plantar sites can be anaesthetised in this manner.

Once a needle has penetrated the skin, stop to determine the degree of pain prior to continuing injection. If pain is significant, partial needle withdrawal or redirection may adequately ease discomfort. Pain experienced during injection can be greatly reduced by extremely slow introduction. Individual plantar sites typically receive 0.5–1.0 ml of anaesthetic solution within 15–45 seconds, depending upon patient tolerance. Patients are usually injected while they are in a seated position, although when apprehension is apparent, they may be reclined with a pillow for added comfort.

Another method of inducing local anaesthesia has been personally investigated since 1989 and used plantarly over 2000 times on some 250 patients. A jet-injection device, designed to inject insulin without a needle (Medi-Jector, Medi-Ject Corporation USA), has been modified to deliver an estimated 0.01 ml, 1–2 mm spot of surface anaesthesia through which

Lorimer, *Neale's Common Foot Disorders, 5th edn*
ISBN 0 443 05258 1

Errata

Figure 22.3 on page 390 has been printed upside down.

In the second paragraph on page 397, the last sentence should read 'Silicone implanted at metatarsal head 2, 3, or 4 may migrate distally or proximally as can a natural *fat pad* under weight bearing'.

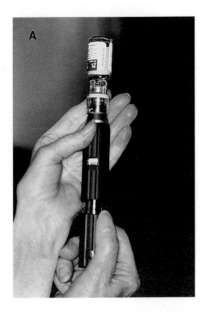

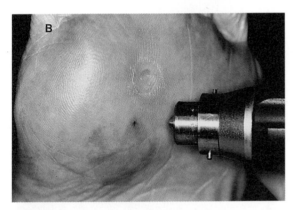

Figure 22.4   A: 10 ml vial of 2% xylocaine attached to nozzle assembly provides several hundred anaesthetic jet-injections. B: Held 5–10 mm from plantar skin, the jet-injector creates a pin-head (1–2 mm) spot of anaesthesia.

local anaesthesia is easily deepened by standard injection (Fig 22.4). A momentary sting may be felt when this instrument is used, but overall pain is considerably reduced. In selected patients, the jet-injector alone permits injection of silicone without additional local anaesthetic solution.

Fluid silicone implantation technique

Calloused tissue is removed prior to implantation, in order to pinpoint readily the exact site of maximum pressure. Using an indelible felt-tipped skin-marking

pen, a 1–2 mm spot serves as a guide during injection. In a sensitive foot, firm pressure directly over the skin mark prior to anaesthesia should coincide with an underlying bony prominence and elicit pain.

Silicone fluid is injected with a disposable tuberculin Luer–Lok syringe measured in hundredths of a millilitre. A 26 or 27 gauge 12 mm ($\frac{1}{2}$ inch) needle is used for lesser toes, a 25 gauge 22 mm ($\frac{7}{8}$ inch) needle for metatarsal head areas or the hallux, and a 25 gauge, 38 mm (1.5 inch) length for the heel. Snap-on, snap-off non-sterile needle guides attach to the syringe and assist in more precise silicone placement (Fig. 22.5).

Whether dorsal, distal or interdigital, corns receive 0.05–0.10 ml per injection with a total of 0.2–0.4 ml. A callus at any plantar site receives 0.1–0.2 ml per injection and a total of 0.5–1.5 ml, averaging 1.0 ml. All injections are made deeply into the existing fatty layer. The frequency of visits does not affect results. Most patients were seen at 1–2 week intervals and some monthly. Rarely, injections were given two to three times weekly. Multiple pressure keratoses can be treated at the same visit depending upon patient tolerance. When mechanical stress is severe, special pads are temporarily applied to be worn with shoes of choice. Foot bathing is suspended on the day of injection. No other activities are altered.

Results

Sensitive feet

Diligent, ongoing patient follow-up has been the hallmark of this study. The most significant findings are long-term pain relief, corn and callus elimination, or marked decreases in the frequency of care (Figs 22.6–22.8). A majority, who had needed near constant or professional palliation every 1–3 months, needed little or no trimming for several to 32 years post-implantation. A small percentage reported improvement after a first implant, with most expressing increased weight-bearing comfort at other stages of treatment. Walking or standing barefooted on hard surfaces also became comfortable for most.

A person's age, sex or duration and location of symptoms had no apparent effect on outcome. When successful, women were able to wear a wider selection of shoes, including stylish fashion shoes which were likely to have been responsible for the original complaint. Up to 90% of flat fibrous calluses were either eliminated or had their associated pain considerably lessened. Sixty-five to eighty-five percent of those with nucleated centres responded favourably, but more slowly. The poorest results, as low as 40–50%, were

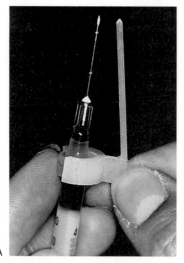
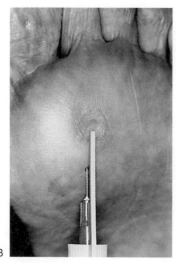
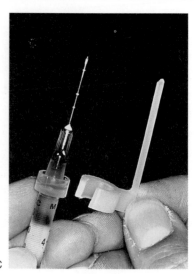

A   B   C

Figure 22.5 A: A needle guide attached to a syringe is equal in length to a silicone implant needle. B: The needle guide tip directs the implant needle to the site of maximum pressure for silicone deposit. C: The re-usable guide is removed following injection.

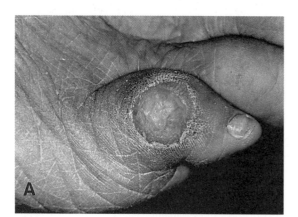
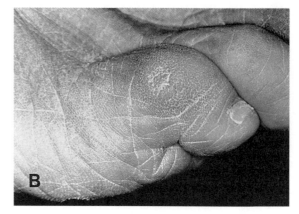

Figure 22.6 A: A 72-year-old man received care once or twice monthly for a large corn of 10 years' duration. B: 0.10 ml of silicone injected at each of six visits (total 0.60 ml) eliminated the corn during a 9-year follow-up.

plantar sites where prior aggressive or invasive treatment had resulted in painful scar formation. Benign skin conditions, such as warts or calluses under weight-bearing bone should be treated with great caution when using electrocautery, laser or excisional procedures, as scar formation may result in pain more severe than the original problem.

Following favourable results lasting several to many years, 50% of plantarly injected sites and 25% of toes, including the hallux, required additional fluid upon return of symptoms. Silicone cushioning had dissipated in these patients and booster injections generally

gave new relief. A few given added fluid at later dates, in amounts equal to or greater than were originally implanted, did not respond a second time.

Very rarely, and for reasons unknown, an initially failed site responded with dramatic improvement 1 or more years later. Careful history could not explain this surprisingly late positive result. For these few, there had been no change to a more appropriate shoe style, custom-made in-shoe devices, a less active life style or significant weight loss to account for the long delay in pain or callus disappearance.

No injected corn or callus is known to have wors-

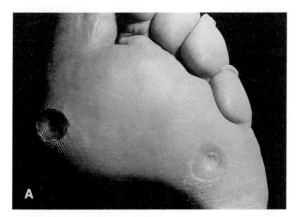
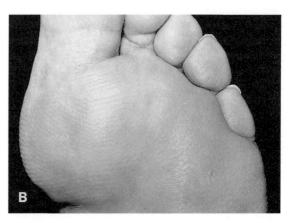

Figure 22.7   A: A 55-year-old man with insulin-dependent diabetes required care at 2–4 week intervals for painful calluses of 15 years' duration. B: In 1965 and 1966, 10 ml of silicone injected under the first metatarsal head, and 5.1 ml beneath the fourth, reduced care to once yearly for years. (Reprinted with permission from Balkin 1972.)

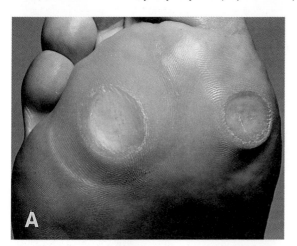
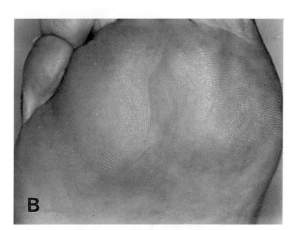

Figure 22.8   A: A 55-year-old woman with calluses of 3 years' duration provided self-care with razor blades three times weekly. B: 1.3 ml of silicone at the first and third metatarsal heads in 1980, and a 0.30 ml booster at the first in 1990, have kept these sites pain-free for 15 years.

ened following implantation, nor have new adjacent plantar keratoses been seen, as may follow shortly after metatarsal surgery to relieve forefoot pressure. Pain encountered during the series of injections was at the keratosis itself, and was due to inadequate trimming. Post-implant pain may also occur at the exact point of anaesthetic or silicone needle entry. If severe, post-treatment needle pain is effectively managed by cold compresses. In a few instances ultrasound was used with benefit.

Insensitive feet

When digital or plantar sensory responses are lacking, as with Hansen's disease (leprosy) or diabetic neuropathy, a painless corn or callus invariably becomes a painless ulcer. It is therefore essential to recognise any decrease in skin sensation, especially when associated with keratoses, and make pressure control mandatory. A small percentage with insensitive skin develop open sores due to ill-fitting shoes, foreign object penetration, or application of harsh chemicals, but elevated pressure in the form of calluses is associated with a 77-fold increased risk of ulceration (Murray & Boulton 1995).

A retrospective study on silicone fluid injected into insensitive diabetic feet has been impressive. It was used for corns and calluses without prior ulceration, as well as for preventing ulcer recurrence when injected after healing. Of 29 healed plantar ulcers, 23 (79%) had no recurrences during 13–201 months of observation (mean 6.3 years). None of 16 painless keratoses recurred or ulcerated over 1–139 months (mean 4.7 years) (Fig. 22.9).

Of seven insensitive digital ulcers, each preceded by corns, there were no recurrences, nor did they require additional silicone over 18–156 months (mean 7.3 years). Follow-up of diabetic patients has been up to 25 years without evidence of any serious adverse complication that could be attributed to the silicone (Balkin & Kaplan 1991; Figs 22.10–22.12; also Plate 11).

Detecting increased plantar pressure

Simple, inexpensive plantar pressure imprints before and after silicone implantation show significant decreases in transmitted forces post-implant (Fig. 22.13). Expensive systems measuring weight-bearing stress (Cavanagh & Ulbrecht 1994), and ultrasound to record plantar tissue thickness in millimetres (Bygrave & Betts 1992), can now be utilised to record pressure reduction and fat pad thickening induced by the silicone fluid.

Callus formation is easily recognisable, but more difficult to detect is a widening of skin lines beneath

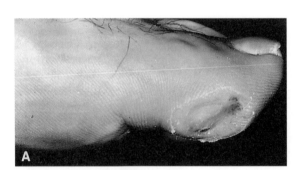
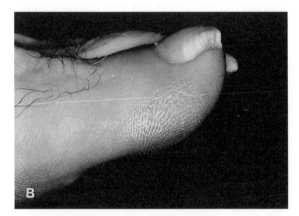

Figure 22.9   A: A 74-year-old woman with a painless pre-ulcerative callus. B: 0.75 ml of silicone injected in 1986 eliminated the callus during 9 years of observation.

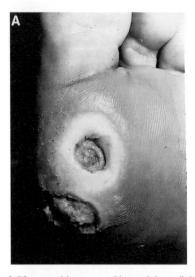
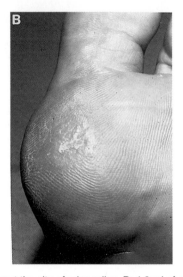

Figure 22.10   A: A 58-year-old woman with a painless diabetic ulcer at the site of prior callus. B: 4.9 ml of silicone implanted after healing in 1966 prevented ulcer recurrence for 16 years, during which time no special shoes or in-shoe devices were worn. (Reproduced with permission from Balkin 1984.)

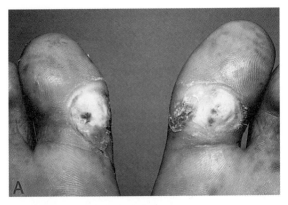 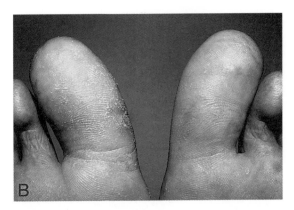

Figure 22.11   A: A 60-year-old male with insulin-dependent diabetes experienced multiple episodes of painless ulceration where calluses had formed. B: 2.3 ml of silicone in the right great toe and 1.9 ml in the left prevented skin breakdown during 20 years of follow-up. (Reproduced with permission from Balkin 1984.)

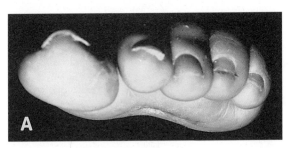 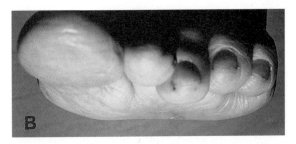

Figure 22.12   A: Multiple ulcerations followed by healing in a 60-year-old woman with insulin-dependent diabetes caused a painless loss of fibro-fatty tissue beneath the second and third metatarsal heads—one period of ulceration persisted for 8 years. B: Upon healing, 5.0 ml of silicone was implanted over 11 visits in 1969, and followed through 9 years of weight-bearing with no further skin breakdown. (Reproduced with permission from Balkin 1984.)

points of abnormal weight-bearing. These are discernible upon close inspection (Fig. 22.14). Separation of dermal ridges at pressure-bearing points may be an early sign of impending ulceration. A painless foot that records high plantar pressure areas, with or without widened skin lines or callus, warrants silicone implants as a prophylaxis against skin breakdown.

Fluid migration

Since silicone injections for the foot and fluid drift were first reported (Balkin 1966), migration of this material remains the singular adverse response of significance. It had been assumed such appearances were due to over-injection; however, even relatively small amounts can migrate, and in rare instances they require surgical excision. Such movement may be seen as a thin silicone skin-tag proximal to weight-bearing metatarsal heads, at times with a fine keratotic leading

edge. These are essentially asymptomatic on bearing weight or direct palpation.

From 1964 to June 1995, 1350 patients, 986 female (73%) and 364 male (27%) aged 17–104 years (mean 60.8 years) received silicone injections. Most were over the soles; however, lesser toes, the hallux, heels, and bases of the first and fifth metatarsals were also implanted. Among this group, 885 received plantar injections beneath 1879 metatarsal heads. Of these 885 patients, 17 (1.92%) developed a soft to firm mass of migrant fibrous silicone tissue over the dorsum at 21 sites. Four patients had a single migratory site bilaterally. These were all observed on pressure-bearing only and were painless upon firm palpation. This unusual response has been reported previously (Balkin 1984). The earliest post-injection appearance was noted at 15 months and the latest at 13 years, an average of 5 years. Four out of 885 patients (0.45%) experienced sufficient discomfort in shoewear to war-

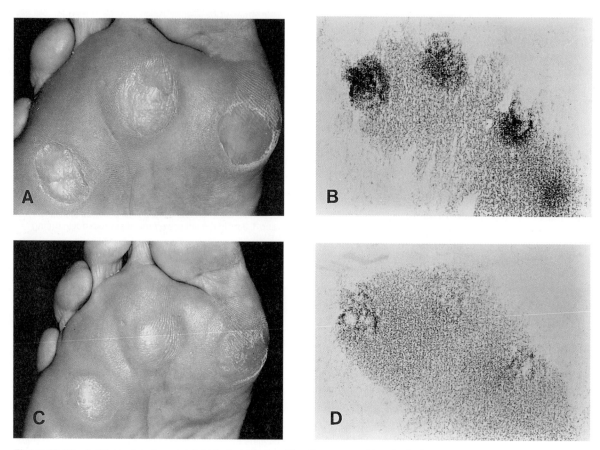

Figure 22.13 A: Plantar keratoses at right first, second and fourth metatarsal heads. B: Simple footprint after keratosis trimming. C: 6 years after silicone implantation, modest callus persists with reduced frequency of care. D: Foot imprint 6 years after silicone implants demonstrate continuing reduction in weight-bearing pressure.

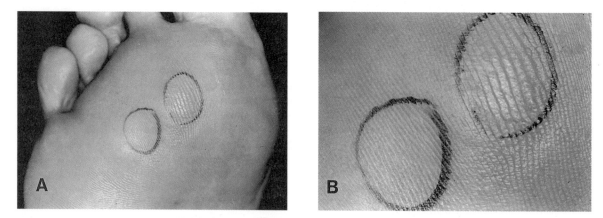

Figure 22.14 A: Widened skin lines (right second metatarsal head) are frequently seen in both painful and painless feet under abnormal pressure. B: Close-up shows separation and decreased number of dermal ridges compared to the third metatarsal head.

rant surgical removal, which was uneventful and without return of symptoms.

Migration from beneath a first or fifth metatarsal head tends to travel proximal medial or proximal lateral, respectively. In all instances where silicone moved from plantar to dorsal, it followed implants beneath a second, third or fourth metatarsal head. What is puzzling about this type of migration is that it was unseen or undetected in earlier cases when larger amounts were injected. The 17 cases reported here received total amounts ranging from 0.4 to 4.1 ml (mean 1.46 ml). Of 17 patients with dorsal migration, 16 (94%) were women. Beyond the role lymphatics play in transporting silicone droplets, altered biomechanics induced by women's shoes, which considerably increase forefoot pressure, appear to be contributory. Silicone implanted at metatarsal head 2, 3 or 4 may migrate distally or proximally as can a natural head under weight-bearing.

Regardless of fluid migration, in most patients the originally injected calluses remained improved or resolved, indicating that a further reduction of injected silicone might be desirable. Considering the inordinate forces to which feet are subjected, it may be impossible to prevent migration in every case.

The most fluid injected into one patient at a single plantar site was 17.8 ml, in 1966. This massive amount was 10–15 times greater than is currently suggested for a callus, and is remarkable for its size and appearance (Fig. 22.15). Over 30 years it has remained asymptomatic.

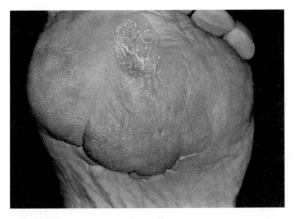

Figure 22.15   A 42-year-old male received care at 2–3 week intervals for a painful callus/scar at the second metatarsal head. During 10 visits from 1965 to 1968, a total of 17.8 ml was injected. On two occasions, 3.0 ml was given in a single injection. Over a 15-year period a massive fibrous silicone pad developed proximally and stabilised. For 30 years, the migrant silicone has remained painless on palpation and weight-bearing. The originally injected site remains free of pain and has required no care.

Silicone migration following lesser toe implantation can also occur. Similar to plantar migration, such movement is infrequent and rarely symptomatic. Injections for a corn may make the toe appear fuller, but never with the characteristics of inflammation, such as heat, redness, swelling and pain. In several hundred treated small toes, a need for surgical excision of migrant silicone due to discomfort was rare, estimated at 0.5% or less. In these rarely seen cases, as with plantar migration, the original painful keratosis often resolved.

Histopathology

Beyond silicone's clinical effects, its morphologic cellular responses and end-fate have been analysed microscopically. Thirty-three surgical biopsies and 124 postmortem specimens from 32 patients were studied. Of these, 58 were digital and 66 were plantar. The earliest post-injection tissue examined was 1 month, and the oldest was 29 years. Regardless of time since injection, each specimen showed the presence of silicone. The fluid was well-retained where deposited by two essentially non-inflammatory tissue responses—histiocytosis and fibrosis. Histiocytes ingest (phagocytise) foreign matter, and are part of the body's scavenger system. The silicone is engulfed and retained within the histiocyte cell body as countless microscopic droplets (Fig. 22.16).

The second key reaction to silicone fluid is that it stimulates the production of collagen fibres. This newly formed mesh of fibrous tissue acts like a web to further entrap and retain silicone fluid where deposited. Microscopic findings also show that numerous droplets envelop microneural and microvascular structures (Fig. 22.17).

By thickening skin and encircling nerves with this resilient fibrous silicone coating, neural impingement by bone is decreased, thereby reducing stress and pain. Similar encirclement of tiny blood vessels at pressure points appears to spare or protect vascularity by this cushioning mechanism. This benefits the patient population where neuropathic skin suffers from pressure due to unrecognised callus or tight shoes. They are less likely to shift body weight as seen when nerves are intact, and these longer periods of unrelieved stress, when standing, walking or at rest, can diminish or stop local circulation.

To determine if an inflammatory process is occurring, pathologists look for cells such as lymphocytes, eosinophils, fibroblasts and plasma cells. These are characteristic of chronic inflammation, but are infrequently seen in silicone-injected tissue.

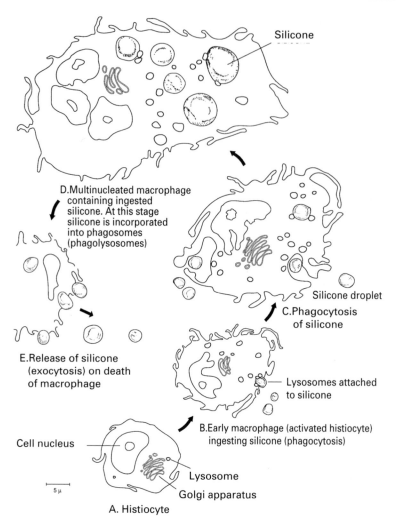

Figure 22.16 Silicone retention through life-cycle of histiocyte seen by electron microscopy. A: Histiocytes with cellular components—lysosomes are packets of enzymes which degrade or confine foreign matter. B: Early macrophage (activated histiocyte) starts the ingestion process as lysosomes attach to silicone. C: Phagocytosis of silicone into cell body. D: Macrophages can enlarge by fusion and are then termed multinucleated macrophages. E: Upon death of the macrophage (1–3 months), its membrane ruptures, releasing silicone droplets which are engulfed by a new generation of histiocytes making silicone retention cyclical and life-long. (Robert L. Van de Velde PhD, Department of Pathology, Cedars-Sinai Medical Center, Los Angeles, California.)

Gathering specimens after death has also afforded an opportunity to study inguinal nodes in 11 patients, including four in whom other lymph node systems were studied, as well as all major viscera. Although the body does not reject silicone fluid, microscopic droplets are transported into the groin lymph nodes without clinical signs or symptoms. Other deep nodal systems and viscera revealed no silicone. Histopathologic findings suggest that medical-quality silicone injected into the foot is a safe procedure.

SUMMARY

Chemical and biomedical engineering advances have

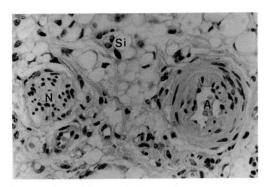

Figure 22.17 Subcutaneous encirclement of small artery (A), arterioles, capillaries and small nerve (N), by microdroplets of silicone (Si) (H & E, × 240). (Reproduced with permission from Balkin & Kaplan 1991.)

provided the health care industry with implantable polymeric biomaterials capable of repairing or replacing body parts. One such polymer, silicone fluid, is an implant material that can augment soft tissue and be remarkably well retained. For the foot, this means that an injectable procedure can control or eliminate history's most common painful affliction—corns and cal-

luses. Thirty-two years of independent evaluation have concluded that this material and procedure are safe and effective as a soft tissue substitute for treating pressure-induced foot disorders. Constant long-term patient review and extensive microscopic analysis have found no serious complications. No tumours, infection, implant rejection, or inflammatory, allergic or systemic responses were noted. Additionally, injected silicone does not impair healing nor impede venous or arterial circulation.

All drugs and medical devices have risks and benefits, and silicone injections into the foot are no different. However, a risk of painless fluid migration or the rare need for surgical removal is far surpassed by weight-bearing pain relief. For patients with diabetes, the fluid can prevent insensitive digital or plantar ulceration, and with that there is the extraordinary potential of preventing toe, foot or leg amputation. Once the chain of events, from increased pressure to ulcer, is broken, disastrous diabetic foot complications and their social and economic costs will lessen dramatically. Confirmation of these most favourable findings through official investigation, followed by silicone approval and appropriate usage, could herald a new and exciting era in the history of foot care.

REFERENCES AND FURTHER READING

Balkin S W 1966 Silicone injection for plantar keratoses: preliminary report. Journal of the American Podiatry Association 56: 1–11

Balkin S W 1984 The fluid silicone prosthesis. In: Weil L S (ed) Clinics in Podiatry. WB Saunders, Philadelphia 1: 145

Balkin S W, Kaplan L 1991 Injectable silicone and the diabetic foot: a 25-year report. Foot 2: 83–88

Boulton A J M 1988 The diabetic foot. Medical Clinics of North America. 72: 1513–1530

Braley S 1965 The silicones as tools in biological engineering. Medical Electronics and Biological Engineering 3: 127–136

Bygrave C J Betts R P 1992 The plantar tissue thickness in the foot: a new ultrasound technique for loadbearing measurements and a metatarsal head depth study. The Foot 2: 71–78

Cavanagh P R, Ubrecht J S 1994 Clinical plantar measurement in diabetes: rationale and methodology. Foot 4: 123–135

Chen T H 1995 Silicone injection granulomas of the breast: treatment by subcutaneous mastectomy and immediate subpectoral breast implant. British Journal of Plastic Surgery 48: 71–76

Ctercteko G C, Dhanendran M, Hutton W C, Le Quesne L P, 1981 Vertical forces acting on the feet of diabetic patients with neuropathic ulceration. British Journal of Surgery 68: 608–614

Delbridge L, Ctercteko G C, Fowler C, Reeves T S, Le Quesne L P 1985 The aetiology of diabetic foot ulceration. British Journal of Surgery 72: 1–6

Edmonds M E, Blundell M P, Morris M E, Cotton L T, Watkins P J 1986 Improved survival of the diabetic foot: the role of a specialized foot clinic. Quarterly Journal of Medicine 232: 763–771

Edmonds M E, Watkins P J 1987 Management of the diabetic foot. In: Dyck P J, Thomas P K, Asbury A K, Winegrad A L, Porte D (eds) Diabetic Neuropathy, WB Saunders, Philadelphia, 208–215

Franz F P, Blocksma R, Brundage S R, Ringler S L 1988 Massive injection of liquid silicone for hemifacial atrophy. Annals of Plastic Surgery 20: 140–145

Frisch E E 1983 Technology of silicones in biomedical applications. In: Rubin L R (ed) Biomaterials in Reconstructive Surgery, C V Mosby, St Louis, 73–90

Gabriel S E, O'Fallon W M, Kurland L T, Beard C M, Woods J E, Melton L J 1994 Risk of connective tissue diseases and other disorders after breast implantation. New England Journal of Medicine 330: 1697–1702

Gott D M, Tinkler J J B 1994 Silicone implants and connective tissue disease: Evaluation of evidence for an association between the implantation of silicones and connective tissue disease. Department of Health, Medical Devices Agency, London

Kagan H D 1963 Sakurai injectable silicone formula – preliminary report. Archives of Otolaryngology 78: 663–668

Murray J H, Boulton A J M 1995 The pathophysiology of diabetic foot ulceration. In: Lavery L A, Kendrick K J (eds) Clinics in Podiatric Medicine and Surgery. WB Saunders, Philadelphia, 12: 1

Nulsen F E, Spitz E B 1952 Treatment of hydrocephalus by direct shunt from ventrical to jugular vein. Surgical Forum 2: 399–403

Sanchez-Guerrero J, Colditz G A, Karlson E W, Hunter D J, Speizer F E, Liang M H 1995 Silicone breast implants and the risk of connective tissue diseases and symptoms. New England Journal of Medicine 332: 1666–1670

Scales J T 1953 Discussion on metals and synthetic materials in relation to soft tissues; tissue reaction to synthetic materials. Proceedings of the Royal Society of Medicine 46: 647–652

Scott J D 1989 Silicone oil as an instrument. In: Ryan S J, Glaser B M, Michaels R G (eds) Retina. C V Mosby, St Louis, 307–315

23

Genetic factors in disorders of the foot

S. J. Ritchie
S. J. A. Raeburn

Keywords

Autosomal dominant
Autosomal recessive
Chromosome defects
Chromosomes
Congenital dislocation of the hip
Gene carriers
Genes
Genetic heterogeneity
Mendelian inheritance
Multifactorial inheritance
Penetrance
Polysyndactyly
Talipes
X-linked disorders

A number of foot disorders are inherited and may therefore occur in several members of a family. Consequently a basic knowledge of genetic principles can help the podiatrist, first in making a complete diagnosis and secondly by awareness that a condition may recur in other family members. Genetic counselling can be arranged by a patient's family doctor to ensure that relevant aspects of inheritance are understood and that the available therapeutic measures are discussed.

The foot deformity may be only one aspect of a more general abnormality, e.g. pes cavus with Charcot–Marie–Tooth disease. An important feature of this condition is muscle weakness and atrophy, particularly in the peroneal muscles. This causes a characteristic abnormality of gait. Thus the podiatrist might suspect that lesions of the feet were part of a more general condition, and, after discussion with the family doctor, further investigation or a specialist referral might be advised in some cases. Not all congenital deformities are inherited, some being attributable to adverse factors operating in utero, such as drug therapy or infections. In addition, pressure on the lower limb or 'amniotic bands' may cause peripheral limb defects. Genetic anomalies fall into three categories:

1. single gene disorders, in which only one gene site is affected (Mendelian disorders)
2. multifactorial disorders, in which both genetic and environmental factors are involved
3. chromosomal defects, e.g. trisomies and monosomies or structural defects such as translocations.

MENDELIAN INHERITANCE

The normal individual has 46 chromosomes, consisting of 22 pairs of autosomes plus two sex chromosomes (two X chromosomes in females and an X and a Y chromosome in males). Except for the sex chromosomes in males and in certain cells of the gonads, all chromosomes occur in pairs, so that at the same location on each of the chromosomes in a pair, a gene exists which directs the development of a particular physical attribute. If both of a gene pair are normal, the individual is normal for that attribute. If there is an abnormality of one of the pair, the abnormal characteristic may be expressed, depending on whether the abnormal gene is dominant or recessive. If an abnormal gene is dominant, the defect is expressed in single dose and the action of the normal gene is suppressed. If an abnormal gene is recessive, the defect is expressed only if *both* the genes are abnormal. The four types of Mendelian inheritance are:

1. autosomal dominant
2. autosomal recessive
3. X-linked recessive
4. X-linked dominant.

Autosomal dominant disorders

Since each parent donates one of the two autosomes in a pair, the child has a 1 in 2 chance of inheriting an autosomal dominant (AD) defect from an affected parent. Conditions caused by autosomal dominant genes therefore commonly occur in each generation of an affected family. In autosomal dominant inheritance, both sexes are equally at risk of involvement. Figure 23.1 shows a typical family tree where autosomal dominance occurs (see also Box 23.1).

Since the diagnosis of one of the syndromes in Box 23.1 does not always imply autosomal dominant inheritance, it is clear that advice from a genetic specialist will often be needed. A difficulty in estimating the risk of others in a family being affected by an AD

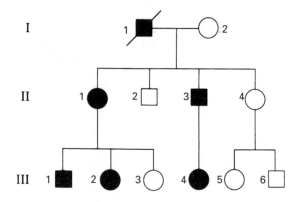

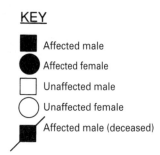

KEY

■ Affected male

● Affected female

□ Unaffected male

○ Unaffected female

◪ Affected male (deceased)

Figure 23.1 An autosomal dominant pedigree. This pedigree shows three generations of a family in which an autosomal dominant disorder occurs. Several orthopaedic disorders which require chiropody are inherited in this way.

Box 23.1 Examples of conditions affecting the feet which are usually autosomal dominant

---

- Lobster claw deformity (ectrodactyly)
- Tarsal fusion syndromes, e.g. calcaneonavicular bar or talocalcaneal coalition
- Some forms of postaxial polydactyly and of syndactyly or brachydactyly
- Tetramelic monodactyly (Somer & Hines 1992)
- Apert's syndrome (acrocephalosyndactyly)

---

disorder is that not all individuals who have the abnormal gene will show any abnormalities. All of the examples in Box 23.1 can occur in such slight forms that the presence of the gene in one subject may be missed. Nevertheless, the risk of that person's offspring inheriting the gene is 50%; consequently, the risk of a child having severe manifestations of the condition may be very high. The percentage of individuals with an abnormal AD gene who manifest the disorder is referred to as the *penetrance* of the abnormal gene. The genetic approach can be complicated by variable penetrance. This may also depend on the sex of the individual. In some conditions, such as the Gordon syndrome characterised by camptodactyly, cleft palate and club foot, the penetrance appears to be more reduced in females than in males (Halal & Fraser 1979).

In many conditions, this phenomenon will be more fully understood if the location of a gene on a specific part of one chromosome, or even the exact structure of the abnormal gene, is identified. Non-manifesting gene carriers could then be recognised by the associated genetic marker patterns or by direct gene probing.

The worldwide Human Genome Project which is currently underway is attempting to localise and specifically identify the function of all genes and may be applicable to this sort of situation in the not-too-distant future.

New mutations occur more frequently in some autosomal dominant conditions, e.g. Apert's syndrome (Mason et al 1990), and may explain an apparently isolated case. However, the risk to the offspring of that individual is then 50%.

Autosomal recessive disorders

To be affected by an autosomal recessive disorder, an individual must have an abnormal gene at the relevant location on both chromosomes of the pair. Autosomal recessive (AR) defects can be expressed in either sex but tend to be seen in one particular sibship and not in several generations of a family. Offspring of a person with an autosomal recessive disorder have a low risk of inheriting the condition, unless the affected person marries a carrier. However, the offspring of that affected person will be 'obligate' carriers of the condition. Both parents of a person with an autosomal recessive disorder are obligate carriers. The risks to the offspring of two such carriers are: 1 in 4 for the child inheriting the condition; 1 in 4 for being clinically and genetically normal; and 1 in 2 for being carriers.

It will be appreciated that if recessive genes occur in a family there may be several healthy carriers in that family. Therefore, if cousins in such families were to marry, their children could inherit one copy of the abnormal gene from each parent. Thus AR diseases occur more often in offspring of consanguineous relationships. Figure 23.2 illustrates such a pedigree, and Box 23.2 contains examples of autosomal recessive disorders.

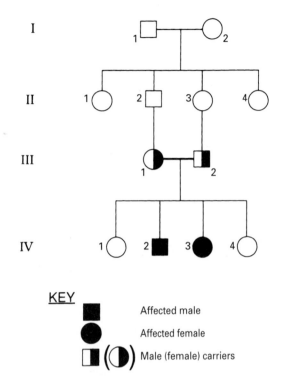

KEY

■ Affected male

● Affected female

◨ (◖) Male (female) carriers

No II: 2 and II: 3 are probable carriers

Figure 23.2 An autosomal recessive pedigree in which the parents of the affected children are consanguineous. As can be seen, III:1 and III:2 are first cousins, their father and mother, respectively, being brother and sister. This consanguinity almost certainly led to the presence of the AR disorder in generation IV, which has affected IV:2 and IV:3.

Box 23.2   Examples of autosomal recessive disorders

- Polysyndactyly plus craniostenosis (Carpenter's syndrome)
- Microcephaly, mental retardation, hypotonia plus syndactyly of the second and third toes (Smith–Lemli–Opitz syndrome)
- Congenital indifference to pain (Charcot's joints may occur)
- Club foot with dwarfism

X-linked disorders

Single gene disorders of the X chromosome account for a large number of conditions of which the best known are haemophilia and Duchenne muscular dystrophy. These two disorders are *X-linked recessive* in nature and this type of inheritance will be considered first.

X-linked recessive disorders (Box 23.3)

Males are almost exclusively affected with these disorders; females have relative protection from the abnormalities caused by an abnormal gene on one X chromosome because of the normal gene on their other X chromosome. In X-linked recessive families, females may be healthy carriers of the disorder. On average, half of the sons of a carrier female will be affected whilst half of the daughters will be carriers.

Detection of carriers of X-linked disorders is difficult, but for many of these conditions there are new techniques based on genetic markers which are identifiable by variations in individual specific segments of DNA or on direct identification of the genetic mutation. Since knowledge has changed very rapidly, it is wise to ensure that patients and their families check up on the developments in their own condition, in case new approaches might be suitable.

Box 23.3 Examples of X-linked recessive disorders

- Haemophilia
- Duchenne muscular dystrophy (pseudohypertrophic)
- Fragile X syndrome (an X-linked recessive form of mental retardation)

X-linked dominant disorders (Box 23.4)

Either sex may be affected with these disorders, but the affected mother may transmit the gene to both sons and daughters, half of whom will be affected. Affected fathers can only transmit the abnormal gene (on the X chromosome) to daughters, all of whom will be affected. With some X-linked dominant disorders, the hemizygous males are thought to have a more severe form of the condition.

Box 23.4 Examples of X-linked dominant disorders

- Hypophosphataemic type of Vitamin D resistant rickets
- Pseudohypoparathyroidism (type 1)

MULTIFACTORIAL INHERITANCE (Box 23.5)

These types of disorder are caused by the combined effects of several genes and environmental factors. The chances of a particular individual inheriting a multi-factorial condition depend on the heritability (i.e. the proportion of the disorder which is due to genetic factors) and on the closeness of relationship to the affected member of the family.

Box 23.5 Examples of multifactorial inheritance

- Diabetes
- Congenital dislocation of the hip
- Arthrogryposis
- Spina bifida and related neural tube defects (e.g. myelomeningocele)
- Talipes deformities

Recognition of multifactorial inheritance is important, because in relevant families, the knowledge of genetic factors operating could help in the identification of increased risk to individuals and families. Then, by modifying environmental aspects, e.g. diet, the condition may be prevented. For example, genetic factors contribute significantly to the cause of neural tube defects. It has recently been shown conclusively that in pregnancies at high risk, the incidence of neural tube defects can be reduced by providing the mother with folic acid supplements from around the time of conception up to the 12-week stage of gestation.

Some studies (Carey et al 1990, Martinez-Fries et al 1992) have suggested an increased risk of pre-axial polydactyly of the feet in infants of diabetic mothers.

CHROMOSOME DEFECTS

Chromosome abnormalities can be due to numerical changes or to structural defects. With numerical changes, there is either an extra or a missing chromosome, although in general those fetuses with an absent chromosome would not survive beyond the early stages of pregnancy. Of live-born chromosome abnormalities, Down's syndrome (trisomy 21) is by far the commonest disorder, and in this condition certain foot defects, including pes planus, can occur. Translocations are examples of structural defects of chromosomes and foot defects can occur as part of the resultant general chromosome imbalance syndrome.

Chromosome defects are very common in early fetuses but most major abnormalities will miscarry before pregnancy is far advanced. Chromosome defects also illustrate another feature of genetic disorders, i.e. that these disorders affect many body systems—brain, cardiovascular system, skeletal system, etc. For example, the Prader–Willi syndrome, which is associated with an abnormality of the short arm of chromosome 15, is characterised by hypotonia, obesity, mental deficiency, hypogonadism and short stature and small hands and feet. However, the small hands and feet are not an invariable finding (Hudgins & Cassidy 1991).

GENETIC HETEROGENEITY

With many clinical abnormalities it has been found that the same apparent syndrome can be due to different genetic causes. For example, in some families, polydactyly can be due to an autosomal dominant gene or it may occur as part of an autosomal recessive syndrome. Polydactyly can also occur in chromosome disorders and certain forms have a multifactorial basis for inheritance. There is also evidence of polydactyly due to an entirely sporadic event which does not recur in a family. Genetic heterogeneity is one reason why caution should be taken in giving genetic advice and information to an isolated patient. To get the correct information, it may often be necessary to take a very careful family history and examine several other members of the family.

CONCLUSIONS

Genetic disorders of the foot are quite common and can be due to a variety of different mechanisms. It is important to realise that the same genetic abnormality might vary in its expression in different members of the family and in the time of onset of complications. It will often be advisable for a podiatrist to ask for advice from an orthopaedic surgeon and a clinical geneticist if clients ask about the risk of genetic recurrence. In general, referral to such specialists is essential for dealing with this type of problem. However, the clinical podiatrist will find a lot of interest in understanding the genetic mechanisms underlying some of the abnormalities he or she treats.

If the treatment is carried out in the patient's home, then family pictures or discussions with others in the family might suggest a genetic element which has not been previously appreciated.

REFERENCES

Carey J C, Hommel M, Fineman R M, Hall B D 1990 Hallucal polydactyly in infants of diabetic mothers: a clinical matter and possible clue to teratogenesis.Proc Greenwood Genetic Centre 9: 95

Halal F, Fraser F C 1979 Camptodactyly, cleft palate, and club foot (the Gordon syndrome). Journal of Medical Genetics 16: 149–150

Hudgins L, Cassidy S B 1991 Hand and foot length in Prader-Willi syndrome. American Journal of Medical Genetics 41: 5–9

Martinez-Fries M L, Bermejo E, Cereijo A 1992 Pre-axial polydactyly of feet in infants of diabetic mothers. American Journal of Medical Genetics 42: 643–646

Mason W H, Wymore M, Berger E 1990 Foot deformities in Apert's syndrome. Journal of American Podiatric Medical Association 80: 540–542

Somer A, Hines J J 1992 Autosomal dominant inheritance of tetramelic monodactyly. American Journal of Medical Genetics 42: 51–52

FURTHER READING

Beighton P 1978 Inherited disorders of the skeleton. Churchill Livingstone, Edinburgh

Wynne-Davis 1973 Heritable disorders in orthopaedic practice. Blackwell Scientific, Oxford

24

Circulatory disorders

P. D. Brash
J. E. Tooke

Keywords

Arteriosclerosis
Lymphatic disease
Macrovascular disease
Microvascular disease
Vasculitis
Vasospastic disease
Venous disease

Circulatory disorders of the foot are caused by arterial (macrovascular) or capillary (microvascular) disease, resulting in ischaemia, or by venous or lymphatic disease which impairs drainage of blood and interstitial fluid.

ARTERIAL DISEASE

Arteriosclerosis

The structure of all arteries alters with advancing age. The intima becomes thickened and fibrosed, and there is replacement of the smooth muscle and elastic fibres of the media with collagen. This results in increased rigidity and tortuosity of the vessels. This contributes to the age-related increase in systolic blood pressure, but is otherwise of little clinical significance as it causes no symptoms.

Macrovascular disease

This term is used to describe atheromatous disease affecting large arteries throughout the body. It is a major cause of morbidity and mortality due to coronary artery disease, cerebrovascular disease and peripheral vascular disease, depending upon which vessels are predominantly affected.

This condition causes progressive narrowing, or stenosis, and occlusion of arteries which results in ischaemia of the tissues supplied by the diseased vessel.

Pathology

The walls of arteries are composed of three layers. The innermost, or intima, is affected first by atheroma. This degenerative condition is extremely common in the Western world. The earliest stage in its development is the appearance of 'fatty streaks'. These are lipid deposits which accumulate on the arterial intima. They are known to occur from childhood onwards. Following the lipid deposition, the intima thickens and smooth muscle cells proliferate, causing a reduction in the lumen of the vessel as it slowly enlarges. It is known as an 'atheromatous plaque' at this stage. The plaque may rupture forming an ulcer upon which secondary thrombosis or haemorrhage into the plaque may occur, the net result being acute vessel occlusion. These segmental lesions cause stenosis or occlusion and affect large or medium-sized vessels throughout the arterial tree, although the coronary, cerebral and lower limb vessels are preferentially affected.

Epidemiology

Intermittent claudication affects approximately 5% of men and 2.5 % of women over the age of 50 years. Approximately 3–6% of these patients will eventually require amputation. Approximately 50% of all claudicants will be dead within 5 years.

Aetiology

Age and sex. Atheroma progresses slowly through adult life. The causal factors exert their effects over a long period and the duration of exposure is of major importance. The lower incidence of atheroma in women until after the menopause reflects the protective effect of female sex hormones.

Genetic predisposition. A strong family history of atheromatous disease is a risk factor in itself.

Hyperlipidaemia. Disorders of lipid metabolism are very common. Both total cholesterol and a fraction of cholesterol known as low density lipoprotein (LDL) are predictive of the risk of atherosclerosis. By contrast, plasma levels of high density lipoprotein (HDL) are inversely related to the risk of atherosclerosis and may be of greater predictive value.

Hypertension. Raised blood pressure (both systolic and diastolic) has been consistently associated with subsequent increased risk of ischaemic heart disease and peripheral vascular disease.

Cigarette smoking. Smoking is a powerful risk factor for atheroma formation. It is directly correlated with the number of cigarettes smoked each day. On giving up smoking, it takes several years for the increased risk to fall.

Diabetes mellitus. Peripheral vascular disease is much more common in diabetes, especially non-insulin-dependent diabetes mellitus (NIDDM). This is related, in part, to the increased incidence of hypertension and hyperlipidaemia.

Clinical features

The three cardinal features of symptomatic peripheral arterial disease are *intermittent claudication*, *rest pain* and *gangrene*, each reflecting an increasing degree of tissue ischaemia.

Intermittent claudication typically causes pain in the leg brought on by exertion and eased by rest, as originally described in 1846 by Sir Benjamin Brodie. The patient complains of a cramp or tightness at the calf, initially on moderate exertion, e.g. walking uphill. The pain becomes more severe with continued exertion, and the patient is forced to stop and rest. Over a period of a few minutes the pain subsides and they are able to continue until the pain returns after a similar amount of exercise. A few patients are able to walk through the pain; possibly, they subconsciously slow down to decrease the load on the ischaemic muscles. As the stenosis worsens, the amount of exercise the patient is able to undertake before the pain develops (exercise tolerance) becomes progressively less. The syndrome commonly affects the calf because the femoropopliteal vessels are the most commonly affected lower limb arteries (60%). More proximal disease affects muscle groups in the thigh, buttocks and lower back in the same fashion.

If the pain is present at rest, this implies that tissue perfusion is inadequate even at rest, and that the limb is critically ischaemic and at risk of gangrene. Classically, the pain is felt in the toes and across the metatarsal heads, initially at night while resting in bed. Relief from pain is derived from hanging the feet out of bed (gravity helps to increase capillary filling). Tissue necrosis (gangrene) occurs when tissue perfusion deteriorates any further.

Physical signs of peripheral arterial disease are:

- decreased or absent pulses
- hair loss
- nail thickening/dystrophy
- smooth shiny skin
- reduced temperature.

Investigation of arterial disease involves clinical assessment, ultrasound Doppler studies and angiography.

Prognosis

Twenty per cent of patients with critical ischaemia will be dead within 1 year, and 50% of amputees will be dead within 3 years of their first major amputation. The usual cause of death is cardiovascular disease, representing the widespread nature of arterial disease (European Working Group on critical leg ischaemia 1991).

Treatment

Conservative management. In patients whose disease does not require intervention, all risk factors should be addressed, especially smoking. They should be encouraged to continue regular activity, as this increases their claudication distance through the development of collateral circulation and adaptive changes in gait and muscle metabolism. Drug therapy has not been shown to be useful.

Angioplasty. Balloon angioplasty is the safest and quickest interventional treatment for short stenoses of the iliac or femoral arteries. It has the advantage that it can be easily repeated if necessary (De Weese et al 1993).

Reconstructive surgery. Bypass procedures in the hands of an experienced vascular surgeon, using venous or Dacron grafts, can save a threatened limb (De Weese et al 1993).

Sympathectomy. This may help relieve rest pain but rarely improves blood flow (Campbell 1993).

Prostanoids. Iloprost is an analogue of the naturally occurring prostaglandin PGI2. It seems a promising if relatively new treatment in patients with critical ischaemia in whom reconstructive surgery is not possible (Loosemore et al 1994). It is very useful in the relief of rest pain.

Amputation. When limb salvage is not possible, amputation is necessary to relieve pain, to prevent access for infection and to enable the patient to begin rehabilitation. The level of amputation must be carefully chosen to enable maximum function and adequate healing. Retention of the knee joint with a below-knee procedure greatly increases potential mobility (European Working Group on critical leg ischaemia 1991).

Acute arterial occlusion

This is usually thrombotic or embolic. Thrombosis of a severely atheromatous artery may cause few or no symptoms. Emboli on the other hand can occlude minimally diseased or normal arteries and are much more likely to be symptomatic. Between 75% and 90% of emboli originate in the heart, usually secondary to atrial fibrillation or from mural thrombosis after myocardial infarction.

Acute arterial embolus causes sudden pain and pallor with loss of pulses below the occlusion. Later, paraesthesiae and paralysis occur. It is a surgical emergency requiring analgesia, heparinisation and prompt embolectomy. The diagnosis is made on clinical grounds, but if there is any doubt an angiogram should be performed without delay to confirm the diagnosis. Thrombolytic therapy has also been used successfully (Campbell 1994).

Vasculitis

This term covers a heterogeneous group of conditions in which there is focal inflammation of the walls of blood vessels, usually arteries or arterioles, but veins and capillaries can also be affected. The two conditions in this group which commonly affect the lower limb are thromboangiitis obliterans (Buerger's disease) and polyarteritis nodosa.

Thromboangiitis obliterans (TAO)

Pathology. Thromboangiitis obliterans is a vasculitis affecting medium and small arteries and veins. Short segments of the affected vessels are occluded by thrombus and there is intense infiltration of the thrombus and the whole thickness of the vessel wall by inflammatory cells. These changes give way to chronic inflammation and finally fibrosis. Different areas of vessels are affected at different times, giving characteristic exacerbations and remissions (Shionoya 1993).

Epidemiology. It is a rare condition which occurs predominantly in young males , although the incidence in women is rising with increasing cigarette consumption. It occurs between 20 and 45 years of age.

Aetiology. The single known important predisposing factor is cigarette smoking. The disease is practically confined to heavy smokers.

Clinical features. Patients develop superficial migratory thrombophlebitis, cool dysaesthetic feet, claudication or rest pain, and gangrene.

Recurrent migratory superficial thrombophlebitis may be present for a year or two before arterial symptoms. A biopsy at this time can confirm the diagnosis, and if patients can be persuaded to stop smoking, the disease can often be stopped at this stage.

Arterial disease causes coldness of the feet, paraesthesiae and trophic changes. Rest pain may be severe. Claudication can occur in the feet as well as the calf.

The foot pulses are lost. A collateral circulation initially develops but this becomes inadequate. Finally ulceration and gangrene develop.

Differential diagnosis. The differential diagnosis is from premature atheromatous disease. Features which distinguish thromboangiitis obliterans from atheroma with super-added thrombosis are:

- early onset
- inflammation
- predilection for small vessels
- involvement of veins as well as arteries
- evidence of ischaemia in the arms as well as the legs.

Prognosis. Prognosis from this condition is good. TAO is not a lethal disease. Most recorded deaths are from complications of surgery.

Treatment

- Total abstinence from tobacco.
- Adequate pain relief.
- Surgical sympathectomy
- Iloprost (PGE1) infusions.

Unfortunately one or more amputations are often required (Shionoya 1993).

Polyarteritis nodosa (PAN)

Pathology. This collagen vascular disease of unknown aetiology is characterised by segmental involvement of the media of medium and small arteries. There is oedema, fibrinoid necrosis of the vessel wall and infiltration of the vessel wall with inflammatory cells. Secondary thrombosis is common. Chronic lesions become fibrosed.

Epidemiology. This is a rare condition which occurs more commonly in men. It occurs at all ages, but is most prevalent between 30 and 50 years of age.

Clinical features. The symptoms and signs of PAN relate to its devastating multisystem inflammatory nature, and vary depending on which organs are predominantly affected. Fatigue, malaise, anorexia and fever are common.

Cutaneous involvement occurs in 25% of cases. The most characteristic finding is the subcutaneous inflammatory nodule. This necrotising vasculitis causes ulceration, subcutaneous haemorrhage and gangrene of the hands and feet (Diaz-Perez & Winkelman 1980, Guillevan et al 1988).

Differential diagnosis. This is mainly from other collagen vascular diseases, which can produce indistinguishable lesions. The diagnosis is usually made on the clinical features. Immunological studies may be useful to exclude other collagen vascular diseases, e.g.:

- hypersensitivity vasculitis—drugs
- Henoch–Schönlein purpura
- cryoglobulinaemia
- vasculitis associated with malignancies.

Prognosis. Without treatment, renal cardiac and cerebral involvement cause death within 5 years in 80–90% of patients. Since treatment with immunosuppressive therapy began, the 5-year survival of this condition has increased to 80% (Guillevan et al 1988).

VASOSPASTIC DISEASE

Primary Raynaud's disease

This condition is characterised by attacks of well-demarcated discolouration of the digits brought on by cold. Between attacks the digits appear normal.

It is a common condition occurring in 5–10% of the population and it is especially common in women aged 20–40 years. The toes are affected in 50% of cases. Classically, the digits become white and numb due to cessation of blood flow. The hands and feet are not involved. As slow blood flow returns, the digits become blue as the blood is desaturated. Finally the digital arteries fully reopen and the digits become red from reactive hyperaemia. There is often a dull throbbing pain at this stage. Primary Raynaud's disease is diagnosed in the absence of other causes. It is mostly a benign condition, but in one study 13% of patients had ulceration, chronic paronychia, scarring, fissuring or necrosis of the skin (Gifford & Hines 1957).

Secondary Raynaud's disease

Raynaud's phenomenon is frequently associated with other medical conditions, especially connective tissue disorders (see Box 24.1).

Treatment

Vasodilator therapy, e.g. nifedipine and alpha-blockers. In severe cases, prostaglandin analogues e.g. iloprost, have been used to good effect (Wigley 1993).

Acrocyanosis

This is characterised by persistent cyanosis and coldness of the digits of the hands and feet, which intensifies with cold and is relieved by warmth. It is a benign condition which is asymptomatic.

Box 24.1 Medical conditions with which Raynaud's phenomenon is associated

- Drugs
  - alpha-blockers
  - ergotamine
- Connective tissue diseases
  - scleroderma
  - systemic lupus erythematosus (SLE)
  - mixed connective tissue disease (MCTD)
- Trauma: vibration injury
- Atherosclerosis
- Thromboangiitis obliterans
- Haemorrheological disorders
- Cryoglobulinaemia—cold agglutinin disease

Microvascular disease

Microvascular disease occurs in insulin-dependent diabetes mellitus (IDDM) and non-insulin-dependent diabetes mellitus (NIDDM), and its development is linked to disease duration. This term refers to damage to the smallest blood vessels, the capillaries, throughout the body. It plays a part in the development of all diabetic complications and plays a role in diabetic foot problems, contributing to the development of peripheral neuropathy. Microvascular disease of the soft tissues of the foot is also very important, because ulcer healing relies on a healthy and adaptable microcirculation to subserve the processes of defence, reconstitution and functional recovery of injured tissue.

It has been estimated that more than 2% of patients attending a diabetic clinic have active foot ulceration. Within the diabetic population, chronic foot ulceration represents the major cause of hospitalisation in the UK, and all too often leads to amputation.

Microscopically, there is thickening of the basement membrane of the capillaries and damage to the endothelial cells. This causes a decrease in blood flow to the tissues and an inability to respond to the stimuli which would normally increase capillary flow, e.g. trauma to the foot. This relative hypoxia of the soft tissues of the foot, and inability to respond appropriately, lead to an impairment of healing. Optimal diabetic control decreases the risk of microangiopathy (DCCT 1996). Once fully developed, microvascular disease is irreversible.

VENOUS DISEASE

Superficial thrombophlebitis

This is a common problem which presents as a tender red swelling, warm to the touch, and the indurated cord of thrombosed vein is usually palpable.

It does not require anticoagulation. Analgesia and non-steroidal anti-inflammatory drugs are usually sufficient. Compression bandages are helpful. Antibiotics are indicated only if there is evidence of infection. Patients should be encouraged to remain mobile.

Deep venous thrombosis (DVT)

DVT poses two problems: first, the impaired drainage of the limb caused by the obstruction, and secondly the risk that the thrombus or a part of it may be dislodged and travel to the lungs. This second problem should not be underestimated as it can cause acute circulatory collapse; it is responsible for 2500 deaths per annum in the UK.

DVT is a common condition, especially amongst hospital in-patients. Most thrombi are small, asymptomatic and usually confined to the calf, in the soleal arcade. Twenty percent of thrombi extend to more proximal vessels and can lead to pulmonary embolism, while 80% of thrombi in symptomatic patients have extended to the popliteal veins or beyond (Anderson et al 1991). The risk factors for the development of DVT are:

- surgery or non-surgical trauma
  - more than 50% of patients develop DVT following hip surgery
  - more than 65% of patients develop DVT following knee replacement
- elderly—decreased fibrinolytic activity
- malignant disease—two- to threefold increased risk
- immobilisation
- heart failure—raised CVP and immobility
- previous DVT—two- to threefold increased risk
- obesity—impaired fibrinolytic activity
- pregnancy
- use of oral contraceptives
- stroke with limb paralysis.

Venous thrombi are generally thought to be secondary to blood coagulation and fibrin formation during venous stasis. An important mechanism of blood clearance from the lower limbs is contraction of the calf muscles, which increases the return of blood to the heart. Thermal dilution studies have shown that during surgery, flow in the iliac and femoral veins decreases by 50% from the induction of anaesthesia and is maintained at this level throughout the operation. Immobility following surgery is a strong risk factor. Patients are at risk for their entire period of immobility (Anderson et al 1991).

Thrombi are removed by endogenous fibrinolysis,

fibrin digestion by leucocytes, organisation of the thrombus and embolisation. Occlusion or recanalisation are the two most common outcomes of venous thrombi. In contrast to arterial thrombi, recanalisation is not uncommon, but may be incomplete.

Clinical diagnosis

This is notoriously difficult. In one study 1000 patients with clinically suspected DVT were examined with venography; 70% of patients had no evidence of thrombus. In another study of 11 000 postmortems, DVT was present in 316 cases. Only 11% of the 316 cases were thought clinically to have DVT (Horowitz & Tatter 1969).

Clinical features

- Swelling
- Warmth
- Tenderness
- Positive Homans' sign (pain in the calf on ankle flexion).

Unfortunately, all of these clinical features are rather non-specific. Diagnosis is confirmed with venography or rheography.

Differential diagnosis

- Muscle injury
- Baker's cyst
- Cellulitis
- Arthritis
- Oedema due to other causes, e.g. congestive cardiac failure (CCF).

Treatment

Bed rest, elevation of the limb, and elastic stockings to reduce swelling of the limb are important, but anticoagulation is the mainstay of treatment. It prevents extension and embolisation of the thrombus and prevents recurrent pulmonary embolism (PE) and DVT.

Heparin should be given by intravenous infusion following a loading bolus as soon as the diagnosis has been confirmed. The activated partial thromboplastin time (APTT) should be maintained at two to three times the laboratory control value to prevent recurrence of venous thromboembolism.

The duration of heparin therapy is still debated; some clinicians give 7 days' therapy, while others discontinue heparin once adequate anticoagulation is achieved with warfarin. Heparin has a short half-life

and can only be administered parenterally. Warfarin, a long-acting dicoumarin anticoagulant, is the preferred agent for longer courses of therapy. Treatment with warfarin can be difficult to manage; its metabolism and excretion vary greatly between individuals, and are significantly affected by diet, drugs and coincidental diseases. The prothrombin time is maintained at twice the control value. Treatment is given for 3–6 months following the thrombosis. For recurrent disease, longer courses of therapy are given, in some cases life-long (Rosenow 1992).

Thrombolysis. Thrombolytic agents are designed to dissolve the thrombus and should only be considered with significant proximal thrombosis where DVT is considered a significant risk. They are not without hazards to the patient, haemorrhage being the main concern. Fatal haemorrhage is twice as common in thrombolytic therapy compared to heparinisation. They have theoretical advantages in that they are more effective at dissolving the thrombus (80%) and, having dissolved the thrombus, there is a reduced chance of postphlebitic syndrome.

Vena caval filters. In cases where anticoagulation is contraindicated or has failed to prevent PE, filters can be placed in the inferior vena cava to mechanically prevent emboli from the legs reaching the lungs.

Chronic venous insufficiency

This condition may result from extensive or repeated venous thrombosis and/or valvular incompetence associated with varicose veins. It is an extremely common problem, increasing in incidence with age, and has been estimated to affect 1% of the adult population at some time during their life (Browse 1983). There is familial clustering of the condition, and recent work suggests a genetic element to its development (Taheri et al 1993).

Following a DVT, the delicate valve leaflets thicken and contract, becoming incapable of maintaining unidirectional flow. There is widespread dilatation of the superficial and deep veins, causing worsening incompetence and a progressive increase in pressure in the venous system.

This increased pressure damages capillaries, which become abnormally permeable, leaking both fluid and large molecules (especially fibrin) into the surrounding tissues. Tissue hypoxia attracts inflammatory cells and macrophages, which worsens capillary damage (Bradbury et al 1993). There is a progressive increase in tissue hypoxia, eventually producing necrosis and ulceration.

Patients complain of a dull ache in their leg, worse

with standing, and eased with elevation of the limb. There are usually signs of swelling, induration and pigmentation. An ulcer may already be present. These can occur anywhere on the leg, but are most commonly seen above the medial malleolus.

Treatment

Untreated venous ulcers will remain unhealed for many years. Almost all venous ulcers can be healed with good medical treatment (Browse 1983). Therapy is aimed at reducing venous hypertension. The foot of the bed should be elevated during sleep, and the feet should be elevated whilst sitting. In the upright position, stretch elastic bandages applied evenly and firmly from toes to knees or thigh, including the heel and malleoli, are of great benefit. Commercially available compression devices, e.g. Flowtron boot, although expensive, may be helpful.

If the chronic venous insufficiency is due to isolated superficial venous incompetence, surgical ligation and stripping of the veins may be a long-term cure.

Ulcers should be cleaned with normal saline and dressed with inert, non-adherent moisture-preserving dressings, e.g. hydrocolloid gels. Antibiotics should be used if there is evidence of infection.

LYMPHATIC DISEASE

The lymphatic system has two main functions:

- to remove large molecules and excess fluid from the interstitial space
- to allow circulation of lymphocytes from lymph nodes to the circulation.

Disease of the lymphatic vessels causes oedema.

Primary lymphoedema

This is caused by either hypoplasia or fibrosis of lymphatic vessels. It is associated with other congenital anomalies, e.g. Turner's syndrome. It causes insidious oedema, usually affecting the lower limbs. There are three different subtypes:

- congenital lymphoedema—appearing at or near birth
- lymphoedema praecox—lymphoedema beginning at puberty
- lymphoedema tarda—lymphoedema after the age of 35 years (Browse & Stewart 1985).

One or both legs may be affected. It may affect the whole limb or be localised, e.g. to the dorsum of the foot. Patients complain of swelling of the limb which fluctuates, being worse at night and better in the morning.

The oedema is pitting, i.e. a depression can be created in the tissues by digital pressure. The chronic oedema causes a fibrotic reaction, leading to induration.

Secondary lymphoedema

Lyphoedema can be acquired from disease obstructing lymphatic drainage:

- *filariasis*—parasitic worms endogenous to West Africa, India and parts of South America cause an intense fibrous reaction when they lodge in lymphatics, causing obstruction, gross swelling and deformity, known as elephantiasis
- *malignant disease*—can cause obstruction due to compression or by metastatic spread to lymph nodes
- *radiotherapy*—causes fibrosis of lymphatics and obstruction
- *trauma*
- *chronic infection.*

Differential diagnosis

This includes all other causes of dependent oedema, but especially:

- venous disease
- heart failure
- hypoproteinaemia, e.g. liver disease
- nephrotic syndrome.

Treatment

- Limb elevation and elastic compression stockings are helpful.
- Pneumatic massaging devices, e.g. Flowtron boots, may be very useful.
- Diuretic therapy is not indicated.
- Recurrent cellulitis can be troublesome and should be treated with appropriate antibiotics.
- Microsurgical techniques have been used to improve lymphatic drainage.
- New research using intra-arterial infusion of the patient's own lymphocytes has been shown to produce a marked and lasting improvement in swelling in refractory cases of lymphoedema (Nagata et al 1994).

REFERENCES

Anderson F A et al 1991 A population based perspective on the incidence and case fatality rates of venous thrombosis and PE; the Worcester DVT study. Archives of Internal Medicine 151: 933

Bradbury A W, Murie J A, Ruckley C V 1993 Role of the leucocyte in the pathogenesis of vascular disease. British Journal of Surgery 80: 1503–1512

Browse N L 1983 Venous ulceration. British Medical Journal 286: 1920

Browse N L, Stewart G 1985 Lymphoedema: pathophysiology and classification. Journal of Cardiovascular Surgery 26: 91–106

Campbell W B 1994 Arterial emboli. In: Morris P J, Malt R A (eds) Oxford textbook of surgery. Oxford Medical, Oxford

Campbell W B 1993 Sympathectomy for chronic arterial ischaemia. European Journal of Vascular Surgery 5(2): 295–297

DeWeese J A, Leather R, Porter J 1993 Practice guidelines: lower extremity revascularization. Journal of Vascular Surgery 18(2): 280–294

Diabetes Control and Complications Trial Research Group 1993

Diaz-Perez J L, Winkelman R K 1980 Cutaneous periarteritis nodosa: a study of 33 patients. In: Wolf K, Winkelman R K (eds) Vasculitis. W B Saunders, Philadelphia

Dormandy J et al Fate of the patient with chronic leg ischaemia. Journal of Cardiovascular Surgery 2 30 1: 50–57

European Working Group on critical leg ischaemia 1991 Circulation 84 (suppl. 4)

Gifford R W Jr, Hines E A Jr 1957 Raynaud's disease among women and girls. Circulation 16: 1012

Guillevan L et al 1988 Clinical findings and prognosis of polyarteritis nodosa and Churg–Strauss angiitis. A study of 165 patients. British Journal of Rheumatology 27: 258

Horowitz R E, Tatter D 1969 Lethal pulmonary embolism. In: Sherry S et al (eds) Thrombosis. Washington DC

Loosemore T M, Chalmers T C, Dormandy J A 1994 A meta-analysis of randomized placebo control trials in Fontaine stages III and IV peripheral occlusive arterial disease. International Angiology 13(2): 133–142

Nagata Y et al 1994 Intra-arterial infusion of autologous lymphocytes for the treatment of refractory lymphoedema. European Journal of Surgery 160(2): 105–109

Rosenow E C 1992 3d venous thrombo-embolism. Postgraduate Medical Journal 68 (suppl. 1): 65–91

Shionoya S 1993 Buerger's disease: diagnosis and management. Cardiovascular Surgery 1(3): 207–214

Taheri S A et al 1993 Genetic alterations in chronic venous insufficiency. Int Angiology 12: 1–14

Tooke J E The microcirculation in diabetes.

Wigley F M 1993 Raynaud's phenomenon. Current Opinion in Rheumatology 5(6): 773–784

FURTHER READING

Bergan J J, Yao J S T 1991 Venous disorders. WB Saunders, Philadelphia

Dormandy J A, Stock G 1990 Critical leg ischaemia. Its pathophysiology and management. Springer-Verlag, Berlin

Young J R, Graor R A, Olin J W, Bartholemew J R (eds) 1991 Peripheral vascular diseases. Mosby, St Louis

25

Metabolic diseases

M. E. Edmonds

Keywords

Diabetes mellitus
Diabetic foot
Hypercalcaemia
Hyperglycaemia
Hyperparathyroidism
Hypocalcaemia
Hypoglycaemia
Insulin-dependent diabetes
Metabolic bone disease
Neuropathy in diabetes
Non-insulin-dependent diabetes
Obesity
Osteomalacia
Osteoporosis
Paget's disease
Renal osteodystrophy
Retinopathy in diabetes
Rickets
Treatment of insulin-dependent diabetes
Treatment of non-insulin-dependent diabetes
Vascular disease in diabetes

Metabolic disorders have a considerable importance with regard to public health and may result in significant disease to the foot. They include diabetes, obesity and metabolic bone disorders, and in this chapter practical aspects that affect the general care of patients as well as the foot will be considered.

DIABETES MELLITUS

The manifestations of diabetes result from a persistently raised blood glucose level as a consequence of reduced production and/or impaired effectiveness of insulin.

Diabetes can be divided into two main groups:

insulin-dependent (IDDM) and *non-insulin-dependent* (NIDDM) diabetes. In addition, there is a small group of *secondary diabetes*.

Insulin-dependent diabetes

Insulin-dependent diabetes (IDDM) indicates that there is almost a complete lack of effective insulin, and in the absence of insulin treatment these patients will usually progress to diabetic ketoacidosis. Most of these patients are children and young people of less than 30 years of age, although it is important to note that IDDM can present in middle age and in the elderly.

IDDM results from damage to the pancreatic beta cells, and genetic, immunologic and probably environmental (e.g. viral) factors are involved, which lead eventually to total destruction of the beta cell. The important genetic risk factor for the development of IDDM is the HLA genes found on the short arm of the sixth chromosome. Two HLA types, DR3 and DR4, are common in patients with IDDM, and these predispose to an immune process which is active at the onset of the disease. Lymphocytes infiltrate the islets of Langerhans, and antibodies against islet cells are present in the sera of 80% of insulin-dependent diabetic patients. There may be certain trigger events, such as viral infections, which precipitate this series of reactions. An increased prevalence of newly diagnosed IDDM has been found in children aged 4–6 and 11–14 years. These coincide with entry to primary and secondary school.

Non-insulin-dependent diabetes

In 25% of cases, a first degree relative has non-insulin-dependent diabetes (NIDDM), and virtually all identical twins of NIDDM patients develop the disease, even if brought up in different environments. In NIDDM, there is a relative, but not an absolute, lack of insulin. Peripheral tissue becomes insulin-resistant, i.e. less sensitive to the effects of insulin.

Patients are usually older than 40 years at diagnosis and are often obese but may have relatively few symptoms. They do not develop ketoacidosis. These patients have normal or increased levels of insulin, but this is associated with relative ineffectiveness of insulin at the cellular level. However, NIDDM patients may nevertheless receive insulin therapy, and indeed, up to 25% of patients do so simply to control their blood glucose. They do not need insulin for survival. However, in certain stressful reactions such as infection and coronary thrombosis, NIDDM patients may also require insulin therapy.

Secondary diabetes

Secondary diabetes occurs when there is direct damage, removal or impairment of action of the mass of beta cells. This type of diabetes is uncommon but causes of a beta cell deficit include:

1. severe malnutrition
2. pancreatic destruction—carcinoma of the pancreas, pancreatitis, cystic fibrosis, haemochromatosis, pancreatectomy
3. antagonism to action of insulin—Cushing's disease, acromegaly or pheochromocytoma
4. drug-induced causes of glucose intolerance— thiazide diuretics, steroid therapy.

Gestational diabetes is impaired glucose tolerance that occurs in pregnancy.

Diagnosis

Diagnosis of diabetes is made on finding a random blood glucose of more than 11 mmol/l. The standard oral glucose tolerance test is rarely required to establish the diagnosis, although the accepted values of capillary blood glucose of a 75 G glucose load to diagnose diabetes is greater than 7 mmol/l fasting and greater than or equal to 11 mmol/l at 2 hours.

Clinical features

The classical symptoms are thirst, polyuria and weight loss combined with pruritus vulvae or balanitis. The intensity of symptoms varies greatly; they tend to be more severe or more acute in IDDM than in NIDDM. The lack of insulin leads initially to hyperglycaemia, and when the glucose concentration in blood reaches a level of 10 mmol/l, the glucose exceeds the tubular reabsorptive capacity and glycosuria results.

In states of severe insulin deficiency, glucose has to be obtained by metabolising amino acids from the breakdown of proteins in a process called gluconeogenesis. Increased breakdown of fat also occurs with the formation of ketone bodies, including acetone, which leads to severe metabolic acidosis, so-called ketoacidotic coma.

The duration of symptoms in IDDM is usually a few weeks. This can lead to wasting and physical weakness, and eventually to vomiting and dehydration. Insulin is needed urgently, and if not given, ketoacidosis will develop, presenting as drowsiness, dehydration and over-breathing (together with acetone in the breath). These are the clinical features of ketoacidosis, which requires urgent admission to hospital and insulin therapy.

The presentation of NIDDM is generally less acute. Patients sometimes complain of only one of the classic symptoms. Symptoms develop over variable periods, frequently over several weeks or months. An increasing number of patients are found to have diabetes at routine screening examinations of either urine or blood. Some older NIDDM patients present for the first time because of diabetic complications. Foot sepsis or ulceration presenting as an emergency almost always indicates a diagnosis of diabetes.

Treatment of insulin-dependent diabetes

IDDM results from the complete absence of insulin, and this can be treated effectively by the replacement of that insulin. Human insulin, commonly prepared by genetic manipulation of yeast, is now used by the majority of patients. Insulin is prepared in four forms: as soluble insulin, isophane (protamine linked) insulin, insulin zinc suspensions and as ready-mixed combinations. The last of these include mixtures of soluble and medium- or long-acting insulins in different proportions. Many are now available in cartridges to fit the several available pen injection devices.

Regular amounts of carbohydrate at fixed times are important in insulin treatment, to reduce the swings of blood glucose and in particular to avoid hypoglycaemia. Thus, the importance of snacks mid-morning, mid-afternoon and before bedtime should be emphasised. During infection or illness, the blood glucose tends to increase. Insulin needs to be increased at these times, particularly when patients stop eating or are vomiting, because hepatic production of glucose in itself often leads to significant hyperglycaemia.

Stress-related 'resistance' to insulin, and the consequent increase in hepatic release of glucose, explains why insulin requirements in the sick patient will be the same or even greater than normal, even if the patient is not eating. One must maintain an adequate fluid and calorie intake with appropriate insulin, all monitored by regular blood glucose measurements.

Treatment of non-insulin-dependent diabetes

Treatment of NIDDM consists of lowering of insulin requirements, together with the use of agents such as sulphonylureas that can increase beta cell production of insulin, biquanides to modify glucose output, and acarbose to reduce the rates of glucose absorption.

Thus, there are three measures available for treatment: diet, hypoglycaemic agents and insulin.

Diet is the cornerstone of treatment, and elimination of simple rapidly absorbed sugars is the minimum necessary requirement. Furthermore, for overweight patients, energy supply must be restricted in order to reduce to ideal weight; 50% of the calorie intake should be from carbohydrates and not more than 35% from fats.

Hypoglycaemia

In the diabetic, a fall in glucose to symptomatic levels represents a temporary mismatch of insulin level to intestinal glucose uptake: a meal may have been missed or delayed, a dose of insulin mismeasured, or unusual exertion undertaken. Symptoms vary from diabetic to diabetic, but remain fairly consistent within the individual.

Patients may experience symptoms of hypoglycaemia when the blood glucose is less than 3 mmol/l, although some who have lost their warning symptoms may pass below this threshold. Others who have suffered previously poor control may be aware of hypoglycaemia at slightly higher levels. With increasing age and duration of diabetes, especially in those who keep their diabetes tightly controlled, there is an increasing tendency towards loss or warning hypoglycaemia.

Symptoms fall into two groups: sympathetic symptoms from activation of the sympathetic nervous system in response to hypoglycaemia; and neuroglycopaenic symptoms which result from a reduction of glucose supply to the brain.

Early warning sympathetic symptoms are shaking, trembling, sweating and pins and needles in the tongue and lips.

Mild neuroglycopaenic symptoms are double vision, difficulty in concentrating, and slurring of speech. Moderate symptoms are confusion, change in behaviour and truculence, and late symptoms are epileptic fits, especially in children, hemiplegia in the elderly and unconsciousness.

Treatment can be as simple as persuading the diabetic to take sugar in some form. If the patient is conscious, then oral glucose as a drink, tablet or gel can be used. The following items contain 10 g of carbohydrate: Lucozade 60 ml, Ribena 15 ml, Coke (not diet) 80 ml. To prevent relapse of hypoglycaemia, this should be followed by more slowly absorbed carbohydrate such as biscuits or sandwiches. The unconscious patient should be placed in the recovery position with the airway maintained, and should be treated with intravenous glucose, usually 20–50 of 50% glucose. If the response is not immediate, then a further dose should be given after 5 minutes, followed by an infusion of 10% glucose.

If intravenous access cannot be obtained, then intramuscular glucagon (1 mg) can be given. When oral hypoglycaemics are the cause of hypoglycaemia, the patient should be admitted to hospital, as these agents can continue to cause hypoglycaemia for up to 48 hours.

COMPLICATIONS AND CONTROL OF DIABETES

Diabetic patients may develop a variety of complications, which include microvascular disease (retinopathy and nephropathy), nervous system abnormalities and macrovascular disease (coronary, peripheral vascular and cerebral vascular disease). It is now known that sustained optimal diabetic control in young insulin-dependent diabetic patients delays the onset and retards the progress of diabetic complications.

Retinopathy, nephropathy and neuropathy are reduced by 35–70%, as demonstrated in the Diabetic Control and Complications Trial (DCCT 1996) in the USA, which compared the effects of tight control with conventional control in 1441 patients. However, hypoglycaemia was three times more common in the tight control group compared with conventional treatments. With regard to macrovascular disease, there is no definite evidence that controlling diabetes can alter the course of the disease.

The microvascular and neurological complications of IDDM are rarely seen before 5–7 years' duration and occur most commonly after 10–20 years. However, in NIDDM patients, 20% have evidence of complications at diagnosis.

Eye disease

Diabetes is the most common cause of blindness under the age of 65 in the UK. Ten percent of diabetic patients who have had retinopathy for 40 years or more become blind, while many more have impaired vision. Eye complications include:

1. Cataracts, which occur earlier and with increased frequency, probably related to repeated osmotic damage of the lens. Cataracts have an increased prevalence in adult diabetics with three- to fourfold increased risk in the age range 50–64 years, with excess risk decreasing in later years.
2. There are transient refractive changes with blurring of vision, which occurs when blood glucose levels are rapidly altered.
3. Retinopathy is a consequence of the microvascular damage, partly ischaemic. This can be divided into background and proliferative retinopathy.

Background retinopathy

There is increased capillary permeability. Dilatation of retinal veins is the earliest recognisable sign. Microaneurysms looking like red dots then develop over the retina and may involve the macula. Haemorrhages, which are large and more irregular in shape than microaneurysms, then occur. Large haemorrhages may extend into the vitreous humour. Hard exudates are yellow-white discrete particles of lipid which can occur in rings around leaking capillaries. They can cause blindness when they develop on the macula and are more common in NIDDM.

Proliferative retinopathy

Proliferative retinopathy reflects capillary nonperfusion. There is new vessel formation, often near the disc, with venous irregularity, cluster haemorrhages and cotton wool spots. Haemorrhages into the vitreous cause sudden blindness, and are followed by fibrosis, leading to retinal detachment. New vessels are treated with laser photocoagulation.

Kidney disease

While insulin-dependent diabetes is responsible for the majority of cases under 50 years of age, there are now more patients with NIDDM in end-stage renal failure, especially in the non-white populations. The development of proteinuria, indicative of nephropathy, is a serious prognostic factor, anticipating not only a decline in renal function but also an increase in cardiovascular disease.

The clinical hallmark of diabetic nephropathy is persistent proteinuria, which is defined as a 24-hour urinary excretion of 500 mg or more of protein on at least three occasions over at least 6 months. An earlier stage, microalbuminuria or incipient nephropathy, is associated with lower levels of albumin excretion. Eighty percent of these patients progress to overt proteinuria. Regular measurement of blood pressure in these patients is crucial and effectively produces progression of renal damage. Renal support treatment is now well established for diabetic patients, comprising dialysis—usually chronic ambulatory peritoneal dialysis (CAPD)—and renal transplantation.

Neuropathy

Peripheral nerves re prone to several different types of damage in dia etes (Watkins 1992), and there are thus highly distin tive syndromes. These include:

1. the common symmetrical sensory neuropathy associated with autonomic neuropathy, which progresses slowly
2. acutely painful neuropathies and mononeuropathies which have a relatively acute presentation and normally recover
3. pressure palsies (especially carpal tunnel syndrome, ulnar nerve compression and lateral popliteal nerve palsy)
4. autonomic neuropathy.

A classification of diabetic neuropathies is summarised in Table 25.1.

Symmetrical sensory and autonomic neuropathy

This is a very common condition affecting 11–50% of diabetic patients, depending on the criteria used or the population selected. Neuropathy is always diffuse and symmetrical (stocking distribution), probably starting with involvement of the smallest fibres (pain, temperature, autonomic) and sometimes but not always progressing to involve all nerve fibre types.

Small non-medullated nerve fibres are the first to be affected and this gives rise to some of the characteristic features of diabetic neuropathy. This small-fibre degeneration leads to loss of pain and temperature sensory modalities, with associated autonomic features, and in these early stages other sensory modalities can remain intact, notably light touch sensation. Early neuropathy is frequently not detected in the clinic because temperature and pain sensation are difficult to assess. Sympathetic failure causes loss of sweating

Table 25.1 Classification of diabetic neuropathies

Progressive	Symmetrical sensory polyneuropathy and autonomic neuropathy
Reversible	Acute painful neuropathies, radiculopathies and mononeuropathies (including proximal motor neuropathy/femoral neuropathy and diabetic amyotrophy)
Pressure palsies	Carpal tunnel syndrome Ulnar nerve depression Foot drops

and denervation of peripheral vessels, leading to vascular rigidity and calcification, with a very high peripheral blood flow, chiefly from opening of arteriovenous anastomoses. These blood flow changes can occur quite early in the course of diabetes, but need sophisticated techniques for their detection.

Small-fibre neuropathies sometimes progress as a selective entity in some patients, leading to symptomatic autonomic neuropathy (causing diarrhoea, gastroparesis, orthostatic hypotension, impotence, neurogenic bladder, gustatory sweating and other problems), often associated with Charcot joints (Stevens et al 1992). These patients sometimes develop iritis as well, and there is some evidence that immune mechanisms may be involved. On the other hand, in some patients, neuropathy progresses to involve all nerve fibre types, and in the worst cases the feet and lower legs become anaesthetic. Major motor involvement is surprisingly uncommon even in the severest cases.

The evolution of sensory and autonomic diabetic neuropathy is extremely slow and very variable, occurring over many years, with the increasing age of the patient and duration of diabetes. It never remits. Study is further complicated by differential rate of progression of the different fibre types and there are only a few observations over periods of 5–10 years.

Neuropathies which recover mononeuropathies, radiculopathies and acute painful neuropathies

Painful neuropathies in diabetes have highly characteristic features, which include constant 'burning', paraesthesiae and shooting pains, together with exquisite contact discomfort caused by clothes and bedclothes. The pains are continuous day and night and cause severe insomnia. They are accompanied by profound weight loss. They occur either in a symmetrical sensory stocking distribution affecting both feet, or they may be confined to a single or adjacent group of nerve roots affecting feet and/or legs, or to one or both thighs, often but not always accompanied by wasting and sometimes debilitating weakness, causing falls. The latter syndrome is known as proximal motor neuropathy, femoral neuropathy or diabetic amyotrophy and is due to either radiculopathy or femoral neuropathy. All of these conditions normally recover in 6–18 months.

Neurological examination of the feet in cases of symmetrical painful neuropathy can be confusing, since abnormalities range from severe sensory neuropathy with major deficits in all modalities (the 'painless painful foot'), to an almost complete lack of neurological abnormalities. This makes assessment and diagnosis of this condition very complex.

Pressure palsies

Median nerve compression in the carpal tunnel syndrome (usually bilateral) may occur in up to 10% of patients. Diagnosis may be difficult in diabetic patients with severe polyneuropathy involving the hands. EMG studies are necessary to measure conduction in the median nerves. Treatment is by surgical decompression. Ulnar nerve compression is less frequent, but again should be investigated by conduction studies. Patients should be advised not to lean on their elbows.

Symptomatic autonomic neuropathy

Autonomic function declines with age in the same way that peripheral nerve conduction progressively slows through life. Deterioration of neurological function is accelerated in diabetes, although this decline is not uniform. Thus, in some patients it is scarcely different from normal, while in others it is accelerated to the point of severe symptomatic autonomic neuropathy (AN), which is associated with an increased mortality. Symptomatic AN is surprisingly uncommon compared to the extremely common finding of abnormal autonomic function tests which can be demonstrated in any diabetic population (Edmonds & Watkins 1994).

Symptoms. Numerous symptoms can be ascribed to diabetic autonomic neuropathy. Dysfunction may be present in the cardiovascular system, causing postural hypotension, and in the gastrointestinal system, causing severe uncontrollable diarrhoea. In the genitourinary system, difficulty with micturition and impotence are important symptoms. A classical symptom of autonomic neuropathy is gustatory sweating, i.e. sweating in the upper third of the body provoked by eating cheese or spicy food.

The presence of autonomic neuropathy may be confirmed by abnormalities in standard autonomic function tests.

Diagnosis. Loss of heart rate variability during deep breathing is the most reliable and simplest test of autonomic neuropathy. It is best assessed using a cardiotachograph during deep respirations (six breaths per minute), taking average readings during six breaths; it can be performed using an ordinary electrocardiograph during a single deep breath (5 seconds in, 5 seconds out). The heart rate difference (maximum rate during inspiration minus minimum rate during expiration) in the under 55s is always greater than 10. Heart rate increase on standing up should be greater than 12 at 15 seconds, and there should normally be an overshoot as well. The Valsalva manoeuvre can be included among the tests; a mercury sphygmomanometer is used, the patient blowing hard through the empty barrel of a 20 ml syringe to maintain the mercury column at 40 mm for 10 seconds. Maximum heart rate during blowing, followed by minimum heart rate after cessation are recorded. There should be a bradycardia after cessation of blowing. The ratio of maximum to minimum heart rate is normally greater than 1.21, and is clearly abnormal when less than 1.10.

Vascular disease

Major arterial disease affecting the coronary circulation, cerebral arteries and causing peripheral vascular disease of feet and legs may represent the most serious of the problems. The prevalence is higher in a diabetic than a non-diabetic population, but it is much greater in those patients who develop proteinuria from diabetic nephropathy. Three-quarters of diabetic patients diagnosed over 60 years of age die from cardiovascular disease, chiefly from myocardial infarction. The proportion is even higher amongst those with nephropathy. Other risk factors are well known, namely smoking, hypertension, hyperlipidaemia and obesity.

The clinical features of major arterial disease are very similar to those in non-diabetic patients, but the following differences should be noted:

- Atheromatous arterial disease has a tendency to a more peripheral distribution in diabetes, especially in the legs, but probably in the coronary vessels as well. Distal lesions are not always amenable to manipulation by angioplasty or arterial surgery, but nonetheless, proximal lesions are still common and often treatable. Diabetic patients should be offered these treatments using exactly the same criteria as those used for non-diabetics.

- Medial arterial calcification (Monckeberg's sclerosis) of distal arteries is a feature of diabetes, and becomes much commoner in those with severe neuropathy. This may result from a medial degeneration in sympathetically denervated vessels. Calcification is further increased and more distal in its distribution in nephropathy patients. Calcified vessels become more rigid than normal, although the effects on blood flow are uncertain (Faris et al 1992).

- Symptomless myocardial infarction is more common in a diabetic population. The presence of autonomic neuropathy is thought to be responsible for the absence of chest pain, but the evidence is conflicting. Mortality in acute myocardial infarction is doubled in diabetic patients.

THE DIABETIC FOOT

The foot in diabetes can be affected by neuropathies and circulatory changes with or without additional problems from trauma and infection, causing potentially serious foot problems (Edmonds & Foster 1994). The clinical abnormalities affecting the lower limb are thus diverse, ranging from permanent abnormalities and symptoms in the feet to the crippling but reversible disorders due to mononeuropathy (proximal motor neuropathy), causing a painful wasting disease of the thigh. A summary of potential disorders affecting the leg is shown in Table 25.2.

The feet are the target of peripheral neuropathy, leading chiefly to sensory deficit and autonomic dysfunction. Ischaemia results from atherosclerosis of the leg vessels, which in the diabetic is often bilateral, multisegmental and distal, involving arteries below the knee. Infection is rarely a sole factor but often complicates neuropathy and ischaemia. Nevertheless, it is responsible for considerable tissue necrosis in the diabetic foot.

For practical purposes, the diabetic foot can be divided into two entities: the neuropathic foot, in which neuropathy predominates and there is a good circulation; and the neuroischaemic foot, where there is both neuropathy and absence of foot pulses. The purely ischaemic foot, with no concomitant neuropathy, is rarely seen in diabetic patients and its management is the same as for the neuroischaemic foot.

The neuropathic foot results in a warm, numb, dry and usually painless foot in which the pulses are palpable. It leads to three complications—the neuropathic ulcer, which is found mainly on the sole of the foot; the neuropathic (Charcot) foot; and, rarely, neuropathic oedema. In contrast, the neuroischaemic foot is cool and the pulses are absent. It is complicated by rest pain, ulceration on the margins of the foot from localised pressure necrosis, and gangrene.

The neuropathic foot

Neuropathic ulcer

Neuropathic ulcers result from noxious stimuli, unperceived by the patient because of loss of pain sensation and causing mechanical, thermal and chemical injuries. This characteristically occurs at sites of high mechanical pressure on the plantar surface of the foot. The presence of neuropathy (even in its earliest stage, with relatively mild sensory defects) may itself disturb the posture of the foot and so predispose to local increases in pressure, which are also commonly caused by deformities such as claw or hammer toes, pes cavus, Charcot joints and previous ray amputations. The high vertical and shear forces under the plantar surface of the metatarsal heads and toes lead to the formation of callosities, of which the patient is often unaware. Repetitive mechanical forces lead to inflammatory autolysis and subkeratotic haematomas, which eventually break through to the skin surface, forming an ulcer. Direct mechanical injuries to the plantar surface result from treading on nails and other sharp objects. However, the most frequent cause of ulceration brought about by mechanical factors is the neglected callosity.

Complications of ulceration. Ulcers can become infected by staphylococci, streptococci, coliforms and anaerobic bacteria. If untreated, cellulitis can develop, with tracking of infection to involve underlying tendons, bones and joints. Staphylococci and streptococci act synergistically when they are present together: streptococci produce hyaluronidase which facilitates spread of necrotising toxins from the staphylococci.

In the deep tissues of the foot, aerobic organisms act synergistically with microaerophilic or anaerobic organisms, leading to necrotising infection, the production of subcutaneous gas and, finally, gangrene.

Management of ulceration. Excess callous tissue should be 'pared' away with a scalpel by the podiatrist to expose the floor of the ulcer and allow efficient drainage of the lesion. The next step is to take a bacteriological swab from the floor of the ulcer and, according to the organisms isolated, prescribe the appropriate oral antibiotics until the ulcer has healed (e.g. amoxy-

Table 25.2 Leg abnormalities in diabetes

	Neuropathy	Ischaemia
Symptoms	None Paraesthesiae Pain Oedema Painful wasted thigh Foot drop	None Claudication Rest pain
Structural damage	Ulcer Sepsis Abscess Osteomyelitis Digital gangrene Charcot joints	Ulcer Sepsis Gangrene

cillin, 500 mg t.d.s., for streptococcal infections; flucloxacillin, 500 mg q.d.s., for staphylococcal sepsis; metronidazole, 400 mg t.d.s., for anaerobic infections; and ciprofloxacin, 500 mg b.d. for Gram-negative infections). If the ulcer is superficial and there is no cellulitis, treatment can take place on an out-patient basis.

Redistribution of weight-bearing forces on vulnerable parts of the foot should be attempted using special footwear, such as moulded insoles with energy-absorbing properties, e.g. plastozote and microcellular rubber. Special shoes may be needed to accommodate the shape of the foot. In cases of severe deformity, it is necessary to construct shoes individually for the patient. However, in most patients, extra depth 'stock' shoes will usually suffice (Chantelau & Leisch 1994).

In the case of large indolent ulcers, total contact plaster casts may be used which conform to all the contours of the foot thereby reducing shear forces on the plantar surface (Mueller et al 1989). Great care must be taken, especially with the fitting of plasters, to prevent chafing and subsequent ulcer formation elsewhere on the foot or ankle.

If cellulitis or skin discolouration is present, the limb is threatened and urgent hospital admission should be arranged. After blood cultures have been taken, intravenous antibiotics are administered to treat possible staphylococci, streptococci, Gram-negative bacteria and anaerobes (flucloxacillin, 500 mg i.v. 6-hourly; amoxycillin, 500 mg i.v. 8-hourly; ceftazidine, 1 g i.v. 8-hourly; and metronidazole, 1 g per rectum 8-hourly). This antibiotic regimen may need revision after the results of bacterial cultures are available. If the toe complicated by ulceration becomes necrotic, then the patient should undergo digital or ray amputation (which includes the metatarsal head). Such wounds usually heal extremely well in the neuropathic foot (see also Ch. 9).

Neuropathic (Charcot's) joint

The precipitating event for a neuropathic joint is usually a minor traumatic episode, such as tripping, which results in a swollen, erythematous, hot and sometimes painful foot. Initially, radiographs are likely to be normal, but subsequently, serial radiographs show evidence of bony fracture, osteolysis, fragmentation, new bone formation, subluxation and joint disorganisation.

This destructive process often takes place over only a few months, and can lead to considerable deformity of the foot. The metatarsal–tarsal joints are most commonly involved (Sanders & Frykberg 1991).

Early diagnosis is essential. The initial presentation of unilateral warmth and swelling in a neuropathic foot is extremely suggestive of a developing Charcot's joint. Bone scans are more sensitive indicators of new bone formation than radiography and should be used to confirm the diagnosis.

Management. This comprises immobilisation of the injured part. This can be achieved by non-weight-bearing, using crutches or a total contact plaster cast, and the immobilisation is continued until the oedema and local warmth have resolved. The foot should then be gradually mobilised using a moulded insole in a special shoe. Recently, bisphosphonates have been used to inhibit osteoclastic activity, leading to a reduction in foot temperature and resolution of symptoms.

Neuropathic oedema

Neuropathic oedema consists of swelling of the feet and lower legs associated with severe peripheral neuropathy; it is extremely uncommon.

Ephedrine, 30 mg t.d.s., has been shown to be useful by reducing peripheral blood flow and increasing renal excretion of sodium.

The neuroischaemic foot

Pathogenesis

The neuroischaemic foot results from atherosclerosis of the vessels of the leg, with neuropathy predisposing it to minor trauma. In diabetic patients, atherosclerosis is multisegmental, bilateral and distal, often involving the popliteal, the tibial and the peroneal arteries.

Presentation

The clinical features of ischaemia are intermittent claudication, rest pain, ulceration and gangrene. However, the most frequent symptom is ulceration. The ulcers present as areas of necrosis, often surrounded by a rim of erythema. In contrast to ulceration in the neuropathic foot, callous tissue is usually absent. Furthermore, ulceration in the ischaemic foot is often painful, although this varies from patient to patient according to the coexistence of a peripheral neuropathy. In the ischaemic foot, the most frequent sites of ulceration are the tips of the toes, the medial surface of the head of the first metatarsal, the lateral surface of the fifth metatarsal head and the heel.

Management

Medical management is indicated if the ulcer is small and shallow and is of recent onset, within the previous month. Ischaemic ulcers may be painful and it may be necessary to prescribe opiates. It is the role of the podiatrist to remove necrotic tissue from the ulcers and, in the case of subungual ulcers, to cut back the nail to allow drainage of the ulcer. Ulcer swabs are taken as with the neuropathic foot and the ulcers are cleaned with normal saline and dressed with a sterile non-adherent dressing. It is important to eradicate infection with prompt and specific antibiotic therapy after consultation with the microbiologist. However, severe sepsis in the ischaemic foot is an indication for emergency admission, first, to control sepsis by intravenous antibiotics and surgical debridement and, secondly, to assess the possibility of revascularisation by either angioplasty or reconstruction. Footwear should be supplied to accommodate the foot, and in most cases an extra depth ready-made shoe to protect the borders of the foot is adequate, unless there is severe deformity, when bespoke shoes will be needed. If any lesion, however small and trivial, in the pulseless foot has not responded to conservative treatment within 4 weeks, then the patient should be considered for arteriography and revascularisation.

One of the most important advances over the last 10 years has been the development of new techniques of revascularisation of the diabetic foot. Patients with relatively localised disease, for example, stenosis or short (<10 cm) occlusions, often do well with angioplasty, particularly in the iliac, superficial femoral and popliteal arteries. However, diabetic patients often have lesions in the calf arteries, but recent advances in catheter techniques and imaging have made it possible to perform angioplasty in these arteries, although the long-term results are still under review. Given the same lesion, a diabetic patient will do equally well as a non-diabetic following femoral popliteal angioplasty, assuming equality of other factors such as inflow and outflow.

Diabetes is not a contraindication to arterial bypass in the leg, and distal bypass to either the tibial or peroneal vessels is often necessary to restore pulsatile blood flow to the diabetic foot, which is vital in cases of severe sepsis and necrosis.

There is a different approach to digital necrosis or gangrene in the ischaemic foot compared with the neuropathic foot. If it is possible to improve the circulation by arterial reconstruction, then digital amputation can be performed in the ischaemic foot. However, if it is not feasible to improve the circulation, then amputation of a necrotic toe should not be performed. It is unlikely to heal. However, successful auto-amputation, in which the necrotic digit drops off to reveal a healed stump, can occur as long as infection is controlled and there is regular debridement by the podiatrist along the demarcation line.

OBESITY

Excess of body fat can only be measured indirectly, and the commonest assessment is weight in relation to height and age. The body mass index (BMI) is commonly used and equals weight (in kg) over height (in metres) and the normal range is up to 25. Genetic, environmental and socio-economic factors are important in the aetiology of obesity. Rarely, endocrine diseases such as hypothyroidism and Cushing's syndrome may be a direct cause of obesity.

Obesity in the human species is a disorder of intake. In animal studies, a defect in thermogenesis has been identified in brown fat cells which limits the ability of these animals to burn off calories, although these findings have not been confirmed in humans. Obese subjects exhibit not low, but high, metabolic rates associated with the extra work involved in the operation of a heavier body mass. They often have a reduced perception of their calorie intake.

Major long-term health hazards of obesity are those affecting the cardiovascular system, including hypertension and coronary artery disease. Osteoarthritis is a very common condition in obese individuals. Excess weight imposes a severe burden on individuals with respiratory disease, and in simple obesity one of the most frequent complaints is breathlessness on mild exertion. Back ache is also common and is induced by ligamentous strain.

Obesity is often linked with increased risk of morbidity and mortality, although when it is considered as an independent variable, obesity itself is of little significance. It is mainly because of its association with risk factors such as hyperlipidaemia, hyperglycaemia, hypertension, hyperuricaemia and lack of exercise that obesity is important.

Specific disorders associated with obesity, such as myxoedema and Cushing's syndrome, should be searched for and treated. However, the cornerstone of treatment is to reduce the calorie intake to below expenditure.

Crash diets may induce severe metabolic disturbances and even cardiac arrest, but their effects are not permanent. The aim of treatment is to achieve a healthy and enjoyable pattern of eating, with the patient in control of her weight reduction. Rapport also is important to improve compliance, and initially weight reduction targets should be modest.

Medical treatments to decrease appetite have a limited role. The most commonly used drugs are diethyl-proprion and fenfluramine. The latter acts on the serotoninergic system. None of the drugs should be given long-term. They should be withdrawn slowly.

There are more radical approaches, such as intestinal bypass, gastric stapling, gastric balloons, wiring of the jaws, prolonged behavioural courses and surgical removal of excess adipose tissue. However, these are not without dangers.

METABOLIC BONE DISEASE

A brief account of bone metabolism will be given and the clinical features of hyper- and hypocalcaemia will be described, followed by short accounts of osteomalacia and rickets, hyperparathyroidism, renal osteodystrophy and Paget's disease.

Bone and calcium metabolism

The connective tissue matrix of bone, the osteoid, consists of collagen fibres in a polysaccharide ground substance. The osteoid is made rigid by the deposition of mineral, mainly of crystalline bone salts of calcium phosphate and carbonate. The mineralisation of osteoid is dependent partly on the chemical concentration at the tissue surface of calcium, phosphate and hydrogen ions, and of the enzyme alkaline phosphatase, and partly on the activity of osteocytes comprising osteoclasts and osteoblasts. Parathormone (PTH) and calcitonin strongly affect the osteoclasts and osteoblasts, and vitamin D acts especially on the chemical environment.

Hormonal physiology

PTH is synthesised in the parathyroid glands and is the main factor in calcium homeostasis. Its secretion increases when calcium levels fall, and it stimulates release from bone and calcium reabsorption by the kidney. Calcitonin is secreted by parafollicular cells (C-cells) of the thyroid gland. When infused at high levels, it diminishes plasma calcium by reducing the rate of osteoclastic resorption of bone and increasing

urinary excretion. Vitamin D, in its active form, influences calcium and phosphate flux in bone, kidney and intestine. Over 90% of the parent hormone is synthesised in the skin, and the level of the critical highly active form $1,25(OH)_2 D_3$ is directly influenced by the concentration of calcium ion and PTH.

HYPERCALCAEMIA

The commonest causes of hypercalcaemia are malignancy and hyperparathyroidism. Any tendency to hypercalcaemia can be aggravated by dehydration, impaired renal function, or circumstances stimulating bone demineralisation such as immobilisation or fracture.

Hypercalcaemia interferes with reabsorption of water by the renal tubules, producing polyuria and causing thirst, eventually producing renal stones. There is decreased neuromuscular excitability, which may lead to general muscular weakness. Decreased excitability also affects smooth muscle, causing constipation. Anorexia and vomiting are also common. Patients with hypercalcaemia may feel generally ill and depressed and may be diagnosed as having some psychological disorder. Calcium deposits may occur at the junction of the cornea and sclera. The deposits have a granular gritty appearance and are associated with increased vascularity. If bone is affected by the primary disease, there may be pain and weakness, perhaps with fractures. Severe hypercalcaemia produces confusion, coma, anuria and death, sometimes through cardiac arrest.

If possible, a specific diagnosis as to the cause of hypercalcaemia should be made, but other general measures are useful as temporary expedients or to achieve symptomatic relief. Rehydration is essential, and diuresis may be further encouraged by the combination of generous intravenous fluid infusion with normal saline and loop diuretics such as frusemide. Steroids (400 mg daily of intravenously infused hydrocortisone or 40–60 mg daily of oral prednisolone) can be effective, especially in malignancy.

HYPOCALCAEMIA

Calcium is an ion of considerable importance in numerous cell systems, but the acute clinical effects of hypocalcaemia and tetany are mainly those of increased neuromuscular excitability, while the long-term effects are mainly ectodermal.

In hypocalcaemia and tetany, there may be peripheral paraesthesia, muscle cramps, epileptic fits, laryngeal spasm in children, occasionally acute hypertension, or psychosis, and the important physical signs, *Chvostek's* and *Trousseau's*.

Chvostek's sign is obtained by tapping over the facial nerve as it emerges from the parotid gland beneath the zygoma. A hemifacial twitch constitutes a positive response. Trousseau's sign is elicited by the application of a cuff to the arm and raising the pressure to above the patient's systolic blood pressure for 3 minutes, by which time the hands should have adopted the classical *'main d'accoucher'* position—wrist and metacarpophalangeal joints flexed and fingers extended.

The signs of long-standing hypocalcaemia may also include a dry, scaly skin; loss of eyelashes, thin eyebrows, patchy alopecia, and scanty axillary and pubic hair; brittleness of nails; (in children) hypoplasia or aplasia of teeth; cataracts; calcification in the basal ganglia; rarely papilloedema; susceptibility to moniliasis, probably due to immune deficiency; and cardiomegaly, with prolonged QT interval on the ECG.

In emergencies, a slow intravenous injection of 10–20 ml of 10% calcium gluconate solution should be instituted until symptoms are relieved or total plasma calcium reaches 1.9 mmol/l.

In the long term, dietary calcium can be supplemented and a vitamin D preparation administered carefully. To avoid overdosage, levels of calcium and phosphate should be monitored, frequently at first, and then at intervals not exceeding 6 months even when the situation is apparently stable. 1-α-hydroxylated derivatives of vitamin D are preferred for their shorter half-life. Usual daily maintenance doses are 1 ug for 1-α-$(OH)D_3$ (alfacalcidol) and $1,25(OH)_2D_3$ (calcitriol).

OSTEOPOROSIS

Osteoporosis is by far the most common metabolic bone disease and is the most difficult to treat. By definition, osteoporosis is the state of less bone being present than is normal for the patient's age and sex. Osteoporosis becomes clinically important only after fracture, but treatment of the disorder after the onset of fractures is less than satisfactory, with prevention being a more effective approach.

Although osteoporosis does occur commonly in the foot and ankle after injury, often to a severe degree, the two forms encountered most often are the senile and the related postmenopausal osteoporosis. Osteoporosis is related to an inequality between the rates of osteoblastic accretion of new bone and osteoclastic removal of old bone. Although the spine and proximal femur are the sites of the most significant fractures in osteoporosis, the foot and ankle are frequent sites for

fractures in an osteoporotic patient. Toe and metatarsal fractures are very common. However, a bone with osteoporosis is not deficient in its response to fracture repair, and thus usually a very active osteoblastic response leads to adequate fracture callus.

A patient with osteoporosis may present for the first time with an injury to the foot, without a prior diagnosis of osteoporosis having been reached. Usually osteoporosis is a diagnosis of exclusion, and osteomalacia, renal pathology and hyperparathyroidism should be excluded by screening for serum calcium, phosphorus and alkaline phosphatase, although the last of these may be slightly increased following fracture (especially of long bones).

The aim of therapy is to reduce the rate of bone loss by adequate calcium intake, female hormone replacement therapy (which prevents menopausal bone loss), regular physical exercise and a diet with a daily intake of 1–1.5 g calcium per day (one pint of milk contains approximately 750 mg of calcium).

OSTEOMALACIA AND RICKETS

Osteomalacia and rickets are conditions in which there is defective mineralisation of the matrix of bone. In rickets, the defect is present in infancy and childhood. Osteomalacia is the adult counterpart of rickets. In children, rickets is rarely seen until the patient is over 1 year old when he presents with abnormal patterns of bone modelling, epiphyseal growth and dentition. Rickets is rarely seen in children today because of the addition of vitamin D to milk.

There are many causes of osteomalacia (and rickets), some of which are very rare. They may be divided into three main groups: nutritional, malabsorptive and renal. Nutritional causes follow from lack of vitamin D by deficient synthesis in the skin or low dietary intake. Malabsorption of vitamin D occurs in coeliac disease, gastric surgery, bowel resection and biliary cirrhosis. With regard to the kidney, osteomalacia and rickets can follow from renal glomerular failure as well as renal tubular failure. The effects of renal glomerular failure on the skeleton are complex and are termed renal osteodystrophy, with excessive bone resorption, defective bone mineralisation and in some cases osteoporosis (see below). Many renal tubular disorders also lead to osteomalacia.

In the adult, osteomalacia may produce bone and muscle and tenderness, often due to subclinical fractures. In the leg, the presenting symptom may be aching pain adjacent to an affected portion of the tibia. An increased blood flow is indicated by the increased warmth in the anterior leg. Deformity results from weight-bearing and gastrocnemious pulling forces on the tibia when the disease is in its lytic and weakened phase. Patients who have developed bowing of the femurs and tibias can then develop degenerative arthritis of both the ankle and knee joints, due to the abnormal wear on the articular surfaces secondary to the bone deformity.

Rickets is not seen until after the patient is 1 year old, when swelling of the ankles and wrists may be an early physical finding. The earliest clinical symptoms are tiredness and muscular weakness. There is bone pain and pain on movement. Dentition is delayed and the teeth may be deformed and quickly become carious. Swelling and tenderness of distal ends of the radius and ulna are common, and so is the rickety rosary (costochondral swellings). Frontal and parietal bossing of the skull occurs and occipitoparietal flattening may result from the softness of the skull (craniotabes). If the child can stand or walk, bowing of the legs may result from weight-bearing, and kyphoscoliosis may appear. Radiographs show widening and decreased density of the line of calcification next to the metaphysis, with irregularity and concavity of the metaphysis itself. In severe cases, there may be rarefaction with deformities in the shaft of the bone.

Rickets and osteomalacia can always be cured by administering vitamin D or one of its potent derivatives—alfacalcidol or calcitriol. Patients will need a long-term maintenance dosage of one of these derivatives. Surgical correction of deformity is occasionally required.

HYPERPARATHYROIDISM

Hyperparathyroidism may present as a form of osteoporosis with a fracture. Very occasionally, the giant cell tumour seen in association with severe hyperparathyroidism may present as a mass in the tibia. The radiological abnormalities are due to bone resorption by osteoclasts, and subperiosteal resorption of the cortices of phalanges in the feet, as well as the hands, is the early bony abnormality.

RENAL OSTEODYSTROPHY

The skeletal disorders found in chronic renal failure are collectively called renal osteodystrophy and may occur singly or in various combinations. It may develop early in the course of chronic renal disease and may persist after renal transplantation. The main bone changes that occur are osteomalacia, caused by the deficiency of active metabolites of vitamin D, and secondary hypoparathyroidism which is associated with increased retention of phosphate by the kidneys. Retention of phosphate with resulting hypocalcaemia stimulates the parathyroid glands to secrete parathormone, which leads to mobilisation of calcium from bone by osteoclastic resorption. Thus, bony pathology includes hyperparathyroidism with osteitis fibrosa, osteomalacia and decreased availability of vitamin D, calcium and phosphates, osteoporosis, osteonecrosis, osteosclerosis and periosteal new bone formation (a radiographic finding) and extra skeletal calcification.

A further abnormality seen in the steroid-treated renal patients is a vascular necrosis of the talus, often in association with a renal transplant.

Management of renal osteodystrophy is according to the mechanisms involved in the pathogenesis of the disease. Treatment with phosphate-binding agents or a low phosphate diet decreases phosphate retention and prevents progressive secondary hyperparathyroidism and soft tissue calcification. Vitamin D therapy is indicated in hypoparathyroidism and in vitamin D deficiency osteomalacia. Parathyroidectomy is indicated in patients with severe forms of secondary hyperparathyroidism.

PAGET'S DISEASE

Paget's disease is a focal disorder of bone remodelling characterised by excessive osteoclastic resorption. Patients with Paget's disease are usually over the age of 40 years, but the prevalence essentially doubles with every decade over the age of 50.

The clinical features are bone pain, which is probably a result of combined increased vascularity and new bone formation which stretches the periosteum. Degenerative joint disease leads to distortion of the articular surface. The abnormal bone texture allows long bones to bend, and fractures commonly develop on the convex margin. Neurological symptoms may result from involvement of the spine, leading to paraplegia. Neuropathies of the cranial and peripheral nerves may occur secondary to entrapment.

The earliest radiological abnormality in a long bone is resorption of a previously normal cortex. Microscopically, osteoclasts are noted within resorption cavities and this is associated with increased osteoblastic activity, with the formation of new osteotrabeculae adjacent to the site of bone resorption.

Serum alkaline phosphatase is a marker for bone formation and provides a simple method of evaluating a patient over the course of time. Indeed, the detection of Paget's disease may be due to the elevated alkaline phosphatase levels obtained during screening examinations. The urinary excretion of hydroxyproline indicates collagen breakdown, and this level is markedly raised in many patients with Paget's disease, often in association with the degree of elevation of the alkaline phosphatase activity.

The biochemical changes are similar in rickets and osteomalacia. The plasma calcium is usually a little low and occasionally considerably reduced. The plasma phosphate level is low but the alkaline phosphatase is frequently increased.

The treatment of Paget's disease is by drugs that inhibit bone resorption. This is reflected by an early fall in urinary hydroxyproline and then serum alkaline phosphatase. Bisphosphonates act directly on osteoclasts to inhibit resorption of bone. Calcitonin appears to be equally effective but must be administered by injection.

REFERENCES

Chantelau E, Leisch A 1994 Footwear, uses and abuses. In: Boulton A J M, Connor H, Cavanagh P R (eds) The foot in diabetes. John Wiley, Chichester, p 99–108

Diabetes Control and Complications Trial Research Group 1993 Effect of intensive treatment of diabetes on the development and progression of long term complications in insulin dependent diabetes mellitus. New England Journal of Medicine 329: 977–986

Edmonds M E, Foster A V M 1994 Classification and management of neuropathic and neuroischaemic ulcers. In: Boulton A J M, Connor H, Cavanagh P (eds) The foot in diabetes. John Wiley, Chichester, p 109–120

Edmonds M E, Watkins P J 1994 Autonomic neuropathy. In: Marshall S M, Home P D (eds) The diabetes annual. Elsevier, Amsterdam, p 389–405

Faris I B, McCollum P, Mantese V et al 1992 Investigation of the patient with atheroma. In: Bell P R F, Jamieson C W,

Ruckley C V (eds) Surgical management of vascular disease. WB Saunders, London, p 131–196

Mueller M J, Diamond J E, Sinacore D R et al 1989 Total contact casting in treatment of diabetic plantar ulcers. Diabetes Care 12: 384–388

Sanders L J, Frykberg R G 1991 Diabetic neuropathic osteoarthropathy: the Charcot foot. In: Frykberg R G (ed) The high risk foot in diabetes. Churchill Livingstone, New York, p 227–238

Stevens M J, Edmonds M E, Foster A V M, Watkins P J 1992 Selective neuropathy and preserved vascular responses in the diabetic Charcot foot. Diabetologia 35: 148–154

Thomas P K 1992 Diabetic neuropathy: a neurologist's view. In: Treatment of diabetic neuropathy: a new approach. Churchill Livingstone, Edinburgh, p 11–20

Watkins P J 1992 Clinical observations and experiments in diabetic neuropathy. Diabetologia 35: 2–11

FURTHER READING

Kumar P J, Clark M L 1994 Clinical medicine, 3rd edn. Ballière Tindall, London

Ress P J, Trounce J R 1988 A new short textbook of medicine. Hodder and Stoughton, London

Rubinstein D, Wayne D 1991 Lecture notes on clinical medicine. Blackwell Scientific, Oxford

Watkins P J, Drury P L, Howell S 1996 Diabetes and its management. Blackwell Scientific, Oxford

26

Rheumatic diseases

I. Haslock

Keywords

Ankylosing spondylitis
Connective tissue disease
Crohn's disease
Crystal arthritis
Disease modifying antirheumatic drugs
Inflammatory rheumatic diseases
Non-steroidal anti-inflammatory drugs
Osteoarthritis
Podagra
Polyarteritis nodosa
Psoriatic arthritis
Reactive arthritis
Rheumatoid arthritis
    Articular features of rheumatoid arthritis
    Non-articular features of rheumatoid arthritis
Septic arthritis
Seronegative spondarthritides
Systemic lupus erythematosus
Systemic sclerosis
Surgery
Team-working
Treatment of rheumatoid arthritis
Vasculitides
Whipple's disease

The speciality of rheumatology embraces the medical disorders of the locomotor system, including bones, joints, tendons, ligaments, bursae and their attendant connective tissue structures. Rheumatic diseases are common in the population, and it is estimated that more than 8 million people in the UK have arthritis that is sufficiently severe to make an impact on their lives. Rheumatic diseases also form a considerable part of the work of the health service. About one in 15 members of the population consult their general practitioner each year regarding a locomotor disorder, accounting for about one-fifth of all consultations. Referrals to hospital rheumatology departments have risen progressively—one recorded instance in South

Cleveland Hospital, UK showed a fivefold increase over the last 20 years—and many referrals to orthopaedic departments relate to rheumatic disorders, especially soft tissue rheumatism and osteoarthritis. The cost of arthritis to the National Health Service (NHS) is over £500 million, and the total cost of arthritis in the UK, including NHS costs, work loss, costs to individuals and expenditure on research exceeds £1.2 billion.

The feet are commonly involved both in the generalised rheumatic diseases and by local disorders. Especially in the case of inflammatory diseases, it is essential that foot problems are not considered in isolation, but are put in the context of the overall problems and needs of the patient. Although many of the simpler rheumatological problems will be treated in general practice, the greater challenges produced by more severe and extensive inflammatory diseases can only be addressed by a multi-professional team. The full extent of the hospital rheumatology team is shown in Box 26.1, although in practice the rheumatologist, specialist rheumatology nurse, physiotherapist and occupational therapist form the core of the team, with others contributing their expertise as required. Rheumatology nurse specialists have taken on ever expanding roles in the past decade, and are now key members of the team, often carrying responsibility for liaison with other professionals and for much of the vital ongoing liaison within the team.

Box 26.1 The multidisciplinary team

- Appliance officer/orthotist
- Dietician
- Nurse specialist
- Occupational therapist
- Patient and carers
- Pharmacist
- Physiotherapist
- Podiatrist
- Psychologist
- Rheumatologist
- Social worker

Team-working

Although it is now impossible to envisage high-quality rheumatological care without a multidisciplinary team, working within such a team is not easy. Three areas produce particular problems. Firstly, communication must be immaculate and must embrace communication not only with the patient but also among the professionals involved. Unless all are fully informed regarding the information received by each of them, and the therapeutic actions each has undertaken, care will be fragmented and disorganised. Secondly, there must be a clear commonality of aims amongst the professionals involved. There is no point in the podiatrist, physiotherapist and nurse putting enormous effort into encouraging the patient to walk while the occupational therapist is telling the patient that walking will not be possible and teaching the use of a wheelchair. True commonality of aims often requires discussion between team members, and some form of multidisciplinary meeting is an essential part of this process. Thirdly, effective team members must bring an educational approach to their work. This means education of the patient and their carers, and also education of other team members about the changing potential of their own profession. It also implies learning from others what they do and how their contribution to patient care is changing. A team member who is neither teaching colleagues nor learning from them is a substandard resource to the rest of the team. Because of their professional structure, podiatrists have made too small an impact on most rheumatology teams in the past and it is hoped that their closer integration into the specialist setting will enhance the contribution they are able to make in the future, to the ultimate benefit of their colleagues and the patients.

INDIVIDUAL RHEUMATIC DISEASES

These will be considered under four headings:

1. inflammatory arthritis including rheumatoid arthritis and the seronegative spondarthritides
2. diffuse connective tissue diseases including systemic sclerosis and the vasculitides
3. osteoarthritis
4. crystal arthritis and sepsis.

INFLAMMATORY RHEUMATIC DISEASES

Rheumatoid arthritis (RA)

This is the most common and severe of the inflammatory rheumatic diseases. The overall prevalence is about 1% in the adult population, with women outnumbering men by 3:1. There are about 600 000 people with RA in the UK, with the prevalence rising to 5% in women and 2% in men over 55 years of age. However, 50% of cases start before the age of 40. This means that the disease often affects people at the peak of their professional and social development, and the disease has long-term economic and sociological problems as well as purely physical ones.

Pathology

Rheumatoid arthritis is an inflammatory disease of unknown aetiology. Within the joints the inflammation predominantly involves the synovial membrane. There is a dense infiltration of cells, including some polymorphs but mainly lymphocytes and plasma cells, emphasising that this is an immuno-inflammatory process. The initial effect is soft swelling of the joint produced by the synovial thickening and increased production of synovial fluid by the inflamed membrane. This swelling stretches the articular capsule which, being relatively inelastic, tends to remain stretched. As the capsule is involved in maintaining joint stability and alignment, this capsular stretching contributes to later instability and deformity. The inflamed synovial membrane adheres to the joints at their margin, and an outpouring of digestive enzymes, especially the proteases, causes destruction of bone and cartilage, producing the characteristic erosions at the edge of the joint, seen on X-ray in Figure 26.1. In addition, the high concentrations of enzymes in the joint fluid cause cartilage digestion from the surface downwards, visualised on X-ray as joint space narrowing (Fig. 26.2).

The inflammation may involve any or all of the joints in the body. Involvement is usually symmetrical, and the small joints of the hands and feet are the most commonly involved, both at the beginning of the disease and during its course. Although the inflammation may last the patient's lifetime, 80% of those joints which will eventually show evidence of destructive change show some erosion within the first 2 years of the disease.

Although conventionally called an arthritis, the inflammation of rheumatoid disease is not confined to the joints. Similar inflammatory changes occur in tendon sheaths, and muscles are involved by inflammation as well as disuse. Inflammation also occurs in non-locomotor sites such as the pericardium and pleura. Inflammation within the lungs leads to pulmonary fibrosis. Inflammation in blood vessels, rheumatoid vasculitis, may cause lesions varying in severity from small nodular vasculitic lesions to large ulcers and even major tissue loss and gangrene. Rheumatoid nodules are pathegnomonic of rheumatoid arthritis, and tend to occur at points of pressure. Although the classical position is at the elbows, they may also occur in the feet, often causing problems with footwear (Fig. 26.3). Anaemia occurs in 80% of the patients with rheumatoid arthritis, and it is the anaemia of chronic disease which fails to respond to any therapy except control of the underlying inflammatory process.

Diagnosis

Although rheumatoid arthritis is a common disease in the community, new cases are relatively infrequent. The incidence rate is about 36 per 100 000 women and

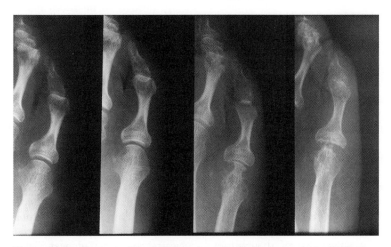

Figure 26.1   Close-up of the little toe of a patient with rheumatoid arthritis at presentation (far left) and after 1, 3 and 5 years (left to right). The proximal phalangeal head has undergone progressive erosive change.

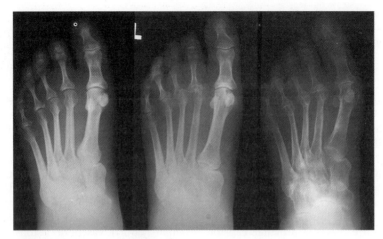

Figure 26.2 X-rays of patient with rheumatoid arthritis taken in 1982 (left), 1984 (centre) and 1986 (right). There is progressive joint space narrowing, joint erosion, subluxation of the joints and osteoporosis.

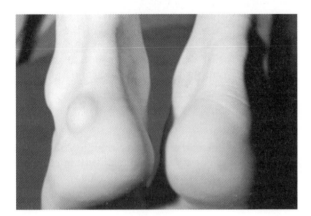

Figure 26.3 Rheumatoid nodule on the left heel, causing difficulty with footwear.

14 per 100 000 men, which means that a general practitioner with a list of 2000 patients will see less than one new case per year on average. The diagnosis is clinical, based on the patient's history of joint pain accompanied by morning stiffness and general fatigue, and the observation of inflammatory joint swelling. Investigations may show anaemia, an elevated erythrocyte sedimentation rate (ESR), plasma viscosity or C-reactive protein, and the presence of rheumatoid factor (RF) in the blood. Rheumatoid factor is an autoantibody found in 80% of patients with rheumatoid arthritis, but also in 7% of the normal population. Although its presence is suggestive of rheumatoid arthritis, it is not diagnostic, and the disease cannot be diagnosed from the presence of RF alone. X-rays of the

hands and feet may show the typical erosions of rheumatoid arthritis, but most rheumatologists would now hope to make the diagnosis, and initiate treatment of the patient, before erosive damage has taken place.

Clinical course

The initial symptoms of pain and stiffness are accompanied by progressive loss of function. This may vary from minor difficulties, such as inability to turn on stiff taps, to total dependence and a wheelchair existence. The ability to use scissors to cut toenails and the dexterity needed to tie shoes may be lost early in the course of the disease.

Rheumatoid arthritis is a disease of exacerbations and remissions, i.e. periods when inflammation is active and times when inflammatory activity is less. However, even in periods of remission, symptoms still arise from joint destruction and deformity which has taken place previously. This tends to be cumulative, so that in late disease, pain and disability may be constant irrespective of inflammatory activity.

Articular features

The most obvious articular signs of RA are in the hands. Swelling of the metacarpophalangeal and proximal interphalangeal joints occurs early. Later, the classical changes of ulnar deviation and volar subluxation at the metacarpophalangeal joints can take place (Fig. 26.4), and may become gross with advanced dis-

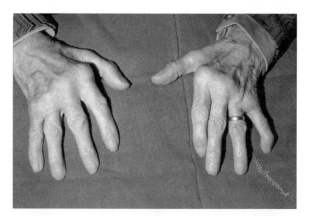

Figure 26.4 Hand deformities in a patient with rheumatoid arthritis. These are associated with significant decrease in function.

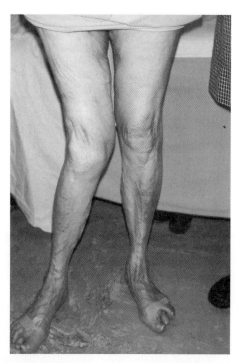

Figure 26.5 Rheumatoid arthritis. Valgus deformity of the right knee causing leg length inequality and abnormal stresses on more distal joints.

ease. Inflammatory disease involving the wrist also has an effect on hand function, and its multiplicity of joints are often the site of severe, progressive erosive damage. The elbows and shoulders may also be the site of inflammatory change and functional limitation. Spinal disease is rarely a problem except in the cervical spine, where RA may cause instability of the atlanto-axial joint or the inflamed synovial mass may cause compression of the cord. Knowledge of the state of the cervical spine is especially important when general anaesthesia is contemplated, as forced positioning of the rheumatoid neck during intubation can lead to cord damage.

In the lower limbs, synovitis of the knee with considerable swelling is quite common. Posterior swelling into the popliteal fossa is called a Baker's cyst, and this may extend into the calf causing obvious calf swelling. Rupture of a Baker's cyst produces symptoms and signs indistinguishable from deep venous thrombosis in the leg. Differentiation is by phlebography and arthrography. Inflammation in the knee may produce loss of full extension, causing a flexion deformity and consequent leg length discrepancy. Destructive arthritis can produce either varus or valgus deformity, which may become severe as the disease progresses. Such deformities inevitably have consequences on the ankles and feet, and an adequate assessment of the rheumatoid foot must take into account the length and alignment of the whole of the lower limb (Fig. 26.5).

The ankle joint may be involved by rheumatoid synovitis with joint destruction. However, much pain described as ankle pain in fact arises from the hindfoot joints. The calcaneum tends to drift into abduction at an early stage in the disease. It has been suggested that

early detection of this deformity and orthotic correction have long-term benefits as far as disability and function of the foot are concerned. The midfoot tends to assume a valgus sag (Fig. 26.6), often early in the course of the disease. Despite this, midfoot joint disease appears to be the least serious part of foot involvement in RA. Clawing of the toes occurs early in the disease. When synovitis causes distension of the metatarsophalangeal (MTP) joints, they move to the position of the least pressure for volume, with consequent clawing of the toes (Fig. 26.7). This is easily seen during intra-articular injection of these joints, where accurate placing of the injection is accompanied by the toes drawing up into a clawed position. When the toes become chronically clawed, the fibro-fatty pad located under the MTP joints migrates distally, leaving the metatarsal heads superficially placed under the skin (Fig. 26.8). Patients often describe this as a feeling of walking on pebbles or marbles. Fibular deviation of the toes is the pedal equivalent of ulnar deviation in the hands. It does occur but is not common except in the great toe, which often adopts a position of gross valgus. This may be coupled with clawing of the lesser toes to give the characteristic appearance of the advanced rheumatoid foot (Fig. 26.9).

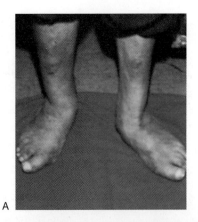

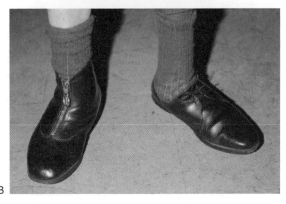

A

B

Figure 26.6 A: Rheumatoid arthritis. Valgus sag at the midfoot. B: The pair of shoes made-to-measure for the patient in A.

Non-articular features

The joint disease in the rheumatoid foot may be complicated both by extra-articular disease and by secondary skin changes. Rheumatoid tenosynovitis may involve any of the tendon sheaths in the foot, with local pain, swelling and obstruction to the smooth function of the tendons. The appearance of rheumatoid nodules has already been mentioned and, rarely, nodules may appear in the sole. Rheumatoid vasculitis may cause not only loss of skin tissue (Fig 26.10), but also, when the vasi nervori are involved, peripheral sensory neuropathy. The small end arterioles at the base of the nail are the same size as the vasi nervorsi. As these are end arterioles, their involvement is associated with tiny areas of local gangrene at the nail bases, most easily seen in the fingers. The appearance of these apparently trivial lesions is a warning to conduct a careful neurological examination, particularly of foot sensation.

Although skin loss may be caused by vasculitis, this

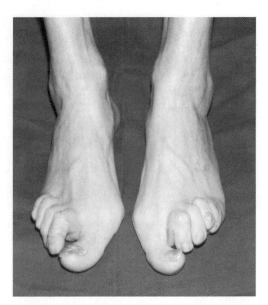

Figure 26.7 Rheumatoid arthritis. Clawing of toes.

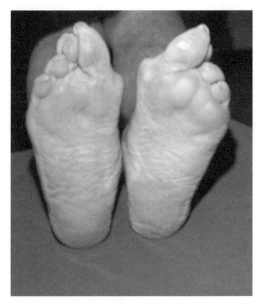

Figure 26.8 Rheumatoid feet from the plantar surface. Clawing of the toes has led to exposure of the metatarsal heads under the skin, with secondary thickening over them.

is much rarer than loss through pressure and abrasion against footwear. This occurs most commonly over the first MTP joint (Fig. 26.11; also Plate 10) and the interphalangeal joints of the toes. In contrast, the skin under the metatarsal heads shows thickening and

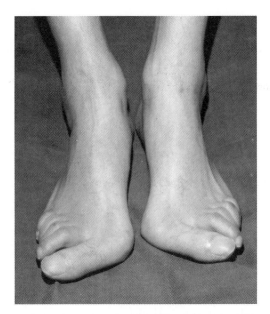

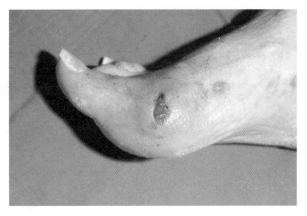

Figure 26.11   Rheumatoid arthritis. Skin loss caused by pressure over the first MTP joint in this case led to sepsis in the underlying joint.

Figure 26.9   Rheumatoid arthritis. Fibular deviation of the toes.

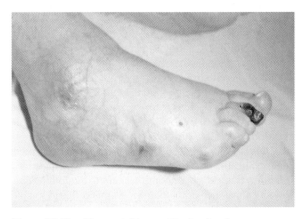

Figure 26.10   Rheumatoid vasculitis, leading to gangrene of the second toe.

cornification, and a similar reaction may occur over the interphalangeal joints before, or instead of, ulceration. These areas of skin damage are important, not only in themselves but also as a potential site of ingress of infection.

Treatment

All the varied skills of the multidisciplinary team must be brought to bear on the problems of RA in a coordinated fashion. Maintenance of function and muscle

strength, and support and help with coping skills, pain management, domestic, financial and employment problems are all necessary. All this must take place in an atmosphere of positive encouragement based on a high degree of specialist professional knowledge. The organisation of the rheumatology department must enable easy access of the patients to the wide range of professionals involved in their care at any time during the evolution of the disease.

Drug treatment is a small but important part of overall management. Relief of symptoms, especially pain, is usually achieved by the use of non-steroidal anti-inflammatory drugs (NSAIDs). Aspirin was the original member of this group, but a large number of newer members of this family now exist. The commonest side-effects are gastrointestinal, with acute or chronic blood loss being the most serious. The podiatrist may obtain information about indigestion, haematemesis or melaena when taking the patient's history or when talking with the patient during treatments. There may be physical evidence of anaemia such as pallor on examination, and rarer signs of drug side-effects such as rashes, including the petechial rash of thrombocytopenia, may be found on inspection (see also Ch. 13). These must be discussed with a doctor, nurse or pharmacist in the patient's treatment team.

NSAIDs are purely symptomatic remedies. Modern treatment aims to introduce drugs designed to control the rheumatoid inflammation and thus decrease joint destruction as early as possible in the course of the disease. These drugs are variously referred to as second line drugs, disease-modifying antirheumatic drugs (DMARDs), slow-acting antirheumatic drugs (SAARDs) or remission-inducing drugs. The drugs concerned are shown in Box 26.2. All have side-effects

---

> **Box 26.2** Disease-modifying antirheumatic drugs
>
> - Auranofin
> - Azathioprine
> - Chloroquine: hydroxychloroquine
> - Cyclosporin
> - D-penicillamine
> - Methotrexate
> - Sodium aurothiomalate (Myocrisin)
> - Sulphasalazine

that are common and may be lethal, and all require careful use and meticulous safety monitoring. As with NSAIDs, the podiatrist may be the first to notice rashes, especially of thrombocytopenia. Both azathioprine, which is particularly effective in vasculitis, and methotrexate, which is rapidly becoming more widely used to treat RA, are immunosuppressive agents. Their safety monitoring includes regular white cell counts, but even where these remain normal they interfere with the body's capacity to ward off infections. This is most commonly seen as an unusual susceptibility to viral infections, such as herpes zoster, but also shows in a failure to deal adequately with bacterial infections. As was mentioned earlier, broken skin on the rheumatoid foot can be a source of infection, and in these patients, immaculate foot hygiene, which may be difficult for the patient with RA, and scrupulous podiatric care are mandatory.

One patient who illustrates the potential problems had advanced, but relatively inactive, RA and his walking ability had been transformed by a left total knee replacement. He had an untreated heloma durum under his left second metatarsal head, and developed an accumulation of pus under it. This produced spread of infection to his knee, with intra-articular sepsis involving his prosthetic joint. Despite local treatment and antibiotics, the infection could not be controlled and his knee prosthesis was removed. The infection was still uncontrolled and he had an above-knee amputation. Despite this, he developed a staphylococcal septicaemia from which he died, the organism all along being the one isolated from under his heloma. In short, this man died from the complication of a corn. His demise illustrates perfectly the need for meticulous observation and multidisciplinary care of patients with RA.

Corticosteroids were widely used in the treatment of RA in the 1950s, soon after their introduction into medical treatment. It was rapidly discovered that, despite their obvious effectiveness as anti-inflammatories, they have severe side-effects which make their use unacceptable except under very specific circumstances. These include disease uncontrolled by any other means, and some of the more severe systemic complications of RA, such as vasculitis. Corticosteroid side-effects of particular importance to podiatrists include skin thinning, which is seen especially over the shins. The skin becomes so friable that it breaks with minimal trauma and is almost impossible to suture. It is also pigmented, making it unsightly, and small subcutaneous bruises, caused by a leakage of blood from capillaries which lack support because of the catabolic effect of corticosteroids on connective tissue, are also an unsightly problem to patients. The moon face of the corticosteroid-treated patient also warns that ineffective control of infections, especially fungal infections, may occur in the feet. Steroid-induced osteoporosis results in easy fractures of long bones as well as vertebrae, and patients taking corticosteroids require boosting of their steroid dose at the time of operation and may heal more slowly afterwards. More modern ways of using corticosteroids include intravenous or intramuscular pulses of high doses, given at the initiation of disease-modifying therapy, to control severe flares of disease activity or to enable attendance at important events such as weddings or holidays. Used judiciously, this can be a valuable and relatively safe way of using corticosteroids. Local inflammation in one or a few particularly inflamed joints may be treated by intra-articular injections of corticosteroids. Provided care is taken to avoid infection by use of a meticulous technique, this is a safe and effective form of treatment, if it is not repeated too often. The MTP joints, in particular, respond well to intra-articular injections, although accurate injection requires skill and practice. Inflamed tendon sheaths also respond to corticosteroid injection, although there is a need for great care to avoid injection into the substance of the tendon, as this can lead to tendon rupture.

Surgery

The lives of many patients with RA have been revolutionised by surgery, especially total joint replacements. In the upper limbs, shoulder and elbow joint replacement give good functional movement and freedom from pain. Wrist replacement is now available, although at present it appears to have a relatively narrow application, and the painless stability offered by wrist fusion is usually preferable. Similarly, fusion of the thumb offering a pain-free stable prop for opposition of the fingers is often the operation of choice in that digit. Silastic metacarpophalangeal joint replacement aids stability and function, although it is prone to failure. No satisfactory interphalangeal joint replacement is yet available. Surgery to the cervical spine aims at stability and reduction in actual or potential cord compression.

Lower limb surgery has generally been dramatically effective. The Charnley total hip replacement was a major technical innovation, combining pain relief with good function. There are now a number of other hip replacements available, using a variety of materials. Non-cement fixation may be advantageous when revision is anticipated, and soft layer surfaces promise to reduce wear dramatically. All prostheses do wear, and wear and loosening are the main indications for re-replacement. This is technically a much more difficult operation, best carried out in specialist centres. Knee replacements are technically more difficult to design and implant, but now give results comparable to those of hip replacements when expertly performed. Both hip and knee replacements may affect the feet by altering leg length and alignment, and the feet and footwear should always be reassessed after their insertion.

Ankle replacements exist, but are not yet sufficiently developed to be widely used, with fusion being the operation of choice. Similarly, fusion of the hindfoot joints is an effective way of restoring alignment and reducing pain. Pain from the subluxed metatarsal heads of RA can be relieved effectively by their excision. Provision of a smooth curve of metatarsal stumps is essential if good results are to be obtained, and lack of alignment is inevitably associated with persistent pain (Fig. 26.12). The first metatarsal joint is usually

treated by fusion, coupled with excision of any associated bunion. Less severe metatarsal disease may be treated by metatarsal osteotomies. Following metatarsal surgery, the clawed toes may drop into reasonable alignment, but often need to be wired into position.

After foot surgery, feet and footwear must be reassessed as a routine. Gait correction and reassessment of walking aids are also important. Despite the accent placed on large joint disease and large joint surgery in RA, the feet remain the most common site of pathology leading to disability, and their assessment and correction are undervalued as a part of both surgical and non-surgical treatment.

The seronegative spondarthritides

This group of diseases, of which ankylosing spondylitis is the prototype, is grouped together because of their clinical similarities and genetic associations, especially a greater or lesser association with the tissue type HLA-B27. The diseases included are shown in Box 26.3 and of them two deserve special consideration.

Box 26.3 The seronegative spondarthriditides

- Ankylosing spondylitis
- Psoriatic arthritis
- Arthritis with inflammatory bowel disease
  — Crohn's disease
  — ulcerative colitis
- Whipple's disease
- Reactive arthritis
  — sexually-acquired
  — enteropathic

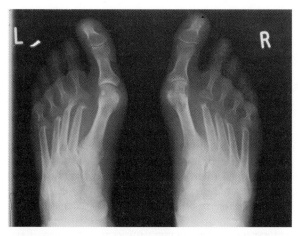

Figure 26.12 Rheumatoid arthritis following excision of the metatarsal heads. This was successful on the right foot, but there was persistent pain under the left second and third metatarsal heads, which had not been trimmed in alignment.

Ankylosing spondylitis (AS)

This is an inflammatory disease affecting especially the sacroiliac joints, the spine, the hips and the knees. Men are affected more than women, in a ratio of about 3:1, and the disease often starts in young adult life. The main characteristic is progressive stiffening of the spine, leading, in advanced cases, to a stooped posture. If the hip joints are flexible, spinal stiffness and even fusion are compatible with the ability to bend forward sufficiently to touch the toes, but the presence of hip disease increases disability significantly. Another characteristic of AS is the presence of enthesitis—that is, inflammation at the entheses, the sites of insertion of tendons into bone. Two common sites of this are the insertion of the Achilles tendon and the plantar fascia at the heel. Inflammatory disease of the joints of the foot may occur in AS but is not common.

Psoriatic arthritis

This is a seronegative inflammatory disease associated with psoriasis. In contrast to RA, it tends to be asymmetric and lacks systemic features. Tendon sheaths are, however, often involved. One characteristic lesion in psoriatic arthritis is the 'sausage' digit. Inflammation in both the proximal and distal interphalangeal joints associated with tendon sheath inflammation gives an appearance which, in the foot, resembles a chipolata sausage. Joints affected by psoriatic arthritis are often the site of severe erosion, and the highly destructive arthritis mutilans was first described in this disease. Foot care is complicated by psoriatic skin and nail involvement.

Although the disease is often more limited in extent, the treatment of psoriatic arthritis is similar to that of RA. With the exception of methotrexate, which has a beneficial effect on both skin and joints, the dermal and locomotor components of psoriatic arthritis are treated separately, and the severity of one component has no effect on the other.

CONNECTIVE TISSUE DISEASES

This is a group of rare conditions which appear to be linked by their association with autoimmunity, i.e. a tendency for the body to produce an inflammatory reaction directed against its own tissues.

Systemic lupus erythematosus is a diffuse disease involving many organ systems, with inflammation in the skin and joints being particularly common. Kidney involvement is particularly serious and may be lethal. Raynaud's phenomenon occurs, in which exposure to cold causes the digits to become sequentially purple then white, with an intense erythematous flush on rewarming. This also occurs in *progressive systemic sclerosis*, in which the skin becomes thickened, tight and inelastic. Loss of digital pulp from avascular necrosis, and deposition of calcium in the subcutaneous tissues are also found in this disease. *Polyarteritis nodosa* is characterised by inflammation of small and medium-sized blood vessels, leading to tissue loss, ulceration and neuropathy. *Polymyositis* and *dermatomyositis* are associated with inflammation in the muscles producing pain and weakness, which may be profound.

Drugs used to treat these conditions are predominantly corticosteroids and immunosuppressives, although the severity of the systemic disease means that the doses may need to be higher than those used in rheumatoid arthritis, with the consequence of increased side-effects. Because of their severity, complexity and wide-reaching consequences, these diseases must be treated by a multidisciplinary team. The podiatrist will be involved in assessing and correcting deformity due to muscle weakness, and coping with the tissue vulnerability and damage produced by impaired blood supply and by peripheral neuropathy.

OSTEOARTHRITIS

Osteoarthritis (OA) is the commonest of the rheumatic diseases, and is the biggest cause of physical debility in the UK. More than 3 million people with OA consult their family doctor each year.

Pathology

The idea that OA is just 'wear and tear' has now been abandoned. Articular cartilage is in a constant state of balance between wear and reconstitution. Osteoarthritis represents a state of imbalance, with failure of the joint to cope with the demands made upon it. The initial change is splitting and roughening of the articular cartilage surface. Secondary changes occur in bone, with increased thickening, or sclerosis, of the subchondral area and bony outgrowth at the joint margins to form osteophytes. Secondary inflammatory changes occur within the joint. The end result is complete loss of articular cartilage, leading to the exposed bone ends rubbing together.

Symptoms

Pain is more usually felt on use, especially in weight-bearing joints, and is usually minimal or absent at rest until the disease is advanced. Pain disturbing sleep is a prime indication for surgical intervention. Stiffness occurs in the mornings, when it is usually short-lived, less than half an hour, in contrast to the prolonged morning stiffness of inflammatory arthritis. Stiffness also occurs after periods of rest, so-called articular gelling. Loss of function is a reflection of both the severity of the disease and the joint or joints involved. Primary generalised osteoarthritis, with involvement of the distal interphalangeal joints of the fingers, usually causes little functional deficit. OA of the carpometacarpal joint of the thumb produces characteristic insinking and is of much greater functional importance, often producing problems with grip. Large joint OA of the hip and knee produces most functional deficit and is the cause of major disability if untreated.

Osteoarthritis of the foot

The main target for OA change is the tarsometatarsal joint of the great toe. This joint is particularly prone to minor trauma due to its important position in load-bearing, both in normal gait and in extra physical activities such as jumping and running, and due to its exposure to the deforming forces of poorly designed or poorly fitting shoes. Shoes which combine high heels and pointed toes are particularly damaging. As the most prominent toe, the great toe is also exposed to trauma in accidental and deliberate kicking or knocking of the foot. Two characteristic deformities may result. Hallux valgus may occur alone or in combination with abduction deformity of the metatarsal (hallux abductovalgus). The development of a bursa over the prominent exposed medial border of the metatarsal head is often called a 'bunion' (Fig. 26.13). Inflammation in the bursa may cause more pain and disability than the associated OA. There is a risk of both skin loss and sepsis in association with this condition. In hallux rigidus, the alignment of the MTP joint may be normal, but its movement is lost. The forces on the plantar surface of the toe often push it into slight dorsiflexion, so the digit is not only stiff but becomes hyperextended at the distal phalanx. This makes footwear uncomfortable and induces trauma to the nail from the toecap of the shoe.

In the foot, the second common site for OA is the hindfoot. This occurs particularly in conjunction with flat feet and a valgus sag—pes planovalgus. Ankle OA is usually related to trauma, primary OA at this site being much less common than in the knee or hip. Careful examination is always essential, as the patient almost always refers to hindfoot symptoms as coming from the ankle.

Treatment

Whenever possible non-drug treatments should be tried first in OA as many patients are elderly and particularly prone to drug side-effects, especially when NSAIDs are used. Weight loss and appropriate exercise to develop good supportive muscles are valuable. Comfortable, well-fitting shoes with good impact-absorbing soles are essential for all patients with lower limb OA; small degrees of leg realignment with wedged insoles have been pioneered in Japan, although the long-term benefits have not as yet been evaluated. Valgus sag should first be treated by exercises, and then by supportive insoles where these fail. Localised OA in the foot requires comprehensive advice regarding footwear, insoles and appropriate appliances (see Ch. 14).

Pain control may require the use of drugs despite these physical measures. Analgesics such as paracetamol are preferred to NSAIDs, but the latter may be necessary in some patients. It has been suggested that the anti-prostaglandin effect of NSAIDs might, in fact, compromise cartilage metabolism. In vitro, there are differences between NSAIDs in their effect on cartilage, but there is little in vivo evidence of differential effects. The term 'chondroprotection' is much in vogue, implying drug treatment capable of preventing or reversing ongoing cartilage damage in OA. This concept is more popular in continental Europe, where drugs which claim such properties are widely used. Their use is not yet considered of proven benefit in the UK.

Surgery

The benefits of surgery mentioned under rheumatoid

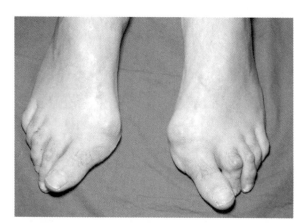

Figure 26.13 Bilateral hallux abductovalgus.

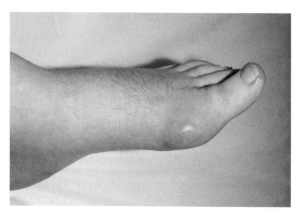

Figure 26.14 Acute gout of the first metatarsal—podagra.

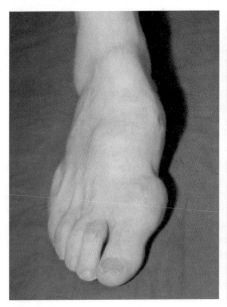 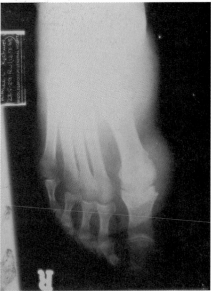

Figure 26.15 A tophus associated with the first metatarsal joint shown clinically (left) and on X-ray (right). Punched-out erosions can be seen radiologically and the tophaceous material can also be seen at an area of slightly increased radiolucency.

arthritis are even more dramatic in OA, as there is less likely to be postoperative restriction by multi-joint disease and the systemic consequences of inflammation. Local surgery to the great toe involves removal of the bunion, trimming the metatarsal head and realignment of the toe to the metatarsal. Usually this is followed by fusion of the MTP joint, but in younger patients with otherwise normal feet a silastic arthroplasty may be used. In the hindfoot and ankle, fusion of the appropriate joints is the surgical treatment of choice. Following all lower limb surgery, the gait, weight distribution and footwear must all be reassessed.

CRYSTALS AND INFECTION

Two of the most dramatic affections of the foot joints are *crystal arthritis* and *infective arthritis*. The classical crystal arthritis in the foot is gout of the great toe MTP joint or *'podagra'* (Fig. 26.14). Gout occurs when the serum level of uric acid, present as a metabolic breakdown product, is excessive. Crystals of sodium urate appear in the joint and excite an intense inflammatory reaction. The great toe MTP joint is the commonest site for gouty attacks, and is involved in 80% of first attacks. Accurate diagnosis is made by aspirating the joint and examining the synovial fluid for crystals

using polarised light microscopy. Treatment of acute attacks is by NSAIDs, and of the underlying condition by uric acid, treatment is by reduction using the xanthine oxidase inhibitor allopurinol or uricosuric agents which increase urate excretion by the kidneys. Gouty material can accumulate at cartilaginous sites, producing tophi either in the joint, where they produce punched-out erosions, or subcutaneously (Fig. 26.15). These occasionally involve the feet, and are diagnosed by identification of urate crystals within them.

Septic arthritis may occur either as a consequence of septicaemia or by direct ingress to the joint. Patients who are immunocompromised either by treatment of RA, connective tissue diseases, malignancy or transplantation, or by diseases such as AIDS, are particularly vulnerable. Direct infection may follow surgery, joint infection or penetration of a foreign body (such as a nail trodden upon accidentally), or may be caused by tracking from a local soft tissue septic site such as a bunion or ulcer. Diagnosis is by aspiration and culture of the organism, sometimes accompanied by surgical removal of local purulent material. When the source is an abnormality such as a bunion or ulceration of a clawed toe, it is important that this is treated, once the infection has been eradicated, to prevent recurrence.

27

Neurological disorders

N. E. F. Cartlidge

Keywords

Cerebral tumours
Degenerative diseases
Demyelinating diseases
Disorders of the spinal cord
Motor disorders
Muscle disorders
Peripheral nerve disorders
Sensory system
Stroke

Neurological disorders encompass a wide variety of clinical syndromes, many of which affect the legs and feet. Amongst the most common disorders are those involving motor and sensory function and these will be considered first. Thereafter, there will be a brief description of some of the other common neurological disorders.

MOTOR DISORDERS

Anatomy and physiology

Voluntary movements

The performance of voluntary movements depends upon the integration of several different descending systems from the brain to the brain stem and the spinal cord, acting ultimately on the motor cells in the anterior horn and thereby stimulating the muscle fibres of the motor unit. Such voluntary movements are achieved predominantly by the activity of the voluntary upper motor neurone cell discharging the lower motor neurone in the anterior horn of the spinal cord or brain stem nuclei. However, this essentially two-neurone system is modified and modulated by other components of the motor system, most notably the basal ganglia, whose reflex activity through the cortex and via the extrapyramidal system is responsible for resting tone in the muscles, and the cerebellum, whose reflex arcs provide for coordination with other neurones and muscle cells in the body. There are thus four important series of structures involved in the transmission of voluntary impulses from the cortex to the muscle.

Upper motor neurone. Cells in the percentral gyrus of the frontal lobe (Brodman area 4) give rise to the fibres which activate muscles on the opposite side of the body. Chief among these cells are the Betz cells in the fifth layer of the cortex, which have synaptic connections with the anterior horn cells of the spinal cord and with cells in the immediately adjacent gyrus. This adjacent cortical area is referred to as the association cortex (Brodman area 6), and interconnections between groups of cells at this level are responsible for the integration of activity in the precentral gyrus and the linking of the primary motor cortex to other neurones in both hemispheres.

The amount of cortex dedicated to each part of the body is proportional not to its size but to its importance in terms of movement. Thus, the areas such as the fingers, lips and tongue, where great precision is required, have a larger representation than the thigh, trunk and shoulder. The cells in the cortex are concerned predominantly with movements rather than with the activity of individual muscles.

The main axons from the cortical neurones converge in the corona radiata and then pass through the internal capsule and the cerebral peduncle into the base of the pons. The fibres continue to the medulla at the lower end of which the corticospinal tracts decussate as the medullary pyramids. The proportion of fibres which cross in these tracts varies, but approximately 75% travel to the contralateral lateral corticospinal tract. These fibres travel in the cord to the level of their destination and then synapse either with the anterior horn cell or with internuncial neurones in the spinal grey matter.

Lower motor neurone. Lower motor neurones are the final common pathway for nervous impulses to the muscles. The anterior horn cells are in the spinal grey matter and the axons leave in the ventral roots and thereafter join the dorsal roots to pass through the intervertebral foramina. The roots travel distally through the various plexuses to become, ultimately, peripheral nerves and to supply voluntary muscles.

The junction between the nerve and muscle is termed the neuromuscular junction, and the major neurotransmitter at this level is acetylcholine.

The basal ganglia. Deep in the structure of the cerebral hemispheres are grey matter nuclei including the caudate nucleus, the putamen and globus pallidus, the claustrum and the subthalamic nucleus. These, together with the substantia nigra in the upper end of the brain stem, make up the structures termed the basal ganglia. The main afferent fibres to the basal ganglia appear to be from the cerebral cortex to the putamen and from the substantia nigra to the putamen. After interconnections within the basal ganglia, the main efferent pathway is to the ventrolateral nucleus of the thalamus and thence to the cortex.

Cerebellum. The cerebellum is concerned with coordination of movement and the maintenance of posture. The cerebellum controls movement by an effect upon the motor cortex. The central connections of the cerebellum are exceedingly complex. It receives input from the motor cortex, the vestibular apparatus and the spinal cord and has efferent connections with the motor cortex via the thalamus.

Damage to the motor system

There are four major identifiable groups of symptoms resulting from damage to the various components of the nervous system controlling movement.

Upper motor neurone weakness (Table 27.1)

Upper motor neurone weakness is characterised by spasticity, increased reflexes and an extensor plantar response. Hemiplegia refers to weakness affecting one

Table 27.1 Differences between upper motor neurone (UMN) and lower motor neurone (LMN) lesions

	UMN	LMN
Pattern of weakness	Extensors of upper limb, flexors of lower limb	Individual muscles affected May affect multiple muscles (see Tables 1.2, 1.3)
Atrophy/wasting	Little—where present due to disuse	Marked loss of bulk
Tone	Spastic	Flaccid
Reflexes	Hyperactive and extensor plantar response	Loss of reflexes
Fasciculation	Absent	Present (in anterior horn cell and proximal lesions)
EMG	No denervation, normal nerve conduction	Denervation potentials Abnormal nerve conduction

side of the body and is characteristic of damage to the contralateral motor cortex or corticospinal tract.

Paraplegia refers to weakness affecting both legs and is typical of damage to the descending cortico-spinal tracts in the mid- or lower spinal cord.

Quadriplegia (tetraplegia) refers to weakness affecting all four limbs and is typical of damage to the descending corticospinal tracts in the upper part of the spinal cord.

Clinical disorders. Damage to the upper motor neurone pathway in the cortex most commonly occurs as the result of stroke, head injury or brain tumour. Typically there will be weakness of the opposite side (hemiplegia), with the other typical signs of an upper motor neurone lesion.

Damage to the descending corticospinal tracts in the brain or spinal cord is seen in multiple sclerosis, motor neurone disease or trauma. Damage to the descending motor pathways in the spinal cord typically produces weakness on both sides of the body.

Lower motor neurone weakness (Table 27.1)

Damage to the lower motor neurones results in flaccid weakness with loss of reflexes and muscle wasting. There may be visible fasciculation in the muscles due to the spontaneous firing of motor units and this is particularly common with damage to the anterior horn cells.

Clinical disorders. Damage to the lower motor neurone may occur anywhere throughout its length between the anterior horn cells and the muscles.

Disorders which damage the anterior horn cells include motor neurone disease and poliomyelitis. A wide variety of disorders may affect the peripheral nerves—the so-called peripheral neuropathies. Myasthenia gravis is a rare disorder which affects the neuromuscular junction and produces symptoms of fatigue. A wide range of disorders may affect voluntary muscles (the so-called myopathies).

Basal ganglia disturbance

Disturbances in this system result in reduced movement, akinesia or bradykinesia, disorders of posture, alterations in muscle tone and involuntary movements.

Clinical disorders. Of the wide variety of clinical disorders seen in damage to the basal ganglia the commonest is Parkinson's disease. This is characterised by slowness of movement, akinesia, stiffness of the muscles (rigidity) and an involuntary movement typically in the hands (tremor). Other basal ganglia disorders

are characterised by involuntary movements such as chorea and dystonia.

Cerebellum

Damage to the cerebellum or its connections results in ataxia and disturbance of balance and coordination. This may affect any aspect of movement. In the eyes, cerebellar disorders are often characterised by jerking movements (nystagmus). Speech is often affected, producing a so-called dysarthria with slurring of speech. Gait is typically disturbed with an ataxia of gait, and incoordination of the limbs results in clumsiness.

Clinical disorders. The cerebellum may be damaged by stroke and multiple sclerosis. The cerebellar degenerations are a familial group of disorders where there is progressive neuronal death within the cerebellum, producing progressive incoordination.

SENSORY SYSTEM

Anatomy and physiology

The four common cutaneous sensations—touch, pain, heat and cold—together with the deep sensations of pressure and proprioception are referred to as the somatic sensations. These are consciously appreciated in all parts of the body and have a common pathway within the nervous system. An appropriate stimulus generates an impulse at the periphery which passes into the central nervous system, is relayed by the thalamus, and thence, by a final relay, is passed to the appropriate part of the cerebral cortex. In simple terms, the pathway for somatic sensation is subserved by three orders of neurones: the first-order neurone is concerned with transmitting information from the periphery to the spinal cord; the second-order neurone transmits information from the spinal cord to the thalamus; and the third-order neurone transmits information from the thalamus to the cerebral cortex.

Patterns of sensory disturbance

Mononeuropathy. Damage to an individual peripheral nerve will produce sensory loss within the distribution of that nerve.

Polyneuropathy. Damage to multiple peripheral nerves as in peripheral neuropathies produces typically a distal sensory loss, affecting the feet and hands in what is called the glove and stocking distribution.

Spinal cord syndromes. Damage to sensory pathways within the spinal cord typically produces loss of sensation below the level of the damage (Fig. 27.1).

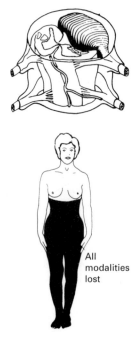

Figure 27.1 Diagrammatic presentation of a spinal cord tumour producing loss of sensation of the lower half of the body.

Damage within the cerebral cortex. Damage to the cerebral cortex, as in a stroke, typically produces impairment of sensation over the opposite half of the body.

SPECIFIC NEUROLOGICAL CONDITIONS

STROKE

Stroke, a common clinical problem, is defined as a rapidly developing focal disturbance of brain function of presumed vascular origin and of more than 24 hours' duration. This includes cerebral infarction and haemorrhage, subarachnoid haemorrhage, brain stem and cerebellar vascular disease, and spinal cord infarction and haemorrhage. Transient ischaemic attacks (TIAs) are also a manifestation of cerebrovascular disease, but the focal deficit is reversed in less than 24 hours.

Epidemiology

Stroke is the third commonest cause of death in the UK, and in most other affluent countries; only heart disease and cancer rank higher. Approximately 100 000 deaths from stroke occur annually in the UK, and about 1 000 000 in Europe as a whole. About 20% of patients die within a month of the stroke, and 50% of survivors are permanently disabled; 70% show obvious neurological deficit. One-third of patients with stroke are younger than 65 years.

Atherosclerotic cerebrovascular disease

This is the commonest type of stroke where the primary pathological process is atheromatous disease of the arteries supplying the brain. Figure 27.2 is a diagrammatic representation of the sequence of events that are thought to be mechanisms of arteriosclerotic cerebral infarction.

Clinical syndromes

Cerebral infarction (Fig 27.3)

Clinical picture. The clinical picture shows great variation, but the hallmark of thromboembolic stroke is the suddenness of onset of the neurological deficit; in some instances the deficit resolves within 24 hours (the so-called transient ischaemic attack) and in others the deficit persists. An arbitrary distinction is drawn between a deficit which persists for less than a week (minor stroke) and a deficit which persists for longer than a week (major stroke).

Specific clinical pictures may result from occlusion of particular arteries.

Investigations. In the majority of cases of cerebral infarction, extensive investigation is not required. When the diagnosis is in doubt then the definitive investigation is the CT or MRI scan (Fig. 27.4).

Management. The patient who has suffered any area of extensive cerebral infarction requires simple basic medical and nursing care and little else. A variety of complications may develop, some early and some late, and the most feared is cerebral oedema which is the commonest cause of death within 48 hours. Basic medical and nursing care is usually given, other than to those patients who are generally feeble or extremely aged, and once the acute stage is passed, physiotherapy and other appropriate rehabilitative measures may be instituted.

Transient ischaemic attacks. A special group of patients are those who suffer transient neurological deficits lasting for less than 24 hours, the majority of whom have resolution of their neurological deficits within a matter of minutes. These transient ischaemic attacks are important markers of cerebrovascular dis-

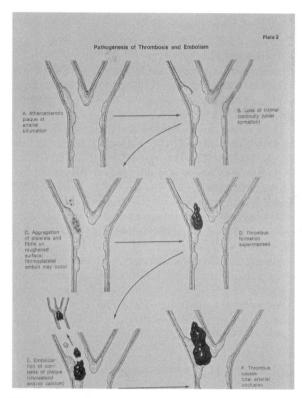

Figure 27.2   Diagrammatic representation of atheromatous disease as it affects the arteries supplying the brain.

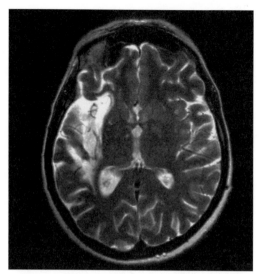

Figure 27.4   Area of cerebral infarction visible on MRI scan.

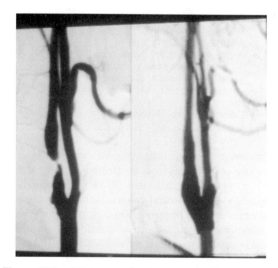

Figure 27.5   Arteriogram showing stenosis of internal carotid artery with postoperative appearance after carotid endarterectomy.

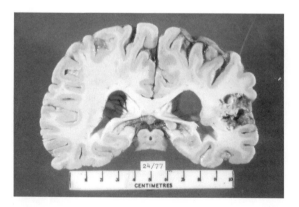

Figure 27.3   Section through brain showing area of cerebral infarction.

ease, and the patients are at significant risk for subsequent stroke, although the commonest cause of death in this group of patients is myocardial infarction.

Studies have now shown that aspirin, when taken by patients who have had transient ischaemic attacks,

reduces the risk of stroke. In patients who can be shown to have arterial narrowing, removal of this by surgery (carotid endarterectomy) may reduce the risk of subsequent stroke (Fig. 27.5).

Non-atherosclerotic causes of cerebral infarction. The causes of this are listed in Box 27.1. The commonest is cerebral embolism of cardiac origin. This should be suspected in any patient with the sudden onset of a presumed cerebral infarct with no other manifestation of atherosclerotic vascular disease, in the context of known cardiac disease or where accompanied by other evidence of emboli-systemic organs.

Box 27.1 Non-atherosclerotic causes of stroke

- *Cardiac causes*
  Cerebral emboli from prosthetic valves, intracardiac clot, intracardiac tumour
  Air or fat embolism
  Foreign body embolism
- *Haematological causes*
  Disorders associated with increased tendencies to thrombosis
  Polycythaemia
  Sickle cell disease
  Thrombotic thrombocytopenic purpura
  Thrombocytosis
- *Vascular causes*
  Arterial causes
    Vasospasm (migraine)
    Trauma
    Miscellaneous arterial disease
    Fibromuscular dysplasia
    Postradiation damage
    Arteritis
    — meningovascular syphilis
    — arteritis secondary to meningitis
    — collagen vascular disorders
    — dissecting aortic aneurysm
  Venous causes
    Cerebral thrombophlebitis

Treatment. There is now good evidence that the long-term use of anticoagulants is effective in the prevention of embolism in cases of atrial fibrillation, myocardial infarction and valve prosthesis. Once cerebral embolism has occurred, the time of institution of anticoagulant therapy must be considered carefully. There is a risk that in some patients early institution of anticoagulants may result in bleeding into the area of cerebral infarction.

Spontaneous intracranial haemorrhage

This is rare in the absence of hypertension, although it may be seen in patients with one of the haemorrhagic diatheses. These haemorrhages usually occur deep within the substance of the brain and are believed to originate from small arterioles damaged as a result of chronic hypertension. There is some evidence to suggest that the haemorrhages result from rupture of so-called Charcot–Bouchard aneurysms. The common sites for haemorrhage are:

- putamen thalamus and adjacent internal capsule

- cerebellum
- pons.

Clinical features. In the majority of cases, the symptoms develop when the patient is active with a sudden headache and a rapidly evolving neurological deficit. Coma supervenes in many cases and 80% of patients die without recovery.

Management. In most instances, patients deteriorate and die before any form of treatment may be instituted, and usually active treatment has little to offer. The exception is in the patient who has an intracerebellar haematoma where surgical evacuation may be life-saving. The diagnosis of an intracerebral haemorrhage may be strongly suspected clinically, but may only be absolutely confirmed by CT or MRI scan (Fig. 27.6).

The more widespread use of CT scanning in patients with stroke syndromes has revealed a number of patients where an unsuspected small intracerebral haematoma has been found to be producing a syndrome that was thought clinically to be due to a localised area of cerebral infarction.

Subarachnoid haemorrhage

This most commonly results from rupture of a berry aneurysm.

Aneurysmal subarachnoid haemorrhage. The berry aneurysms which are a common cause of subarach-

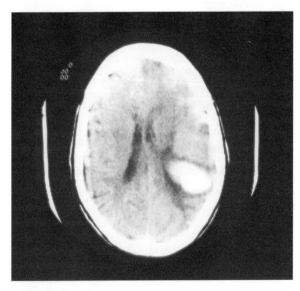

Figure 27.6 CT scan showing a small intracerebral haematoma.

noid haemorrhage are a not uncommon incidental finding at autopsy and are though to be developmental in nature. Their enlargement and rupture are believed to result in most instances from hypertension.

The aneurysms are usually asymptomatic before they rupture, although in some people they enlarge to considerable dimensions and produce neurological symptoms as a result of compression on the intracranial structures. The commonest deficit to result from compression of such an aneurysm is a third nerve palsy resulting from an aneurysm developing on the posterior communicating artery.

When the aneurysms rupture, blood at arterial pressure exits into the subarachnoid space and produces an immediate headache, the suddenness of onset of which often makes the patient think that he has been struck a blow to the head. In many instances, immediate vasospasm occurs causing cessation of the bleeding. If such vasospasm does not develop then rapid death ensues, resulting from massive increase in intracranial pressure. In patients who survive the initial bleed, the vasospasm may reach such a degree as to result in cerebral infarction and this is a common cause of death within the first 48 hours of the initial bleed.

Management. Unfortunately, nothing can be done in the early stages and the survival of the patient during the first few days is out of the hands of the attending physician. In most instances, the diagnosis may be made clinically and the presence of blood in the subarachnoid space may be confirmed by lumbar puncture or CT scan. The important principle of management of subarachnoid haemorrhage is the prevention of re-bleeding. As many as one-third of the patients will die of the first bleed and nothing can be done to save these. Of the survivors, as many as 50% will re-bleed and in the majority this will occur within 2 weeks of the initial episode. The management of such patients involves the identification of the aneurysm that has ruptured by angiography and surgical treatment of the aneurysm to prevent the risk of further bleeds.

CEREBRAL TUMOUR

Primary brain tumours account for only 1% of all tumours. However, in adults, at least 50% of tumours occurring within the brain are metastatic in nature, and furthermore in some series as many as 70% of patients dying of malignant disease have metastasis demonstrable in the brain at autopsy.

Moreover, brain tumours are important because they are one of the commonest causes of raised intracranial pressure. This will be discussed later.

Aetiology

Table 27.2 lists some of the common types of brain tumour with the incidence of such tumours in children and adults.

Metastatic tumours. These are the commonest intracranial tumour in adults and are frequently multiple. Metastases may occur in any site but most often are seen in the cerebral hemispheres or cerebellum. The common tumours to spread to the brain are the common cancers such as carcinoma of the breast and carcinoma of the bronchus.

Gliomas. These are the commonest form of primary intracranial tumour. They are derived from the cells which form a glia and a number of classifications have been attempted. The terms applied to the tumours relate to the putative cells of origin. Gliomas are found in many different sites in the brain; in adults they are most common in the cerebral hemispheres, whereas in children they are most common in the cerebellum and brain stem.

Meningioma. These tumours are thought to arise from the arachnoid cells of the arachnoid villi and tend to show slow growth developing initially over the surface of the brain.

Miscellaneous tumours. Numerous other intracranial tumours occur but most, numerically, are relatively

Table 27.2 Frequency of primary intracranial tumours

	Child (%)	Adult (%)
Neuroepithelial		
Medulloblastoma	25	5
Spongioblastoma	26	8
Oligodendroglioma	1	9
Astroglioma	3	7
Glioblastoma	<1	14
Ependymoma	12	<1
Choroid plexus papilloma	3	<1
Pinealoma	<1	<1
Mesodermal		
Meningioma	2	21
Angioblastic	<1	1
Sarcoma	3	4
Chordoma	<1	<1
Ectodermal		
Craniopharyngioma	6	4
Pituitary	<1	9
Glomus	<1	<1
Maldevelopment		
Dermoid/epidermoid	<1	2
Vascular		
Arteriovenous malformation	6	4
Other	7	7

uncommon. Of the remainder only a few deserve mention.

Haemangioblastomas are tumours developing from angioblasts and are most commonly seen in the cerebellum. Pituitary tumours are an important group as they may readily threaten vision by compression of the optic chiasma. Acoustic neuromas growing on the eighth cranial nerve, though uncommon, are an important tumour as they may present in the early stage simply with unilateral hearing impairment.

Clinical features of brain tumours

Symptoms and signs resulting from brain tumours occur as a result of either (1) local effects of the tumour; or (2) the effects of raised intracranial pressure. In many instances both sets of signs and symptoms may occur. The rapidity of onset of symptoms depends on the rate of growth of the tumour, or the site of the tumour.

Local effects. Overall, one of the commonest local effects of a tumour is epilepsy. Seizures may be either focal or generalised and tumours in certain sites are most likely to produce seizures. Tumours of the temporal lobe commonly present with fits, and tumours growing over the surface of the brain, such as meningiomas, commonly have fits as an early symptom.

Raised intracranial pressure. The brain is enclosed within the box of the skull, within which is contained the 1500 g of brain, 75 ml of blood and 75 ml of cerebrospinal fluid. Any expanding mass within the skull very readily leads to an increase in the intracranial pressure; the term for such expanding lesions is 'space-occupying lesion' and tumours are one type of several such lesions.

Any space-occupying lesions which impinge upon the substance of the brain, and tumours in particular, are likely to be associated with oedema of the surrounding cerebral tissue, which acts as an additional space-occupying effect. Indeed, with some tumours, the degree of cerebral oedema produces a greater space-occupying effect than does the tumour itself (this has important therapeutic implications, see below). The sequence of symptoms and signs that develop in increasing intracranial pressure tends to be relatively stereotyped. With tumours in silent areas, such as the non-dominant frontal temporal lobes, symptoms of raised intracranial pressure, and false localising symptoms in particular, may present before any local effects of the tumour. Death from brain tumour usually results from the progressive increase in intracranial pressure, resulting in herniation with brain stem compression, either in the region of the tentorium or in the foramen magnum.

Investigation

The intensity of investigation of a brain tumour suspect depends on the index of clinical suspicion. As many intracranial tumours in adults are metastatic in origin, routine haematological, biochemical and radiological investigations should be performed before resorting to specific neurological investigations. There is no place nowadays for the use of skull X-rays, EEG or technetium brain scan in the investigation of patients thought to have a brain tumour. Lumbar puncture is absolutely contraindicated. The investigation of choice is a CT scan. In some instances, angiography may be required to delineate the blood supply of the tumour and its vascularity, but it is excessively rare nowadays to need to use any other neuroradiological investigation. The role of MRI scans has yet to be determined.

Treatment

The treatment of choice of cerebral tumours is complete surgical removal. In patients with metastatic cerebral tumours, this is rarely feasible or advisable, although occasionally it may be justifiable to consider removal of a single secondary when the patient's life expectancy otherwise from any primary tumour can be measured in more than a few months. Many patients with cerebral secondaries show quite dramatic improvement with high-dose corticosteroid therapy, which produces significant improvement in the associated cerebral oedema. There is considerable controversy about the treatment of patients with gliomas, although surgical biopsy may be necessary to confirm the diagnosis. High-dose corticosteroid treatment may produce temporary improvement, and in some centres radiotherapy and chemotherapy are used enthusiastically.

The treatment of choice for benign tumours, such as meningiomas, or acoustic neuromas, is complete surgical removal, and in most instances this will lead to a cure. High-dose corticosteroids may be used in the pre-operative period to reduce cerebral oedema, and Mannitol and other dehydrating agents may produce similar improvement.

DEMYELINATING DISEASES

The demyelinating diseases are a group of central nervous system disorders in which the brunt of the damage is to the myelin sheaths. Multiple sclerosis is by far the commonest such disorder.

Multiple sclerosis

Multiple sclerosis (MS) is now the most common

potentially crippling disease of young adults in the UK, with a prevalence of 50–100 per 100 000 population in England, 127 per 100 000 in north-east Scotland and over 300 per 100 000 in the Shetlands and Orkneys. Most family practitioners will have one or two patients with MS on their list. The prevalence in northern Europe, southern Australia and the northern part of the USA is approximately the same as in the UK. In southern Europe, it is probably lower, but this is controversial. In contrast with temperate countries, the prevalence is very low in the tropics.

MS is more common in women, with a male:female ratio of 3:2, and the peak age of onset is around 30 years; onset below the age of 10 years is exceedingly uncommon and the incidence of new cases declines rapidly after the age of 45 years. MS is sometimes found at autopsy in elderly patients who have died from quite different causes and in whom there is no history of relevant symptoms.

Pathology

MS is a primary demyelinating disease, meaning that, initially, myelin is destroyed while the axons remain intact. Demyelination occurs in plaques scattered throughout the brain, spinal cord and optic nerves. Sites of predilection are the cervical spinal cord, the optic nerves and periventricular structures. Plaques are often almost symmetrically distributed, but MS is not a systematised disease and the lesions are not restricted by anatomical boundaries.

Clinical features

Onset is monosymptomatic (i.e. with evidence of disease at a single site) in about 80% of patients. In the remainder, there is immediate evidence of multiple lesions. Many different symptoms may occur at the onset, as plaques can develop in any part of the CNS. The commonest modes of onset and some of the symptoms that may cause diagnostic confusion are:

- optic neuritis
- weakness of one or both lower limbs
- impairment of cutaneous sensation in the lower limbs and trunk
- brain stem symptoms (e.g. diplopia, vertigo).

Course

The disease pursues a relapsing and remitting course in about 85% of patients, while in the remainder it is progressive from the onset. In a typical case, the rate of relapse is about once in 2 years, and initial relapses are followed by complete recovery. After a succession of relapses, however, some disability persists and this increases in subsequent attacks. Eventually the disease enters the progressive stage without further remission. Deterioration may be imperceptible for a number of years and a reasonable level of activity can be continued, but eventually walking becomes increasingly difficult and other symptoms add to the disability.

Mean survival is of the order of 30 years and death occurs due to effects of severe paralysis and resulting infections in the form of pneumonia.

Treatment

There is no effective curative treatment for MS, although well-conducted, rational, therapeutic trials of many forms of treatment are reported with increasing frequency. Claims of therapeutic benefit from different regimens seldom go beyond the reduction of relapse rate or slowing of deterioration. Even if such claims can be substantiated, they do not promise a cure, but any advance may indicate the path to future progress.

The use of the corticosteroid drugs at the time of acute attacks may be of benefit, but the cornerstone of management is symptomatic treatment and rehabilitation.

DEGENERATIVE DISEASES (Box 27.2)

The degenerative diseases encompass a wide range of disorders characterised by a progressive neuronal death. The clinical features are determined by which neurones are damaged. For example, when the loss of neurones occurs within the cerebellum, the clinical features are those of a progressive cerebellar syndrome with unsteadiness and incoordination. The progressive cerebellar degenerations are often familial and are presumed to occur on the basis of a genetic defect.

Parkinson's disease is the commonest of the basal ganglia degenerative disorders, and in this instance there is progressive neuronal loss within a number of the basal ganglia, notably the substantia nigra.

Progressive loss of neurones within the cerebral cortex produces a clinical syndrome of dementia and is characteristic of Alzheimer's disease.

In most instances the cause of the progressive degenerative process within neurones is unknown, and almost all of the degenerative diseases are progressive to death without effective treatment.

PERIPHERAL NERVE DISORDERS

A wide variety of disorders may damage peripheral

Box 27.2 Some of the commonest degenerative diseases

- *Disorders in which dementia is prominent*
  Alzheimer's disease
  Pick's disease
  Huntington's chorea

- *Disorders in which extrapyramidal features are prominent*
  Parkinson's disease
  Wilson's disease
  Progressive supranuclear palsy
  Shy–Drager syndrome
  Striatonigral degeneration
  Hallervorden–Spatz disease
  Basal ganglia calcification
  Dystonias
  Essential tumour
  Progressive myoclonus epilepsy
  Tic syndrome

- *Spinocerebellar degenerations*
  Hereditary ataxias of metabolic origin
  Hereditary ataxias of unknown cause
  Sporadic late onset cerebellar degeneration

- *Motor system degenerations*
  Hereditary spastic paraparesis
  Motor neurone disease
  Spinal muscular atrophy

Box 27.3 Clinical classification of peripheral neuropathy

- *Inherited neuropathies*
  Mixed sensory motor neuropathies
  — idiopathic
  — metabolic
  Sensory neuropathies

- *Acute acquired neuropathies*
  Guillain–Barré syndrome
  Porphyria
  Toxic
  Diphtheric

- *Subacute acquired neuropathies*
  Deficiency states
  Heavy metals
  Drug intoxication
  Uraemic
  Diabetic
  Arteritic

- *Chronic acquired neuropathies*
  Carcinoma
  Paraproteinaemia
  Uraemic
  Beri-beri
  Diabetic
  Hypothyroid
  Connective tissue
  Amyloid
  Leprosy

---

nerves to produce the clinical picture of a peripheral neuropathy (polyneuropathy) (Box 27.3). Damage to individual peripheral nerves (mononeuropathy) most commonly occurs as a result of trauma, and the causes of mononeuropathy are listed in Table 27.3.

The clinical features of peripheral neuropathy include weakness which most commonly begins distally and sensory loss, which again typically begins distally in the feet and hands. Aside from weakness there is often muscle wasting and loss of tendon reflexes. In patients with sensory loss, there may be trophic ulcers (Fig. 27.7).

MUSCLE DISORDERS

Disorders of muscle are termed myopathies and are characterised by weakness most often occurring in proximal muscles.

Genetically determined myopathies

The disorders in this group are commonly known as the muscular dystrophies (Box 27.4). They include Duchenne muscular dystrophy, which is a disorder seen only in males and characterised by progressive

Table 27.3 Causes of mononeuropathies

Entrapment	Constriction of a nerve by fibrous bands, or in a fibro-osseous tunnel, e.g. carpal tunnel syndrome
Compression	Sustained pressure on a nerve, e.g. Saturday night radial palsy
Nerve injury	Blunt or sharp trauma
Stretch of nerves	Usually associated with trauma; may be a factor in entrapment or occupational palsies
Infarction	May affect multiple nerves, e.g. polyarteritis nodosa
Predisposition to mononeuropathies	Susceptibility to compression or entrapment, e.g. diabetes mellitus
Tumours of nerves	Schwannomas in neurofibromatosis, and malignant invasion of lymph nodes
Infections	Leprosy, herpes zoster

weakness beginning in childhood leading to death in the second or third decade of life.

Acquired myopathies

Polymyositis and the other inflammatory myopathies

Box 27.4 Muscular dystrophies

- X-linked muscular dystrophies
  — Duchenne muscular dystrophy
  — Becker muscular dystrophy
- Limb-girdle muscular dystrophy
- Facio-scapulohumeral muscular dystrophy
- Scapuloperoneal muscular dystrophy
- Myotonic dystrophy

Box 27.5 Inflammatory myopathies

- Idiopathic polymyositis/dermatomyositis (adult onset)
- Childhood-type dermatomyositis
- Dermatomyositis/polymyositis associated with autoimmune disorders
- Dermatomyositis/polymyositis associated with malignancy
- Sarcoid myopathy
- Inclusion body myositis
- Polymyositis due to infections and infestations

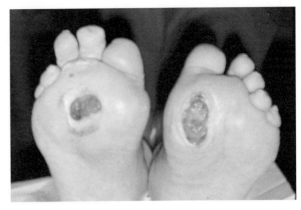

Figure 27.7 Typical trophic ulcers on the soles of the feet in a patient with a peripheral neuropathy, with sensory loss in the feet.

Box 27.6 Disorders of the spinal cord

- *Developmental disorders*
  Spina bifida
- *Spinal degenerative disorders*
  Cervical and lumbar spondylosis
  Disc disease
- *Spinal cord tumours*
- *Infections*
  Bacterial
  Syphilis
  Tuberculosis
- *Deficiency disorders*
  Pernicious anaemia

(Box 27.5) are the commonest acquired forms of myopathy. The damage to the muscle fibres results from an inflammatory process probably mediated by an autoimmune mechanism.

DISORDERS OF THE SPINAL CORD

Damage to the spinal cord may produce deficits due to involvement of the descending motor pathway, the ascending sensory pathways, the pathways concerned with autonomic function, and the nerve roots. Complete transection of the cord at a single level will produce paralysis of all motor function below that level (paraplegia or tetraplegia), complete anaesthesia below that level, loss of bowel and bladder function, impairment of sweating and vasomotor control and, due to damage to the anterior horn cells, segmental lower motor neurone motor dysfunction.

Damage to the spinal roots typically produces pain which is referred in the distribution of the sensory supply of the root. The commonest such pain is so-called sciatica

resulting from lumbar disc disease with compression of either the fifth lumbar or the first sciatic root. Disc disease and degenerative spondylosis in either the lumbar or cervical regions are the commonest causes of spinal cord dysfunction. In general, cervical and lumbar spondylosis can be regarded as processes related to ageing and are a normal radiological finding in those over 60.

A wide variety of other disorders may affect the spinal cord (Box 27.6). In young adults, multiple sclerosis is the commonest cause of spinal cord damage.

FURTHER READING

Chadwick D, Cartlidge N E F, Bates D 1989 Medical neurology. Churchill Livingstone, Edinburgh

Bradley W G, Daroff R B, Fenichel G M, Marsden D C 1996 Neurology in clinical practice, 2nd edn. Butterworth-Heinemann, Oxford

Swash M, Schwartz M S 1989 Neurology: a concise clinical text. Baillière Tindall, London

28

Leprosy

H. A. Cross

Keywords

· Anaesthesia
Autonomic impairment
Complications of ulceration
Epidemiology
Hansen's disease
Infection control
Mal perforans
Motor paralysis
Neuropathy
Orthotic options
Tarsal disintegration

Hansen's disease (HD), or Hanseniasis, are preferred terms for leprosy as they do not evoke the connotations that leprosy does. Once an individual is diagnosed as having leprosy, his or her role in society will lead to an inevitable social death. The patient's experience of the disease is profoundly affected by the social beliefs and expectations of the society of which the individual is a part. Leprosy is not simply a dysfunction of physiological order but it has psychosocial manifestations that profoundly affect the patient's family and community.

THE MEANING OF LEPROSY

Ironically, the tragedy of leprosy has little to do with the bacillus. The general perception of leprosy within a community is confined to conditions associated with characteristic secondary deformities. Thus it is possible that long after Hansen's disease may have been cured, the sequelae of the disease, unless controlled, may continue to deform and disable the patient. It is such patients who will then continue to be perceived as having leprosy. Impairment control is a practicable objective, but it demands life-long vigilance. The podiatrist has a specialised approach to chronic pedal disorders. Podiatric training is, therefore, particularly appropriate for the implicit needs of impairment control. The podiatrist is trained to accept the challenge posed by incurable conditions and is uniquely facilitated to develop a provider/receiver relationship that can protect the patient physically and rehabilitate him or her socially.

Epidemiology

Hansen's disease is essentially a problem in the developing countries. Findings published by the World Health Organization (WHO) in 1991 demonstrated that India, grouped with Indonesia, Brazil, Nigeria and Myanmar, contributes 82% of all registered cases of leprosy. Prevalence figures demonstrating registered cases in India were recorded as 2–2.9 per 1000 (Noorden 1992). These figures are disputed, and prevalence rates of 5–6 per 1000 have also been cited (Weis et al 1992). The extent of the problem is difficult to assess, due to social, demographic and political factors.

Endemicity is shown to vary markedly between regions where the disease is prevalent. However, in India alone, with a population approaching 900 million there are between 1.8 and 5.4 million people suffering from Hansen's disease, or its secondary effects. Of this number, 33.3% suffer foot pathology secondary to the disease (Brand 1991). These figures suggest that between 600 000 and 1.8 million people in India present with feet that are compromised as a consequence of Hansen's disease. After diabetes mellitus, leprosy is the most common cause of sensory neuropathy globally and is probably the major cause of neuropathy in Asia and Africa, where it affects predominantly the lower socio-economic groups.

The mode of transmission remains a topic of investigation and the three possible routes are the respiratory tract, the skin and the gastrointestinal tract. Direct skin to skin contact is no longer considered the most likely form of transmission, as it appears that *Microsporum* (*M.*) *leprae* is not capable of penetrating the papillary zone of the dermis. However, transmission through skin abrasions has not been excluded (Jopling & McDougal 1988).

Aerosol contamination remains the most likely form of transmission and there is evidence which demonstrates that infected droplets can be expelled during sneezing, coughing and even talking. Droplets may also be absorbed by dust and viable *M. leprae* have been identified in desiccated secretions a week after expectorating. The principal theory of transmission is that contaminated droplets are inspired, *M. leprae*

enter the capillaries around the alveoli and then continue to target cells via a haematological route. It has also been suggested that damage to the nasal mucosa provides an accessible portal of infection from the same source. The most significant target cell is the Schwann cell but *M. leprae* is also found in significant numbers in macrophages, endothelium, chondrocytes and melanocytes.

The bacillus is not virulent and infected subjects can host vast numbers without feeling any ill effect, and chemotherapy rapidly compromises the viability of the bacillus. It is therefore from undiagnosed, multibacillary hosts that the threat of infection is greatest.

Classification

Host resistance to the bacillus will determine the classification of the disease type. The Ridley Jopling classification is the most widely used system. It describes the spectrum of disease from tuberculoid (TT), which demonstrates vigorous resistance and low infection (pauci bacillary, PB), to lepromatous (LL), which demonstrates severely compromised resistance and massive infection (multibacillary, MB). Borderline (BB) describes resistance that lies between the two polar responses. Further subdivisions are made which represent responses that lie between the principal responses (Jopling & McDougal 1988).

Neuropathy in tuberculoid leprosy

The most significant changes in tuberculoid leprosy involve the cutaneous and subcutaneous nerves. Nerve damage is an inherent effect of host response and is not related to massive proliferation of bacilli. Infected nerves are invaded and destroyed beyond recognition by epithelioid granuloma. An intense response to infection may lead to necrosis and the development of nerve abscesses. Where a nerve trunk is affected, the sensori-motor deficit will be superimposed, giving rise to the localised mixture of neurological defects characteristic of tuberculoid leprosy. The destruction of dermal nerves explains the localised anaesthetic patches, sometimes the only indication of polar tuberculoid leprosy. Autonomic loss is a feature of tuberculoid lesions, where axon reflex and sweating are found to be absent. Involvement of nerve trunks, being in proximity to skin lesions, is probably secondary to cutaneous nerve involvement. The nerves most frequently affected are the common peroneal, the saphenous and the sural nerves.

Neuropathy in lepromatous leprosy

Due to depressed cell-mediated immunity in lepromatous leprosy, the haematogenous spread of the bacilli allows the unchecked proliferation of bacilli. Nerve damage is slower to become apparent than in other forms of leprosy. Whilst bacilli continue to multiply within Schwann cells and perineurium, others are dispersed with the destruction of the same. Liberated bacilli are engulfed by histiocytes in which they are not destroyed, and the histiocyte becomes a vehicle that transports multiplying bacilli to other regions of the nerve or other tissues. It is these cells that are known as lepra cells, carrying masses of bacilli collectively called globi.

Symmetrical and bilateral sensory loss of lepromatous leprosy is explained by the massive and widespread distribution of bacilli and is clearly related to body temperature. Sabin & Swift (1984) presented repeated patterns of surface temperature obtained by thermographic scanning of normal subjects. By comparing gradients between different body temperatures and the evolution of neurological deficit, a clear relationship between the usual distribution of surface temperatures and sensory loss was demonstrated.

Neuropathy in borderline (dimorphous) leprosy

Whilst nerve damage in borderline leprosy is essentially limited to the same sites as those common in lepromatous leprosy, the potential for uncharacteristic neurological defects is greater. Cases of borderline leprosy demonstrate the greatest potential for catastrophic peripheral nerve damage. This is explained by a dual effect. An inadequate host response ensures that an initial haematogenous spread of disease is not prevented. However, unlike lepromatous leprosy, there is a degree of resistance, resulting in a prompt and radical response when bacilli are detected. As a result, widespread, tuberculoid-type nerve damage is demonstrated early in the disease.

Where a borderline case demonstrates a tendency to fall closer to the tuberculoid pole (BT), paralysis and sensory loss are always asymmetrical. Where borderline cases lie at the midpoint of the spectrum (BB), involvement is asymmetrical and indicates intracutaneous nerve dysfunction as the borders of insensitivity do not conform to dermatomes. In a low resistance borderline case (BL), there will be numerous lesions, symmetrically distributed. Areas of insensitivity may exceed the borders of lesions, and temperature-linked patterns of sensory loss become apparent. However,

the spread of involvement is less diffuse than in lepromatous leprosy and is not as symmetrical (Sabin & Swift 1984).

THE LOWER LIMB IN HANSEN'S DISEASE

Anaesthesia

The integrity of the foot is dependent on safety information relating to current conditions of the substratum. The high density of Vater–Pacini corpuscles in the subcutaneous fat chambers provides an acute sense of deep pressure and vibration. These modalities are associated with high frequency shock and tissue displacement, whereas it is postulated that the Meissener's corpuscles register low frequency shock. The dual effect of these modalities is that the foot's movement against the ground and the character of the weight-bearing surface may be perceived. The ability to register pressure coupled with withdrawal and postural reflexes is essential for self-protection (Jorgensen & Bosjen-Moller 1991). The major factor compromising the foot in Hansen's disease is anaesthesia. Denied the benefits of sensory feedback, the undesirable effects of pathomechanical forces are undetected. Tissue may be strained by mechanical stress, beyond its threshold of competence, in which case it breaks down.

Factors associated with plantar ulceration

- Motor paralysis
- Pre-existing pathomechanical foot function
- Tarsal disintegration
- Absorption and pathological fractures
- Autonomic impairment
- Social and behavioural variables.

Motor paralysis. It has been suggested that only 6% of ulcerated feet display anaesthesia alone; when the foot was further compromised by intrinsic muscular paralysis this figure was increased 10-fold (Brand 1991). It is probable that paralysis of the intrinsic muscles increases the vulnerability of the foot by creating instability during propulsion. The extent to which pre-existing functional abnormalities could exacerbate this condition has not been widely considered.

Claw toes. Claw toe deformity is a common feature of the neuropathic foot in Hansen's disease and is generally considered to indicate intrinsic muscle paralysis. (The development of the deformity should not be taken as a qualification for muscle paralysis per se, as muscle imbalance due to other mechanical factors is also a cause of claw toe deformity (Root et al 1977).) The extension of the proximal phalanges results in the plantarflexion of the metatarsal heads and anterior drifting of the fibro-fatty pad. Compromised by the loss of digital stabilisation, the metatarsal heads are exposed to abnormally directed, excessive forces, focused on a reduced area of loading. Extreme peak pressure readings have been reported under the ulcerated metatarsal heads of leprosy-impaired subjects (Bauman et al 1963).

Extrinsic muscle paralysis. M. leprae, with a predilection for cooler sites such as the peroneal nerve as it winds around the fibular neck, where it is particularly vulnerable to infiltration. Peroneal and anterior compartment paralysis are not uncommon. The resulting foot drop deformity can severely compromise the patient. Excessive lateral and forefoot loading predisposes the patient to ulceration, particularly under the fifth metatarsal head. The plantarflexors and posterior tibialis have not been found to be affected by neuropathy in Hansen's disease.

Pre-existing pathomechanical foot function. Factors of a congenital and/or developmental origin affecting foot function are probably implicated in the development of plantar ulceration. It has been reported that 85% of plantar ulcers occur in the forefoot, with the remaining 15% occurring in the heel (10%) and lateral border (5%) (Brand 1991). The predilection for forefoot ulceration suggests that standing pressure and injury are less likely to be causative factors than walking.

Of first ulcers that occur on the forefoot, the most common sites are:

- between the first metatarsal head and proximal phalanx of the hallux
- the second metatarsal head
- the hallux.

The frequency of occurrence at these sites suggests an association with excessive or abnormal loading, which is generally associated with compensatory subtalar pronation for rearfoot or extrinsic abnormalities.

Tarsal disintegration. In late lepromatous leprosy, a complication may be the massive infiltration of bacilli into the bones of the foot. Such infiltration may cause rarefaction of cancellous bone and some loss of trabeculae. Mechanical stress, during phases of acute infiltration, can result in fracture and disintegration of tarsal bones. In most cases of this nature, the acute phase is followed by a period of recalcification. During this period, the skeleton either returns to normal, if undamaged, or is reorganised following disintegration or fracture. Tarsal disintegration as a direct consequence of infiltration is unusual (about 1% of all cases of leprosy).

A more common cause of disintegration and absorption is a periosteal osteoclastic action which occurs as a consequence of hyperaemia following ulceration (Kulkarni & Mehta 1983). It is, however, the combination of neuropathy and pathomechanical foot function that most disadvantages the HD patient. Talonavicular and calcaneocuboid instabilities have been implicated as major compromising features, as tarsal disintegration most commonly begins from either of these joints. Excessive calcaneal eversion, with subtalar pronation, may result in the impingement of the lateral process of the talus into the crucial angle of the calcaneus. A splitting of the calcaneus at this location is also a common early feature of tarsal disintegration.

Absorption and pathological fractures. Brand (1991) recorded that just over 33.3% of patients with Hansen's disease show distinct radiological changes in the bones and joints of the feet. These changes are caused either by infiltration of *M. leprae* (4%) or by secondary changes, including periostitis, osteoporosis and sequestration with associated pathological fractures and disintegration of bone. *M. Leprae* has been described as a specific pathogen with a predilection for infecting bone (in multibacillary disease). However, the more common invasive and destructive nature of non-specific osteomyelitis is attributed to secondary infection. Active secondary infection of ulceration may lead to periostitis and osteomyelitis, which commonly leads to sequestration.

Hyperaemia, associated with chronic plantar ulceration, and active infection of bone can also cause osteoporosis. The osteoporotic state of bone predisposes it to pathological fractures, particularly when pain sensation in the joints is lost. Fracture and infection may lead to absorption of bone, giving rise to short foot or tarsal disintegration. The gross organisation of such feet predisposes them to further ulceration due to the vulnerability of tissue beneath bony prominences.

Autonomic impairment. The impairment of dermal sympathetic nerve function may result in the loss of sweat and axon reflexes. Dehydration of the epidermis results in the loss of keratin flexibility and elasticity. The integrity of the skin is therefore compromised and tensile stress causes fatigue and breakdown. Apart from being a contributory factor affecting ulceration, anhidrosis very commonly causes fissures, which are a potentially serious complication for patients as they provide a portal for infection (Fig. 28.1).

Social and behavioural variables. Hansen's disease is predominantly a problem amongst lower socio-

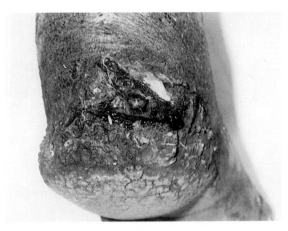

Figure 28.1   Anhidrotic fissure on the posterior aspect of the heel extending to the calcaneus.

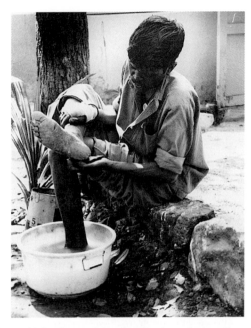

Figure 28.2   Appropriate education to motivate self-care is the mainstay of impairment control for HD patients. A midday break provides a good opportunity for this man to wash his feet in soapy water and rub away hardened skin with a stone. Such diligence is rare.

economic groups. Patients are constrained to continue working to avoid dependence on family members and loss of dignity. Very often the employment opportunities available to sufferers are limited to manual labour and agricultural occupations, where patients are compelled to submit their feet to excessive demands and are unable to rest (Fig. 28.2). Poverty dictates that such patients are unable to purchase suitable footwear, if indeed they can purchase any at all. Podiatry has mainly focused therapeutic developments around the interaction between the foot and footwear. Treating underprivileged, unshod populations is a daunting challenge.

Complications of ulceration

Secondary infection. Common causative organisms implicated are *Staphylococcus aureus*, *Streptococcus haemolyticus*, *Pseudomonus aeruginosa*, *Proteus mirabilis* and *Escherichia coli*. Aggravated by continuous mechanical forces in the absence of pain, infection spreads rapidly along tendon sheaths and into synovial joint spaces.

Squamous cell carcinoma. The chronic irritation of regenerating epithelium around an ulcer and osteomyelitis with chronic discharging sinuses are two of the predisposing factors thought to influence the development of squamous cell carcinoma. Hyperplasia, influenced by chronic irritation, initiates the regeneration of cells which manifest as papillomatoses adapted to irritation. Continued irritation leads to dysplasia with decreasing cell differentiation and, ultimately, carcinoma (Sane & Mehta 1988).

Treatment of pedal pathologies

When treating Hansen's disease-related foot problems in developing countries, the availability of materials and medications will dictate management options. A sound understanding of therapeutic principles, a pragmatic philosophy and imaginative resourcefulness will be the key attributes of the successful clinician in such circumstances.

Ulceration

The treatment of neuropathic ulceration should aim to enhance the normal response to trauma. The physiological response to wound healing follows a recognised sequential pattern. The biochemical and cellular responses, demonstrated as inflammation, proliferation and maturation, demonstrate a continuous process that aims to restore continuity and tissue strength. Where the overlapping phases of inflammation, epithelialisation, contraction and connective tissue formation are continuously disrupted, the process of resolution or organisation is confounded by the effects of chronic inflammation. Chronic inflammation is perpetuated by foreign body irritation and repeated microtrauma. A prolonged inflammatory response is associated with a delay in tissue regeneration and consequent retarded development of tissue tensile strength.

The normal physiological response to ulceration demonstrates three phases:

1. the active phase
2. the proliferative phase
3. the maturation or remodelling phase.

The active phase of ulceration. The leucocytic migration to a traumatised location results in the active debridement and solubilisation of devitalised tissue. Complementing phagocytic activity is the monocytic production of collagenase and proteoglycan-degrading enzymes. Associated with the increased migration of macrophages and plasma proteins is the accumulation of transudate. The normally clear, straw-coloured serous exudate displays discolouration and odour, reflecting its altered status as a cellular aggregate. The viscous and purulent aggregate of cells and debris which drains from an opened wound is a sterile exudation. Within a week, the cells and plasma constituents of the exudate cease to function and become incorporated into a necrotic coagulum. Necrotic tissue (slough) may remain relatively fluid or dehydrate to become a hardened eschar. In the active phase of ulceration, discharge is copious. The volume of exudate inhibits the consolidation of materials to form an eschar. Oedema and infection can contribute considerably to the amount of exudate expressed.

Unresolved disruptive forces perpetuate haemostatic mechanisms. The occlusion of microcirculation serves to exacerbate the anoxic necrosis of tissue. Where pressure is implicated as a precipitating factor, endothelial cells lining the microcirculation become separated. The resultant separation of junctional complexes allows contact between procoagulants of the blood and subendothelial tissues, notably collagen, causing an aggregation of platelets. Platelet aggregation leads to vascular occlusion and further tissue necrosis (Barton 1976, Cruickshank 1976).

The pathological process during the destructive phase of ulceration causes the lesion to spread inwards, thereby destroying subcutaneous tissue faster than the overlying skin. The undermined edges of active ulcers are a characteristic feature (Fig. 28.3; also Plate 8). Recently formed and active ulcers have been described as exhibiting a mobile relationship with deeper tissues. The organisation of fibrous tissue associated with chronicity results in the lesion being tied to deeper structures, thereby reducing its mobility. The

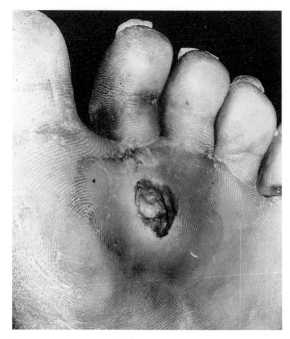

Figure 28.3 The undermined edges of active ulcers are a characteristic feature. The second metatarsal head is a common site for the first ulcer.

indurated and punched-out edges of chronic ulceration are the manifestation of the accumulation of collagen (Kloth & Miller 1990).

The proliferative phase of ulceration

Granulation. A primary indication of ulcer resolution is the appearance of granulation tissue at the base of an ulcer. Granulation tissue is a vascular and lymphatic system in a gel-like matrix, contained within a fibrous collagen network. The matrix is composed of hyaluronic acid and fibronectin, with other salts and colloidal materials. The vascular network carries nutrients to macrophages and fibroblasts, whilst the lymphatics prevent oedema. Granulation tissue is produced until the wound cavity is filled, reducing the depth of the ulcer almost to the level of the surrounding skin (Thomas 1990).

Re-epithelialisation. The spread of granulation to the level of the skin stimulates the activation of the epithelium which begins to proliferate over the wound (Thomas 1990). It has been suggested that wounded tissue does not produce chalones, and therefore that the separated surfaces at a free edge would not be subject to the inhibitory effect of chalone on biological events. This hypothesis may explain the common occurrence of hyperkeratinisation around the periphery of ulcers (Daly 1990).

Factors influencing healing during the active and proliferative phases. Vitamin C and oxygen are fundamental factors influencing the hydroxylation of proline and lysine. When there is a deficit of these factors, there follows an inhibition of collagen synthesis. Vitamin A deficiency has been recorded as delaying re-epithelialisation. Protein deficiency results in an amino acid deficit, causing a consequent lack of availability of material to structure granulation tissue. Protein deficiency may have on inhibiting effect on host defence against infection. Deficiency of trace elements, particularly zinc and copper, has been implicated as a cause of delayed healing (Westaby 1982, Zederfeldt et al 1986, Daly 1990).

Other factors recorded as inhibiting wound healing include systemic and topical steroids, antineoplastic drugs, haemostatic agents, non-steroidal anti-inflammatory drugs, nicotine and many systemic antibiotics. Local conditions may be compromised by the effects of antimicrobial toxicity, whilst dressings may adversely affect healing by creating an unsuitable environment for this process (Westaby 1982, Daly 1990).

The maturation or remodelling phase of ulceration. An outline of events characterising this phase includes the decline in concentration of fibroblasts and the complex reorientation of collagen fibres. The result is eventual consolidation of scar tissue, which displays a maximum strength of 20% less than that of intact skin. The realignment of collagen fibres is thought to be a response to pressure. When pressure is applied, collagen releases piezoelectric substances. It is postulated that these stress-generated voltages are responsible for the realignment and general maintenance of collagen (Price 1990).

Mal perforans

Complicated ulcers (Fig. 28.4; also Plate 9) extend to involve tendons, synovial sheaths, joint capsules and bone. Pyogenic infection of bone may result from the localisation of infection via a haematogenous route or from abscesses. Infection may lead to chronic osteomyelitis with multiple sinus formation (Enna 1988). A more common causative factor contributing to involvement of deeper tissue is secondary infection of an uncomplicated ulcer. Sequestration, remodelling of bone and copious periosteal reaction are associated with pyogenic infection. In such cases, restoration of tissue stability is dependent on overcoming infection and the removal of necrotic bone and soft tissue. In the absence of compromising factors, complicated ulcers proceed to heal by secondary intention.

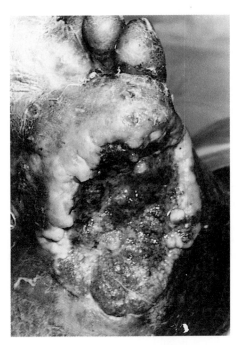

Figure 28.4 Complicated ulcer. The hypergranulating surface suggests the involvement of necrotic bone.

Enhancing the healing process

Factors that should be taken into account include:

- infection control
- maintaining an optimal wound environment
- rest.

Infection control. Hansen's disease is not associated with generally compromised immunological defences. Where other variables are addressed, healing is usually faster than diabetic ulceration because Hansen's disease is not complicated by vascular disease. The immune system may, however, be suppressed by systemic and topical steroid therapy, malnutrition and nicotine. These factors should be considered when planning infection control. The choice of antiseptic medicaments should be balanced between the perceived threat of infection and the cytotoxicity of available medicaments.

Maintaining an optimal wound environment. The general principles of ulcer management are that the lesion should be kept clean and clear of slough, avascular or necrotic soft tissue (see Ch. 9); overlying callus and epidermis should be excised to reduce stress and encourage healing by secondary intention; excessively discharging complicated lesions or hypergranulating lesions indicate investigation for sequestrae or other foreign bodies, which must be removed.

The lesion should be kept moist at all times. During the active phase dressings capable of absorbing exudate are indicated. During the proliferative and remodelling phases, there is greater danger from the wound becoming too dry; the choice of dressings should be considered accordingly.

Other criteria for the ideal wound environment include:

- thermal stability (exposure to cold or heat will impede healing)
- unimpeded gaseous exchange
- inaccessibility to microorganisms, arthropods and foreign bodies (including fibres from dressings).

Strike-through of gauze type dressings can provide access to the lesion by microorganisms. Removal of adherent dressings traumatises delicate granulation or epithelium. Incorrect dressings can counteract the healing process by compromising the wound environment.

Rest. Wherever possible, patients with acute ulceration should be treated with bed rest and medication. Where this is possible, after a week oedema and discharge will have diminished and a walking plaster can be applied. Plaster casting is contraindicated for profusely discharging ulcers. If after a week the ulcer continues to discharge copiously, involvement of bony tissue should be considered. Swelling subsides rapidly when the foot is immobilised, and unless the plaster is removed after the first week, the cast may become loose and problematic. Further plaster casts can be applied and changed depending on the rate of discharge from the ulcer, looseness of cast and the extent of wear. Although ulcers have been known to heal within 3 weeks, the patient should be advised not to expect healing before 6 weeks. Attention to plaster casting technique cannot be overemphasised. Well-applied plaster, appropriately placed padding, and either a rubber heel or wooden rocker will immobilise the foot and distribute weight-bearing over the foot and up the leg.

Debate continues as to the efficacy of *window casting*. The advantage is that direct access is given to the ulcer for dressing and assessment. The major disadvantage is that oedema results in the protrusion of the ulcer into the window, which delays healing and renders the ulcer vulnerable to further trauma.

Orthotic options

Simple ulcers of 1 cm diameter have been shown to heal using appropriate appliance therapy (Cross et al 1995). Appliance therapy is also particularly useful for the preservation of the foot after healing by plaster casting. The recurrence of ulceration after cast removal is a common problem.

Resource availability will dictate orthotic prescription and manufacture. There is no substitute for a thorough grounding in functional anatomy, biomechanics and the therapeutic rationale supporting appliance therapy.

Note. Neither palliative nor functional orthoses should be supplied unless the patient can be monitored diligently.

Orthotic prescription is based on:

- footwear
- availability of the patient for monitoring
- biomechanical examination of the foot
- gait analysis.

Detailed screening and examination may indicate patients at risk of ulceration or tarsal disintegration. Timely orthotic intervention may be a valuable adjunct to other disability prevention measures (Watson 1986, ILEP 1993).

REFERENCES

Barton A A 1976 The pathogenesis of skin wounds due to pressure. In: Kenedi R M, Cowden J M (eds) Bed sore biomechanics. Macmillan, London

Bauman J H, Girling J P, Brand P W 1963 Plantar pressures and trophic ulceration. Journal of Bone and Joint Surgery 45B: 652

Brand P 1991 The insensitive foot (including leprosy). In: Jahss M H (ed) Disorders of the foot and ankle. WB Saunders, Philadelphia

Cross H, Sane S, Dey A, Kulkarni V N 1995 The efficacy of podiatric orthoses as an adjunct to the treatment of plantar ulceration in leprosy. Leprosy Review 66: 144–157

Cruickshank C N D 1976 The micro anatomy of the epidermis in relation to tissue trauma. In: Kenedi R M, Cowden J M (eds) Bed sore biomechanics. Macmillan, London

Daly M D 1990 The repair phase of wound healing – re-epithelialisation and contraction. In: Kloth L C, McCulloch J M, Feedar J A (eds) Wound healing: alternatives in management. FA Davis, London

ILEP Medical Commission 1993 Guidelines for leprosy control programmes. ILEP, London

Jopling W H, McDougal A C 1988 Handbook of leprosy, 4th edn. Heinemann, Oxford

Jorgensen U, Bosjen-Moller F 1991 The plantar soft tissues:

functional anatomy and clinical applications. In: Jahss M H (ed) Disorders of the foot, vol 1. WB Saunders, Philadelphia

Kloth L, Miller K 1990 The inflammatory response to wounding. In: Kloth L C, McCulloch J M, Feedar J A (eds) Wound healing: alternatives in management. FA Davis, London

Kulkarni V N, Mehta J M 1983 Tarsal disintegration (T.D.) in leprosy. Leprosy in India 55(2): 338–370

Noorden S K 1992 Estimated numbers of leprosy cases in the world. Bulletin World Health Organization 70(1): 7–10

Price H 1990 Connective tissue in wound healing. In: Kloth L C, McCulloch J M, Feedar J A (eds) Wound healing: alternatives in management. FA Davis, London

Root M L, Orien W P, Weed J H 1977 Normal and abnormal function of the foot. In: Clinical Biomechanics, Vol. 11. Clinical Biomechanics Corporation, Los Angeles

Sabin T D, Swift T C 1984 Leprosy. In: Dyck P J, Thomas P K, Lambert E H, Bunge R (eds) Peripheral neuropathy, vol 2. WB Saunders, Philadelphia

Sane S B, Mehta J 1988 Malignant transformation in trophic ulcers in leprosy: a study of 12 cases. Indian Journal of Leprosy 60: 93–99

Thomas S 1990 Wound management and dressings. Pharmaceutical Press, London

Watson J 1986 Disability prevention in leprosy patients. Leprosy Mission International, London

Weis M G, Doongaji D R, Siddharatha S et al 1992 The explanatory model interview catalogue. Contribution to cross cultural research methods: from a study of leprosy and mental health. British Journal of Psychiatry 160: 819–830

Westaby S 1982 Wound care no. 8 – wound infection: causes and prevention. Nursing Times 16(suppl): 29–32

Zederfeldt B, Jacobsson S, Ahonen J 1986 Wounds and wound healing. Wolfe Medical, London

Appendices

APPENDIX 1
Orientation and terminology

THE CARDINAL BODY PLANES

The anatomical relationships of parts of the body to each other, and also their movements and positions, are denoted in terms which relate them to the three cardinal body planes, which correspond to the three dimensions of space. These are the *sagittal, frontal* and *transverse* planes which intersect at the centre of gravity of the body, located at the level of the pelvis. Planes parallel to these cardinal planes are then imagined at any desired point in order to aid descriptions of movements or positions (Fig. A1.1).

A *sagittal plane* is an anteroposterior vertical plane which divides the body into right and left sections and divides the foot into medial and lateral sections. Movement of the foot (or toes) in this plane hinges on a horizontal axis either upwards or downwards from the horizontal (or transverse) plane, i.e. dorsiflexion of the foot at the ankle joint, and extension or flexion of the toes at the metatarsophalangeal joints.

A *transverse* (or *horizontal*) *plane* is a plane parallel to the horizon (or floor) which divides the body into upper (superior) and lower (inferior) sections, and divides the foot into upper (dorsal) and lower (plantar) sections. Movement of the foot (or part) in this plane turns on a vertical axis either towards (adduction) or away from (abduction) the midline of the body, the cardinal sagittal plane.

An exception to this general rule applies to the muscles and movements of the toes, which are related to the sagittal plane bisecting the second metatarsal segment. This makes no difference to the terminology applicable to the muscles and movements of the three lateral toes. In the case of the hallux, however, *abduction* denotes movement away from the second metatarsal line and towards the midline of the body, and *adduction* denotes the opposite movement. The corresponding muscles are denominated as *abductor hallucis* and *adductor hallucis*, respectively.

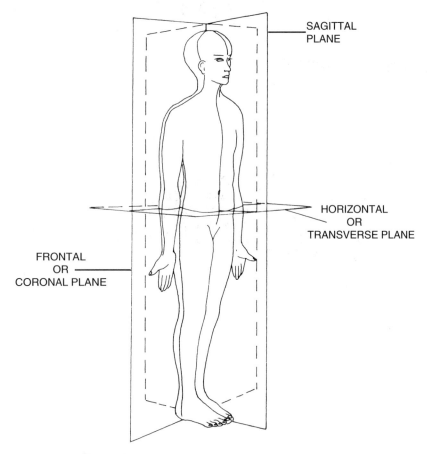

Figure A1.1 The cardinal body planes.

A *frontal* (or *coronal*) *plane* is a side-to-side vertical plane which divides the body into front (anterior) and back (posterior) sections, and divides the foot into hindfoot (proximal) and forefoot (distal) sections. Movement of the foot (or part) in this plane turns on a longitudinal axis and is either towards (inversion) or away from (eversion) the midline of the body.

JOINT MOVEMENTS

Movements in a joint are determined by its intrinsic structure, which may permit motion in one, two or three planes. Such motion is depicted as occurring around axes perpendicular to the plane of motion. The knee and the ankle are hinge-like joints, allowing movement only in the sagittal plane and around a single axis for each joint (Fig. A1.2). The first metatarsophalangeal joint moves in both the sagittal and transverse planes around two axes, while the hip, being a ball-and-socket joint, allows movement in all

three planes around three axes. The peritalar joints (ankle, subtalar and midtarsal joints) also provide collectively for movements in all three planes.

Joint movements may thus be *simple* (motion in one plane) or *complex* (motion in two or three planes simultaneously).

Simple movements in each of the three planes result in *positions*, which are denoted in the following summary in both traditional and biomechanical terminology (Table A1.1). *Fixation* of any such position which prevents the foot (or part) from assuming a normal attitude indicates a structural abnormality.

Complex movements of the foot or its parts occur on all three planes simultaneously and are denoted by the terms *supination* and *pronation*.

Supination denotes a compound movement of inversion, adduction and plantarflexion of the foot or parts of the foot taking place at the peritalar joints. Pronation denotes the compound movement of eversion, abduction and dorsiflexion of the foot or parts of

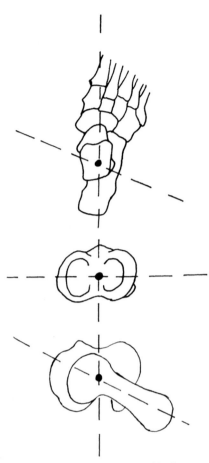

Figure A1.2 Frontal plane axes of the hip, knee and ankle joints. With the knee axis aligned on the frontal plane as shown, the head and neck of the femur are externally rotated on the shaft to a variable extent (the angle of anteversion). The ankle axis is also externally rotated because of the normal torsion in the lower end of the tibial shaft. This also varies in extent between individuals, and at different ages in the same subject.

the foot taking place at the peritalar joints. Both of these movements turn on an oblique axis which passes through the foot from the posterior, lateral and plantar aspects to the anterior medial and dorsal aspects of the tarsus (Figs A1.3 and A1.4).

The midtarsal joint, being compounded of the talonavicular and the calcaneocuboid joints, is regarded as having two resultant axes, providing for reciprocal longitudinal torsion of the forefoot on the hindfoot in order to maintain the metatarsus in a correct relationship to the ground as the hindfoot supinates/pronates in locomotion. The position of the subtalar joint dictates the range of movement in the midtarsal joint. In eversion, the axes of the separate components become parallel, thereby facilitating movement and hence flexibility in the foot for shock absorption. In inversion, the separate axes diverge, thus restricting movement and inducing greater rigidity in the foot for purposes of leverage (Fig. A1.5).

The five metatarsal segments (or rays) distal to the midtarsal joint provide dorsoplantar movement for the metatarsal heads, enabling them to adjust to the surface as required by motions within the foot or by varying and irregular terrain. The three medial segments comprise both cuneiforms and metatarsals; the lateral two comprise metatarsals only. While each is capable of some independent movement, their function of adapting to the ground surface is essentially a collective one. The first and fifth have the greatest range of movements about their respective oblique axes (Fig. A1.6), including some capacity for inversion and eversion.

TERMINOLOGY

Traditionally, the terms *valgus* and *varus* have been applied to fixed positions of the lower limb and its parts in relation to *both* the vertical and horizontal dimensions of the cardinal sagittal plane, i.e. to devia-

Table A1.1 Summary of orientation terminology

	Sections of body	Sections of foot	Simple movement of foot or part	Traditional terminology	Biomechanical terminology
Sagittal plane	Right	Medial	Dorsiflexion (extension of toes)	Calcaneus	Calcaneus
	Left	Lateral	Plantarflexion (flexion of toes)	Equinus	Equinus
Transverse (horizontal) plane	Superior Inferior	Dorsal Plantar	Adduction Abduction	Varus Valgus	Adductus Abductus
Frontal (coronal) plane	Anterior Posterior	Distal Proximal	Inversion Eversion	Inverted (varus) Everted (valgus)	Varus Valgus

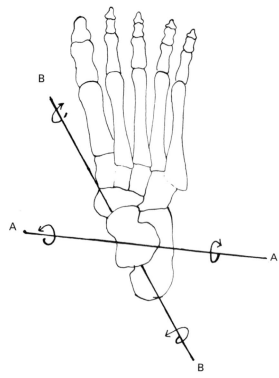

Figure A1.3 The axis of the ankle (AA) and the subtalar joint (BB) (dorsal view).

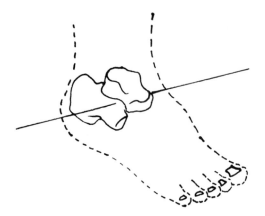

Figure A1.4 The subtalar joint axis around which the foot pronates and supinates. It is normally angled at 42° to the transverse plane and 16° to the sagittal plane, but this varies between individuals.

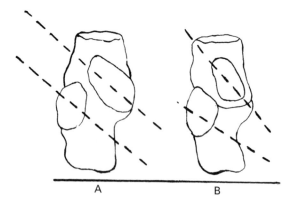

Figure A1.5 The articular facets of talonavicular and calcaneocuboid components of the midtarsal joint. In eversion (A), they are more congruent with each other, thereby facilitating flexibility for shock absorption. In inversion (B), they are less congruent, thus 'locking' the joint and imparting rigidity to the foot for leverage purposes.

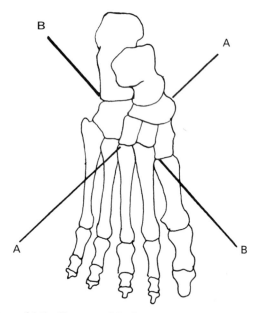

Figure A1.6 The axes of the first (AA) and fifth (BB) metatarsal segments (dorsal view).

quinti varus have all denoted variations from the normal, towards (varus) or away from (valgus) the cardinal sagittal plane.

Current biomechanical usage departs from the traditional in confining *varus* and *valgus* to positional deviations of the foot or its parts in the frontal plane only. Thus hindfoot valgus and hindfoot varus denote positions of eversion and inversion of the hindfoot,

tions in *both* the frontal and transverse planes. Hence, the terms coxa valga and vara, genu valgum and varum, talipes equinovarus and calcaneovalgus, pes valgus, hallux valgus, metatarsus varus and digiti respectively, and similarly for the forefoot. Hence, also, metatarsus adductus and hallux abductus are preferred to metatarsus varus and hallux valgus. When applied to the toes, these terms denote axial rotations, varus in an inverted direction and valgus in an everted direction, corresponding to similar frontal plane movements of the foot. This usage leads logically to hallux abductovalgus (lateral deviation of the hallux with an everted axial rotation) instead of hallux valgus, and to digiti quinti adductovarus (medial deviation of the fifth toe with an inverted axial rotation) instead of digiti quinti varus.

Although entirely logical, this usage may initially be confusing, particularly in the case of the hallux, where it conflicts with the traditional anatomical nomenclature which relates movement of the hallux and actions of its abductor and adductor muscles to the sagittal plane bisecting the second metatarsal segment. If the term *hallux abductovalgus* is used, it must be remembered that the abduction element is in relation to the *midline of the body* and not to the line through the second metatarsal segment from which the muscles are denominated. Similarly, the *valgus* element refers to the everted axial rotation of the hallux and not to its abduction from the midline of the body.

It should be borne in mind that terms are often descriptive rather than specifically diagnostic. For example, *pes cavus* describes the main clinical feature of a deformity which has various causes, and similarly with *pes planovalgus*. Both traditional and biomechanical forms of terminology have their uses and will coexist. Both forms are given where necessary, the biomechanical terminology being given preference in the general text.

For ease of reference, a list of the main terms which are related, though not necessarily interchangeable, is given in Table A1.2.

Compensations

The degree of compensation depends in each case on the degree of the primary skeletal deformity:

Table A1.2 Traditional and biomechanical forms of terminology

Traditional terms	Related biomechanical terms
Pes planus, flat foot, congenital flat foot	Calcaneovalgus, hindfoot valgus
Talipes equinus, short tendo Achilles	Ankle equinus
Pes valgus, valgus foot, acquired flat foot, supinated forefoot	Pronated foot
Pes cavus	Forefoot valgus, plantarflexed first metatarsal
Metatarsus varus	Metatarsus adductus
Metatarsus primus varus	Metatarsus primus adductus
Hallux valgus	Hallux abductovalgus
Digitus quintus varus	Digitus quintus adductovarus

- Calcaneovalgus is usually compensated by supination of the forefoot, resulting in a low-arched foot.
- Ankle equinus is usually compensated by pronation of the hindfoot to permit additional dorsiflexion at the midtarsal joint.
- Calcaneovarus is usually compensated by sufficient pronation of the foot to enable the heel and forefoot to reach the horizontal plane.
- Forefoot varus is usually compensated by pronation of the hindfoot to enable the forefoot to reach the horizontal plane.
- Forefoot valgus, when it is an intrinsic deformity, is usually compensated by supination of the hindfoot, resulting in a high-arched foot. It may, however, be caused for other reasons, particularly neuropathies (see Ch. 27).

APPENDIX 2
Ossification timetable

Bone	Appearance of centres of ossification		Fusion	Remarks
	Primary centres	Secondary centres		
Tibia—diaphysis	7th week			
Tibia—upper epiphysis	—	At birth	20th year	
Tibia—lower epiphysis	—	2nd year	18th year	Sometimes a separate centre for the medial malleolus appears at the same time
Fibula—diaphysis	8th week	—	—	
Fibula—upper epiphysis	—	4th year	25th year	
Fibula—lower epiphysis	—	2nd year	20th year	
Calcaneum—body	6th month	—	—	
Calcaneum epiphysis	—	6th–10th year	13th–15th year	
Talus	7th month	—	—	
Cuboid	At birth	—	—	
Lateral cuneiform	1st year	—	—	
Medial cuneiform	3rd year	—	—	
Intermediate cuneiform	4th year	—	—	
Navicular	4th year	—	—	
First metatarsal shaft	8th–9th week	—	—	
First metatarsal base	—	3rd year	17th–20th year	Sometimes a separate centre for the head appears at the same time
Other metatarsal shafts	8th–9th week	—	—	Sometimes a separate centre for the base of the fifth metatarsal appears at the same time
Other metatarsal heads				
Proximal phalanx shafts	12th–14th week			
Proximal phalanx bases	—	3rd–6th year	17th–18th year	
Intermediate phalanx shafts	4th–9th month	—	—	That for the fifth toe does not appear until shortly after birth
Intermediate phalanx bases	—	3rd–6th year	17th–18th year	Distal phalanx of hallux
Distal phalanx shafts	8th week	—	—	
Distal phalanx bases	—	6th year	17th–18th year	

APPENDIX 3
Clinical emergencies

Emergencies are relatively rare in podiatric practice and most of these situations can be prevented by good practice, careful preparation and close monitoring of the patient's state and reactions. The good practitioner should be prepared to deal effectively with any such problems and this section is designed to outline the best procedures to be followed.

The most common emergency situation is a faint, which is often attributable to the patient's apprehension of the clinical situation; therefore it is important to put patients at their ease, consider their problems with interest and explain the treatment to be followed clearly but not too graphically. During treatment, it is better if the patient can be semi-recumbent and patients' chairs which allow this are of considerable value, as is a well ventilated surgery maintained at a comfortable temperature. An essential preparation which must be made when using local anaesthetics is the provision of oxygen apparatus for resuscitation, which should also be checked regularly to ensure its effective function if it is needed.

This account of emergency resuscitation will be confined to the management of unconsciousness in patients. For a more comprehensive review of the provision of first aid procedures the reader is recommended to refer to one of the many standard texts on first aid.

ASSESSMENT OF CONSCIOUSNESS

There are four main levels of consciousness to be considered:

1. Full consciousness—the patient is fully orientated, usually able to speak and to answer questions sensibly.
2. Drowsiness—this is the first level of unconsciousness. At this stage the patient can be roused easily, is usually orientated but can lapse back into the unconscious state.

3. Stupor—in this second level of unconsciousness, the patient can only be aroused with difficulty and with painful stimuli; the patient is usually disorientated and not able to answer questions sensibly.
4. Coma—the patient is deeply unconscious and cannot be roused using any means.

The Glasgow Coma Scale

This is an internationally recognised and highly valuable method of recording the conscious state of a patient and can be used for both initial and continuous assessment. It is based upon eye opening, verbal and motor responses.

For first aid in clinical emergencies, an adaptation of the Glasgow Coma Scale may prove useful, and the initial assessment will accompany the patient to hospital if this is necessary (Table A3.1).

RESUSCITATION

This is a series of procedures which can be taken to support the process of breathing and circulation or restore them if they cease. Asphyxia is due to a decrease in the amount of oxygen and an increase in the amount of carbon dioxide in the body as a result of some interference in the respiratory process.

A clear airway

Any foreign object in the mouth must be removed, e.g.

Table A3.1   Glasgow Coma Scale (adapted)

Name of patient:		Date:
Time:		
Eyes open	Spontaneously To speech To pain No response	
Movement	Obeys commands To painful stimulus No response	
Verbal responses	Normal Confused Nonsensical words No response	
Pulse		
Respiration		
Pupil size	R L R L R L R L	

dentures, broken teeth, blood, saliva, etc. Neckwear must be loosened and the neck placed in the fully extended position (Fig. A3.1). The lower jaw of the patient is held in a forward position by the pressure of the thumb behind the angle of the jaw. This forces the tongue into a forward position and so maintains a clear airway. Should the tongue fall to the back of the throat, it would obstruct the airway.

Very often, clearing the airway will lead to the return of spontaneous breathing. Cyanosis and asphyxia will improve and consciousness will frequently return. Thereafter, the patient is kept comfortable and his condition monitored. Should spontaneous respiration not occur, artificial respiration must be commenced.

Artificial respiration

This is the maintenance of respiratory movements and oxygenation of the lungs by artificial means. The most effective procedure is mouth-to-mouth breathing (Fig. A3.2).

Mouth-to-mouth method

1. The airway is cleared and the patient is put on his back.
2. The soft lower part of the patient's nose is pinched in order to prevent escape of air.
3. The operator gives five short pants with her mouth over the mouth of the patient. This, in itself, may initiate spontaneous breathing.
4. If not, air is breathed directly into the mouth of the patient at a rate of 20 breaths per minute, the operator having sealed her lips over the mouth of the patient and ensuring that the patient's head is rotated so that the airway is open. After each exhalation, the operator should check to see whether the patient's

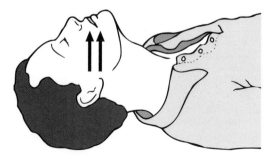

Figure A3.1   Resuscitation. Fully extended position of neck.

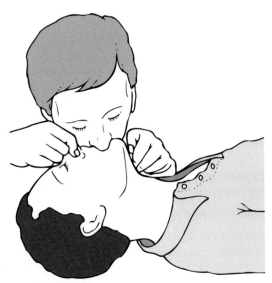

Figure A3.2   Resuscitation. Mouth-to-mouth lung ventilation.

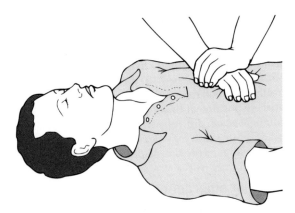

Figure A3.3   Resuscitation. External cardiac massage.

lungs have expanded, which indicates that air has entered them.

5. If the patient is a young child, the nostrils need not be pinched, since the area of the adult mouth easily covers the mouth and nostrils.

Artificial respiration may be required for a considerable period of time, and should be continued until a doctor or ambulance arrives or until the patient is certified dead by a doctor. Since the procedure may be long and tiring, it is important for the operator to be comfortable, removing her jacket or coat and loosening her neckwear.

External cardiac massage

When the heart has stopped beating, the pupils of the eyes remain dilated, the carotid and femoral pulses cannot be palpated and cyanosis persists despite artificial respiration.

In such cases, external cardiac massage should be started immediately to maintain circulation of oxygenated blood:

1. The patient should be placed on a firm base. The legs are raised to 90° for 10 seconds in order to help venous return to the heart.

2. A sharp blow should be given to the lower left third of the sternum. This sometimes stimulates the heart to beat spontaneously.

3. If this does not occur, the heels of the hands should be placed one over the other on the lower third of the sternum and the sternum depressed 4 cm (1.5 inches) at a rate of 60 times per minute (Fig. A3.3).

External cardiac massage must be continued until:

- the carotid pulse returns
- the resuscitation is taken over by the medical team
- the operator is asked to discontinue by a doctor.

Mouth-to-mouth ventilation and cardiac massage combined

In this instance, it is preferable that there be two operators maintaining one lung inflation to five sternal depressions. If one operator only is present, two lung inflations to 10 sternal depressions should be performed.

Cardiac arrest

When the heart stops beating suddenly, with immediate loss of consciousness, cyanosis, absence of pulses and dilatation of the pupils, a cardiac arrest has occurred. The most common causes are heart attack, severe shock or anaphylactoid reaction. The patient is rested supine on a firm support and the airway cleared. In external cardiac massage, the heart is compressed between the operator's hands from above and the vertebral column from below in order to pump blood forward to maintain the circulation. Artificial ventilation (mouth-to-mouth) must also be administered.

UNCONSCIOUSNESS

In podiatric practice, the loss of consciousness is likely

to be caused through faints, cerebrovascular accidents, epilepsy, hyper- or hypoglycaemic coma, anaphylaxis, heart conditions, etc. The major consideration is to ensure the patient's ability to breathe, and tight clothing should be loosened. If the patient continues to breathe without trouble, he should be placed in the recovery position or three-quarters prone (Fig. A3.4).

If there is any difficulty in breathing, oxygen should be administered. It may be necessary to use resuscitative measures as previously described.

Vascular emergencies

Cerebral haemorrhage, clot, embolus or subarachnoid haemorrhage can lead to unconsciousness with shock. Resuscitation may be required. If breathing is stable, place the patient in the three-quarter prone recovery position. Partial paralysis is usually present and medical attention is essential.

Faints

A faint occurs when there is a temporary inadequate supply of blood to the brain. Commonly, people faint in hot airless rooms, but in podiatric practice they may do so from anxiety. The patient may have forewarning, feeling hot and clammy with yawning or nausea. This is followed by giddiness and fainting. The patient may, however, turn ashen grey and drop down without any warning.

Treatment

Lay the patient flat, loosen neckwear and ensure a clear airway. Recovery will usually occur in 1 or 2 minutes, but an older person may take longer due to poorer cerebral circulation. On recovery, rest the patient and administer sips of water or tea. A check-up by the family doctor is a wise precaution.

Epilepsy

Fits indicate a disturbance of brain function and are of two types. In a *minor* fit, the patient stares into space and appears to be in a daydream. One part of the body may quiver, e.g. a hand or arm. Such a fit usually lasts about a minute and on recovery the patient has no recollection of the event. In a *major* fit, the patient loses consciousness and falls to the ground. The face becomes congested and foaming occurs at the mouth together with general muscle convulsions, and incontinence may occur. On recovery, the patient is exhausted and falls into a deep sleep.

Treatment

During a fit, the patient has to be protected from inadvertent injury by the removal of any sources of danger from the vicinity. The mouth should not be forced open, but all neckwear should be loosened and the breathing monitored. All such patients should be advised to consult their doctor, particularly if they have not had a fit before, and should be escorted home.

Diabetic emergencies leading to unconsciousness

Insulin excess resulting in hypoglycaemia

This can occur when the patient has missed a meal or inadvertently had too much insulin. The signs and symptoms are profuse sweating and a feeling of hunger, followed by nausea and confusion which may lead to unconsciousness.

Treatment. If a patient is conscious, administer a sugary drink, but beware of a tendency to vomit and only give sips at a time. Never attempt to give an unconscious patient anything to eat or drink. Obtain medical help or arrange transport to hospital. While waiting for an ambulance, maintain a clear airway, loosen neckwear and maintain the patient in the three-quarter prone recovery position (Fig. A3.4).

Insulin lack resulting in hyperglycaemia

This can occur when the patient has had insufficient insulin or has failed to comply with the prescribed diet. It also occurs in diabetics with an infection, e.g. a carbuncle or pneumonia. The skin is dry and the patient smells of acetone.

Treatment. Such patients must go to hospital immediately. If there is doubt as to whether the patient is hyperglycaemic or hypoglycaemic, a sugary drink can be given provided he is not unconscious. If the patient

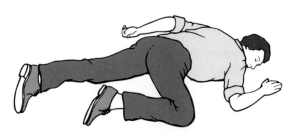

Figure A3.4 Unconsciousness. Three-quarter prone recovery position.

is hypoglycaemic he will improve, but if he is not then no harm will be done

Medi-alert bracelets or chains

Patients who are on special treatment may have a bracelet or chain giving this information. They may also carry cards giving details of their condition, treatment and the name of their family doctor.

APPENDIX 4
Treatment list relating to Chapter 11

Activity modification

1. Hard walk programme
2. Walk/run programme
3. Daily activity only (walking only)
4. Reduce stair/hill walking
5. Reduce running partially
6. Discontinue speed work
7. Discontinue hill work
8. Prolonged rest
9. Bicycle/swim alternative
10. Wheelchair or bed rest
11. Crutches or cane

Ice/heat therapy

12. Contrast baths
13. Ice pack after activity
14. Ice massage
15. Hot water soaks/heat packs
16. Deep heat lotion massage

Shoes

17. Change to shoes which limit pronation
18. Change to shoes with more shock absorption
19. Modify shoes with built-in changes
20. Special shoes
21. Stay with same shoes
22. Biven shoe, wooden sole shoe

Taping, supportive strapping, wraps

23. Rest strapping for the midtarsal joint
24. Rest strapping for the ankle
25. Combination of both
26. Figure-of-eight strapping
27. Special area taping (digits, etc.)

28. Removable ankle wrap
29. Removable knee wrap
30. Knee immobiliser
31. Tubular grip bandage
32. Tubular grip bandage with horseshoe padding
33. Orthoplast or air cast splints
34. Lateral ankle splints

Foot inserts/orthoses

35. Spenco padding
36. Sorbothane padding for the heel
37. Foot accommodation (e.g. Korex)
38. Felt arch padding or 'D' pads
39. Metatarsal support
40. Metatarsal bar
41. Runner's varus heel wedge
42. Heel cup
43. Forefoot/rearfoot wedge
44. Spenco or arch support
45. Cuboid padding
46. Heel lifts
47. Morton's extension
48. Latex shields
49. Bunion splints/digital splints
50. Biomechanical examination and casting for orthoses
51. Dispense orthoses
52. Modification of orthoses, if necessary

Stretching exercises

53. Static stretching programme for use at home
54. Contracting and relaxing programme for home use
55. Contracting and relaxing therapy programme
56. Spray and stretch techniques
57. Forty-five minute programme of heat/ice stretch
58. Cryostretch programme; stretching after application of cold

Stretching and range of movement

59. Isometric strengthening
60. Theraband or elastic rubber tubing techniques
61. Isotonic strengthening
62. Isokinetic strengthening
63. Upper body sotonic programme
64. Range of motion exercises
65. Muscle stimulator for home use

Physical therapy treatment

66. Ultrasound therapy
67. Electrogalvanic stimulation
68. Electro-acupuncture probe therapy
69. Dynamometer muscle test
70. Deep friction massage
71. Electro-accuscope therapy
72. Transcutaneous nerve stimulation

Medication

73. Aspirin
74. Strong anti-inflammatory medication
75. Oral steroid therapy for 6 days
76. Vitamins
77. Oral calcium supplements
78. Iron supplements
79. Vitamin B_{12} injection
80. Short-acting cortisone injection
81. Long-acting cortisone injection
82. Hyaluronidase injection
83. Local anaesthesia diagnostic injection
84. Local anaesthesia therapeutic injection
85. Diet evaluation

Special tests

86. X-rays
87. Bone scan
88. Computed tomography scan (CT scan)
89. Xerogram—reverse X-ray for soft tissues
90. Arthrogram
91. Nuclear magnetic resonance

Surgery

92. Surgical discussion
93. Surgical intervention

Casts

94. Standard below-knee cast
95. Removable below-knee casts
96. Above-knee cast
97. Unaboot cast—calamine lotion compressive bandage

Miscellaneous

98. Foot manipulation techniques

99. Referral to an orthopaedic surgeon
100. Referral to a neurologist
101. Referral to a physician
102. Referral to a chiropractor
103. Referral to a dietician
104. Referral to a rheumatologist
105. Referral to a vascular specialist
106. Evaluation

Index